AF886419

Antibodies
Applications and New Developments

Edited By

Eline P. Meulenberg

Ambachtsweg 5, 6581 AX Malden
The Netherlands

CONTENTS

FOREWORD

This book is intended to familiarise the reader with the history, development, terminology and theoretical considerations associated with the development, production and use of Immunoassays. The reader will be led through the theoretical and practical considerations associated with antibody, production and then into the practical applications and complications of antibody's use in assays. Finally there are a series of chapters on specific applications and future technologies, ending with a chapter on Aptamers which may represent an alternative to antibodies and the future of assay development.

This foreword will recount the theories and discoveries which have led to the explosion in commercial immunoassays and to their development as powerful research tools.

The chapters provide details of the development of immunoassays establishing an "evolutionary tree", the path of events and the stages which have been reached and possible directions for future research and developments. The relationship between immunoassays and other analytical techniques is presented clearly and there are indications as to potential future developments.

Modern immunoassays have arisen from the desire to detect and quantify complex biological molecules under conditions for which chemical and physical analytical techniques were either unsuitable or not available. Current methodologies are based firmly in classical immunology. The theoretical high sensitivity and high specificity of the antibody-antigen interaction attracted the attention of workers wishing to exploit these properties in this search for improved analytical techniques. Indeed, modern trends are towards the development of increasingly sensitive assays; expanding the range of analytes being detected: to an increasing variety of substances which can be analysed in new and developing fields; to increasing rapidity of results and to simplicity of use in terms of the intervention needed and the skills of the operator in carrying out and interpreting the results.

The driving force for these developments has changed as assays have been shown to be successful and the methods have become more established. Originally immunoassays were developed to facilitate the study of the immune system, particularly the role of antibody-antigen interactions as a defence against disease. The original assays were therefore used in clinical research and areas are closely related to medicine (Chapter **1**).

As an increasing usefulness of the assays was demonstrated the demand for greater sensitivity and accuracy increased. This has generated a greater knowledge of these type of assay outside the clinical field and their use in a wider variety of fields began to increase.

As part of this demand there has been the development of a greater understanding of the nature of antibodies and their production. Despite earlier historical references to protection against disease by the injection of live organisms from smallpox pustules into healthy patients, the generally accepted beginnings of Immunology as a science are Jenner's observations on and use of cowpox as a protection against smallpox. This then was the first scientifically reported observation of an antibody-antigen reaction, although not realised as being such at the time. What Jenner had observed was a clinically useful incidence of cross-reactivity. However it was not until over a hundred years, later that in 1897, Rudolph Kraus in Vienna reported that the interaction between a soluble antigen and the corresponding soluble antibody resulted in the formation of a precipitate. Thus the use of antibodies in assays systems was initiated and the production of these useful antibody molecules as a part of scientific study became a study in its own right (Chapter **2**).

Much of the development of immunoassays is dependent upon knowledge of the structure of antibodies. The gradual development of information regarding the structure of antibodies has been the key to the establishment of immunoassays. The fact that immunoglobulins are proteins initially allowed researchers to measure the concentration of immunoprecipitates by simply determining the concentration of nitrogen in the dried precipitate and then calculating the concentrations of antibody and antigen in the precipitate. This, obviously, was a time consuming and technically demanding procedure and hence the aim of research in one important aspect as to develop alternative methods for determining antigen concentration. In the aftermath of the development of radioisotope development and detection the application of such isotopes to the monitoring of the antibody antigen reaction was one of many attempts to use such material peacefully. However, despite considerable initial success the health and safety issues combined with the high costs of using radioactivity drove the search for yet another alternative method of detection. Thus returning to the structure of antibodies as a source of inspiration resulted in the use of protein biochemistry to carry out reactions linking labels to the antibody. The additional knowledge that IgG has a Y-shaped structure with the specific binding region at the ends of the arms, F_{ab}, binding region and the stem, F_c, crystallisable, forming a region on which chemistries can be conducted without interfering with the specific binding reactions provided a basis for future developments, labelled antibodies which retained their specific binding capabilities.

Simultaneously the methods of separating the bound and unbound enzyme labelled antibody were being developed. A significant step was the description of the use of reagents, either antibody or antigen, bound to solid phases, including glass, plastic, latex and metals, which allowed the rapid and easy separation of the reactants in immunoassay systems. Thus the ELISA, Enzyme Linked Immunosorbent Assay was developed, using the F_c region to bind the antibody to solid substrates being one of the alternative models of immunoassay.

There are now numerous immunoassay types; however what all the immunoassayists have to understand is that the systems in all their forms consist of a molecule with a highly specific binding capacity and a system for detecting the reaction between this binding molecule and a specific analyte. Specifically for immunoassays the molecules concerned are conventional antibodies and antigens or haptens. Provided the reader remembers that all immunoassays are based on the measurement of antibody-antigen interactions and the variations attempt is only to provide more sensitive, accurate, reliable or robust means of achieving this, little misunderstanding will occur.

However it is essential to standardise these assays. Without consistency in the results obtained when using any form of analytical method, the method is worthless. Thus having demonstrated the ability of techniques based on immune reactions to monitor concentrations of particular analytes in a highly specific and extremely sensitive format the immunoassayist must also consider reliability, reproducibility, simplicity of assays and assay formats. These aspects are dealt with in detail in (Chapter **3**).

The final important development in application of immunoassays to Food samples has been the consideration of matrix effects on the assay results. In essence, immunoassays were developed by the clinical researchers, who used the techniques as the means of rapid diagnosis. Such clinical studies routinely detected antibody or antibody's level in body fluids, particularly the serum, under physiological conditions. This application of the assays in a single, or very limited number of matrices, with very similar characteristics simplifies the importance of matrix effects. However once the assays began to be applied to systems which are not simple, do not have physiological characteristics such as pH, ion balance and temperature. The effects of the matrix becomes significant. Thus in food systems the matrix has an important function and the variable effects on immunoassays. For the immunoassayist using the techniques in food related applications it is important to consider the matrices in which such reactions may occur and how the matrix may interfere with the reaction. In (Chapter **4**) these matrix effects are discussed in detail and the options available in order to provide standardised, reliable assays are suitable for routine usage described.

Having established the essentials of producing antibodies, developing assays and standardising these assays to provide reliable analytical tools, the second section of the text provides examples of the application of immunoassays in the field of food analysis. This is a very wide field and at one end can include aspects which might be more appropriately considered at environmental analysis and at other supportive clinical diagnosis for allergy. The first step is to understand how and when antibodies can be used in the analysis of food and food materials. The myriad of formats, ELISA, Transverse Flow, Lateral Flow, *etc.* and the varieties of arrangements, direct, indirect, competitive, non-competitive, sandwich *etc.* and the possibilities for single and multiple tests and multi-arrays, all need to be described and discussed in order to provide the analyst with information on which decisions will be based as to how to select a suitable assay for the particular analyte and matrix (Chapter **5**).

The adulterants and contaminants found in food can be considered myriad. Many bacterial and chemical contaminants are found in food purely as a result of accident but in other cases these, chemical contaminants may be found in the food as the consequence of the use of these in the environment or as treatments in food animals. One specific group of food contaminants which may be found in food are the antibiotics. These are used to treat diseases in animals but they and their residues may be found in the foods derived from those animals and may have unforeseen consequences. Older readers will recall Rachel Carson's "The Silent Spring" as ground-breaking text defining the adverse consequences of the use of pesticides and the transfer of these materials along with the food chain. There is a similar progression of antibiotics along with the food chain which has potentially greater consequences for the human population. Simple financial consequences may be demonstrated by the example of the use of antibiotics to treat mastitis in cattle. This can if controls are ignored lead to the presence of antibiotics in milk; if this milk is used in cheese making the antibiotic can prevent the growth of the starter culture and lead to significant losses in terms of Cheese production. The presence of antibiotics in milk, it was at one time, considered to be the cause of various maladies in people, especially young children. Hence its detection in the food chain of antibiotics has a particular relevance for both human health and industrial profitability (Chapter **6**).

In a similar vein the treatment of animals with growth promoters results in the transfer of these materials and their residues along with the food chain as well as their release into the environment where they may, in the case of oestrogen-like agents, cause changes such as feminisation of fish and the modification of population ratios (Chapter **7**).

Immunoassays have other applications and one opportunity is in environmental analysis. This type of analysis develops simply and obviously from the detection of pesticides and other chemical agents, *e.g.* growth promoters, in food matrices to the detection of the same pesticides and their residues in the environmental samples, especially potable water (Chapter **8**). A significant feature of antibody-based immunoassays is the specificity of the ligand and the application of this specificity to the detection of a single analyte; however in many instances the analyst requires a methodology which detects more than one analyte. The development and application of immunoassays, which have multi-analyte detection capabilities, is a major research aim. Having established the criteria for the single analyte assay in many formats and in numerous matrices the option for the development of multi-analyte assays was to return to a simple matrix and begins their development with the simplest of all matrices, water (Chapter **9**).

This foreword opens the section of the book which provides descriptions of novel and alternative assay methodologies and provides an indication as to the future development of immunoassays. There are many different alternative routes along which immunoassays that may develop. These four chapters demonstrate the lines of development which have been investigated. A specific chapter is dedicated to each because of the impact of these techniques that it may have had on the field. The importance of the method of separation of the reactants and non-reactants following the reaction of antibody with antigen was stated in the initial stages of immunoassay development. The interaction of the two large molecules often results in the formation of an insoluble precipitate which easily solves the problem of separation as unreacted components remain in solution allowing filtration or centrifugation, physical methods, to be used to separate the components. However when the analyte is a small molecule the reaction with antibody may not produce a precipitate necessitating the use of other methods for separating the antibody-analyte product from the unreacted antibody and analyte in the reaction mixture. Binding one or other of the components to a solid phase that allows the simplified separation of the bound materials. Thus the use of systems such as latex bound antibody allows the development of agglutination assays, provided the antigen was multivalent and thus allowed cross-linking of the latex beads *via* the bound antibody. If alternatively the analyte is monovalent and hence cross-linking is not possible and the alternatives are the use of magnetic beads, which can be separated from the solution very simply or the binding of one component of the reaction to another solid matrix which allows easy separation. A problem of these options is the matrix effect which can interfere with or totally prevent the reaction. Such problems can be reduced or eliminated by using a method which combines a separation technique and an immunological reaction. An important example of this type of technique is Immunoaffinity chromatography (Chapter **10**). This technique is also important in establishing the use of chromatography in immunoassay systems. In chemistry the separation of components by chromatography began with the use of paper as the separation medium across which the liquid solvent carried solutes at different rates, separating Indian ink into its component colours, for example. To achieve greater and more complex separations chemists moved from paper to glass plates coated with other inert substances through which liquid might diffuse. Eventually the concepts were combined and plastic backed nitrocellulose "paper" sheets were developed. Immunoassayist eventually took this development in the form of Mylar-backed nitrocellulose and used it to produce lateral flow immunoassays, basis for both rapid diagnostic and simple "dipstick" immunoassay techniques (Chapter **11**). Finally, the use of alternative methods of detecting the immune reaction has led to the development of some interesting alternative assays. As it has been described. One of the major problems which immunoassayists have been attempting to overcome is how to detect the reaction between the antibody and the antigen. The detection methods have in many cases been by means of secondary reaction, i.e. those reactions such as precipitation which occur as a result of the "primary" reaction, i.e. binding of the antibody to the antigen or hapten, however the requirements of the assay are that the "primary" reaction be measured directly. Two examples, amongst an increasing number, are immunosensors (Chapter **12**) and immunoelectrochemistry (Chapter **13**).

All of these chapters provide considerable areas for research and development, however if this is not sufficient then in the final chapters the reader is given information as to other possibilities. The intention is for this book to lead the reader through the story of immunoassays and to suggest fields of current interesting research and potential future significant developments. In attempting to predict the future there is considerable room for error and hence the last three chapters describe current research with considerable potential rather than developing speculative ideas.

In completing the story of immunoassays the research has now moved to considering alternatives to the antibody molecule. Antibodies are molecules which are normally developed *in vivo* by "challenging" the immune system of an animal with a "foreign" molecule. Simplistically the immune system is a defence mechanism which recognises "foreign" or "non-self" molecules and responds by producing antibodies which bind to and assist in the removal of these "threatening" molecules. Scientists have taken advantage of this natural defence mechanism to induce animals to produce antibodies to specific molecules. Again simplistically, the injection of the "foreign" molecules into animals results in an immune response and thus produces antibodies in the blood which will specifically bind to this molecule. By collecting the blood, it is possible to recover the antibody molecules and have these available for use in assays. Such a natural system of production results in a plethora of antibody molecules with a range of specificities and affinities. The first steps in moving away from this methodology were the development of antibodies from single cell clones, monoclonal antibodies. Monoclonal antibodies are identical antibody molecules produced from a clone of cells which have artificially been created by fusing an antibody producing cell with an "immortal" cell line to yield cells which can be grown *in vitro* and thus make the antibody more akin to a standard chemical reagent. Monoclonal antibodies are only one development in the attempts to modify or replace the conventional, animal-derived, polyclonal antibodies used in early immunoassays. One possibility is to use only parts of the antibody molecule, the F_{ab}, antigen binding fragment. These type of modifications are refered to as "antibody engineering" (Chapter **14**). Such techniques may currently be confined to the field of medical diagnostics, but it is possible that they may be increasingly useful to the food scientist.

Similarly the modification of the antibody molecule to provide reagents which can be used in specialist situations as a matter of fact. Specifically antibodies which can be used as therapeutic reagents are being generated. Whether such techniques can be moved from the field of medical diagnosis to food analysis may simply depend upon the ingenuity of the researchers working in these fields (Chapter **15**).

Finally there is a possibility that the antibody molecule may be removed completely and that assays will use an alternative. Some may suggest that the use of molecules derived from animals or involving the use of animals is ethically and morally questionable. Whether or not this is the case, science is moving on and the discovery of short sections of nucleotides which bind specifically, with high affinity to proteins and peptides, aptamers, has provided a potential alternative to the antibody molecule over a period of time. In the last two decades, since their discovery aptamers have been shown to have the potential to be more specific, have superb affinity and to function in a wider range of matrices than antibodies. Aptamers are short nucleotide sequences which can be produced without the use of animal, thus obviating the moral and ethical objections which are associated with antibodies. Further, Aptamers can be selected from a naïve DNA library. Specificity and affinity relates not only to proteins but may extend to a variety of other molecules. Significantly once the aptamer has been identified it can be reproduced very simply by cloning into E. coli and with sufficient quantities available sequence can be identified and further amounts produced by chemical synthesis. The final Chapter (Chapter **16**) describes the capabilities and possibilities of aptamers and thus provides a range of potential future applications.

For the student and the established research it is hoped that the text, prepared by authors of considerable standing in the field, would provide significant interest and suggestions for future research.

Christopher Smith

Professor, Food Science

Co-Director, Manchester Food Research Centre

Manchester Metropolitan University

UK

PREFACE

This book has been accomplished with the contribution of several high-standing researchers in the field of immunochemical techniques. It illustrates the diverse aspects of antibodies, antibody engineering, immunoassays, immunoaffinity chromatography, immunosensors and immunotherapeutics, and the application in the various fields of analysis. I wish to thank all the contributors for their cooperation and their willingness to share their knowledge and expertise. In addition, I would like to thank the referees to review the various chapters and give useful comments.

Eline P. Meulenberg
Ambachtsweg 5, 6581 AX Malden
The Netherlands

List of Contributors

Amerongen van, Aart

Wageningen UR Food & Biobased Research, Biomolecular Sensing & Diagnostics, P.O. Box 17, 6700 AA Wageningen, The Netherlands.
aart.vanamerongen@wur.nl

Baty, Daniel

INSERM U624, GDR2352, 163 avenue de Luminy - case 915, 13288 Marseille Cedex 09, Centi, Sonia Università degli Studi di Firenze, Dipartimento di Fisiopatologia Clinica, Viale G. Pieraccini, 6 - 50139 Firenze.
daniel.baty@inserm.fr

Chames, Patrick

INSERM U624, GDR2352, 163 avenue de Luminy - case 915, 13288 Marseille Cedex 09, France.
patrick.chames@inserm.fr

Hage, David S.

Department of Chemistry, University of Nebraska, Lincoln, NE 68588-0304, USA.
dhage@unlserve.unl.edu

Delahaut, Ph.

CER Groupe, Rue du point du jour, 8 – B-6900 Marloie, Belgium.
p.delahaut@cergroupe.be

Dodig, Slavica

Department of Clinical Laboratory Diagnosis, Srebrnjak Children's Hospital, Srebrnjak 100, 10000 Zagreb, Croatia.
slavica.dodig@zg.t-com.hr

Eyer, Ludek

Veterinary Research Institute, Hudcova 70, 62100 Brno, Czech Republic.
eyer@vri.cz

Franek, Milan

Veterinary Research Institute, Hudcova 70, 62100 Brno, Czech Republic.
franek@vri.cz

Haasnoot, Willem

RIKILT-Institute of Food Safety, Wageningen UR, Wageningen, the Netherlands.
willem.haasnoot@wur.nl

Hall, Christopher

School of Environmental Sciences, University of Guelph, 50 Stone Road East, Guelph, Ontario, Canada, N1G 2W1.
jchall@uoguelph.ca

Houwen , Frans

ScienceLynk B.V., Heuvelsestraat 5, 5976 NG Kronenberg, The Netherlands.
info@sciencelynk.eu

Jackson Abby J.

Department of Chemistry, University of Nebraska, Lincoln, NE 68588-0304, USA.
ajackson@unlserve.unl.edu

Kage, Andreas

TU-Berlin, Institute of medical biotechnology, Berlin, Germany & Aptares AG, Am Scheunenviertel 1, 15749 Mittenwalde, Berlin, Germany.
a.kage@aptares.de

Crean, Carol

School of Biotechnology and Biomedical Diagnostics Institute, National Centre for Sensor Research, Dublin City University, Dublin 9, Ireland.
c.crean@surrey.ac.uk

Mahlknecht, George

Weizmann Institute of Science, Department of Immunology, 76100 Rehovot, Israel.
georgmahlknecht@gmx.at

Mascini, Marco

Università degli Studi di Firenze, Dipartimento di Chimica, Polo Scientifico, *via* della Lastruccia 3, 50019 Sesto Fiorentino, Firenze, Italy.
marco.mascini@unifi.it

Meulenberg, Eline P.

ELTI Support VOF, Ambachtsweg 5, 6581 AX, Malden, The Netherlands.
E.Meulenberg@eltisupport.nl

Morris, H.A.

School of Pharmacy and Medical Sciences, University of South Australia, Adelaide, South Australia 5001 and Chemical Pathology, SA Pathology, Adelaide, South Australia 5000 Australia.
howard.morris@imvs.sa.gov.au

O'Kennedy, Richard

School of Biotechnology and Biomedical Diagnostics Institute, National Centre for Sensor Research, Dublin City University, Dublin 9, Ireland.
richard.okennedy@dcu.ie

Posthuma-Trumpie, Geertuida A.

Wageningen UR Food & Biobased Research, Biomolecular Sensing & Diagnostics, P.O. Box 17, 6700 AA Wageningen, The Netherlands.
truus.posthuma@wur.nl

Proll, G.

Institute of Physical and Theoretical Chemistry (IPTC) Eberhard Karls University of Tuebingen, Germay.
guenther.proll@ipc.uni-tuebingen.de

Richard, Gabrielle

School of Environmental Sciences, University of Guelph, 50 Stone Road East, Guelph, Ontario, Canada, N1G 2W1.

Sonia Centi

Università degli Studi di Firenze, Dipartimento di Fisiopatologia Clinica, Viale G. Pieraccini, 6 - 50139 Firenze Sobansky, Italy.
sonia.centi@unifi.it

Sobansky, Matthew R.

Department of Chemistry, University of Nebraska, Lincoln, NE 68588-0304, USA.
msobansky@unlserve.unl.edu

Viguier, Caroline

Enfer Scientific Unit T, M7 Business Park, Newhall, Naas, Co. Kildare, Republic of Ireland.
carolineviguier@yahoo.com

Wood, William Grahem

retired (INSTAND e.V. Düsseldorf, Germany), Lärchenredder 1, D-23627 Groß Grönau, Germany.
wood@instand-ev.de

Xie, Xuemei

School of Environmental Sciences, University of Guelph, 50 Stone Road East, Guelph, Ontario, Canada, N1G 2W1.

CHAPTER 1

The Discovery and Development of the Antigen-Antibody Reaction

Part 1: A Brief History

William Graham Wood*

Lärchenredder 1, D-23627 Groß Grönau, Germany

Abstract: This chapter deals with the discovery and application of the antibody-antigen reaction in the form of inoculation, variolation and vaccination to induce immunity - at first to smallpox, later to other diseases and common afflictions such as rabies, anthrax and cholera, caused by microorganisms.

The work of the pioneers in this field and their discoveries is briefly described here.

The *in vitro* applications of the antibody-antigen reaction - mainly in the form of radioimmunoassays - is covered and includes the early development of this technique both in assay design and data reduction, which allowed the rapid acceptance of radioimmunoassay in clinical diagnostic procedures, especially in the fields of endocrinology, microbiology and pharmacology.

The successors to radioimmunoassay which use non-radioisotopic labels have also been described in detail as well as listing the pioneers in immunoassay development.

The above topics have been considered in the context of antigen-antibody reactions and some of the persons who can be termed pioneers in this area of predominantly medically-related research.

Keywords: Antibody, Immunoassay, History.

FIRST STEPS - FROM ORIENT TO OCCIDENT

The practical application of antigen-antibody reactions in preventive medicine was possibly already in use for smallpox over 3000 years ago in India [1], although some Sanskrit scholars deny that the sources cited refer to the process of variolation, insufflation or inoculation, used to induce immunity [2].

The first written reference to smallpox inoculation was made by the Chinese author Wan Quan (1499-1582) in his *Douzhen xinfa* (痘疹心法) (or "Secret methods for treatment of pox and rashes") published in 1549 [3] during the reign of the Ming Emperor Zhu Houcong, (also known as Jiajing). Dried smallpox scabs were blown up the noses of healthy individuals, who developed a mild form of the disease around one week later, recovered after two or three days and were immune thereafter. The mortality rate was less than 2% compared with up to 30% mortality of the disease itself.

Variolation was performed routinely in countries under Islamic influence (Persia, Turkey and North Africa) in the 17th Century. In 1714 and 1716 two reports of the Turkish method of inoculation were made to the Royal Society in England, by Emmanuel Timoni, a doctor affiliated with the British Embassy in Istanbul [4], and Giacomo Pylarini. Lady Mary Wortley Montagu (1689-1762), the wife of the British ambassador to the Ottoman Empire, is widely credited with introducing inoculation to Great Britain in 1721 after investigating the procedure in Turkey [5], although she met with unfounded and injudicious opposition from prominent members of the medical profession of the time.

THE DAWN OF REASON - RENAISSANCE AND REVOLUTION

With the founding of The Royal Society by Charles II in 1660 in Gresham College, London, the age of

***Address correspondence to William Graham Wood:** Lärchenredder 1, D-23627 Groß Grönau, Germany; E-mail: wood@instand-ev.de

Eline P. Meulenberg (Ed)

experimentation began, first in physics, chemistry and astronomy, then in biology and medicine. Early members included Robert Boyle, Isaac Newton, Robert Hooke, John Flamsteed and Christopher Wren to name but a few.

Jan Ingenhousz (1730-1799), a Dutch physicist, biologist and chemist and member of the Royal Society, who also discovered photosynthesis, was an active supporter of inoculation against smallpox [6] and inoculated the British royal family of George III - after successful inoculation of criminals as test-persons had shown the procedure to be effective against the disease! He also became the court physician to Maria Theresia, Empress of Austria, in Vienna.

Edward Jenner (1749-1823), an English surgeon and general practitioner, has been credited with the introduction of mass-inoculation using vaccination (from the Latin: vacca = cow) with cowpox virus, a more reliable form of treatment, after observing that milkmaids who contracted cowpox were immune to smallpox [7]. In 1803 the Jenner Institute was opened, which offered vaccination for the general public which ensured the national acceptance of vaccination in Great Britain and Europe. Some 20 years before, Benjamin Jesty (1736-1816), a farmer inoculated his family against smallpox using material from cowpox pustules, after he had also noticed that his milkmaids who had been infected with cowpox did not contract smallpox in a local epidemic [8].

The 19th Century brought more light into how and why things happened and here the name of Louis Pasteur (1822-1895) must be mentioned. Pasteur revolutionised the field of immunisation and expanded its field of operation by developing vaccines for chicken cholera [9], rabies and anthrax, (having learned of its importance from Robert Koch) [10]. He also further developed the theory of germs [11] and worked on the attenuation (producing weakened strains) of bacteria and viruses [12], a vital point in the further development of inducing immunity against recurrent endemic diseases, finally resulting in the founding of one of the world's leading authorities on vaccines, the Institut Pasteur.

THE RISE OF THE LABORATORY - FROM *IN VIVO* TO *IN VITRO*

Robert Koch (1843-1910), one of the founders of modern microbiology renowned for his work on tuberculosis [13], suffered a setback with his "Tuberculin" vaccine, which did not come up to expectations as it did not lead to long-term prevention of the disease. This was to change his scientific life permanently, but led to the establishment of the Königlich Preußisches Institut für Infektionskrankheiten, (the predecessor of the Robert-Koch-Institut) in Berlin.

The introduction of systematic analysis of biological phenomena in the 19th Century led to the definition of basic units which are still used in immunology.

The term antibody (Antikörper) was first used by Paul Ehrlich (1854-1915) in 1891 [14], although the word as such was first accepted internationally several years later. He was also famous for his "side-chain" theory of antigen-presentation and antibody production [15]. This was the forerunner of the modern selection theory of immune defence.

The term antigen was first used in 1899 by Lásló Detre (also known as Ladislas Deutsch) (1874-1939) [16]. The term antigen (a shortened form of antibody-generator or antisomatogen) is usually defined as: Any substance which, when recognized as non-self by the adaptive immune system of an organism, triggers an immune response, thus stimulating production of an antibody which specifically reacts with the substance.

The word "hapten" was first used in 1921 by Karl Landsteiner (1868-1943) to define the portion of a complex antigen which determines its specific reactivity rather than the ability to function as an antigen [17].

The study of the reaction of haptens with different antibodies was carried out by Michael Heidelberger (1888-1991) and Forrest Kendall (1899-1987) in their experiments on the precipitin reaction in the early

1930s [18]. This can be seen as the beginnings of immunochemistry, which has become an integral part of laboratory medicine.

The concept of epitopes (and paratopes) was first described by David W. Talmage (b. 1919) in 1959 [19]. A similar concept was also developed by Frank Macfarlane Burnet (1899-1985) [20] and published in 1957. An epitope (or antigenic determinant) is defined as: The distinct molecular surface features of an antigen capable of being bound by an antibody. Large molecules can have several epitopes, haptens, just a single epitope.

The following table summarises the development up to the discovery of immunoassay.

Table 1: Discoveries in antigen-antibody reactions from ca. 1000 BC to 1960 AD.

Date	Pioneer/Country	Field of Research
ca. 1000 BC	Indian healers	Variolation against smallpox
1549 AD	Wan Quan-China	Treatment of pox and rashes
17th Century	Medical practitioners-Ottoman Empire	Inoculation against smallpox
1714, 1716	Emanuel Timmoni-Turkey, Great Britain	Lectures on inoculation against smallpox at the Royal Society
1721	Lady Mary Wortley Montagu-Great Britain	Introduction of smallpox inoculation from Turkey to England
1768	Jan Ingenhousz-Netherlands/Great Britain	Inoculation of the British and Austrian Royal Families against smallpox
1774	Benjamin Jesty/Great Britain	Inoculation against smallpox
1794	Edward Jenner/Great Britain	Vaccination against smallpox
19th Century	Louis Pasteur/France	Development of vaccines against rabies, anthrax and chicken cholera
19th Century	Robert Koch/Germany	Development of vaccine against tuberculosis
1891	Paul Ehrlich/Germany	Introduction of the term "antibody"
1899	Lásló Detre/Hungary	Introduction of the term "antigen"
1921	Karl Landsteiner/Austria	Introduction of the term "hapten"
1930s	Michael Heidelberger and Forrest Kendall/USA	Experiments on the precipitin reaction
1957	Frank Macfarland Burnett/Australia	Concept of epitopes
1959	David W. Talmage/USA	Concept of paratopes

Antibodies or immunoglobulins form the majority of the gamma globulin fraction in electropherograms of human serum. There are five classes of immunoglobulins [21], which bear the abbreviations: IgA, IgD, IgE, IgG and IgM; four of which play an active role in immune defence. The role of IgD is still not fully understood, but appears to enhance immune surveillance [22]. IgA and IgM are the immunoglobulins of the early immune reaction, IgA being produced at endothelial surfaces such as lung, intestine and bladder and IgM in response to direct somatic infiltration. IgE is typical for allergic reactions such as asthma or eczema. IgG gives "long term" protection and is a secondary response. IgM production usually leads to induction of IgG antibodies of higher avidity and specificity. In contrast to IgM production, IgA production does not appear to lead to direct induction of IgG [23] and continues over long periods of time, which explains the efficacy of oral vaccines such as those used against poliomyelitis.

A RADIANT FUTURE - THE BIRTH OF IMMUNOASSAY

The commercial production of radioisotopes started soon after the second world war and iodine 131 was already supplied to selected medical institutions in Canada in 1949 from the National Research Experimental (NRX) project started in 1943/44 [24].

The continued studies on radioiodination during the 1950s [25, 26] led to a relatively effective and simple method for radioiodination of proteins was published by McFarland in 1958 [27] using labelled iodine monochloride (^{131}ICl).

The substitution of radioisotopes in natural substances such as ^{131}I-labelled thyroxine led Roger Ekins in 1959 to develop his Competitive Protein Binding Assay (CPBA) for the determination of thyroxine (T_4) in serum [28, 29]. In the same year, Rosalyn Yalow and Solomon Berson used radioiodinated insulin, together with an insulin antibody to measure insulin in human blood plasma [30, 31]. This was the interim result of many years investigation in *in vivo* and *in vivo* studies on the distribution and fate of radioiodinated proteins [32]. As radioimmunoassay was not patented, it became available to thousands of researchers which encouraged its rapid development and implementation, especially in the field of laboratory diagnostic procedures.

Early radioimmunoassays were not easy to perform and were purely manual procedures with complicated separation of bound and free antigen and resulting quantitation of radioactivity. The half-life of ^{131}I was short (8.02 days), which meant that labels had to be prepared regularly. The high energy beta- (606 keV) and gamma-emission (364 keV) resulted in radiolysis, which could change the antigen structure. The relative ease of production (^{131}I is a fission product of ^{235}U, with an efficiency of around 2.83%) made it the isotope of choice. It has been replaced by ^{125}I for *in vitro* use such as in immunoassays [33]. ^{125}I is a relatively "soft" gamma-emitter (35 keV) with a half life of 59.4 days and is produced by neutron bombardment of ^{124}Xe gas. ^{125}I produces less radiolysis and its longer half-life leads to the less-frequent need for radioiodination. ^{125}I decays *via* electron capture to ^{125m}Te, which in turn reverts to stable ^{125}Te with gamma emission (145 keV) and a half-life of 57.4 days. This second decay can also lead to increased radiolysis in the tracer.

The majority of methods of iodination involve the oxidation of iodide (I^-) anions to iodinium (I^+) cations which then react with tyrosyl- (or histidyl-) residues of proteins or peptides. Molecules without such moieties must have a tyrosyl residue introduced before iodination can take place. Iodination agents include ^{125}iodine monochloride [27], chloramine-T [34, 35] or 1,3,4,6-tetrachloro-3α,6α-diphenyl glycoluril (better known as Iodogen) [35, 36], the latter two requiring $Na^{125}I$ as source of iodine.

Conventional liquid-phase radioimmunoassay used a diluted native polyclonal antiserum as a binding agent, defined amounts of unlabelled antigen as standard and radiolabelled antigen as tracer, whereby the antibody was limited, with a capacity to bind usually between 10-50% of the label. The antigen in the sample to be measured competed with the fixed amount of tracer for the binding sites on the antibody, (hence the name "competitive (immune)assay"). After reaction, the antibody-bound fraction of the radioactive-labelled antigen [tracer] together with antigen bound from the sample (the so-called "bound" fraction) was separated from the incubation mixture using a separation agent. The latter could be a specific reagent such as a liquid [37] or solid-phase [38, 39] "second antibody" directed against the antigen-specific (first) antibody, or a non-specific solid-phase adsorbent (charcoal [40], ion-exchange resin [41]) or a precipitant (polyethylene glycol) [42], ethanol [43]). Combinations of the above techniques were also developed, for example the combination of polyethylene glycol and second antibody [44].

In the case of the non-specific adsorbant based separation, either the precipitate (free-fraction) or the supernate (bound-fraction) was counted. In the case of the precipitant, the precipitate (bound-fraction) was usually counted after centrifugation and aspiration of the supernatant. For ^{125}I-labelled assays this was performed directly, with beta-emitters such as ^{14}C or ^{3}H, often used in early steroid immunoassays, after transfer of the supernate to a scintillation cocktail, an organic mixture, which emitted (blue) light on atomic decay.

Immunoassay design has continually improved, the first step being the development of immune(radio)metric assays with either two antibodies, both directed against different epitopes on the antigen and thus limited to larger molecules, or with two antigen molecules bridged by a specific antibody [45]. Such assays are known as "sandwich assays" and are based on solid-phase technology, where one of the "sandwich halves" is attached to a macro- or micro support. Classic examples of immunoradiometric assays are those for hepatitis B surface antigen (HBsAg) and antibodies to HBsAg (Anti HBsAg) [46].

An immunometric assay is more specific than a competitive immunoassay and potentially has a lower limit of detection (= better analytical sensitivity) [45-48]. Immunometric assays are always associated with a solid-phase, whereas competitive immunoassays may be liquid or solid-phase based. Solid phases used for immobilisation of assay components include: the vessel wall (coated-tubes [49]), macro-solid phases (coated balls [44]), particulate solid-phases (coated magnetic-particles [50], cellulose [51], polymer-granulate [52]) and micro-solid phases (polystyrene latex particles [53], gold nanoparticles [54]).

ROBOTS AND COMPUTERS - ADVANCES IN AUTOMATION - 1

With the advent of computers, the tedious calculation of results, usually as counts in the sample read off a calibration curve manually drawn on (semi-logarithmic) graph paper. There were many "ideal" algorithms used, which were based rather on theory (the law of mass-action) than practice. Linearisation of the curve was one aim, as it made the programming easier! Such an approach was the so-called weighted [55, 56] or unweighted logit-log plot [57, 58] developed by Rodbard. An empirical and more flexible approach was applied by Marschner in the 1970s, which used a smoothed cubic spline function [59, 60]. Comparison of spline, logistic-log and logit-log has also been performed [61]. There has rarely been an area of immunoassay which has so fiercely been contested as that concerning the "correct" processing of assay data [56-61].

The first phase of linking assays with computerisation dealt more or less completely with the data processing [55-61]. Setting up and running assays remained at this time a manual procedure, with the exception of semi-automatic micropipettes [62]. For newcomers to immunoassay it is hard to visualise that the first desktop computers in the 1970s had 4kB RAM and a cassette for data storage, Microsoft DOS 2.11 came on a 3.5 inch 1.44 MB floppy disk and a Siemens 404/3 computer (originally the Zuse Z43, renamed after the takeover by Siemens) [63], which needed an air-conditioned room, weighed a couple of tons complete with endless-paper printer, punch tape reader, magnetic tape storage and a unit with removable 10 MB hard disks each protected in its own cassette [64].

ELECTROMAGNETIC ALTERNATIVES - NON-RADIOISOTOPIC IMMUNOASSAY

The disadvantages of a radioisotopic label were obvious from the beginning, but were accepted as long as the advantages outweighed the disadvantages. The main disadvantages were the large volumes of low-active radioactive waste, the increased risk of personal contamination with ^{125}I, especially in the thyroid, the relatively short shelf-life and the low efficiency of the label related to the decay constant as only a small number of molecules decayed within the counting period and the need for special laboratories in which radioisotopes could be used.

Alternative labelling methods were desirable, but were themselves fraught with disadvantages. The first steps were visible some 10 years after the introduction of radioimmunoassay, when enzyme-labelling was shown to be possible. The "new" labels were often patented, so that their freedom of use became more limited.

The first alternatives were the solid phase heterogeneous assay which was christened ELISA (Enzyme Linked Immunosorbent Assay), thus issuing in the era of "female" assays (in more than one sense, as this assay was published by Eva Engvall and Peter Perlmann [65]) The homogeneous EMIT (Enzyme Multiplied Immunoassay Technique) [66] was published around the same time as well as the first attempts at using fluorescent labels [67].

The enzymes used had to be robust and remain biologically active after coupling to antigens or antibodies, as well as having a high turnover and giving rise to an intensely coloured product. Alkaline phosphatase, ß-galactosidase and horseradish peroxidase were usually chosen for ELISA techniques [68], whereas EMIT systems tended to use dehydrogenases [66, 69], which together with NAD(P) could be measured at 334/340 nm in conventional clinical chemistry analysers [70].

The first fluorescent labels were derivatives of fluorescein isothiocyanate [68]. The problem with fluorescent labels was quenching by the sample [analogous to that in radioimmunoassay with β-emitters such as ^{14}C, ^{3}H, ^{32}P or ^{35}S using liquid scintillation counting] which made solid-phase systems preferable [71].

The 1980s saw the advent of luminescent labels either in combination with enzyme labelling (alkaline phosphatase [72, 73] or peroxidase [74] with continuous signal or "glow" luminescence) or chemiluminescence with luminol and acridinium derivatives (flash luminescence). The advantage of glow luminescence is that a signal re-measurement is possible, which is not the case for flash luminescence.

The first commercial luminescence immunoassays were those of the Amerlite range from Amersham [74]. The early attempts with charcoal separation in luminescence immunoassays [75] were soon replaced by robust solid phase assays [76, 77] which are still in use in commercial immunoassays over 25 years later. Luminescent labels were the first to achieve and even surpass radioisotopic labelling in term of the lower detection limits possible [77].

Further development of luminescent signals has led to the Boehringer-Mannheim/Roche Elecsys immunoassays using ruthenium electrochemiluminescence combined with magnetic particles [78].

An alternative to chemiluminescence was the time-resolved fluorescence method [79, 80] developed at the same time by Wallac in Finland [DELFIA] and later introduced in a modified form by CIS/Brahms as the Kryptor method [81]. Time resolved fluorescence has the advantage of being long-lived (200-600 ms) compared with conventional fluorescence (ns range) so that any interfering natural fluorescence signal can be eliminated by changing the time measuring window [79].

Most hormone immunoassays offered today have luminescent signal detection in order to achieve the necessary analytical sensitivity. Where this is not necessary, enzyme labelling without signal amplification is the method of choice.

ROBOTS AND COMPUTERS - ADVANCES IN AUTOMATION - 2

The introduction of non-radioisotopic labelling has produced a large number of immunoassay techniques, many of which are patented and intended to circumvent existing patents. This has led to unnecessary complications and development of specialised equipment, automation and closed-systems in which only "company-reagents" can be used and which often makes academic research difficult or even impossible with such devices.

One of the earliest and most successful of these novel systems were the Abbott FLx/TDx Fluorescence-Polarisation Immunoassays (FPIA) [82] introduced in 1981 and IMx microparticle enhanced immunoassays (MEIA) [83] introduced in 1988 both of which are still in routine use today. Both principles were combined in the fully automated system AxSYM [84] in 1993.

The EMIT homogeneous immunoassays, patented by Syva [85] could be performed on conventional clinical chemistry analysers, thus facilitating drug monitoring without the need for additional equipment (= investment) [86].

Solid-phase enzyme immunoassays using conventional colorimetric measurements were adapted to microtiter plate or strip format, thus keeping an open-system on which assays from different manufacturers could be performed. Microtiter plates were first introduced in 1951 by a Hungarian, Dr. G. Takatsky [87], who machined 6 rows of 12 "wells" in Lucite (polymethylmethacrylate), although their popularity first increased with the introduction of microtiter plate readers in the 1980s. Microtiter plates were first used in microbiology and virology for cultures [87].

Fully automatic enzyme immunoassays were developed either as modular systems (pipetting station, incubator unit, microtiter plate reader, data-processing unit, printer) [88], where each unit was connected to a central computer or as integrated partially open systems such as the Bio-Rad Coda [89], although the latter have not become as popular as was expected. The availability of cheap desktop computers has supported the modular design approach. Complete analyser systems using coated tubes were developed by Boehringer-Mannheim in their ES-600 and ES-300 devices [90, 91]. These had the advantage that the exact number of reaction vessels could be chosen which is not possible with microtiter plates and only partially possible with strips. At this time, experiments with one-point recalibration (instead of a standard curve) were published as a proposed rationalisation step with cost-optimisation [92].

The introduction of luminescent labels opened the market for further open and closed systems. The pioneer of luminometers suitable for routine use was Berthold, who first developed the LB 950 T [93] for research and then the LB 952 [94] for routine use, the latter being offered as OEM-device by many kit-producers.

Whether potential new labels for immunoassay become commercially available depends upon the investment costs to a large degree. Examples here include Nuclear Magnetic Resonance (NMR) [95], which has been possible for a couple of decades, but has not seen a breakthrough due to the enormous costs of instrumentation and surface plasmon resonance [96], which has a better chance, as commercial interest has been shown. Electrochemical luminescence [78] is an example, where commercial interest has resulted in the introduction of an expensive technology into the routine laboratory.

The most important developments in immunoassay are shown in the following table:

Table 2: Pioneers of immunoassay and related procedures.

Date	Pioneer/Country	Assay Development
1960	R.P. Ekins/Great Britain	CPBA for thyroxine
1960	R. Yalow, S. Berson/USA	RIA for Insulin
1968	L.E.M. Miles, C.N. Hales/Great Britain	IRMA for Insulin
1969-1972	D. Rodbard/USA; I. Marschner/Germany	Development of computer programmes for processing immunoassay data
1971	E. Engvall, P. Perlmann/Sweden; B.K. Van Weeman , A.H.W.M. Schuurs/Netherlands	ELISA for proteins and haptens
1972	K.E. Rubenstein, R.S. Schneider, E.F. Ullmann/USA	EMIT for drugs
1972	Foundation of the National Institute of Biological Standards and Control [formerly NBSB]/Great Britain	International reference preparations/reagents and standards for immunoassay [IRP; IS; RR]
1975	G. Köhler, C. Milstein/USA	Discovery and production of monoclonal antibodies [MAbs]
1981	M.E. Jolley/USA	FPIA for haptens
1981	M. Passagli, M.Serio/Italy	LIA for progesterone
1983	T. Lövgren, E. Soini/Finland	TRFIA - DELFIA for haptens and peptide hormones
1983	I. Rönnberg/Sweden	Surface plasmon resonance

This terminates the historical overview of antigen-antibody reactions in medical science and the development of the various forms of immunoassay. Further developments, applications and considerations are to be found in the next part of this chapter.

REFERENCES

[1] Bourzac K. "Smallpox: Historical Review of a Potential Bioterrorist Tool". JYI 2002; 6(3). www.jyi.org/volumes/volume6/index.html.

[2] Wujastyk D. "Medicine in India". In: Oriental Medicine: An Illustrated Guide to the Asian Arts of Healing. Eds. van Alphen, J; Aris, A; London: Serindia Publications, 1995. pp. 19-38. ISBN 0-906026-36-9; 271 pages.
[3] Needham J. In: "Part 6, Medicine". Science and Civilization in China: Volume 6, Biology and Biological Technology. Cambridge: Cambridge University Press, 1999. 134 pages.
[4] Behbehani AM. The smallpox story: life and death of an old disease. Microbiol Rev 1983; 47: 455-509.
[5] In: Letters of the Right Honourable Lady Mary Wortley Montagu: Written during her Travels in Europe, Asia and Africa to Persons of Distinction, Men of Letters &c. in different Parts of Europe. Which contain, among other Curious Relations, Accounts of the Policy and Manners of the Turks. Drawn from Sources that have been inaccessible to other Travellers. Berlin: 1781. (First Edition) Sold by August Mylius.
[6] von Wiesner J, Escherich T, Mach E, von Töply R, Wegscheider R. Jan Ingen-Housz: Sein Leben und sein Wirken als Naturforscher und Arzt. Verlag Carl Konegen, Vienna, 1905; 252 pages.
[7] Jenner E. An inquiry into the causes and effects of the variolae vaccinae, a disease discovered in the western counties of England, particularly Gloucestershire and known by the name of the cow pox. Second edition, Printed by Sampson Low, London, 1800; 183 pages.
[8] Hammarsten JF, Tattersall W, Hammarsten JE. Who discovered smallpox vaccination? Edward Jenner or Benjamin Jesty? Trans Am Clin Climatol Assoc 1979; 90: 44-55.
[9] Pasteur L: Sur les maladies virulentes, et en particulier sur la maladie appelée vulgairement cholera des poules. Comptes Rendus Hebdomadaires des Séances de l' Academie des Sciences 1880; 90: 249-248. .
[10] Koch R: Die Aetiologie der Milzbrand-Krankheit, begründet auf die Entwicklungsgeschichte des Bacillus anthracis. Beitrage zur Biologie der Pflanzen 1876; 2: 277-310.
[11] Pasteur L, Joubert JF, Chamberland C: La théorie des germes et ses applications à la médicine et a la chirurgie. Comptes Rendus Hebdomadaires des Séances de l' Academie des Sciences 1878; 86: 1037-43. .
[12] Pasteur L, Chamberland C, Roux PPE: De l'attenuation des virus et de leur retore à la virulence. Comptes Rendus des Séances de L'Academie des Sciences 1881; 92: 430-5. .
[13] Koch, R. Die Aetiologie der Tuberculose, Berliner Klinische Wochenschrift. Organ für practische Ärzte, 1882; 19: 221-230.
[14] Lindenmann J. Origin of the Terms 'Antibody' and 'Antigen'. Scand J Immunol 1984; 19: 281-5.
[15] Ehrlich P: Zur Kenntnis der Antitoxinwirkung. Fortschritte der Medizin 1897; 15: 41-3.
[16] Eichmann K. The Network Collective Rise and Fall of a Scientific Paradigm - Part III Science between Fact and Fiction, Chapter 16, Fiction turned fact - The case of antibodies. Birkhäuser Basel, 2008; pp. 213-224; ISBN 978-3-7643-8372-5: 274 pages.
[17] Landsteiner K. Über heterogenetisches Antigen und Hapten XV. Mitteilung Über Antigene. Biochem Z 1921;119: 294-306.
[18] Heidelberger E, Kendall FM: Studies on the precipitin reaction: Precipitating haptens; species differences in antibodies. J Exp Med 1933; 57: 373-9.
[19] Talmage, DW: Immunological specificity: An alternative to the classical concept. Science 1959; 129: 1643-8.
[20] Burnet FM. A modification of Jerne's theory of antibody production using the concept of clonal selection. Aust J Sci 1957; 20: 67-9.
[21] Market E, Papavasiliou FN (2003) V(D)J Recombination and the Evolution of the Adaptive Immune System. PLoS Biol 1[1]: e16. doi:10.1371/journal.pbio.0000016.
[22] Chen K, Xu W, Wilson M, *et al.* Immunoglobulin D enhances immune surveillance by activating antimicrobial, proinflammatory and B cell-stimulating programs in basophils. Nat Immunol 2009; 10: 889-98.
[23] Scavone P, Sosa V, Pellegrino R, Galvalisi U, Zunino P. Mucosal vaccination of mice with recombinant Proteus mirabilis structural fimbrial proteins. Microbes and Infection 2004; 6: 853-60.
[24] Ullyett B. In: Chapter 5 Radioisotopes, Canada enters the nuclear age; a technical history of Atomic Energy of Canada Limited as seen from its research laboratories. Atomic Energy of Canada Limited, Eds. Hurst DG *et al.*, McGill-Queen's University Press, Montreal, Québec, 1997; pp. 97-116: ISBN 0-7735-1601-8, 448 Pages.
[25] Joiner CL, Pearson JD. V. Studies with Insulin Labelled with Iodine 131. Br J Radiol 1959; 32: 657-60.
[26] McFarlane AS. Labeling of plasma proteins with radioactive iodine. Biochem J 1956; 62: 135-43.
[27] McFarlane AS. Efficient trace-labelling of proteins with iodine (Letter). Nature 1958; 182: 53.
[28] Ekins RP. Estimation of protein bound ^{131}I in plasma. Phys Med Biol 1959; 4: 182-4.
[29] Ekins R.P. The estimation of thyroxine in human plasma by an electrophoretic technique. Clin Chim Acta 1960; 5:453-9.
[30] *Berson SA, Yalow RS.* Quantitative aspects of the reaction between insulin and insulin-binding antibody. J Clin Invest 1959; 38: 1996-2016.

[31] *Yalow RS, Berson SA.* Immunoassay of endogenous plasma insulin in man. J Clin Invest 1960; 39: 1157-75.
[32] Berson SA, Yalow RS, Schreiber SS, Post J. Tracer experiments with I-131 labeled human serum albumin: Distribution and degradation studies. J Clin Invest 1953; 32: 746-68.
[33] Yalow RS, Berson SA. Labeling of proteins - problems and practices. Trans NY Acad Sci 1966; 28: 1033-44.
[34] Greenwood FC, Hunter WM. The preparation of ^{131}I-labelled human growth hormone of high specific radioactivity. Biochem J 1963; 89; 114-23.
[35] Wood WG, Wachter C, Scriba PC. Experiences using Chloramine-T and 1,3,4,6-Tetrachloro-3α, 6α-diphenylglycoluril (Iodogen®) for Radioiodination of Materials for Radioimmunoassay. J Clin Chem Clin Biochem 1981; 19: 1051-6.
[36] Paus E, Bormer O, Nustad K. Radioiodination of proteins with the Iodogen method. In: RIA and Related Procedures in Medicine, IAEA, Vienna 1982; pp. 161-171.
[37] Burrell CJ, Leadbetter G, Black SH, Hunter WM. Rapid detection of hepatitis B surface antigen by double antibody radioimmunoassay. J Med Virol 1978; 3: 19-26.
[38] Gardner J, Bailey G, Chard T. Observations on the use of solid-phase-coupled antibodies in the radioimmunoassay of human placental lactogen. Biochem J 1974; 137: 469-76.
[39] Cocola F, Genazzani AR, Neri P. New radioimmunoassay technique using second antibody to solid phase applied to assays of human chorionic somatomammotropin. J Nucl Biol Med 1973; 17: 14-21.
[40] Wool MS, Selenkow HA. Charcoal-dextran radioimmunoassay of human growth hormone. Acta Endocrinol (Copenh) 1968; 57: 109-14.
[41] Lazarus L, Young JD. Radioimmunoassay of human growth hormone using ion exchange resin. J Clin Endocrinol Metab 1966; 26: 213-8.
[42] Desbuquois B, Aurbach GD. Use of polyethylene glycol to separate free and antibody-bound peptide hormones in radioimmunoassays. J Clin Endocrinol Metab 1971; 33: 732-8.
[43] Letchworth AT, Boardman R, Bristow C, Landon J, Chard T. A rapid radioimmunoassay for human chorionic somatomammotrophin. Br J Gynaecol 1971; 78: 535-41.
[44] Wood WG, Stalla G, Müller OA, Scriba PC. A rapid and specific method for separation of bound and free antigen in radioimmunoassay systems. J Clin Chem Clin Biochem 1979; 17: 111-4.
[45] Miles LEM, Hales CN. Labelled antibodies and immunological assay systems. Nature 1968; 189: 26.
[46] Bond WW, Petersen NJ, Favero MS, Schable CA, Murphy BL, Berquist KA, Maynard, JE. Evaluation of a finger prick blood collection method for the seroepidemiology of hepatitis B. Bull WHO 1978; 56: 791-6.
[47] Rodbard D, Weiss GH. Mathematical theory of immunometric (labeled antibody) assay. Anal Biochem 1973; 52: 10.
[48] Jackson TN, Marshall MJ, Ekins RP. Optimization of immunoradiometric (labeled antibody) assays. Immunoassays Clin Chem 1983; 557-75.
[49] Baumann JB, Girard J, and Vest M. Solid-phase radioimmunoassay for human growth hormone: Experience with antiserum-coated assay-tubes. Immunochemistry 1967; 6: 699-713.
[50] Birkmeyer RC, Diaco R, Hutson DK, Lau HP, Miller WK, Neelkantan NV, Pankratz TJ. Application of novel chromium dioxide magnetic particles to immunoassay development. Clin Chem 1987; 33: 1543-7.
[51] Sutherland RM, Ratcliffe JG, Chapman RS. Immunoassay of blood spot TSH; development of a rapid two-site immunoradiometric assay and comparison with radioimmunoassay as a screening method for neonatal hypothyroidism. Clin Chim Acta 1982; 124: 1-11.
[52] Johansen L, Nustad K, Orstavik TB, Ugelstad J, Berge A, Ellingsen T. Excess antibody immunoassay for rat glandular kallikrein. Monosized polymer particles as the preferred solid phase material. J Immunol Methods 1983; 59: 255-64.
[53] Bernard AM, Vysko A, Lauwerys RR. Determination of β_2-microglobulin in human urine and serum by latex immunoassay. Clin Chem 1981; 27: 832-7.
[54] Khlebtsov BN, Khanadeev VA, Bogatyrev VA, Dykman LA, Khlebtsov NG. Use of gold nanoshells in solid-phase immunoassay. Nanotech Russia 2008; 3: 442-55.
[55] Rodbard D, Bridson W, Rayford PL. Rapid calculation of radioimmunoassay results. J Lab Clin Med 1969; 74: 770-81.
[56] McDonald M. Calculator program for weighted logit-log radioimmunoassay data reduction. Clin Chem 1981; 27: 1946.
[57] Fischer L. Logit-log radioimmunoassay data reduction: weighted vs unweighted. Clin Chem 1983; 29: 391-2.

[58] Rodbard D. Data processing for radioimmunoassay -:An overview. Clinical Immunochemistry: Chemical and Cellular Bases and Applications in Disease, S. Natelson *et al.*, Eds., AACC, Washington, DC, 1978, pp 477-94.

[59] Marschner I, Erhardt F, Scriba PC. Calculation of the radioimmunoassay standard curve by "spline function". Radioimmunoassay and related procedures in medicine, Vol. 1. IAEA, Vienna, 1974; pp. 383-97.

[60] Marschner I, Dobry H, Erhardt F, Landersdorfer T, Popp B, Ringel C, Scriba PC. Berechnung radioimmunologischer Meßwerte mittels Spline-Funktionen. Ärztl Lab 1974; 20: 184-91.

[61] Plikaytis BD, Turner SH, Gheesling LL, Carlone GM. Comparisons of standard curve-fitting methods to quantitate neisseria meningitidis group a polysaccharide antibody levels by enzyme-linked immunosorbent assay. J Clin Microbiol 1991; 29: 1439-46.

[62] Lasky FD, Al Razi J, Karmen A. Improved approach to sequential addition immunoassay. Clin Chem 1978; 24: 1381-5.

[63] Müller OA, Braun J, Fröhlich R, Scriba PC. Eine mechanisierte kompetitive Proteinbindungsanalyse für Cortisol im Serum ohne vorherige Extraktion mit organischen Lösungsmitteln. J Clin Chem Clin Biochem 1974; 12: 276-8.

[64] Kurz C, Richter M. Feature-Skript: Konrad Zuse - Der rechnende Raum. Erste Aufführung: 11. Oktober 2006 im Hermann-von-Helmholtz-Zentrum für Kulturtechnik der Humboldt-Universität zu Berlin anläßlich der Tagung 70 Jahre Zuse Z1 - 25 Jahre IBM-PC des Berliner Stiftungsverbundkollegs der Alcatel SEL Stiftung. www.46halbe.org/zuse.html.

[65] Engvall E, Perlman P. Enzyme-linked immunosorbent assay [ELISA] Quantitative assay of immunoglobulin G. Immunochemistry 1971; 8: 871-4.

[66] Rubenstein KE, Schneider RS, Ullmann EF. "Homogeneous" enzyme immunoassay. A new immunochemical technique. Biochem Biophys Res Commun 1972; 47: 846-51.

[67] Curry RE, Heitzman H, Riege DH, Sweet RV and Simonsen MG. A systems approach to fluorescent immunoassay: general principles and representative applications. Clin Chem 1979; 25: 1591-5.

[68] Nosoda H, Wataru T, Tsukamoto R, Nambara T. Sensitivity of steroid enzyme immunoassays. Comparison of alkaline phosphatase, β-galactosidase and horseradish peroxidase as labels in a colorimetric assay system. Chem Pharm Bull 1987; 35: 3336-42.

[69] Van Weemen B, Schuurs A. Immunoassay using antigen-enzyme conjugates. FEBS Lett 1971; 15: 232.

[70] Scharpé SL, Cooreman WM, Blomme WJ, Laekeman GM. Quantitative enzyme immunoassay: Current Status. Clin Chem 1976; 22: 733-8.

[71] Phillips DJ, Galland GG, Reimer CB, Kendal AP. Evaluation of a solid-phase immunoassay with fluorescein isothiocyanate-conjugated heterogeneous or monoclonal antibodies for identification of virus isolates, with influenza virus as a model. J Clin Microbiol 1982; 15: 931-7.

[72] Adam W, Reinhardt D, Saha-Möller CR. From the firefly bioluminescence to the dioxetane-based [AMPPD] chemiluminescence immunoassay: a retroanalysis. Analyst 1996; 121, 1527-31.

[73] Janda I, Jaensch H, Braun J, Wood WG. A comparison of four immunometric assays for myeloperoxidase using luminescent and colorimetric signal detection. J Clin Chem Clin Biochem 1990; 28: 475-80.

[74] Whitehead TP, Thorpe BHG, Carter TJN, Grocutt C, Kricka U. Enhanced luminescence procedure for sensitive determination of peroxidase labelled conjugates in immunoassay. Nature 1983; 305:158-9.

[75] Pazzagli M, Kim JB, Messeri G, Martinazzo G, Kohen F, Franceschetti F, Tommasi A, Salerno R, Serio M. Luminescent immunoassay (LIA) for progesterone in a heterogeneous system. Clin Chim Acta 1981; 115: 287-96.

[76] Wood WG, Fricke H, Haritz J, Gadow A, Krausz HS, Tode B, Strasburger CJ, Scriba PC. An evaluation of four different luminescence immunoassay systems: CELIA (chemiluminescent immunoassay), SPALT (solid-phase antigen luminescence technique), ILMA (immunoluminometric assay) and ILSA (immunoluminometric labelled second antibody). A critical study of macro solid phases for use in immunoassay systems, Part III. J Clin Chem Clin Biochem 1984; 22: 349-56.

[77] Weeks I, Sturgess M, Siddle K, Jones MK, Woodhead JS. A high sensitivity immunochemiluminometric assay for human thyrotrophin. Clin Endocrinol (Oxf) 1984; 20: 489-95.

[78] Forest JC, Massé J, Lane A. Evaluation of the analytical performance of the boehringer mannheim elecsys® 2010 immunoanalyzer. Clin Biochem 1998; 31: 81-8.

[79] Soini E, Kojola H. Time-resolved fluorimeter for lanthanide chelates. A new generation of non-isotopic immunoassays. Clin Chem 1983; 29: 65-8.

[80] Lövgren T, Hemmilä I, Pettersson K, Halonen P. Time-resolved fluorimetry in immunoassay. In: Alternative Immunoassays, Ed. Collins W, John Wiley & Sons, Chichester UK, 1985; pp. 203-17.

[81] Bauer T, Charl S, Sturm G. Comparison of the test methods (KRYPTOR, ES 600 and CIS-RIA) for CEA, CA 15-3 and CA 125 follow-up and ONCOCHECK quality control. Anticancer Res 2000; 20: 5245-7.

[82] Jolley ME. Fluorescence polarization immunoassay for the determination of therapeutic drug levels in human plasma. J Anal Toxicol 1981; 5: 236-40.

[83] Flare M, Mitchell J, Doan T, *et al.* Abbott imx^{tm} automated benchtop immunochemistry analyzer system. Clin Chem 1988; 34: 1726-32.

[84] Smith J, Osikowicz G. Abbott AxSYM random and continuous access immunoassay system for improved workflow in the clinical laboratory. Clin Chem 1993; 39: 2063-9.

[85] US Patent 3880715 : Immunoassay for haptens, Syva Company, Palo Alto CA, Apr. 29, 1975.

[86] Orsulah PJ, Haven MC, Huth JA, Studts DJ. EMIT Quantitative tricyclic antidepressant assays applied to the Hitachi 705 chemistry analyzer. Clin Chem 1987; 33: 1471.

[87] Sever JL. Application of a microtechnique to viral serological investigations. J Immunol 1962; 88: 320-9.

[88] Jaklevic JM, Garner HR, Miller GA. Instrumentation for the genome project. Annu Rev Biomed Eng 1999; 1: 649-78.

[89] Kim YK, Suh IB, Kim H, *et al.* The plasma levels of interleukin-12 in schizophrenia, major depression, and bipolar mania: effects of psychotropic drugs. Mol Psychiatry 2002; 7: 1107-14.

[90] Gässler N, Wood WG. Evaluierung und Methodenvergleich des ES 600 Enzymun-Test®-Systems zu anderen immunologischen Routinemethoden. Lab Med 1990; 14: 93-101.

[91] Camara PD, Velletri K, Krupski M, Rosner M, Griffiths WC. Evaluation of the Boehringer Mannheim ES 300 immunoassay analyzer and comparison with enzyme immunoassay, fluorescence polarization immunoassay, and radioimmunoassay methods. Clin Biochem 1992; 25: 251-4.

[92] Meyer HD, Keller H. One-point recalibration of heterogeneous enzyme immunoassays with non-linear calibration curves. Clin Chem 1988; 3: 113-7.

[93] Braun J, Schultek T, Tegtmeyer KF, *et al.* Luminometric assays of seven acute-phase proteins in minimal volumes of serum, plasma, sputum, and bronchioalveolar lavage. Clin Chem 1986; 32: 743-7.

[94] Missler U, Wood WG. Ein neuer immunoluminometrischer Festphasen-Sandwich-Assay zum quantitativen Nachweis von Antikörpern gegen das Hepatitis B-Oberflächen (HB_s)-Antigen. J Clin Chem Clin Biochem 1988; 26: 569-72.

[95] Lucchese A, Mittelman A, Lin M-S, *et al.* Epitope definition by proteomic similarity analysis: identification of the linear determinant of the anti-Dsg3 MAb 5H10. J Transl Med 2004; 2:43.

[96] Jönsson U, Malmqvist M, Rönnberg I. Immobilization of immunoglobulins on silica surfaces: stability. Biochem J 1985; 227: 363-71.

CHAPTER 1

The Discovery and Development of the Antigen-Antibody Reaction

Part 2: Commercial Immunoassay Development and Applications

William Graham Wood*

Lärchenredder 1, D-23627 Groß Grönau, Germany

Abstract: The second chapter continues the history of immunoassay and mainly deals with the commercialization and automation of immunoassays, the impact of monoclonal antibodies and their potential role in standardization and the continued development towards microformats and multianalyte immunoassays.

This chapter also includes the terminology used in immunoassays and schematic representation of assay design in the form of diagrams, as well as a brief look into the possible future development of immunoassay techniques and their application and impact in clinical *in vitro* diagnostic procedures.

Keywords: Antibody, Immunoassay, Design, Labelling.

COMMERCIALISATION - ECOLOGICALLY FRIENDLY ASSAYS FOR EVERYONE

This chapter deals with practical questions raised in conjunction with immunoassays as well as the possible future of such techniques.

The first radioimmunoassays had to be performed in special laboratories equipped for working with radioisotopes. Often, special permission had to be obtained from local or government authorities with the same regulations applicable to atomic power stations, cyclotrons and similar establishments. Those performing radioimmunoassays were expected to receive special education in the use and dangers of radioisotopes. Radioactive waste had to be stored in designated areas for ten half-lives of the isotopes (for example: with ^{125}I this was 600 days). It was no wonder, that the majority of clinically relevant radioimmunoassays were performed in nuclear medicine departments and institutes under the direction of radiologists and endocrinologists, who used ^{125}I and ^{131}I for routine *in vivo* thyroid scans and treatment of thyroid cancers.

Immunoassays with non-radioisotopic labels can be performed in normal clinical diagnostic laboratories, which led to their rapid introduction and spread into routine use. Furthermore, such immunoassays could be automated, without the danger of widespread radioisotopic contamination, which had prevented a successful automation of the radioimmunoassay.

DO WE KNOW WHAT WE REALLY MEASURE? - MONOCLONAL ANTIBODIES AND EPITOPES

The specificity of immunoassays depends upon the antibodies used. In the first immunoassays, these were raised in animals such as rabbits, goats, sheep and guinea-pigs, which produced a mixture of antibodies raised against the purified immunogen, which itself was usually a mixture [1, 2]. These polyclonal antisera (arising from many natural T-cell/B-cell interactions) were often relatively unspecific which led to the often non-optimal comparison of results from assays using such antisera [3]. The immunoassay of autoantibodies, such as those directed against thyroid tissues or tissue components [4, 5] reflects this heterogeneity in the bad comparison between numerical results from different kits, despite "standardisation" with internationally accepted standard preparations (although these are often over 40 years old!). This highlights the fact, that immunoassays cannot be standardised simply by using WHO-

***Address correspondence to William Graham Wood:** Lärchenredder 1, D-23627 Groß Grönau, Germany; E-mail: wood@instand-ev.de

Eline P. Meulenberg (Ed)

standards for calibration, even if these have been produced by recombinant techniques and are thus well defined. The comparability of results between different immunoassays for the same analyte can be seen in the results from external quality control programmes [4, 5]. This can be a problem, especially if the recipient of immunoassay results has only the reference ranges for the assays used in "his own laboratory" and a patient brings results from another method and another laboratory, or if "his own laboratory" changes the reference ranges due to changes in production (new kit, new antibodies, re-standardisation). Possibilities for assay standardisation are given below in the section on monoclonal antibodies.

The production of antibodies to haptens [6, 7] allowed immunoassay of small molecules such as steroids [8] and drugs [9], thus greatly enlarging the scope of immunoassay.

The discovery of how to produce monoclonal (=monospecific) antibodies by Köhler and Milstein [10] radically changed the approach to immunoassay inasmuch as assay-design became possible by defining the epitopes recognised by the antibody, thus defining the molecule measured [11-15]. Although monoclonal antibodies often suffered the disadvantage of having low affinities and avidities, continual improvement in their production and selection has made them the antibody of choice for many assays.

The idea of measuring moles of epitopes or epitope-pairs was seen early on by Ekins, although this simple but brilliant concept has not caught on with kit producers, except for the tumour marker Cyfra 21-1 [16], where the analyte measured is determined by the two monoclonal antibodies used.

The improvement in specificity of immunometric assays is seen in peptide analysis, especially in molecules which exist in several forms such as human choriongonadotropin (hCG) [14] and human growth hormone (hGH) [15]. The specificity of such assays is now employed to detect synthetic peptides often used in doping, both in humans and animals. Despite such standardisation, other components in the sample, such as binding proteins may affect results [15].

The disadvantage of immunometric assays is that they cannot be used for haptens, so that interference - for example with metabolites, still presents problems, as is often seen in steroid and drug immunoassays, despite the use of monoclonal antibodies [17], although such cross-reactivity has been put to use in detecting biologically active metabolites of digoxin in patient monitoring [18].

FROM MACRO TO NANO - VISIBLE TO INVISIBLE

The developments in the field of immunoassays with respect to the lowering of the limits of detection and quantification have improved their clinical use in many selected cases. Examples here are the development of assays for thyrotropin (TSH) [19] and C-Reactive Protein (CRP) [20]. Kit manufacturers have emphasised these improvements with terms such as "3rd or 4th generation" TSH assay [21, 22] or "high-sensitive CRP" [23], with the catastrophic effect that erroneous "new analytes" appear such as "hs-CRP" [24], "supersensitive-TSH" [25] or "microalbumin" [26] due partly to the ignorance of the user of such terms or as a result of advertising purposes of those offering the analyses. Some authors have warned against the misuse of such terms and assays [29].

The improvement in the analytical sensitivity has led to miniaturisation of immunoassays - the so-called lab-on-a-chip methodology [23, 27, 28] now used in laboratory diagnosis and genetic screening [28, 29]. Theoretically, hundreds of analytes can be measured with a few microlitres of serum [30], thus making routine laboratory diagnosis possible in sick newborns, without the need for a subsequent blood transfusion.

Improvements in technology and micronics have led to the application of phenomena known for many years, but which remained as exotic curiosities until recently. Examples include surface plasmon (=quantum of plasma) resonance [31-34], discovered in 1983 by Inger Rönnberg [31] and which is now being used in non-labelled immunoassay on different devices offered by Biacore and Texas Instruments (Spreeta^{TM}) [34]; time-resolved fluorescence, which was observed and published by the Russian physicist Sergey Vavilov 70 years ago [35] marketed by Wallac/Perkin-Elmer and CIS/Brahms: and polarisation fluorescence, known since 1926 [36], but first put into practice over 50 years later by Abbott.

Miniaturisation in both test-geometry and electronics has led to the increase in the number of Point of Care Testing (POCT) devices using antigen-antibody reactions [37-40] thus allowing testing to be transferred from the laboratory to the doctor's office [39] or to the patient's home [40]. POCT has become important in providing medical care both in urban [41] as well as in isolated areas such as the Australian outback [42, 43], Sahel Zone [44], South Pole [45], in holiday resorts [46] or after natural catastrophies [47, 48]. In the days of Internet and USB there is no problem of data transfer [49] to centres which are able to interpret the results and prescribe treatment should this be necessary. The acceptance of POCT devices by the general public is reflected by their overall availability in supermarkets or *via* the Internet, *i.e.* no longer from medically qualified personnel.

A prerequisite for use of POCT is the quality and comparability of results both between POCT-devices and with established methodology [50, 51] and where available, with reference method procedures [52]. POCT has been dealt with in more detail than the centralised health-care system we are used to, as it is the direction in which medical diagnosis will take in the near future [53], with an estimated 30% of all tests performed according to modern trend analysis in worldwide health care [54]. The choice for POCT may be more of a psychological nature than in reducing time in hospital, as has been shown by a study in an emergency department [55]. The introduction of the detection of important infectious bacteria and viruses [56] by POCT using Lab-on-a-chip technology [57] further increases its potential in decentralised monitoring. Further reading in this area, as well as for specific immunoassays has been published in a recent review [58].

THE FUTURE - QUO VADIS?

The development of future technologies depends upon many interacting factors, so that it is difficult to predict what will happen in the next decade. The transfer of novel scientific advances will depend even more than previously upon a cost-benefit analysis before commercial development. The results will be that not everything which is possible (or perhaps desirable) will be realised. Two things are certain; the role of antigen-antibody reactions will continue to play an important role and the process of miniaturisation will continue. It may be expected that non-invasive technologies will be developed in this area, although progress in this direction has been somewhat disappointing, probably due to the poor cost-benefit analysis results of current methodologies.

As stated above, current medical laboratory diagnostics will continue to be moved into decentralised surroundings, which can range from medical centres through general practitioners and medical specialists to home-care monitoring. This does not mean that a central laboratory in a hospital will cease to exist. It does mean that the current transition to POCT on the wards and out-patient clinics will continue, only the non-POCT tests being performed centrally.

The use of new POCT devices in combating endemic diseases in underdeveloped areas will depend on the priority set by governing bodies in the respective countries, as well as upon the engagement and monetary support from central organisations such as the United Nations or World Health Organisation. The development of new commercial tests in this area of health care and disease prevention will depend directly upon the degree of commitment of such worldwide bodies, again based on cost-effectiveness.

A major, and as of yet unsolved problem is the external quality control of POCT devices and services as the testing will be performed by lay-persons, *i.e.* the patients themselves, or from medical auxiliary personnel without specific training in laboratory methods. This is further highlighted by the general availability of such devices for "home-use", which is expected to increase in future and not only for glucose monitoring.

The use of unlabelled immunoassays especially techniques such as surface plasmon resonance and reagent coated gold sol nanoparticles will form part of new miniaturised devices requiring less external calibration and thus leading to more reliability and better quality in both reagent production and patient results. This will be coupled by simple online connections for data analysis and therapeutic feedback from a central advisory unit, which may or may not be a hospital or healthcare centre.

The beauty of new inventions and situations is their spontaneous appearance, which tends to confuse the best oracles of future development, which is probably a good place to terminate this short review on the use of antigen-antibody reactions and turn to the final section on terminology used in immunoassay and schematic portrayal of the different assay formats behind the often impressive names.

TERMINOLOGY, ABBREVIATIONS AND ASSAY DESIGN

As in the case of most specialist fields a "secret code" mentality has developed, in which abbreviations have come to play an internationally accepted role for those initiated! There are however a series of non-standard abbreviations, which have mainly been developed by commercial companies for advertising purposes, some of which may even be confusing, for example MIA, which has at least seven different meanings! This section deals with "generic" terminology and abbreviations used in immunoassay and related procedures and is presented in tabular form, with references for further reading. There are also a few figures to show basic concepts.

i. Basic immunoassay abbreviations.

Abbreviation [References]	***In full***	***Incubation/Principle***
Ag/Ag*	Antigen/Labelled Antigen	
Ab/Ab*	Antibody/Labelled Antibody	
RIA	Radioimmunoassay	Competitive, one-site, liquid or solid-phase
IRMA	Immunoradiometric assay	Usually sequential and two-site, solid-phase
EIA	Enzyme immunoassay	Competitive, one-site and usually solid-phase
IEMA [61]	Immunoenzymometric assay	Usually sequential and two-site, solid-phase
FIA	Fluorescence immunoassay	Competitive, one-site, may be solid-phase
IFMA [62]	Immunofluorimetric assay	Usually sequential and two-site, solid-phase
LIA	Luminescence immunoassay	Competitive, one-site and usually solid-phase
ILMA	Immunoluminometric assay	Usually sequential and two-site, solid-phase

ii. Expanded basic immunoassay abbreviations.

Abbreviation [References]	***In full***	***Explanation***
FEIA [63]	Fluorescence enhanced enzyme immunoassay	Immunoassay with enzyme label but fluorescent substrate and detection
FIEMA	Fluorescence enhanced immunoenzymometric assay	Immunometric assay with enzyme label, fluorescent substrate and detection
LEIA	Luminescence enhanced enzyme immunoassay	Immunoassay with enzyme label but luminescent substrate and detection
LIEMA	Luminescence enhanced immunoenzymometric assay	Immunometric assay with enzyme label, luminescen substrate and detection

iii. Generally accepted abbreviations with wider application.

Abbreviation [References]	***In full***	***Explanation***
CPBA [59]	**C**ompetitive **P**rotein **B**inding **A**ssay	General term for all immunoassays
CEDIA [60]	**C**loned **E**nzyme **D**onor **I**mmuno-**A**ssay	Homogeneous EIA using recombinant enzyme fragments on Ab and Ag
DELFIA	**D**issociation **E**nhanced **L**anthanide **F**luorescence **I**mmuno **A**ssay	FIA/IFMA using europium chelate fluorescence

TRFIA	**T**ime **R**esolved **F**luorescence **I**mmuno **A**ssay	See DELFIA
ELISA	**E**nzyme-**L**inked-**I**mmuno-**S**orbent **A**ssay	Solid-phase EIA or IEMA with colorimetric detection
EMIT	**E**nzyme-**M**ultiplied-**I**mmunoassay **T**echnique	Homogeneous liquid-phase EIA with UV or visible signal detection
FPIA	**F**luorescence-**P**olarisation **I**mmuno-**A**ssay	FIA with molecular rotation signal polarisation
MEIA	**M**icroparticle **E**nzyme **I**mmuno-**A**ssay	EIA or IEMA based on microparticulate solid phase
NIA [64]	**N**ephelometric **I**mmuno-**A**ssay	Turbidimetric measure-ment at 180° [through the cuvette]
TIA [65]	**T**urbidimetric **I**mmuno-**A**ssay	Turbidimetric measure-ment at 90° [at right angles to the light source]
CLIA [66]	**C**hemiluminescent **L**uminescence **I**mmuno-**A**ssay	LIA with "flash-type" luminescence
ECLIA	**E**lectro-**C**hemical-**L**uminescence-**I**mmuno-**A**ssay	LIA or ILMA based on Ruthenium electrochemi-luminscence
ICMA	**I**mmuno-**C**hemilumino-**M**etric-**A**ssay	ILMA with "flash-type" luminescence
SPALT	**S**olid-**P**hase **L**uminescent-**A**ntigen-**T**echnique	One-site ILMA with immobilized antigen

iv. Other abbreviations in use.

Abbreviation [References]	***In full***	***Explanation***
BIA [67]	**B**iosensor **I**mmuno-**A**ssay	Used in conjunction with surface plasmon resonance
BIA [68]	**B**io **I**mmuno **A**ssay	Used for measuring bioactive components in coagulation
CASSIA [69]	**C**olorimetric **A**ctive-**S**ite **S**pecific **I**mmuno-**A**ssay	EIA used in study of coagulation factors
CIA [70]	**C**arbon **I**mmuno **A**ssay	Protein-coated India-ink particle agglutination immunoassay
CIA [71]	**C**hemiluminescent **I**mmuno-**A**ssay	LIA/ILMA with flash-type luminescence
CLIA [72]	**C**hemiluminescence-**L**inked **I**mmuno **A**ssay	LIA with flash-type luminescence
ECLIA [73]	**E**nhanced **C**hemi-**L**uminescence **I**mmuno **A**ssay	Synonymous with LEIA and LIEMA
ELFA [74]	**E**nzyme **L**inked **F**luorescence Immuno-**A**ssay	Synonymous with FEIA and FIEMA
LIA [75]	**L**ine **I**mmuno-**A**ssay	Analogous to Western Blot
MIA [76]	**M**ultiplex **I**mmuno-**A**ssay	Simultaneous analytical measurement of multiple protein biomarkers
MIA [77]	**M**icroarray **I**mmuno-**A**ssay	Chip-based immunoassay for detecting several analytes simultaneously
MIA [78]	**M**agnetic **I**mmuno-**A**ssay	Immunoassay with magnetic solid phase
MIA [79]	**M**agneto **I**mmuno **A**ssay	Immunoassay with ferromagnetic label and transduction detection
MIA [80]	**M**icrosphere based **I**mmuno-**A**ssay	Immunoassay based on Ag/Ab coated [latex] particles
MIA [81]	**M**embrane **I**mmuno-**A**ssay	Ag/Ab attached to such membranes as liposomes or flow-cells
MIA [82]	**M**icrobead **I**mmuno-**A**ssay	Immunoassay based on Ag/Ab coated microbeads
NIA [83]	**N**anofluidic **I**mmuno-**A**ssay	Used in identifying components in proteomics

NIA [84]	**N**ano-**I**mmuno-**A**ssay	Term used for submicro-liter immunoassays
PIA [85]	**P**in **I**mmuno-**A**ssay	Ag/Ab adsorbed to pins for microtiterplate EIA
PIA [86]	**P**CR-Enhanced **I**mmuno-**A**ssay	PCR-amplification prior to the immunoassay
PIA [87]	**P**ulse **I**mmuno-**A**ssay	High Voltage Pulsing coupled with latex agglut-ination immunoassay
SIA [88]	**S**pin **I**mmuno-**A**ssay	Electron-Spin-Resonance labeled immunoassay
SPIA [89]	**S**ol-**P**article **I**mmuno-**A**ssay	Ab/Ag coated polymer microparticle-EIA or FIA coupled to flow cytometry
SIA [90]	**S**trip **I**mmunoblot-**A**ssay	Analogous to Western Blot
SIA [91]	**S**trip **I**mmuno **A**ssay	Test-strip based on the enzyme-channelling technique
TIA [92]	**T**hin Layer **I**mmuno **A**ssay	Immunoassay on plastic solid-phase
VIA [93]	**V**isual **I**mmuno-**A**ssay	Bacterial culture in micro-titer plate coupled to EIA
ZIA [94]	**Z**one **I**mmuno-[electrophoresis]**A**ssay	Combination of immuno-assay with electrophoresis

v. Basic immunoassay principles-standard curve data presentation.

Data	**Competitive Assay**		**Two-Site Immunometric Assay**	
Concentration (Units)	Signal (mean counts)	Counting Error (± 2 SD)	Signal (mean counts)	Counting Error (± 2 SD)
2	9808	345	197	23
5	9422	286	504	60
10	8890	200	1217	97
20	7900	163	2780	140
50	5822	197	5006	162
200	3285	166	7831	150
500	2222	120	9067	204
1000	1497	134	9608	244

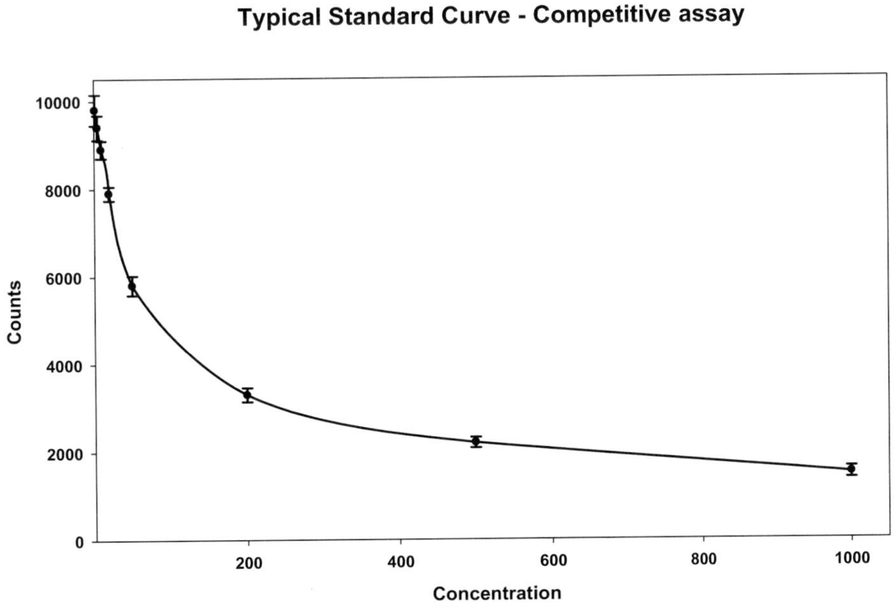

Figure 1: Linear-Linear plot of results from a competitive assay.

If the counts (=signal units) from a competitive immunoassay are plotted on the ordinate (y-axis) and the concentration on the abscissa (x-axis) a similar graph is produced to that above, where all the low values are crammed together (Fig. **1**). Early on, before computers became available, a log-transformation of the x-axis improved the situation for manual calculation of results (Fig. **2**). The analyte concentration was read directly off the calibration or standard curve. The data used for Figs. **1-4** are shown in the table below. For different methods for data-plots see references 51-57 in the previous chapter.

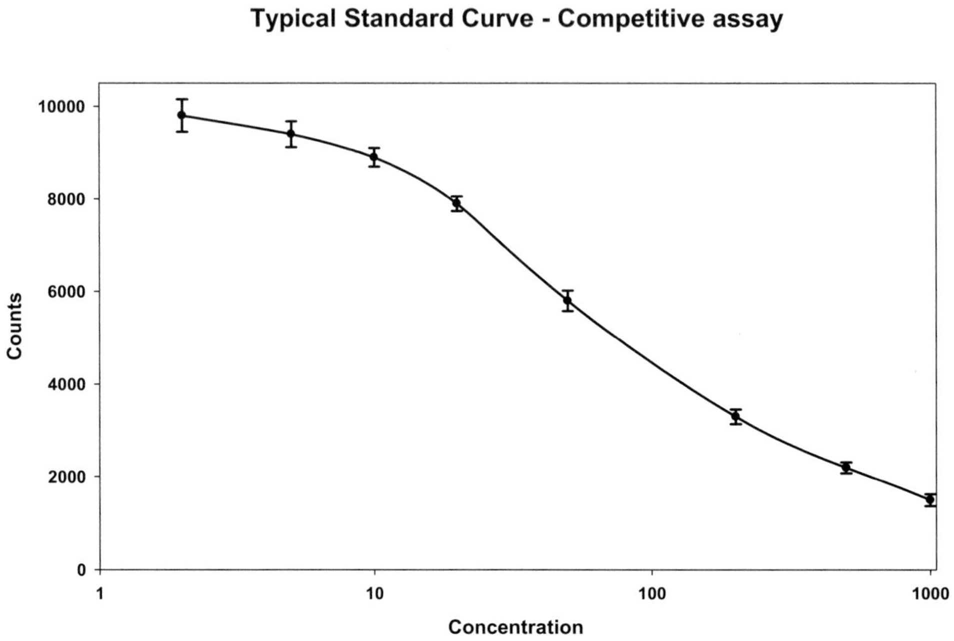

Figure 2: Semi logarithmic plot of results from a competitive assay.

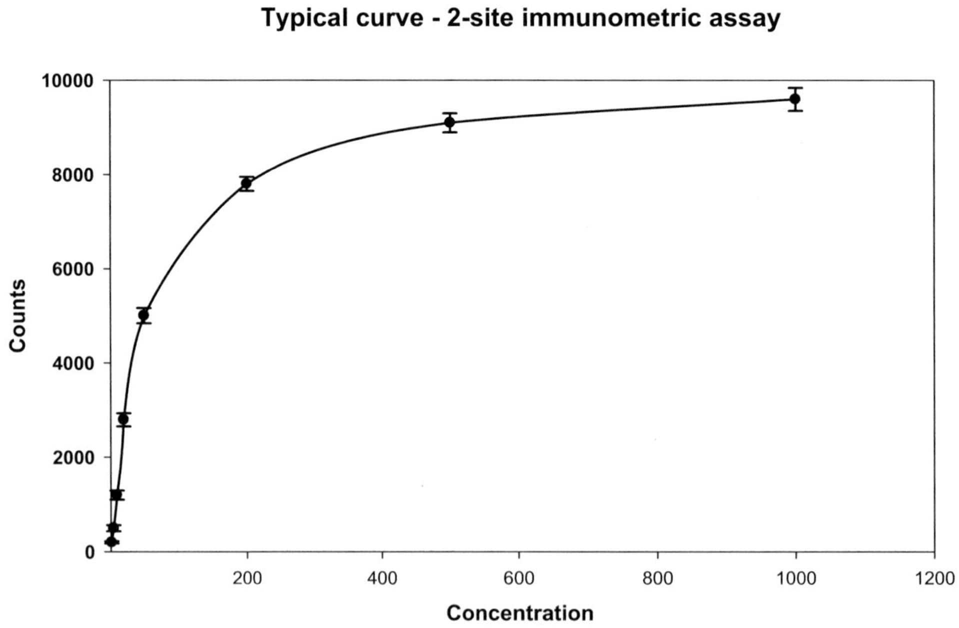

Figure 3: Linear-Linear plot of results from a two-site immunometric assay.

The analogous cases for a two-site immunometric assay are shown in Fig. **3** which shows a linear plot of the data (lin-lin), and Fig. **4**, which shows the semi logarithmic plot (log-lin).

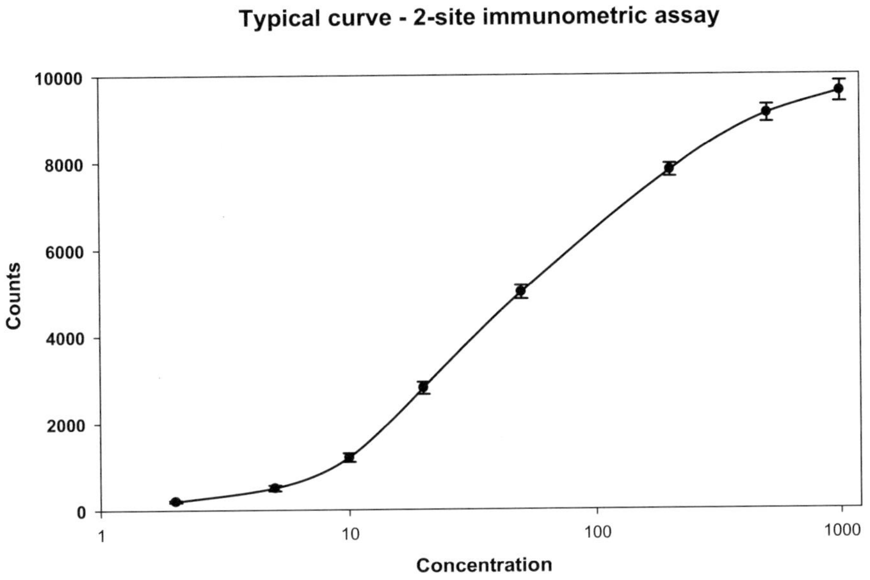

Figure 4: Semi logarithmic plot of results from a two-site immunometric assay.

The data from a competitive assay shows high counts at low concentration if the bound fraction is counted. If the free fraction is counted, then the lower concentrations have the lower counts. Conventionally, the bound fraction is preferred for counting.

In a two-site immunometric assay the counts are directly proportional to the concentration. Only the bound fraction is counted as the labeled antibody is present in excess.

In a one-site immunometric assay with immobilized antigen, the standard curve is similar to that from a competitive assay. Examples of one-site immunometric assays are microtiter plate assays used to detect autoantibodies or antibodies to viruses and bacteria.

Figs. **2** and **4** were plotted using a cubic-spline function with maximal one inflection point.

vi. Immunoassay design.

Figs. **5-8** below show the basic designs of immunoassays. As can be seen, there are three types of immunoassay construction.

In the competitive immunoassay (Fig. **5**), there is a fixed and limited amount of antibody and labeled antigen, the one variable being the antigen in the sample to be measured. The antibody can be either in liquid form or immobilized on a macro or micro solid phase.

After reaction between antibody and antigen, the bound and free fractions are separated and (usually) the bound fraction counted and the data processed, either in the counter or off-line in a computer. This principle is independent of the labeled used, except that a signal-development step is necessary in enzyme and enzyme-enhanced immunoassays.

The two-site immunometric assay (Fig. **6**) has two antigen-specific antibodies, one bound to a solid phase, the second being labeled. Both are in excess. The antigen in the sample and standard are limited. After an incubation step between sample/standard antigen and bound antibody, the unbound components are separated and the labeled antibody allowed to react in a second step. After separation of unbound label, the signal bound to the solid phase is detected directly or after development. The first and second incubations can sometimes be combined, although the risk of a "high-dose hook effect" is thereby increased [95, 96].

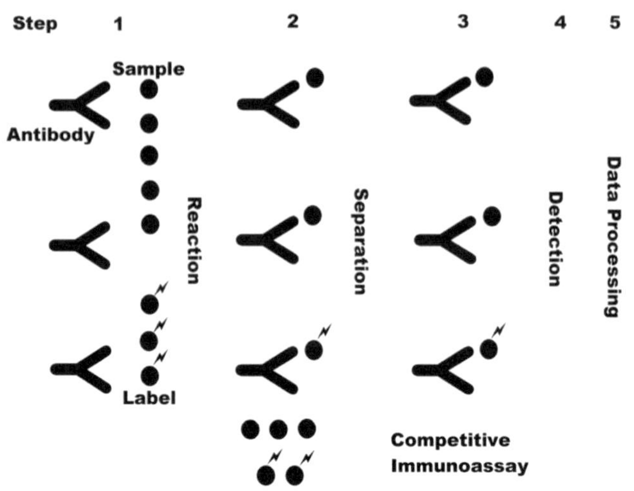

Figure 5: Schematic portrayal of a competitive immunoassay.

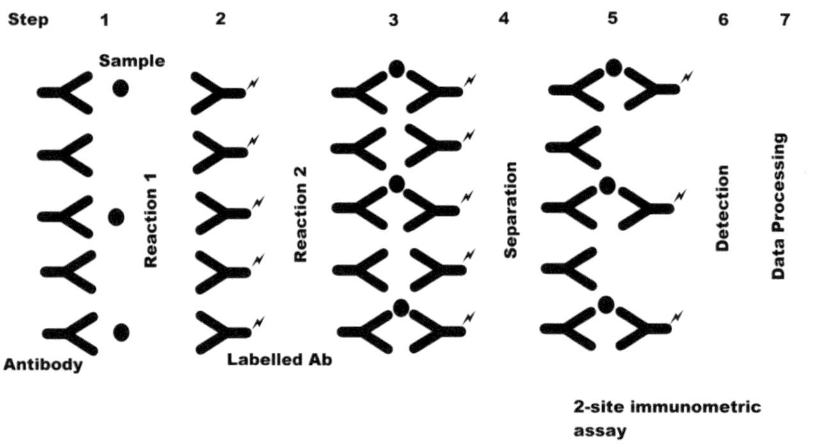

Figure 6: Schematic portrayal of a two-site immunometric assay.

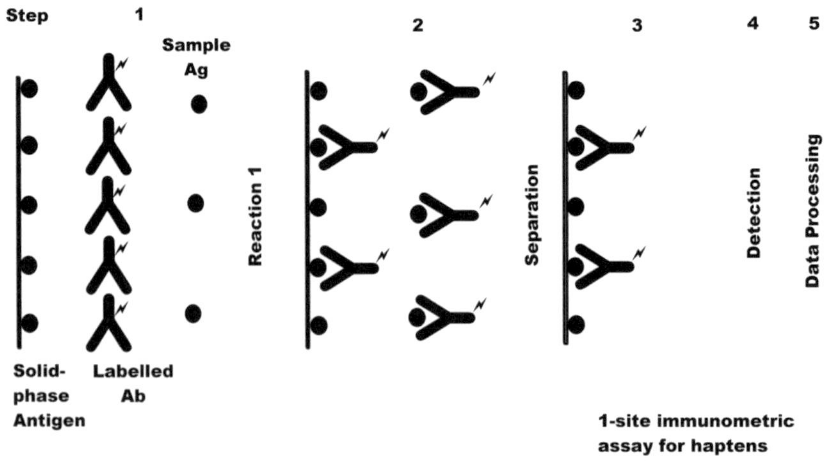

Figure 7: Schematic portrayal of a one-site immunometric assay for small molecules.

The one-site immunometric assay (Fig. 7) uses an immobilized antigen instead of the immobilized antibody in the above two-site immunometric assay. Analogous to the competitive immunoassay above, solid-phase and labeled antigen compete for a limited amount of antibody in a first reaction, after which the unbound components are removed and the signal detected directly or after a development step. This type of assay is usually used for haptens, therefore the antibody is depicted as only having one binding site. This type of assay is probably the most difficult to set up and keep stable.

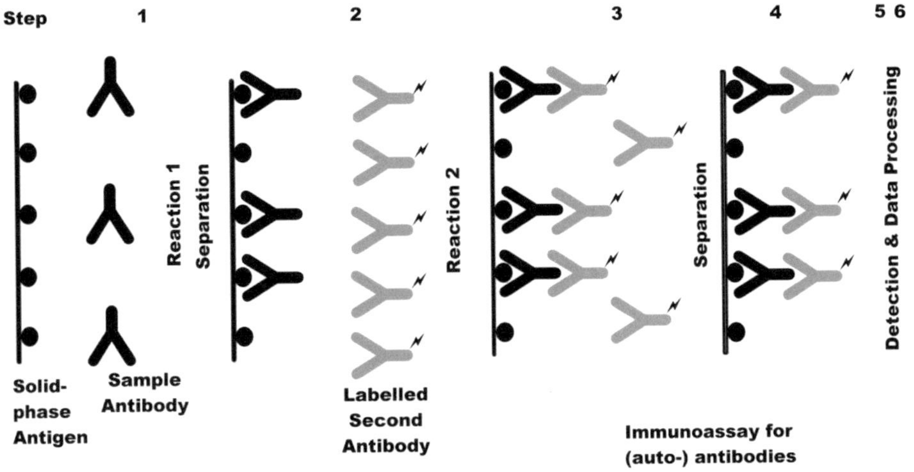

Figure 8: Schematic portrayal of a modified one-site immunometric assay for auto antibodies or antibodies to bacterial or viral agents.

The final assay scheme shown in Fig. **8** is that for detection of antibodies in a sample. This type of assay is usually used to detect autoantibodies, for example in autoimmune diseases [97] and allergies [98], or for antibodies to fungal [99], bacterial [100] or viral agents [101]. The antibody in the sample reacts with an excess of immobilized antigen. After separation a labeled second antibody raised against human immunoglobulin is allowed to react with the bound antibody. After separation of excess label the signal is measured directly or after generation. The label depends on the assay used. For allergens, the labeled antibody is usually an anti-human immunoglobulin [Ig] E (Anti-IgE) [102, 103], although Anti-IgG [104] and Anti-IgA may be used in special cases. For early antibodies an Anti-IgM label is used [105] and for antibodies against epithelial tissue an anti IgA [106] may be the label of choice.

The second antibody can be varied depending upon the animal species in which the antibody is to be detected, for example anti-dog [107] and anti-cat [108] immunoglobulins for veterinary patients.

This type of assay, especially for autoimmune diseases is almost exclusively the domain of the "ELISA" type assays [109]. This assay design is also used in the indirect (IFT, IIFT) [109] or direct (DFT, DIFT) [110] immunofluorescence techniques [109] used in immunohistochemistry where the labeled second antibody is usually labeled with a fluorescent molecule such as fluorescein isothiocyanate [111] or rhodamine [112].

The four assay designs shown above can be used to describe almost all immunoassays, independent of label or solid-phase, in macro- or micro-format.

Finally, it is to be noted that the references given in these two chapters are to aid the reader in intensifying his or her interest in specific areas of immunoassay and related techniques as it is impossible to list all variations of immune reactions in two short chapters. The majority of the references is made to original contributions and covers a period of several decades. All references can be found on the internet for further follow-up using search engines such as PubMed and Google.

The text, all Figures and Tables are exclusive to this manuscript.

REFERENCES

[1] Odell WD, Wilber JF, Paul WE. Radioimmunoassay of thyrotropin in human serum. J Clin Endocr Metab 1965; 25: 1179-88.

[2] Wood WG, Sokolowski G. Radioimmunoassay in theory and practice. Schnetztor-Verlag Konstanz, 1981; 231 pp.

[3] Marschner I, Wood WG, van Thiel D, Habermann J, König A, Scriba PC. Vergleich dreier Ringversuche zur radioimmunologischen Thyrotropin-Bestimmung nach dem Münchner Modell". J Clin Chem Clin Biochem 1983; 21: 301-11.

[4] Wood WG, Hanke R, Reinauer H. Comparability of method results and performance in a national external quality assessment scheme between 1993 and 2003 using thyroid associated analytes as examples. Clin Lab 2004; 50: 333-46.

[5] Wood WG. Sample commutability in external quality assessment surveys [EQAS] for thyroid-related antibodies - state of the art. Clin Lab 2007; 53: 217-22.

[6] Brown BL, Ekins RP, Ellis SM, Reith WS. Specific Antibodies to Triiodothyronine Hormone (Letter). Nature 1970; 226, 359.

[7] Benacerraf B, Paul WE, Green I. Hapten-Carrier Relationships. Ann NY Acad Sci 1970: 169; 93-104.

[8] Chamberlain DA, White RJ. The application of the radioimmunoassay techniques for determining serum levels of digoxin. Clin Sci 1969; 37: 572.

[9] Ekins RP, Brown BL, Ellis SM, Reith WS. The radioimmunoassay of serum triiodothyronine. Clin Sci 1970; 38: 27P.

[10] Köhler G, Milstein C. Continuous cultures of fused cells secreting antibody of predefined specificity. Nature 1975; 256: 495-7.

[11] Stenman UH. Immunoassay standardization: is it possible, who is responsible, who is capable? Clin Chem 2001; 47: 815-20.

[12] Ealey PA, Valente WA, Ekins RP, Kohn LD, Marshall NJ. Characterization of monoclonal antibodies raised against solubilized thyrotropin receptors in a cytochemical bioassay for thyroid stimulators. Endocrinology 1985; 116: 124-31.

[13] Ekins RP. Ligand assays: from electrophoresis to miniaturized microarrays. Clin Chem 1998; 44: 2015-30.

[14] Stenman UH. Standardization of assays for human chorionic gonadotropin. Clin Chem 2004; 50: 798-800.

[15] Bidlingmaier M, Strasburger CJ. Growth hormone assays: current methodologies and their limitations. Pituitary 2007; 10: 115-9 .

[16] Stieber P, Hasholzner U, Bodenmüller H, Nagel D, Sunder-Plassmann L, Dienemann H, Meier W, Fateh-Moghadam, A. CYFRA 21-1: A new marker in lung cancer. Cancer 1993; 72: 707-13 .

[17] Gosling JP. Standardization of immunoassays for hapten analytes. Scand J Clin Lab Invest 1991; 51: 95-104.

[18] Miller JJ, Straub RW Jr, Valdes R Jr. Digoxin immunoassay with cross-reactivity of digoxin metabolites proportional to their biological activity. Clin Chem 1994; 40: 1898-1903 .

[19] Nicoloff JT, Spencer CA. The use and misuse of the sensitive thyrotropin assays. J Clin Endocr Met 1990; 71: 553-558.

[20] Rifai N, Tracy RP, Ridker PM. Clinical efficacy of an automated high-sensitivity c-reactive protein assay. Clin Chem 1999; 45: 2136-41 .

[21] Claus DR, Osmand AP, Gewurz H. Radioimmunoassay of human C-reactive protein and levels in normal sera. J Lab Clin Med 1976; 87: 120-8.

[22] Taimela E, Aalto M, Viikari J, Nuutila P, Irjala K. Third generation time-resolved immunofluorometric TSH assay for automatic immunoassay system evaluated. Scand J Clin Lab Invest 1995; 55: 537-41 .

[23] Wu AHB. Quality specifications in thyroid diseases. Clin Chim Acta 2004; 346: 73-7.

[24] http://www.micromedical.de/downloads_cholestech_ldx/hsCRP%20Datenblatt.pdf.

[25] Lavin N. In: Manual of Endocrinology and Metabolism - 4th Edition. Section X: Special topics in clinical endocrinology, F. Thyroid stimulating hormone [TSH], p 730. Wolters Kluwer Health, Lippincott, Williams & Wilkins, Baltimore, Philadelphia, 2009; ISBN 0-7817-6886-1.

[26] http://www.labtestsonline.org/understanding/analytes/microalbumin/glance.html.

[27] Ekins RP, Chu F. Developing multianalyte assays, [Review]. Trends Biotechnol 1994; 12: 89-94.

[28] Nature Insight: Lab on a chip (Suppl.) Nature 2006; 442; No. 7101 pp. 367-418.
[29] Byrne M , Reynolds JV, O'Donnell JS, *et al.* Long-term activation of the pro-coagulant response after neoadjuvant chemoradiation and major cancer surgery. Brit J Cancer 2010; 102: 73-9.
[30] Di Serio F, Amodio G, Ruggieri E, *et al.* Proteomic approach to the diagnosis of acute coronary syndrome: Preliminary results. Clin Chim Acta 2005; 357: 226-35.
[31] Jönsson U, Malmqvist M, Rönnberg I. Immobilization of immunoglobulins on silica surfaces. Stability. Biochem J 1985; 227: 363-71.
[32] Raether H. [1988]. Surface plasmons on smooth and rough surfaces and on gratings, Springer Verlag, Berlin, 136 pages. ISBN 3-5401-7363-3.
[33] Lee S, Mayer KM, Hafner JH. Improved localized surface plasmon resonance immunoassay with gold bipyramid substrates. Anal Chem 2009; 81: 4450-5.
[34] Marchesini GR, Koopal K, Meulenberg E, Haasnoot W, Irth H. Spreeta-based biosensor assays for endocrine disruptors. Biosens Bioelectron 2007; 22: 1908-15.
[35] Vavilov SI, Sevchenko AN. Dokl Akad Nauk SSSR 1940; 27: 541-6 Cited by: Puko RA, Mit'kina NN, Kuznetsova VV, Kotlo VN, Khomenko VS. Polarisation of luminescence of some rare earth diketonates. Zhurnal Prikladnoi Spektroskopii 1974; 21: 736-8 .
[36] Perrin F. Polarization de la Lumière de Fluorescence. Vie Moyenne de Molecules dans L'état Excité. J Phys Radium 1926; 7: 390-401.
[37] Lepage R, Albert C. Fifty years of development in the endocrinology laboratory. Clin Biochem 2006; 39: 542-57.
[38] George S. Position of immunological techniques in screening in clinical toxicology. Clin Chem Lab Med 2004; 42: 1288-309.
[39] Ahn JS, Choi S, Jang SH, *et al.* Development of a point-of-care assay system for high-sensitivity C-reactive protein in whole blood. Clin Chim Acta 2003; 332: 51-9.
[40] Bissell M, Sanfilippo F. Empowering patients with point-of-care testing. Trends Biotechnol 2002; 20: 269-70.
[41] Mastrovitch TA, Bithoney WG, DeBari VA, Nina AG. Point-of-care testing for drugs of abuse in an urban emergency department. Ann Clin Lab Sci 2002; 32: 383-6.
[42] Shephard MD, Mazzachi BC, Shephard AK, *et al.* The impact of point of care testing on diabetes services along Victoria's Mallee Track: results of a community-based diabetes risk assessment and management program. Rural Remote Health 2005; 5: 371. Epub 2005 Jul 15.
[43] Shephard MD, Gill JP. The analytical quality of point-of-care testing in the 'qaams' model for diabetes management in Australian aboriginal medical services. Clin Biochem Rev 2006; 27: 185-90.
[44] Mshelia DS, Buba AA. Point of care testing: a delight or a dilemma in the developing world? an overview. Niger Postgrad Med J 2005; 12: 136-9.
[45] www.dsls.usra.edu/20060425.pdf [Slide 15/62].
[46] Hortas ML, Montiel N, Redondo M, *et al.* Quality assurance of point-of-care testing in the Costa del Sol Healthcare Area [Marbella, Spain]. Clin Chim Acta 2001; 307:113-8.
[47] Kost GJ, Tran NK, Tuntideelert M, Kulrattanamaneeporn S, Peungposop N. Katrina, the tsunami, and point-of-care testing: optimizing rapid response diagnosis in disasters. Am J Clin Pathol 2006; 126: 513-20.
[48] Kost GJ, Hale KN, Brock TK, *et al.* Point-of-care testing for disasters: needs assessment, strategic planning, and future design. Clin Lab Med 2009; 29: 583-605.
[49] Toffaletti J. Wireless POCT data transmission. Med Lab Obs 2000; 32: 44-8, 50-1.
[50] Möckel M, Danne O, Schmidt A, *et al.* Reference values for cardiac troponins I and T in a goal-oriented concept of health: cardiac marker values in a series of outpatients without acute coronary syndromes. Clin Chim Acta 2004; 342: 83-6.
[51] Hallani H, Leung DY, Newland E, Juergens CP. Use of a quantitative point-of-care test for the detection of serum cardiac troponin T in patients with suspected acute coronary syndromes. Intern Med J 2005; 35: 560-2.
[52] Altinier S, Zaninotto M, Mion M, *et al.* Point-of-care testing of cardiac markers: results from an experience in an Emergency Department. Clin Chim Acta 2001; 311: 67-72.
[53] Melo MR, Rosenfeld LG Meeting the challenges of globalisation and miniaturisation in laboratory services. Malays J Pathol 2007; 29: 57-61.
[54] Point of Care Diagnostic Testing World Markets. Vol. TMRPOC 09-1101 Publication Date: Nov, 2009, Trimark Publications: 388 Pages.

[55] Plerhoples W, Zwemer FL Jr, Bazarian J. Point of care pregnancy testing provides staff satisfaction but does not change ED length of stay. Am J Emerg Med 2004; 22: 460-4.

[56] Prod'hom G, Bille J. Diagnostic des maladies infectieuses: place des "point of care tests" [POCT]. Rev Med Suisse 2008; 4: 908-13.

[57] Do J, Ahn CH. A polymer lab-on-a-chip for magnetic immunoassay with on-chip sampling and detection capabilities. Lab Chip 2008; 8: 542-9. Epub 2008 Feb 28.

[58] Wood WG. Immunoassays & co.: past, present, future? - A review and outlook from personal experience and involvement over the past 35 years. Clin Lab 2008; 54: 423-38.

[59] Murphy BE, Pattee CJ. Determination of plasma corticoids by competitive protein-binding analysis using gel filtration. J Clin Endocrinol Metab 1964; 24: 919-23.

[60] Henderson DR, Friedman SB, Harris JD, *et al.* CEDIA, a new homogeneous immunoassay system. Clin Chem 1986; 32: 1637-41.

[61] Bersinger NA. Enzyme immunometric assay for the determination of pregnancy associated plasma protein A (PAPP-A) with the antigen as solid phase (conjoint IEMA). Experientia 1984; 40: 1022-4.

[62] Hierholzer JC, Phillips DJ, Humphrey DD, Coombs RA, Reimer CB. Application of a solid-phase immunofluorometric assay to the selection of monoclonal antibody specific for the adenovirus group-reactive hexon antigen. Arch Virol 1984; 80: 1-10.

[63] Parinaud J, Blanc M, Fournié A, Biermé S, Grandjean H. A fluorimetric enzyme-linked immunoassay (FEIA) for measurement of anti-D antibodies. Nouv Rev Fr Hematol 1984; 26: 299-302.

[64] Macintyre SS. C-reactive protein. Methods Enzymol 1988; 163: 383-99.

[65] Van Munster PJ, Hoelen GE, Samwel-Mantingh M, Holtman-Van Meurs M. A turbidimetric immuno assay (TIA) with automated individual blank compensation. Clin Chim Acta 1977; 76: 377-88.

[66] Bagazgoitia FJ, Garcia JL, Ibarra JM, *et al.* Chemiluminescent immunoassay (CLIA) for urinary albumin. J Biolumin Chemilumin 1989; 3 :169-74.

[67] Poiesi C, Albertini A, Ghielmi S, *et al.* Kinetic analysis of TNF-alpha oligomer-monomer transition by surface plasmon resonance and immunochemical methods. Cytokine 1993; 5: 539-45.

[68] Mahmoud M, Gaffney PJ. Bioimmunoassay (BIA) of tissue plasminogen activator [t-PA] and its specific inhibitor (t-PA/INH). Thromb Haemost 1985; 53: 356-9.

[69] Lundblad RL, Bergstrom J, De Vreker R, Bray G, Gomperts E, Baker D, Kingdon HS, Mann KG, Hartshorn J, Jenny RJ. Measurement of active coagulation factors in Autoplex-T with colorimetric active site-specific assay technology. Thromb Haemost 1998; 80: 811-5.

[70] Bergquist NR, Waller T. A novel simple immunoassay for rapid detection of human IgG antibodies to Toxoplasma gondii. J Immunol Methods 1983; 61: 339-44.

[71] Pinzani P, Franceschetti F, Magini A, Orlandini A, Pazzagli M. A chemiluminescent immunoassay for the direct measurement of urinary 5 alpha-androstane-3 alpha, 17 beta-diol-glucuronide in urine. J Biolumin Chemilumin 1989; 4: 575-9.

[72] Konishi E, Iwasa S, Kondo K, Hori M. Chemiluminescence-linked immunoassay for detection of mumps virus antibodies. J Clin Microbiol 1980; 12: 140-3.

[73] Guo JX, Ma HB, Li YL, *et al.* (Evaluation of the ELISA and the enhanced chemiluminescence immunoassay in use to determine the serum markers for liver fibrosis) Zhonghua Shi Yan He Lin Chuang Bing Du Xue Za Zhi 2009; 23: 71-3. (In Chinese).

[74] Yolken RH, Stopa PJ. Enzyme-linked fluorescence assay: Ultrasensitive solid-phase assay for detection of human rotavirus. J Clin Microbiol 1979; 10(3): 317-21.

[75] Ijsselmuiden OE, Beelaert G, Schouls LM, *et al.* Line immunoassay and enzyme-linked line immunofiltration assay for simultaneous detection of antibody to two treponemal antigens. Eur J Clin Microbiol Infect Dis 1989; 8: 716-21.

[76] Roos P, Skinner CD. A two bead immunoassay in a micro fluidic device using a flat laser intensity profile for illumination. Analyst 2003; 128: 527-31.

[77] Ekins RP. Ligand assays: from electrophoresis to miniaturized microarrays. Clin Chem 1998; 44: 2015-30.

[78] Tsai HY, Jian SJ, Huang ST, Fuh CB. Competitive magnetic immunoassay for protein detection in thin channels. J Chromatogr A 2009; 1216: 7493-6. Epub 2009 May 19.

[79] Kriz K, Gehrke J, Kriz D. Advancements toward magneto immunoassays. Biosens Bioelectron 1998; 13: 817-23.

[80] Johnson AJ, Cheshier RC, Cosentino G, *et al.* Validation of a microsphere-based immunoassay for detection of anti-West Nile virus and anti-St. Louis encephalitis virus immunoglobulin M antibodies. Clin Vaccine Immunol 2007; 14: 1084-93. Epub 2007 Jul 3.

[81] Chan SW, Tan CT, Hsia JC. Spin membrane immunoassay: simplicity and specificity. J Immunol Methods 1978; 21: 185-95.

[82] Syrjälä MT, Tölö H, Koistinen J, Krusius T. Determination of anti-IgA antibodies with a flow cytometer-based microbead immunoassay (MIA). J Immunol Methods 1991; 139: 265-70.

[83] Fan AC, Deb-Basu D, Orban MW, *et al.* Nanofluidic proteomic assay for serial analysis of oncoprotein activation in clinical specimens. Nat Med 2009; 15: 566-71. Epub 2009 Apr 12.

[84] Lee KB, Kim EY, Mirkin CA, Wolinsky SM, The Use of Nanoarrays for Highly Sensitive and Selective Detection of Human Immunodeficiency Virus Type 1 in Plasma. Nano Lett 2004; 4: 1869-72.

[85] Uchimura H, Aono Y, Suzuki K, *et al.* (Basic and clinical evaluation of EIA (pin immuno assay, PIA) kit for antithyroglobulin antibody (TGAb) and antimicrosomal [antiperoxidase] antibody (TMAb)) Rinsho Byori 1993; 41: 1031-6. (In Japanese).

[86] Aspholm R, Zuo S, Fohlman J, Frisk G, Friman G, Blomberg J. A novel serological technique: polymerase chain reaction enhanced immunoassay. Application to enterovirus IgM diagnosis. J Virol Methods 1999; 80: 187-96.

[87] Tamiya E, Watanabe N, Matsuoka H, Karube I. Pulse immunoassay for human immunoglobulin G using antibody bound latex beads. Biosensors 1987-1988; 3: 139-46.

[88] Montgomery MR, Holtzman JL, Leute RK, Dewees JS, Bolz G. Determination of diphenylhydantoin in human serum by spin immunoassay. Clin Chem 1975; 21: 221-6.

[89] Leuvering JH, Thal PJ, van der Waart M, Schuurs AH. Sol particle immunoassay (SPIA). J Immunoassay 1980; 1: 77-91.

[90] Van Doornum GJ, Slomka MJ, Buimer M, *et al.* Comparison of a monoclonal antibody-blocking enzyme-linked immunoassay and a strip immunoblot assay for identifying type-specific herpes simplex virus type 2 serological responses. Clin Diagn Lab Immunol 2000; 7: 641-4.

[91] Litman DJ, Lee RH, Jeong HJ, *et al.* An internally referenced test strip immunoassay for morphine. Clin Chem. 1983; 29: 1598-603.

[92] Elwing H, Nilsson LA, Ouchterlony O. A simple spot technique for thin layer immunoassays [TIA] on plastic surfaces. J Immunol Methods 1977; 17: 131-45.

[93] Sorell Gómez L, Rojas G. A simple visual immunoassay [VIA] for rapid identification of high lipoprotein(a) blood levels. Clin Chim Acta 1997; 260: 65-71.

[94] Vesterberg O. Zone immunoelectrophoresis assay (ZIA) of alpha-fetoprotein (AFP) using one antiserum. Clin Chim Acta 1983; 135: 99-101.

[95] Rodbard D, Feldman Y, Jaffe ML, Miles LE. Kinetics of two-site immunoradiometric ['sandwich'] assays-II. Studies on the nature of the 'high-dose hook effect'. Immunochemistry 1978; 15: 77-82.

[96] Wood WG. A comparison of eleven commercial kits for the determination of serum ferritin levels. J Clin Chem Clin Biochem 1981; 19: 947-52.

[97] Whittingam S, Mackay IR. Laboratory methods for diagnosis of autoimmune disease. Med J Aust 1969; 1: 1200-5.

[98] Eriksson NE, Ahlstedt S. Diagnosis of reaginic allergy with house dust, animal dander and pollen allergens in adult patients. V. A comparison between the enzyme-linked immunosorbent assay (ELISA), provocation tests, skin tests and RAST. Int Arch Allergy Appl Immunol 1977; 54: 88-95.

[99] Sepulveda R, Longbottom JL, Pepys J. Enzyme linked immunosorbent assay (ELISA) for IgG and IgE antibodies to protein and polysaccharide antigens of Aspergillus fumigatus. Clin Allergy 1979; 9: 359-71.

[100] Carlsson HE, Lindberg AA, Hammarström S. Titration of antibodies to salmonella O antigens by enzyme-linked immunosorbent assay. Infect Immun 1972; 6: 703-8.

[101] Voller A, Bidwell DE. A simple method for detecting antibodies to rubella. Br J Exp Pathol 1975; 56: 338-9.

[102] Hogarth-Scott RS, Johansson SG, Bennich H. Antibodies to Toxocara in the sera of visceral larva migrans patients: the significance of raised levels of IgE. Clin Exp Immunol 1969; 5: 619-25.

[103] Gleich GJ, Averbeck AK, Swedlund HA. Measurement of IgE in normal and allergic serum by radioimmunoassay. J Lab Clin Med 1971; 77: 690-8.

[104] Lindström P, Wager O. IgG autoantibody to human serum albumin studied by the ELISA-technique. Scand J Immunol 1978; 7: 419-25.

[105] Locarnini SA, Coulepis AG, Stratton AM, Kaldor J, Gust ID. Solid-phase enzyme-linked immunosorbent assay for detection of hepatitis A-specific immunoglobulin M. J Clin Microbiol 1979; 9: 459-65.

[106] Volta U, Bonazzi C, Bianchi FB, *et al.* IgA antibodies to dietary antigens in liver cirrhosis. Ric Clin Lab 1987; 17: 235-42.

[107] Campbell KL, George JW. Application of the enzyme-linked immunosorbent assay to detect canine erythrocyte antibodies. Am J Vet Res 1984; 45: 747-50.

[108] Horzinek MC, Ederveen J, Egberink H, *et al.* Virion polypeptide specificity of immune complexes and antibodies in cats inoculated with feline infectious peritonitis virus. Am J Vet Res 1986; 47: 754-61.

[109] O'Beirne AJ, Cooper HR. Heterogeneous enzyme immunoassay. J Histochem Cytochem 1979; 27: 1148-62.

[110] Tokumaru T. A kinetic study on the labeling of serum globulin with fluorescein isothiocyanate by means of the gel filtration technique. J Immunol 1962; 89: 195-203.

[111] Sugenoya A, Silverberg J, Trokoudes K, Row VV, Volpé R. Macrophage-lymphocyte interaction in Graves' disease and Hashimoto's thyroiditis. Acta Endocrinol (Copenh) 1979; 91: 99-108.

[112] Bottazzo GF, Pouplard A, Florin-Christensen A, Doniach D. Autoantibodies to prolactin-secreting cells of human pituitary. Lancet 1975; 2(7925): 97-101.

CHAPTER 2

Production of Antibodies for Immunoanalytical Methods

Ludek Eyer and Milan Franek*

Veterinary Research Institute, Hudcova 70, 62100 Brno, Czech Republic

Abstract: Fundamental immunological principles and factors influencing production strategies for antibodies used as reagents in analytical and diagnostic methods are highlighted. A role of the peptide-protein design for an antibody formation, covering particularly epitope selection, peptide and protein chemistry, carrier-protein conjugation including multiple antigen protein approach are described. Special attention is paid to hapten design and production of antibodies against molecules having low-molecular character. Critical stages in polyclonal and monoclonal antibody development as well as practical hints for their production are discussed.

Keywords: Antibodies, Production, Hapten, Immunogens.

1. INTRODUCTION

In this chapter, we first discuss proteins as immunogens, then peptides and small organic compounds as antigens, and finally the use of antigens and immunogens in antibody production. Antigen design, carrier protein conjugates and critical factors for polyclonal and monoclonal antibody production, are described. The immunochemical properties of produced antibody reagents are important for their analytical and diagnostic applications.

2. IMMUNOGENS, ANTIGENS AND EPITOPES

At the beginning of the chapter, some immunological terms that are important for an understanding of antibody specificity, antigen complementarity and antibody production will be defined. The term immunogen refers to a molecule that is capable of eliciting an immune response by an organism's immune system. An antigen refers to a molecule that is capable of binding to the product of the immune response, *i.e.* antibody. The immunogen is always an antigen capable of binding, but an antigen may not necessarily be an immunogen capable of eliciting immune response. Peptides and haptens are small molecules (less than 1 000 - 3 000 Da) and they need to be conjugated to a carrier protein in order to elicit an immune response. Therefore, low-molecular compounds may always be antigens, but not immunogens. An epitope is defined as the specific sequence of amino acids on an antigen entity to which the respective antibody binds. Epitopes that are easily accessible to the antibody binding site are optimal for antigen design. Native proteins are good immunogens as well as good antigens capable of producing specific immune response by themselves and binding to the formed antibody.

2.1. Proteins as Immunogens

Native proteins are excellent immunogens and have traditionally been used to raise antibodies for immunochemical applications [1, 2]. However, some proteins are not easy to isolate in sufficient amount in a pure form for animal immunization, and thus they cannot be used as immunogens for antibody production. Gene protein products are often available only in extremely low concentrations, however, information on their nucleotide and corresponding amino acid sequences can be utilised for peptide antigen design to generate sequence-specific antibodies. In other instances, the protein has not yet been uncovered, but the gene sequence is described or a new protein has been discovered but only a partial sequence is determined [3-5]. Sometimes, the protein of interest cannot be successfully expressed by recombinant techniques.

***Address correspondence to Milan Franek:** Veterinary Research Institute, Hudcova 70, 62100 Brno, Czech Republic; Tel: +420 5 3333 1901; Fax: +420 5 4121 1229; E-mail: franek@vri.cz

Eline P. Meulenberg (Ed)

2.2. Selection of Peptides as Protein Epitopes

Antibodies against native proteins have traditionally been produced by methods of animal immunization, however, in many cases these methods do not satisfy the requirements for fine specificity or selectivity of the antibody to complex protein molecules. Improving specific properties of antibodies raised against protein antigen of interest, such as enhanced antibody specificity, reduced or enhanced cross-reactivity as well as formation of antibodies against different epitopes of the same protein or against proteins with post-translation modifications can be accomplish using a strategy based on low-molecular peptides derived from the native protein sequences. Thus, optimal antigenic sequences (epitopes) must be selected from available data in order to achieve the expected parameters for produced antibodies.

Epitopes (amino acid sequences) can be classified by their molecular character into several groups. *Linear (continuous) peptide sequence* (also called *linear epitope*), is derived from a linear sequence in a protein. An antibody will bind to these epitopes in the native protein when the sequence is not buried in the interior of the protein. On the other hand, *conformational (discontinuous) peptide sequence,* also called *discontinuous epitope,* corresponds to a three-dimensional (3D) antigen conformation in a particular protein and covers a group of amino acids that are not necessarily continuous in the sequence of the protein molecule however, they are positioned together by folding of the respective peptide chain or using the juxtaposition of two different polypeptide chains [6, 7]. *The unique peptide sequence* enables to raise antibodies, which are highly specific to only one member of the protein family or to one characteristic protein, *e.g.* for a particular pathogen strain [8, 9]. Information on the specific sequence can be found in the NCBI database [10] and selected for epitope design using BLAST scanning procedure [11]. *Homologous peptide sequence* enables a single antibody to recognize multiple proteins. The homologous sequences in protein molecule are characterized by a significant level of sequence amino acid similarity (usually higher than 50%) [8, 9]. Homologous motifs can be selected using the multiple sequence alignment methods [12, 13].

2.3. Epitope Selection and Protein Structure

Knowledge of the 3D structure of the protein molecule can be utilised in choosing the exposed epitopes. Antigenic epitopes of proteins soluble in the natural environment are hydrophilic and flexible and tend to be located on the surface of the proteins thus having the most optimal location with respect to molecular accessibility. In contrast with the hydrophilic sequences, hydrophobic sequence regions tend to stay in the interior of the protein. If a 3D structure is unknown, sequences can be chosen using various predictive algorithms [9, 14-16]. The accessible surface area of residues and other important molecular factors such as protein hydrophilicity, flexibility, and reduction of potential cross reactivity can be calculated and incorporated in an optimized form into antigen design. Practical experience shows that at least 30% immunogenic (external) amino acids such as Lys, Arg, Glu, Asp, Gln, Asn are required for functional design. Peptide sequences of 10 to 20 amino acids in length are used in most designs. Fifteen amino acids can be recommended as an average peptide length, with slightly longer sequences being preferred to shorter sequences [17]. With regard to covalent attachment of the selected sequence to carrier proteins, terminal cysteines located at the N-terminal or C-terminal position are usually preferred. A terminal cysteine allows maximum exposure of the respective peptide sequence and usually produces a biologically stable thioether bond [8].

2.4. Technical Aspects of Peptide Synthesis

Selection of the sequences is not a matter of routine approach and therefore the design for the peptide synthesis should consider not only conformation and other structural factors but also technical attainability with respect to peptide chemistry. The inclusion of unstable amino acids or peptide sequences should be minimized because the peptide antigen should be stable during synthesis, purification and conjugation steps including the immunization process [18]. Stretches of amino acids that require bulky protecting groups during peptide synthesis (*e.g.* Arg, Asn, Gln, Cys, His) are usually problematic during synthesis. Sequences containing long stretches of hydrophobic residues may be difficult to dissolve whereas sequences with multiple Cys may form covalent aggregates. Undesirable sequences such as Cys, Asp-Gly, Asn-Gly, Asp-Pro, N-terminal Gln or N-terminal Asn should be eliminated because they make the peptides chemically unstable [8, 17].

With regard to the conjugation of the peptide to carrier protein, a potential charge in the peptide antigen that was not present in the native protein, from which the peptide sequence was derived, should be eliminated. Thus, the sequence should be capped on one terminus and conjugated on the other. N-terminal epitopes should be amidated or conjugated on the C-terminus, while C-terminal epitopes should be acetylated or conjugated in the C-terminus [19, 20].

2.5. Carrier Protein Conjugation

To prepare functional immunogens for animal immunization, small peptide sequences as well as hapten structures are conjugated to protein macromolecules using various coupling reactions and strategies [21]. With regard to chemical composition of the small molecules and proteins, the common conjugation methods link antigens to the protein carriers mostly *via* free amino and carboxyl or sulfhydryl groups. The procedure chosen for a given conjugation should result in a stable covalent bond and an appropriate conjugation yield. Ovalbumin, albumin, thyroglobulin and keyhole limpet hemocyanin are conventional immunogens of different molecular weight and structure and most often used as carrier proteins. All these carriers enable antibody formation against small molecules if the conjugation procedure ensures spatial accessibility of bound peptide or hapten for interaction with B-cell receptors (see section 2.5.). A parallel conjugation of a small hapten structure with two or more different carrier proteins is recommended to prepare conjugates with optimal properties in order to increase the probability of successful antibody production [22-24]. The chemistry of three traditional reactions, commonly used for the conjugation of small molecular structures to a carrier protein, is presented in the following paragraphs.

a) Attachment of the Peptide to Carrier Protein Using m-Maleimidobenzoyl-N-Hydroxysuccinimide Ester

Heterobifunctional coupling reagent, m-Maleimidobenzoyl-N-hydroxysuccinimide ester (MBS), enables to link peptides to carriers through cysteine sulfhydryl and free amino groups. The MBS reagent contains N-hydroxysuccinimide (NHS) ester on one end and maleimide group on the MBS enables to link peptides to carriers through cysteine sulfhydryl and free amino groups. The conjugation reaction using this reagent proceeds in two steps (Fig. **1**). In the first step, ε-amino groups of lysine residues of carrier protein are activated by reaction with the succinimide moiety of MBS to form a stable amide bond. In the subsequent reaction, the sulfhydryl groups of cysteine residues of the peptide react with the maleimide moiety of the activated carrier protein to create a stable thioether linkage. The advantage of this MBS method is that this conjugation chemistry is well characterized and that it provides chemically stable conjugates for immunological applications [25-27].

b) Conjugation of Small Molecules to Carrier Proteins Using Carbodiimides

1-ethyl-3-(dimethylaminopropyl) carbodiimide (EDC) is one of the most commonly used carbodiimide water-soluble reagents for peptide/hapten-protein conjugation. As shown in Fig. **2**, the EDC activates in the first stage of the reaction the carboxyl group of aspartic or glutamic acid or the terminal carboxyl group in peptide to make them the reactive sites for conjugation with primary amines. The activated structure interacts in the second reaction step with amino groups of lysine in the carrier protein resulting in formation of the final peptide-protein conjugate product [21, 28]. NHS or its water-soluble analog (sulfo-NHS) is often included in EDC procedures to improve the conjugation yields [29]. EDC couples NHS to carboxyl groups (NHS ester formation) while allowing for efficient conjugation to primary amines under common conjugation conditions. If the carrier protein is activated first, the EDC method will couple the carrier protein through the N-terminal alpha-amine and possibly through the amine in the side-chain of lysine, if present in the sequence. EDC is being successfully used for the conjugation of proteins requiring aqueous medium [30]. EDC conjugation creates a well-characterized and stable peptide bond, which makes this method reliable, versatile, and widely dispersed among investigators. The reaction does not introduce any other linker into the conjugate, and so minimizes the changes of antigenic properties of the peptide or hapten [31]. For hydrophobic hapten structures, water insoluble N, N'-dicyclohexylcarbodiimide (DCC) is employed for the activation reaction in formamide solvent [22, 32, 33]. The activated hapten is conjugated to the proteins under conventional conditions.

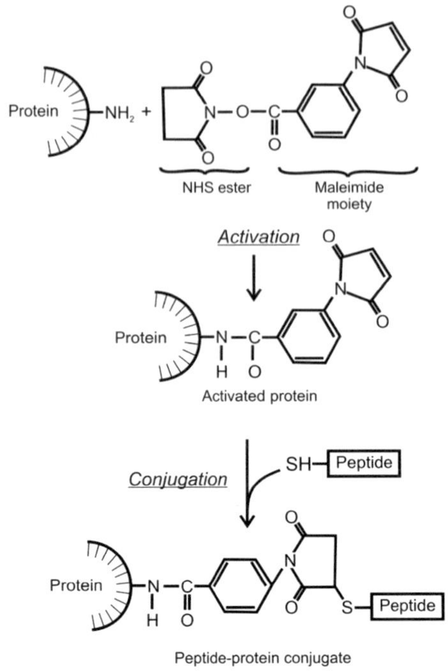

Figure 1: Scheme of conjugation reactions using MBS heterobifunctional reagent.

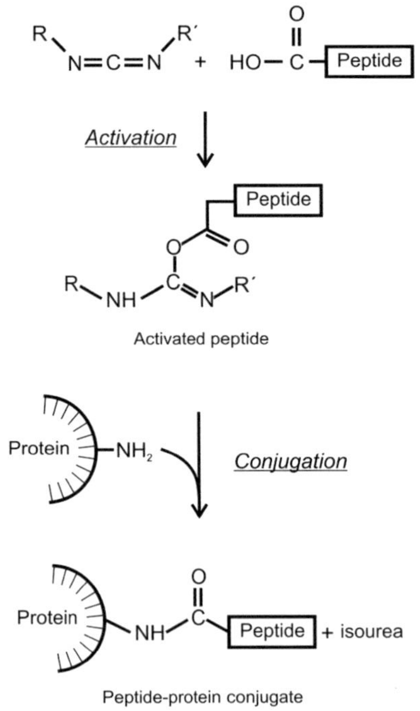

Figure 2: Scheme of conjugation reactions using carbodiimide.

c) Conjugation of Small Molecules to Carrier Protein Through Glutaraldehyde

A homobifunctional cross-linker glutaraldehyde enables to link peptides to carriers especially through the amino groups of lysine. The procedure covers three reaction steps (Fig. **3**): The incubation of peptide with glutaraldehyde forms Schiff base with a free terminal aldehyde, which is then available for the reaction with amino groups of the carrier protein. The excess of non-reacted aldehyde groups is inactivated in the next step by glycine or ethanolamine. To increase stability of the formed bonds, reduction of Shiff bases is possible in the presence of borohydride. The method is attractive because of its simplicity, speed and effectiveness. The glutaraladehyde also provides a highly flexible spacer between a small molecule and a carrier protein for favorable presentation to the immune system. However, the reaction mechanisms of glutaraldehyde conjugation methods and formed chemical spacer structures remain to be characterized. If a high degree of reproducibility is necessary, in either product performance or substitution level, then other methods should be considered [34, 35].

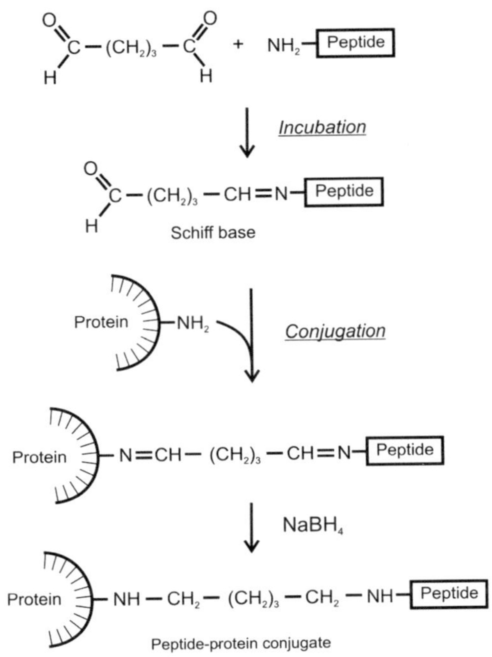

Figure 3: Scheme of conjugation reactions using glutaraldehyde.

3. ANTIGEN DESIGN FOR ANTIBODY PRODUCTION

In this section, important immunochemical concepts and principles influencing production strategies for antibodies used as reagents in analytical and diagnostic methods will be highlighted. A role of the peptide-protein as well as hapten design for antibody production, covering particularly epitope selection, peptide and protein chemistry, carrier-protein conjugation including multiple antigen protein approach will be discussed.

3.1. Antigen-Peptide Carrier Protein Design

Peptide sequences conjugated to carrier proteins can generate highly specific antibodies for a target protein of interest. Sequences with minimum homology to others are selected to decrease non-specific binding. The immunochemical strategy is often focused on the production of capture and detection antibodies applicable to subsequent sandwich assay development. An essential consideration in this approach is that the capture and detection antibodies must recognize two non-overlapping antigenic epitopes on protein surface. When one antigen (epitope sequence) binds to the capture antibody, another epitope intended for the detection antibody must not be buried or obscured in the native protein conformation. Capture and detection antibodies that do not interfere with one another and can bind simultaneously to protein antigen are immunoreagents suitable for use in sandwich assay.

An example of the antigen design for antibodies against clinical biomarker procalcitonin is given in Fig. **4** [36]. This protein molecule is a 116 amino acid polypeptide precursor (and prohormone) of calcitonin consisting of two regions belonging to calcitonin and katacalcin. The design aimed to select unique peptide sequences that would raise specificity to the target protein to produce capture and detection antibodies. Five selected peptide sequences of different domain structures were conjugated with carrier proteins to produce effective immunogens capable of generating high-affinity antibodies. The produced monoclonal antibody reacting with a peptide within the N-terminal region of the procalcitonin was specific for a 19 amino acid oligopeptide and was employed as the capture antibody. Other monoclonal antibodies recognizing a motif of 14 amino acid sequence of the katacalcin area were cross-reactive and were examined as detection antibodies. The results illustrate the fact that careful structural assessment of target protein antigen at the initial phase is desirable for successful antibody production.

It should be noted that, although the probability of success using proposed sequences is relatively high, there is always some risk comparable with any antibody production. There may be obtained high antibody levels against peptide sequences that were synthesized, however, it is not possible to ensure in advance how antibodies raised against selected peptide will work in a real assay.

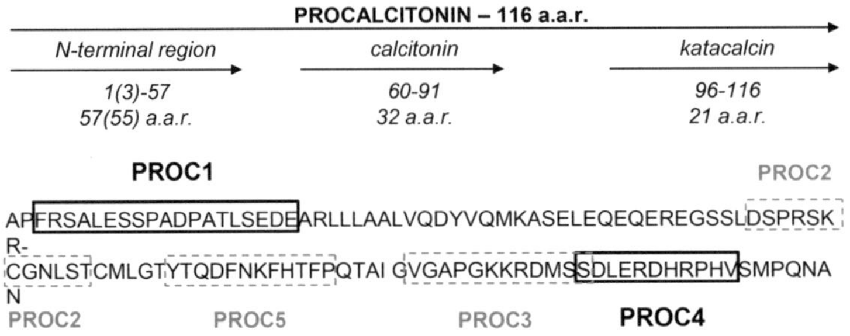

Figure 4: Schematic representation of human procalcitonin molecule and five sequence positions selected for the immunogen preparation and antibody production. According to Kramer *et al.* [36].

3.2. Design of Multiple Antigen Peptide System

An alternative way to conjugate a peptide sequence to a protein carrier is the possibility of producing antigenic immunogens based on the Multiple Antigen Peptide (MAP) system. The concept was introduced in the 90´s to avoid chemically undefined structural details of a peptide-carrier protein conjugate to prepare specific antibodies for vaccines. The MAP system utilizes a small peptidyl core matrix bearing radially branching synthetic peptide sequences as dentritic arms [37]. This MAP scaffold containing (n) sequential lysine levels provides 2^n reactive amino ends to which peptide sequences can be conjugated using a conventional solid-phase chemistry [38, 39]. The typical MAP product is a macromolecular structure consisting of a heptalysine core matrix that links to eight dendritic arms of peptide copies (Fig. **5d**). It can be noted that MAP should not be used when the peptide sequence is derived from the C-terminus of the target protein. The MAP structure of 10-15 kDa has a high molar ratio of peptide antigen to core molecule and can be directly used for immunization without requirement of further conjugation to a carrier protein.

Although the high molar ratio and dense packing of multiple copies of the epitope sequence has been shown to elicit strong immune response in many instances, some laboratories have not found MAP antigens to be as effective as peptides conjugated to carrier proteins [40]. Thus, the MAP approach can rather be employed in situations when no other antigen or conventional immunization has produced the required antibody.

3.3. Hapten Design

Low-molecular organic structures (*e.g.* steroid hormones, pesticides, mycotoxins, drugs, environmental pollutants), called haptens in immunology must be covalently attached to a carrier protein *via* an optimal spacer position in order to elicit a specific immune response in the experimental animal. In this sense, the peptide sequences of proteins selected for specific antibody production may be considered as haptens because they are usually not able to generate antibodies without attachment to carrier protein. Historically speaking, classical studies by Landsteiner [41] in the twenties and thirties became the basis of knowledge on current hapten immunochemistry. After the advent of immunoassays to clinical laboratories [42], steroid hormones became suitable model compounds for the study of hapten-antibody specificity and immunochemical concepts in terms of structural details such as the position of the chemical bridge (spacer) in the hapten structure, spacer binding effect, possible conformational and chemical changes in a linked hapten structure as well as electronic charge distribution across the surface of hapten structure [24, 43]. When tailor made antibodies are intended to be developed, all of the above factors need to be considered whereas the priority role in the hapten design plays the position and chemical character of the spacer introduced to the hapten structure [23].

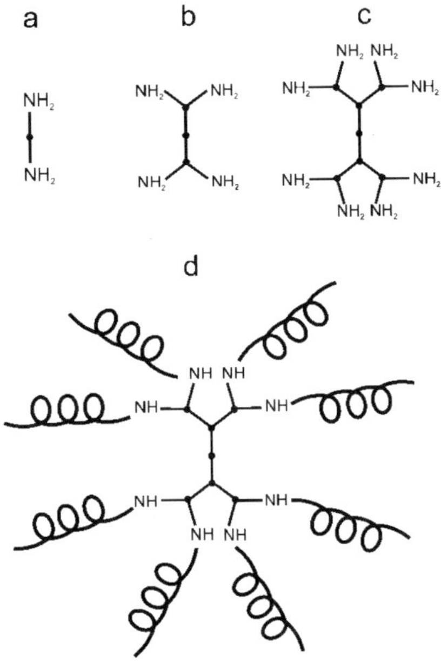

Figure 5: Schematic depiction of the MAP core matrix at divalent level **(a)**, tetravalent level **(b)**, octavalent level **(c)** and an octameric MAP containing three branching levels of lysine and eight amino groups used for conjugation with peptides **(d)**. According to Tam [37].

It is common experience that hapten areas removed from the spacer mostly exhibit a high degree of specificity, whereas the vicinity of the spacer is typified by low specificity. The low degree of specificity (or high cross-reactivity) means that an antibody does not recognize chemical changes in this area of the hapten structure. An example of the hapten design for highly specific antibodies against biologically active testosterone metabolite, 5α-dihydro-testosterone (5α-DHT), is shown in Fig. **6**.

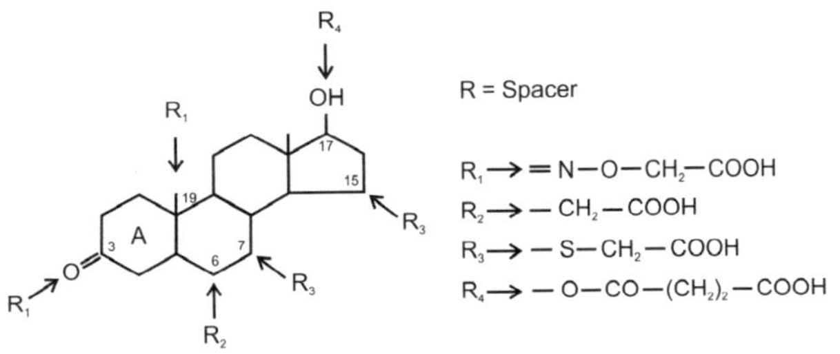

Figure 6: Various positions of the spacers in the steroid (5α-DHT) hapten structure.

The parent (testosterone) and metabolite (5α-DHT) structures are differing from each other only in two stereoatoms of hydrogen (double bound) in the A-ring. In order to distinguish these very small chemical differences by antibodies, numerous hapten syntheses were designed to introduce a spacer into various positions in the steroid skeleton (Fig. **6**). As expected, the C-3 position of the spacer in 5α-DHT resulted in a high cross-reactivity between testosterone and 5α-DHT, whereas placing a spacer in the 15β position was optimal and improved dramatically the specificity of the antibody towards 5α-DHT [44].

On the other hand, antibodies with a broad cross-reactivity pattern are required to detect simultaneously many compounds of interest within a single assay. Such antibodies, referred to as class/group specific or generic antibodies, were used for development of broad-specificity immunoassays for sulfonamides [24], s-triazines and sulfonylurea herbicides [45], O, O-dimethyl organophosphorus pesticides [46] and other groups of low-molecular analytes. The generic haptens based on the molecular "fragments" or special spacer chemistry and heterology were synthesized and used for conjugation with carrier proteins to produce class-selective antibodies [24].

Recently, antibodies against very small hapten molecules were generated and functional immunoassays established. The extremely low immunogenicity of aliphatic molecules such as semicarbazide or acrylamide was overcome by derivatization of the analyte molecules with larger aromatic moiety in order to enlarge hapten structure for conjugation with carrier proteins [29, 47, 48]. This approach offers new possibilities of producing analytical antibodies against small aliphatic structures that cannot be generated by conventional immunochemical procedures.

The methods of molecular modelling have been used to recognize potential structural, stereochemical and electronic changes after the introduction of the spacer substituent into a hapten molecule [24, 33, 49-52]. Although various molecular parameters obtained by computer-assisted molecular modelling were employed for the interpretation of cross-reactivity and binding interactions, the use of methods for the hapten design to predict antibody properties prior to immunization is rather limited. The computer models do not provide an adequate explanation for steric aspects and the location of the hapten in 3 D structure of the carrier protein.

3.4. Spacer Binding Effect and Assay Sensitivity

Analytical sensitivity in antibody based-assays is determined predominantly by intensity of the detection signal coming from the labelled detection compound (most often analyte or the second detection antibody) and by antibody affinity raised against analyte structure. It is useful to know that overall antibody affinity is not always formed only towards hapten structure but the binding energy can also be distributed between the hapten group itself and the respective spacer substituent. The existence of the spacer binding effect in steroid haptens was demonstrated experimentally by homologous spacer substituents introduced into testosterone at the C-3 position [53]. This hapten phenomenon is illustrated in the diagram in Fig. **7c**.

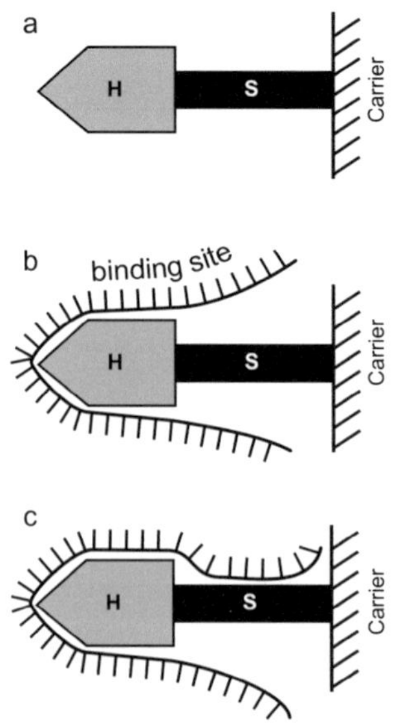

Figure 7: Schematic demonstration of the spacer binding effect. **a)** hapten-conjugate (hapten(H)-spacer(S)-carrier) **b)** antibody without the spacer binding effect **c)** antibody with spacer binding effect. Structural and chemical aspects of the spacer (bridge) binding are discussed in details elsewhere [43].

As depicted in Fig. **7**, the binding interaction between the antibody and hapten takes place predominantly *via* the shape complementarity of the binding site towards antigenic determinant which covers either the hapten structure itself (Fig. **7b**) or the hapten structure plus binding contribution of the spacer (Fig. **7c**). It should be stressed here that hapten design itself cannot eliminate automatically the spacer binding in polyclonal and monoclonal antibodies produced, because immune response towards the same immunogen is varying in each experimental animal. Thus, a higher number of immunized animals is important in order to obtain a broader spectrum of antibody affinities for selection of the optimal reagent. In this laboratory, ten or more rabbits are taken for immunization to select at least one antibody free of spacer binding with high affinity to the target analyte [24, 29].

The spacer binding phenomenon decreases or completely eliminates the sensitivity of the competitive immunoassay systems, such as conventional ELISA formats, working with homologous hapten-spacer-immunoreagents [43]. Since hapten immunoassays are driven by competition between the labelled hapten (or coating hapten-protein conjugate) and target analyte for the antibody binding site, the competitive strength of the target analyte should be the same or higher than the labelled analogs in order to reach the highest possible assay sensitivity. It can be mentioned that haptens (*e.g.* steroids) labelled with tritium are released from the spacer binding effect because no spacer chemistry is being employed in this type of labelling. In real hapten assays, improvement in assay sensitivity can be achieved by structural alteration of the spacer region or even the hapten structure in coating or enzyme conjugate. Different types of hapten/spacer heterology enable manipulation of the antibody affinity in the assay system to get sensitivity in the required concentration range.

3.5. Clonal Selection Theory and Antibody Production

It will be shown in this section that the commonly accepted concept of immunity, called as the clonal selection theory, can be a useful tool for antibody developers to manipulate the immune response during the immunization process. In a simple form, the clonal selection theory of immunity states that an antigen selects from a variety of lymphocytes those with receptors capable of reacting with a specific part of the antigen (antigenic determinant) (Fig. **8**). In other words, the specificity and affinity of antiserum towards the antigen is formed by the selection of the B-lymphocyte (B-cell) repertoire in an experimental animal, *i.e.* those lymphocytes with which the antigen enters into a binding interaction following immunization [54].

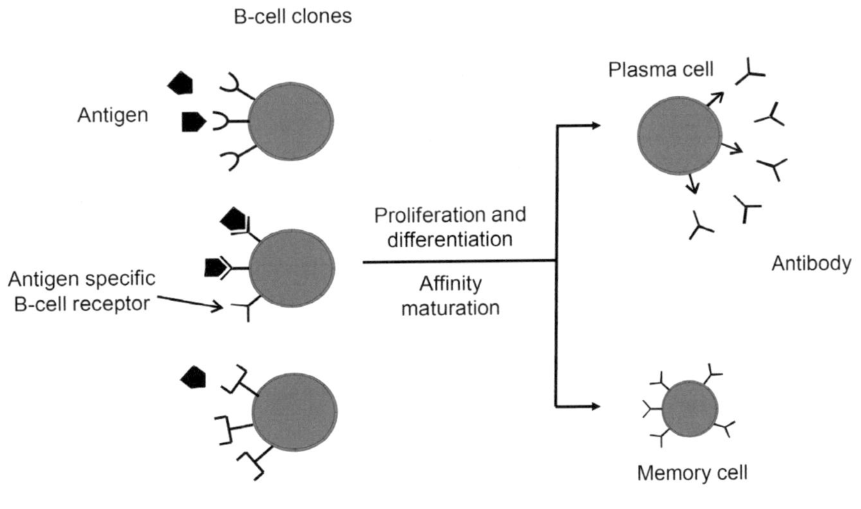

Figure 8: Schematic depiction to explain the mechanism of antigen-driven clonal selection during the immune response. An antigen binds to B-cell receptor (preferring receptors with high binding affinity) and triggers proliferation and differentiation of two different cell types: plasma cells secreting specific antibody (the antibody binding site structurally identical with the activated receptor) and memory cells providing long term memory of the acquired immunity.

Importantly, the clonal selection theory offers practical hints for animal immunization to improve affinity of the antibodies raised towards the antigenic determinant of the immunizing antigen. It has been proved that selection of high affinity lymphocytes will be most effective when the concentration of antigen in an immunized animal is limited [55, 56]. Thus, the lymphocytes possessing the highest affinity receptors will bind the greatest amount of antigen and will consequently be triggered to produce high-affinity antibodies. In addition to the size of antigen dose used for immunization, the length of the rest period between booster immunizations influences the antibody affinity. An effective way of improving antibody properties using clonal theory can be well demonstrated by an immunization scheme differing in immunogen dose and periods between booster immunizations [47]. A reduction of the hapten-protein immunogen dose from 0.3 to 0.05 mg, and lengthening of the rest periods between booster immunizations from 2 to 8 weeks resulted in the increase of antibody sensitivity to the hapten determinant from 3.8 to 0.3 μgL^{-1}. These results can be interpreted in terms of antibody affinity maturation (based on somatic hypermutation of B-cells) frequently resulting in the formation of antibodies with higher specificity and affinity towards the antigen [57, 58]. In this process, the concentration of circulating antigen diminishes over time, therefore the antigen-driven selection will continue to increase antibody affinity. Longer periods between booster injections will enable better clearance of the circulating antigen, stimulating production of the highest affinity antibodies. Moreover, the extended rest immunization periods allow the circulating level of antibody to drop sufficiently to prevent rapid clearance of the newly injected antigen [58]. In another experiment, an 8-week rest period improved significantly the sensitivity of polyclonal antibodies towards semicarbazide in comparison to conventional immunization [29].

4. PRODUCTION OF POLYCLONAL ANTIBODIES

A large number of antisera (polyclonal antibodies) is being used in a variety of immunoanalytical systems because they often allow to reach lower detection limits or broader cross-reactivity pattern than the monoclonal or recombinant antibody reagents [23, 24, 59, 60]. Because the production of polyclonal antibodies (pAbs) is inexpensive compared to the cost of hybridoma technology, such antibodies are utilized in many ELISA kits for screening or determination of environmental and food contaminants.

Polyclonal antibodies (or antisera) are antibodies that are produced from different B-cell lines and are therefore a heterogeneous mixture of antibody species of varying binding affinities, specificities, concentrations and isotypes (see Fig. **8**). An average affinity and specificity of particular polyclonal antiserum consist of many partial contributions from the constituent antibodies differing in their binding sites. Antisera contain not only specific antibodies against an antigen of interest, but also other immunoglobulins of unknown specificity that were present in blood of an animal before immunization [61]. These native immunoglobulins usually do not interfere with binding properties of the specific antibodies in real assays and therefore they may not be separated from the specific antibodies in antiserum. With regard to antiserum production, it is necessary to inject an immunogen into animals as pure as possible in order to reduce undesirable interferences originated from immunizing inoculum. Polyclonal antisera tend to have a broader cross-reactive binding pattern because they contain antibodies to different epitopes, antigens or antigenic subdeterminants such as a hapten spacer that were present in the immunizing inoculum [62].

4.1. Critical Stages in Polyclonal Antibody Production

Antigen design and subsequent immunogen preparation are steps having a crucial importance in the production of antibodies. The chemical purity as well as conformational and chemical stability of the immunogen are particularly important in pAb production because the antibodies will be generated in response to any immunogenic epitope in the injected material including contaminants. Therefore, a high degree of purity is important in the synthesized hapten derivatives and peptide antigens that are employed for the conjugation with carrier proteins. The quantity of injected immunogen as well as length of rest period between booster immunizations influence the immune response that is evoked during the immunization process (see section 2.5.). Depending on the animal size, micrograms to milligrams of immunogen are needed to elicit high titer responses in the experimental animals [58]. It should be noted that the antibody titer, usually defined as the antiserum dilution in the assay system, comprises not only the affinity to the target antigen, but is also influenced by the concentration of the antibody in antiserum.

Rabbits are the most commonly used animals for production of pAb with regard to animal size. Up to 100 mL of antiserum can be obtained from one animal and this is usually a sufficient volume to perform thousands of assays using an antibody typical dilution of 1:10 000. When larger amount of antibodies is required, sheep, goats, llamas and pigs can be used for immunization. The big animal species can generate at least ten times larger volumes of antisera in comparison to rabbit production. The big animals, however, are more difficult and expensive for housing and handling [63]. Generally, for any production strategy, a high number of animals is desirable, because the immune response of each animal is different, even in the case of genetically identical animals. A minimum of three to four animals are recommended for a single immunogen to have a chance of obtaining at least one antiserum of high affinity and selectivity [64].

Chickens can be used as an alternative to the rabbit and big animal antibody production. As a nonmammalin species, chickens offer certain advantages, *e.g.* the ability to easily harvest antibodies from the yolk (IgY) of the egg instead of blood collection and bleeding. Another advantage is that the cost of feeding and handling is considerably lower for chicken than for rabbit. The crude egg yolk may be used as an antibody material, but the lipids in the yolk may interfere with the antibody binding activity. Therefore, avian antibodies are usually purified from the yolk prior to use. A single chicken can produce 10-20 times more antibodies (in total) than a rabbit which can be beneficial for industrial applications requiring large amounts of antibody material [65, 66]. Additionally, chickens are phylogenetically divergent species from mammals, therefore a better immune response to mammal protein antigens can be achieved [67].

4.2. Adjuvants for Immunization

Adjuvants are substances injected together with an immunogen to an experimental animal in order to enhance the humoral and/or cell-mediated immune response to the antigenic determinant [68]. For pAb production, adjuvants are primarily used for increasing intensity and duration of immune response in order to obtain a sufficient amount of antibodies against the given antigen. In common adjuvants, immunomodulators and immunostimulators, such as microbial cells, microbial cell components, or chemically modified microbial products, are used in order to activate and improve differentiation of cells of the immune system [69]. Although numerous adjuvant preparations have been described [70], only a few of them are routinely utilized for immunization of animals.

Freund´s adjuvant is most often used for the production of pAbs because high antibody titers are induced towards almost all types of antigens. Freund´s Complete Adjuvant (FCA) is generally used only for initial (priming) immunization, whereas Freund´s Incomplete Adjuvant (FIA) is utilized for subsequent booster immunizations. FCA is composed of a light mineral oil, an emulsifying agent (mannide monooleate), and heat-killed and dried mycobacterial cells, whereas FIA lacks the mycobacterial components, being just a water-in-oil emulsion. The heat-treated mycobacterial cells are essential for increased humoral antibody response and delayed-type hypersensitivity reaction. The mineral oil facilitates keeping an antigen depot with slow release of antigen transport throughout the lymphatic system to cells of the immune system. Emulsification of an antigen in an aqueous solution with the equal volume of adjuvant and the formation of a stable water-in-oil emulsion is a crucial step in the effectiveness of any adjuvant including Freund´s adjuvant [68].

Although Freund´s adjuvants are potent stimulators of the immune response, their use can sometimes cause serious side effects in laboratory animals, *e.g.* ulceration, granuloma formation or untimely ascites production. In certain cases, Freund´s adjuvants can be replaced by alternative adjuvants which may evoke antibody responses with less tissue destruction. [68, 71, 72]. However, their use for antibody production is not too widespread, especially because of their difficult preparation and higher costs.

4.3. Immunization Procedures

Although many immunization schemes are described in literature, a common immunization protocol comprises a primary immunization, preferring the use of FCA, and several repeated (booster) immunizations with FIA, usually with a month rest period between each one [64]. The antigen/adjuvant emulsion is being administered as a single injection or as multiple injections of low inoculum volumes. In this laboratory, five booster injections using Freund´s adjuvant are proved to be sufficient to produce antibodies against hapten determinants with sufficient affinity and concentration [22, 49]. In routine antibody production, an immunizing inoculum is being administered subcutaneously, intradermally, intramuscularly, intraperitoneally or intravenously, depending on the animal species, antigen properties and long-term experience. The immunized animals are tested for antibody response after the third booster injection and subsequently every four weeks after the following immunization [63].

4.4. Antibody Response Monitoring

Because the immune response is not constant the during immunization process, it is desirable to monitor both qualitative and quantitative characteristics of the antibody response by collecting and evaluating blood samples. In rabbits, the commonly used vessel for blood collection is the middle ear artery running down the centre of the external ear. In sheep, goats and other larger animals, the blood collection is performed usually from the jugular vein, whereas in mice and rats, the commonly used vessel is the tail vein. In chickens, antibody formation in eggs can be studied without the use of invasive methods [64]. Several techniques such as immunoassays, radial immunodiffusion and western blot analysis are routinely used for antibody response monitoring. Using these methods, it is possible to quantitate basic immunochemical parameters and to monitor their changes in time.

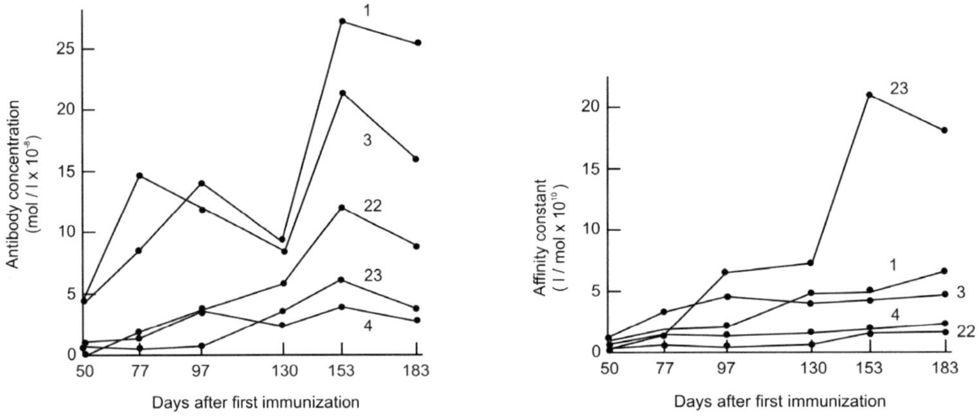

Figure 9: Monitoring of antibody affinity and concentration during long-term immunization of rabbits. According to Franek and Hruska [73].

Dynamic changes in antibody level, affinity and specificity (cross-reactivity) were demonstrated by Franek and Hruska [73] in rabbits immunized in a period of 183 days. Plasma samples were collected at 10-15 days after each booster injection and subsequently analysed by a radioimmunoassay method. It is shown in Fig. **9** that the plasma concentrations of antibodies raised against estron-azo-hapten structure fluctuated within two orders of magnitude and peaked on day 153 after the initial immunization. In compliance with the theory of antibody maturation during a long-term immunization, there was a moderate upward trend in the values of the calculated affinity constants. The highest affinity constant (2.1×10^{11} $Lmol^{-1}$) was observed in the antibody produced by rabbit 23, whereas five to ten times lower values were determined for other antibodies. At the same intervals the changes were examined in cross-reactions using various estron derivatives. During this period covering 8 immunizations, only small changes were observed in the cross-reactivity between estron and methyl estron in all the pAbs whereas the great differences in cross-reactivity values among the tested antibodies were retained (Fig. **10**).

In the end of the immunization procedure, the animals are killed and the maximum antiserum collected. The terminal bleeding of rabbits must be performed under general anesthesia using an approved technique obtaining blood directly from the heart (heart puncture) or by cannulation of large vessels in the proximity of the heart. Properties of the bleeded antiserum are evaluated using conventional immunoanalytical or serological methods.

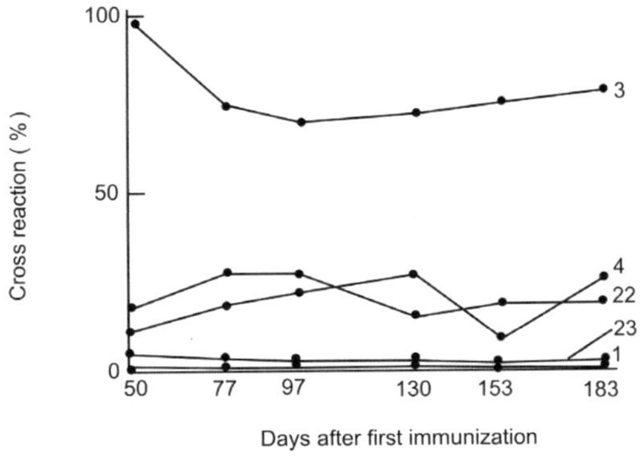

Figure 10: Monitoring of cross-reactivity between estron and methyl estron during long-term immunization of rabbits. According to Franek and Hruska [73].

5. PRODUCTION OF MONOCLONAL ANTIBODIES

Monoclonal Antibodies (mAbs) are produced by hybridoma technology developed in 1975 by Köhler and Milstein [74]. The technology is based on fusion of activated, antibody-forming B-cell lines with a cancerous plasma cells (myeloma cells) resulting in hybridomas, which have the immortal growth properties of the myeloma cells and the antibody secretion capability originated from the B-cells. The clone of such hybridoma cells can be cultured indefinitely and can secrete unlimited amount of mAb. The fact, that mAbs can be produced in large amounts as standard homogenous and chemically defined immunoglobulin entities being consistent over time, makes these antibodies attractive candidates for both research and diagnostic/industrial sphere. When compared with polyclonal antisera, the affinity of mAbs is sometimes inferior but the specificity of the monoclonal reagents is often superior because the binding site of mAb is always formed against one antigenic determinant. This is particularly important for protein antigens where a high degree of specificity towards the peptide subunits is required to recognize only a single epitope.

The mAb development is associated with a higher costs compared with pAbs because a relatively low predictability of the results of hybridoma technology increases the initial costs of antibody production [62, 75]. However, once the hybridoma clone is established, overall production costs may be considerably reduced.

General representation of the hybridoma technology methods used for production of mAbs is shown in Fig. **11**. In this section, the crucial steps of the technology, the obtaining spleen B-cells from the an immunized animal, hybridoma cell production by fusion of the B-cells with myeloma cells, clone selection/isolation and screening of hybridoma clones with immunochemical methods will be discussed.

5.1. Production of B-Cells for Fusion

Activated B-cell material is traditionally obtained by immunization of BALB/c mice because the BALB/c animal strain is syngeneic for the myeloma cells that are most frequently used for fusion. In most situations, mice or rats are chosen for immunizations but mice are usually preferred due to their common convenience and availability of suitable myeloma lines. Rat advantage is their larger size, allowing to obtain bigger volumes of ascetic fluid [75, 76]. The B-cells from LOU/C rats were utilized for the cell fusion [36].

Freund´s adjuvant or alternatively other adjuvants are used for immunization of mice and rats. In general, three to four booster immunizations are sufficient to achieve reasonable antibody titres, with intervals of 14 to 28 days between booster injections, but the immunization protocols may vary among investigators [63]. After the third immunization, blood samples are collected from mouse tail vein to monitor antibody formation prior to a fusion. For antibodies raised against haptens, both competitive indirect and direct ELISA methods can be utilized to test antiserum for titre and sensitivity towards the analyte [29]. Mice showing the best characteristics are euthanized and their spleens removed for cell fusion [77]. To enhance the success of the fusion, the animals are sometimes immunized with a lower antigen dose without adjuvant few days before they are sacrificed. This may ensure that the relevant lymphocytes are at their peak of proliferation [61].

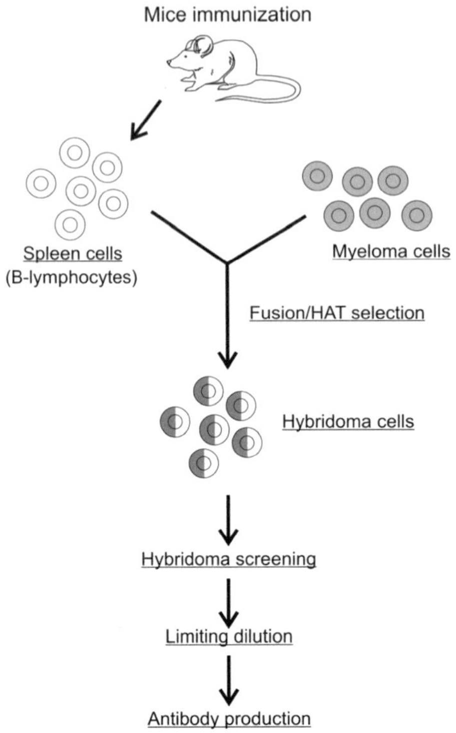

Figure 11: A general representation of the methods used for production of monoclonal antibodies.

5.2. Myeloma Cell Lines

As shown in Fig. **11**, myeloma cells are the second key elements for the fusion experiments. These neoplastic cells are derived from lymphocyte precursors and available from commercial sources. Myeloma cells lack the ability of immunoglobulin formation and have an enzyme deficiency which makes them impossible in to survive poor nutrient conditions during hybridoma selection. Most of the commercially available myeloma cell lines, such as 653 or SP-2, have a deficiency of hypoxanthine-guanine phosphoribosyltransferase (HGPRT) and therefore they are applicable for fusion experiments. Moreover, myeloma cells are advantageous for the hybridoma technology as they are easy to grow in a suspension tissue culture in special growth media with 10% fetal calf serum [61].

5.3. Fusion and Hybridoma Selection

A fusion of myeloma cell with an antibody producing lymphocyte is the most crucial stage in the mAb production. This process results in a hybridoma cell formation with two important properties: unlimited proliferation and production of antibody with constant immunoanalytical properties. The fusion is performed in the presence of polyethylen glycol (PEG) by mixing of B-lymphocytes and myeloma cells. PEG is a cell fusion agent allowing the fusion of cell membranes. When a fusion is completed, the cell suspension is transferred to the HAT (hypoxanthine-aminopterin-thymidine) medium which is used to select the hybridoma cells from unfused B-lymphocytes and myeloma cells [78]. The obtained hybridoma cells are then grown in microtiter plates together with mouse feeder cells (thymocytes, peritoneal macrophages or splenocytes) which supply growth factors promoting growth of the hybridoma cells [79]. The hybridomas are continuously screened for antibody-antigen binding using ELISA or related immunoanalytical methods. The hybridoma screening is a key step for a successful generation of high-affinity and analyte-specific mAbs, particularly when the analyte is a low-molecular weight compound. Automated antibody systems accelerate screening result, which is important for a rapid hybridoma selection because several risk factors, such as genetic instability in hybridoma clones, overgrowth of non-producing cells or bacterial contamination can negatively affect hybridoma cultivation at this early stage [80]. Only some of the antibody-producing hybridomas survive during the first weeks after fusion and these are used for a final clone isolation [81].

5.4. Isolation of Hybridoma Clones

After the fusion and HAT selection the cells grow in wells of microtiter plates forming colonies which contain different hybridoma clones. The isolation of a single hybridoma clone is subsequently performed by a procedure called "cloning by limiting dilution". In this method, the cells are diluted with a complete growth medium across the plate in order to reach a concentration of one or no cell per well whereas the rest of the wells may contain two or more cells. The number of cells in the wells is determined by the density function of the Poisson distribution [82]. For a successful clone isolation, two or more consecutive cloning procedures are usually performed to maximize the proportion of wells that contain only a single clone. Thus, the cloning by limiting dilution may ensure that cells of the hybridoma clone will originate from one cell line and that the produced antibody is monoclonal. The isolated hybridoma clones are stored at -196 °C in liquid nitrogen.

5.5. Methods of Monoclonal Antibody Production

To produce the desired mAbs, hybridoma clones must be grown in ascites fluid in mice or *in vitro* tissue culture. The method based on the mouse ascites is usually available in laboratories involved in hybridoma development, however, in this case mice should be treated with caution during the ascites growth to reduce the pain induced by accumulation of fluid in the abdomen cavity. The *in vitro* tissue-culture method can be employed if anticipated application, *e.g.*, the production of immunoassay kits or immunoaffinity columns, will require medium or large amounts of mAb. *In vitro* methods are more expensive and time-consuming procedures and sometimes may fail to produce the antibody due to a low concentration in culture medium. It should be taken into account that each hybridoma responds differently to the given *in vitro* environment. Today, custom *in vitro* production is easily available in many commercial laboratories.

a) In Vivo Ascites Induction

The traditional way in which mAb is generated in ascites fluid is based on the administration of hybridoma injections into the abdominal cavity of animal (BALB/c mice, LOU/C rats) and collection of the formed ascites fluid from the animal. To improve ascites yields, the animals are first given an intraperitoneal injection with a priming agent, usually pristane or FCA [83], which irritates the peritoneum resulting in ascites fluid secretion [84]. Hybridoma cell-suspension is injected into the peritoneal cavity typically 7 to 10 days after priming. This leads to the production of ascites with an average yield of 2 to 4 mL/mouse. Ascites fluid is usually collected 7 to 14 days after hybridoma cells administration [63, 85]. As this method affects seriously the animal welfare, it can only be used with regard to the valid legislation. Every attempt should be made to obtain material already available or to use an *in vitro* method for production of mAbs. Therefore, any proposed production of mAbs using the ascites method requires justification by the investigator to the animal care committee [86].

b) In Vitro Tissue-Culture Methods

Currently, two types of *in vitro* systems, batch tissue-culture devices and semipermeable-membrane-based systems, are predominantly used for *in vitro* mAb production. The simplest way to produce mAb *in vitro* is to grow the hybridomas in batches containing a culture medium with or without fetal bovine serum [87-89]. The fetal bovine serum is used in tissue culture media as growth supplement because of its high content of embryonic growth promoting factors. The technology is cheap and relatively easy to perform, but it generates mAb of relatively low concentrations (typically below 20 μgmL^{-1}) [90].

The second approach, the semipermeable-membrane-based system, employs a barrier, either a hollow fiber or a membrane, which divides the device into two compartments. In a small chamber, hybridoma cells are cultured to produce antibodies whereas a larger compartment contains the culture media. In the system, nutrients and cell waste products diffuse easily across the membrane barrier but cells and antibodies are retained in the smaller chamber. The technology permits to grow cells at high densities and to replace media without losing cells or antibodies. The major advantage of membrane-based systems is that a total yield of mAb (10-160 mg) can be generated in a relatively low volume of the medium [91].

5.6. Purification and Characterization of mAbs

When the desired amount of hybridoma medium (supernatant) or ascites fluid has been produced, one of several types of purification methods may be chosen. The ascetic fluids are purified usually by quick, single step protein A/G chromatography [22]. Other methods such as ion exchange chromatography, sodium/ammonium sulphate precipitation or affinity chromatography can be combined to purify effectively supernatants containing unwanted impurities, *e.g.* ballast proteins. To achieve maximum purity in a single purification step, affinity purification can be performed to provide superior specificity for the antibody. In this approach, the antigen (peptide-carrier protein) attached to an agarose support is used as an affinity capture element for the corresponding antibody. The final purity can be analyzed using electrophoretic or chromatographic methods (SDS-PAGE, SEC-HPLC). The purified mAb is characterized by determination of immunoglobulin class, subclass and isotype [92].

ACKNOWLEDGEMENTS

This work was supported by the AdmireVet project No. CZ. 1.05/2.1.00/01.0006-ED00060101 (Ministry of Education, Youth and Sports of the Czech Republic) and by the Grant No. MZE00027 (Ministry of Agriculture of the Czech Republic). The authors wish to thank Prof. K. Hruska for careful reading of the manuscript.

REFERENCES

[1] Benjamin DC, Berzofsky JA, East IJ, *et al.* The antigenic structure of proteins - a reappraisal. Annu Rev Immunol 1984; 2: 67-101.

[2] Kahn F, Morgelin M, Shannon O, *et al.* Antibodies against a surface protein of Streptococcus pyogenes promote a pathological inflammatory response. Plos Pathog 2008; 4.

[3] Bennett MK, Garciaarraras JE, Elferink LA, *et al.* The syntaxin family of vesicular transport receptors. Cell 1993; 74: 863-73.

[4] Johannes L, Lledo PM, Roa M, *et al.* The Gtpase rab3a negatively controls calcium-dependent exocytosis in neuroendocrine cells. Embo J 1994; 13: 2029-37.

[5] Shapiro J, Sciaky N, Lee J, *et al.* Localization of endogenous furin in cultured cell lines. J Histochem Cytochem 1997; 45: 3-12.

[6] Van Regenmortel MH. Structural and functional approaches to the study of protein antigenicity. Immunol Today 1986; 10: 266-72.

[7] Van Regenmortel MHV. Mapping epitope structure and activity: from one-dimensional prediction to four-dimensional description of antigenic specificity. Methods 1996; 9: 465-2.

[8] Angeletti RH. Design of useful peptide antigens. J Biomol Tech 1999; 10: 2-10.

[9] Lindskog M, Berglund L, Uhlen M, Sterky F. Selection of antigenic protein fragments for antibody-based proteomics. Mol Cell Proteomics 2005; 4: S63.

[10] National Center for Biotechnology Information; [cited 2011 Jan 10]. Available from: http://www.ncbi.nlm.nih.gov/

[11] BLAST search program. National Center for Biotechnology Information; [cited 2011 Jan 10]. Available from http://www.ncbi.nlm.gov/BLAST/.

[12] Clustal: Multiple Sequence Alignment; [cited 2011 Jan 10]. Available from: http://www.ibc.wustl.edu/service/clustal.html.

[13] Multiple Sequence Alignment program. Institute for Biomedical Computing; [cited 2011 Jan 10]. Available from http://expasy.hcuge.ch/cgi-bin/protscale.pl.

[14] ProtScale program. Swiss Institute of Bioinformatics; [cited 2010 Dec 21]. Available from: http://expasy.hcuge.ch/cgi-bin/protscale.pl.

[15] Joyce S, Nathenson SG. Methods to Study Peptides Associated with Mhc Class-I Molecules (Vol 6, Pg 24, 1994). Curr Opin Immunol 1994; 6: 334.

[16] Kyte J, Doolittle RF. A simple method for displaying the hydropathic character of a protein. J Mol Biol 1982; 157: 105-32.

[17] GenScript, The Biology CRO. The specialized Information Services: Peptide Antigen Design; [cited 2010 Dec10]. Available from: http://www.genscript.com/peptide_design_guideline.html.

[18] Burdick DJ, Stults JT. Analysis of peptide synthesis products by electrospray ionization mass spectrometry. Method Enzymol 1997; 289: 499-519.

[19] Chakrabartty A, Doig AJ, Baldwin RL. Helix capping propensities in peptides parallel those in proteins. P Natl Acad Sci USA 1993; 90: 11332-6.

[20] Presta LG, Rose GD. Helix signals in proteins. Science 1988; 240: 1632-41.

[21] Hermanson GT. Bioconjugate Techniques. Academic Press. San Diego, California 1996.

[22] Cernoch I, Schleicher E, Franek M. Production and analytical characterization of neopterin immunoreagents for biosensor developments. Anal Bioanal Chem 2011; 399: 979-86.

[23] Franek M, Deng AP, Kolar V, Socha J. Direct competitive immunoassays for the coplanar polychlorinated biphenyls. Anal Chim Acta 2001; 444: 131-42.

[24] Franek M, Diblikova I, Cernoch I, Vass M, Hruska K. Broad-specificity immunoassays for sulfonamide detection: Immunochemical strategy for generic antibodies and competitors. Anal Chem 2006; 78: 1559-67.

[25] Lateef SS, Gupta S, Jayathilaka LP, *et al.* An improved protocol for coupling synthetic peptides to carrier proteins for antibody production using DMF to solubilize peptides. J Biomol Tech 2007; 18: 173-6.

[26] Madison LD, Rosenzweig SA, Jamieson JD. Use of the heterobifunctional cross-linker meta-maleimidobenzoyl n-hydroxysuccinimide ester to affinity label cholecystokinin binding-proteins on rat pancreatic plasma-membranes. J Biol Chem 1984; 259: 4818-23.

[27] Peeters JM, Hazendonk TG, Beuvery EC, Tesser GI. Comparison of 4 bifunctional reagents for coupling peptides to proteins and the effect of the 3 moieties on the immunogenicity of the conjugates. J Immunol Methods 1989; 120: 133-43.

[28] Deen C, Claassen E, Gerritse K, Zegers ND, Boersma WJA. A novel carbodiimide coupling method for synthetic peptides - enhanced antipeptide antibody-responses. J Immunol Methods 1990; 129: 119-25.

[29] Vass M, Diblikova I, Cernoch I, Franek M. ELISA for semicarbazide and its application for screening in food contamination. Anal Chim Acta 2008; 608: 86-94.

[30] Shan YM, Wang LP, Shi YH, *et al.* NHS-mediated QDs-peptide/protein conjugation and its application for cell labeling. Talanta 2008; 75: 1008-14.

[31] Carter JM. Conjugation of peptides to carrier protein *via* carbodiimide. In: Walker JM, Ed. The Protein Protocol Handbook. Totowa, Humana Press, 2010; pp. 693-94.

[32] Liu A, Zhou Y, Zhank Y, Chen F, Wang X. Preparation of CIT-protein conjugates using a novel citrinin derivative as hapten. Eur Food Res Technol 2010.

[33] Xu ZL, Shen YD, Zheng WX, *et al.* Broad-specificity immunoassay for O,O-Diethyl organophosphorus pesticides: application of molecular modeling to improve assay sensitivity and study antibody recognition. Anal Chem 2010; 82: 9314-21.

[34] Carter JM. Conjugation of pepides to carrier proteins *via* glutaraldehyde. In: Walker JM, Ed. The Protein Protocol Handbook. Totowa, Humana Press, 2010; pp. 679-87.

[35] Zegers N, Gerritse K, Deen C, Boersma W, Claassen E. An improved conjugation method for controlled covalent coupling of synthetic peptides to proteins using glutaraldehyde in a dialysis method. J Immunol Methods 1990; 130: 195-200.

[36] Kramer PM, Gouzy MF, Kess M, Kleinschmidt U, Kremmer E. Development and characterization of new rat monoclonal antibodies for procalcitonin. Anal Bional Chem 2008; 392: 727-36.

[37] Tam JP. Synthetic peptide vaccine design - synthesis and properties of a high-density multiple antigenic peptide system. P Natl Acad Sci USA 1988; 85: 5409-13.

[38] Posnett DN, Tam JP. Multiple antigenic peptide method for producing antipeptide site-specific antibodies. Method Enzymol 1989; 178: 739-46.

[39] Tam JP, Zavala F. Multiple antigen peptide - a novel-approach to increase detection sensitivity of synthetic peptides in solid-phase immunoassays. J Immunol Methods 1989; 124: 53-61.

[40] Briand JP, Barin C, Vanregenmortel MHV, Muller S. Application and limitations of the multiple antigen peptide (map) system in the production and evaluation of antipeptide and antiprotein antibodies. J Immunol Methods 1992; 156: 255-65.

[41] Landsteiner K. The specificity of serological reactions. Dover Publications. New York, US 1962.

[42] Yalow RS, Berson SA. Immunoassay of endogenous plasma insulin in man (Reprinted from J Clin Invest, vol 39, pg 1157-1175, 1960). Prog Obes R 1996; 4: 583-600.

[43] Franek M. Structural aspects of steroid antibody specificity. J Steroid Biochem 1987; 28: 95-108.

[44] Rao PN, Moore PH. Synthesis of new steroid haptens for radioimmunoassay .1. 15beta-carboxyethyl-mercaptotestosterone-bovine serum-albumin conjugate - measurement of testosterone in male plasma without chromatography. Steroids 1976; 28: 101-9.

[45] Kolar V, Deng AP, Franek M. Production and characterization of generic antibodies against s-triazine and sulfonylurea herbicides. Food Agr Immunol 2002; 14: 91-105.

[46] Liu Y, Lou Y, Xu D, *et al.* Production and characterization of monoclonal antibody for class-specific determination of O,O-dimethyl organophosphorus pesticides and effect of heterologous coating antigens on immunoassay sensitivity. Microchem J 2009; 93: 36-42.

[47] Cooper KM, Caddell A, Elliott CT, Kennedy DG. Production and characterisation of polyclonal antibodies to a derivative of 3-amino-2-oxazolidinone, a metabolite of the nitrofuran furazolidone. Anal Chim Acta 2004; 520: 79-86.

[48] Preston A, Fodey T, Elliott C. Development of a high-throughput enzyme-linked immunosorbent assay for the routine detection of the carcinogen acrylamide in food, *via* rapid derivatisation pre-analysis. Anal Chim Acta 2008; 608: 178-85.

[49] Franek M, Diblikova I, Cernoch I, Vass M, Hruska K. Broad-specificity immunoassays for sulfonamide detection: Immunochemical strategy for generic antibodies and competitors. Anal Chem 2006; 78: 1559-67.

[50] Muldoon MT, Holtzapple CK, Deshpande SS, Beier RC, Stanker LH. Development of a monoclonal antibody-based cELISA for the analysis of sulfadimethoxine. 1. Development and characterization of monoclonal antibodies and molecular modeling studies of antibody recognition. J Agr Food Chem 2000; 48: 537-44.

[51] Xu ZL, Shen YD, Beier RC, *et al.* Application of computer-assisted molecular modeling for immunoassay of low molecular weight food contaminants: A review. Anal Chim Acta 2009; 647: 125-36.

[52] Franek M, Pouzar V, Kolar V. Enzyme-immunoassays for polychlorinated biphenyls: structural aspects of hapten-antibody binding. Anal Chim Acta 1997; 347: 163-76.

[53] Edwards SR, Gilby ED, Jeffcoate SL. Iodine-125 tracers in steroid radioimmunoassay. Radioimmunoassay and related procedures in medicine, IAEA, Vienna: Austria 1974.

[54] Burnet FM. The Clonal Selection Theory of Acquired Immunity. Cambridge University Press. Cambridge, UK 1959.

[55] Goidl EA, Paul WE, Siskind GW, Benacerr B. Effect of antigen dose and time after immunization on amount and affinity of anti-hapten antibody. J Immunol 1968; 100: 371-75.

[56] Siskind GW, Benacerraf B. Cell selection by antigen in the immune response. Adv Immunol 1969; 10: 1-50.

[57] Berek C, Milstein C. Mutation drift and repertoire shift in the maturation of the immune-response. Immunol Rew 1987; 96: 23-41.

[58] Harlow E, Lane D. Antibodies: a Laboratory Manual. Cold Spring Harbor Laboratory Press. New York, US 1988.

[59] Franek M, Kolar V, Eremin SA. Enzyme immunoassays for s-triazine herbicides and their application in environmental and food analysis. Anal Chim Acta 1995; 311: 349-56.

[60] Franek M, Kolar V, Deng AP, Crooks S. Determination of sulphadimindine (sulfamethazine) residues in milk, plasma, urine and edible tissues by sensitive ELISA. Food Agr Immunol 1999; 11: 339-49.

[61] Lidell E. Antibodies. In: Wild D, Ed. The Immunoassay Handbook. London, Nature Publishing Group, 2001; pp. 118-34.

[62] Lipman NS, Jackson LR, Trudel LJ, Weis-Garcia F. Monoclonal versus polyclonal antibodies: Distinguishing characteristics, applications, and information resources. Ilar J 2005; 46: 258-68.

[63] Leenaars M, Hendriksen CFM. Critical steps in the production of polyclonal and monoclonal antibodies evaluation and recommendations. Ilar J 2005; 46: 269-79.

[64] Bean ES. Polyclonal Antibodies. In: Howard GC, Bethell DR, Eds. Basic Methods in Antibody Production and Characterization. Boca Raton, CRC Press LLC, 2001; pp. 31-51.

[65] Lee YI, Surzycki SS, Young IL. Production of egg yolk antibody (igy) against human placental dna-dependent rna polymerase ii. J Biochem Mol Biol 1995; 82: 27-32.

[66] Schade R, Staak C, Hendriksen C, *et al.* The production of avian (egg yolk) antibodies: IgY - The report and recommendations of ECVAM Workshop 21. Atla-Altern Lab Anim 1996; 24: 925-34.

[67] Gassmann M, Thommes P, Weiser T, Hubscher U. Efficient production of chicken egg-yolk antibodies against a conserved mammalian protein. Faseb J 1990; 4: 2528-32.

[68] Stills HF. Adjuvants and antibody production: Dispelling the myths associated with Freund's complete and other adjuvants. Ilar J 2005; 46: 280-93.

[69] Victoratos P, Yiangou M, Avramidis N, Hadjipetrou L. Regulation of cytokine gene expression by adjuvants *in vivo*. Clin Exp Immunol 1997; 109: 569-78.

[70] Vogel FR. Immunological adjuvants for modern vaccine formulations. Ann Ny Acad Sci 1995; 754: 153-60.

[71] Beck I, Gerlach H, Burkhardt E, Kaleta EF. Investigation of several selected adjuvants regarding their efficacy and side effects for the production of a vaccine for parakeets to prevent a disease caused by a paramyxovirus type 3. Vaccine 2003; 21: 1006-22.

[72] Shu Q, Bird SH, Gill HS, *et al.* Antibody response in sheep following immunization with Streptococcus bovis in different adjuvants. Vet Res Commun 2001; 25: 43-54.

[73] Franek M, Hruska K. Specificity of the immune-response to the estrone-azo-hapten structure. J Steroid Biochem 1985; 22: 341-7.

[74] Kohler G, Milstein C. Continuous cultures of fused cells secreting antibody of predefined specificity. Nature 1975; 256: 495-7.

[75] Franek M, Kolar V, Granatova M, Nevorankova Z. Monoclonal elisa for 2,4-dichlorophenoxyacetic acid - characterization of antibodies and assay optimization. J Agr Food Chem 1994; 42: 1369-74.

[76] Bazin H, Cormont F, Xhurdebise LM. Rat Monoclonal-Antibodies. Fresen Z Anal Chem 1982; 311: 347.

[77] Monoclonal Antibody Production; A Report of the Commitee on Methods of Producing Monoclonal Antibodies, Institute for Laboratory Animal Research; National Research Council. National Academy Press, Washington, DC; 1999.

[78] Pohanka M. Monoclonal and polyclonal antibodies production - preparation of potent biorecognition element. J Appl Biomed 2009; 7: 115-21.

[79] Quinlan N, O'Kennedy R. Enhanced cloning efficiencies of murine hybridomas using human plasma supplemented medium. J Immunol Methods 1994; 171: 253-8.

[80] Rieger M, Cervino C, Sauceda JC, Niessner R, Knopp D. Efficient hybridoma screening technique using capture antibody based microarrays. Anal Chem 2009; 81: 2373-7.

[81] Vass M, Kotkova L, Diblikova I, *et al.* Production and characterisation of monoclonal antibodies for the detection of AOZ, a tissue bound metabolite of furazolidone. Vet Med-Czech 2005; 50: 300-10.

[82] Brichta J, Franek M. Identification of monoclonal antibodies against 2,4-D herbicide by ELISA and DNA sequencing. J Agr Food Chem 2003; 51: 6091-7.

[83] Gillette RW. Alternatives to pristane priming for ascitic fluid and monoclonal-antibody production. J Immunol Methods 1987; 99: 21-3.

[84] Moore JM, Rajan TV. Pristane retards clearance of particulate materials from the peritoneal-cavity of laboratory mice. J Immunol Methods 1994; 173: 273-8.

[85] Hendriksen CFM, de Leeuw WA, Falkenberg FW, *et al. In vivo* and *in vitro* production of mAbs - Discussion. Res Immunol 1998; 149: 611-20.

[86] Canadian Council on Animal Care, 2002. Guidelines on: antibody production; (cited 2011 Jan 10). Available from: http://www.ccac.ca.

[87] Federspiel G, Mccullough KC, Kihm U. Hybridoma antibody-production invitro in type-ii serum-free medium using nutridoma-sp supplements - comparisons with invivo methods. J Immunol Methods 1991; 145: 213-21.

[88] Tarleton RL, Beyer AM. Medium-scale production and purification of monoclonal-antibodies in protein-free medium. Biotechniques 1991; 11: 590-8.

[89] Velez D, Reuveny S, Miller L, Macmillan JD. Kinetics of monoclonal-antibody production in low serum growth-medium. J Immunol Methods 1986; 86: 45-52.

[90] Lullau E, Heyse S, Vogel H, *et al.* Antigen binding properties of purified immunoglobulin A and reconstituted secretory immunoglobulin A antibodies. J Biol Chem 1996; 271: 16300-9.

[91] Falkenberg FW, Weichert H, Krane M, *et al. In-vitro* production of monoclonal-antibodies in high-concentration in a new and easy to handle modular minifermenter. J Immunol Methods 1995; 179: 13-29.

[92] Harkins KR. Antibody purification methods. In: Howard GC, Bethell DR, Eds. Basic methods in antibody production and characterization. Boca Raton, CRC Press LLC, 2001; pp. 142-66.

CHAPTER 3

Standardization of Immunoassays

H.A. Morris*

School of Pharmacy and Medical Sciences, University of South Australia, Adelaide, South Australia 5001 and Chemical Pathology, SA Pathology, Adelaide, South Australia 5000 Australia

Abstract: While immunoassays are now used in a variety of fields including medical, food technology and environmental protection because of their high sensitivity, high specificity and ease of automation to provide highly cost effective analyses, it has been in medical testing that their standardization has been most intensely developed. The use of internationally agreed clinical protocols, common reference intervals or decision limits and even electronic health records across health-care institutions are all dependent on medical testing laboratories performing assays that are traceable to internationally recognized reference measurement systems. The application of metrological principles to achieve traceability and standardization for immunoassays is being pursued to this end. Comprehensive measurement systems are available for the total serum hapten assays currently measured in the clinical laboratory by immunoassay. Current research is investigating the usefulness of developing defined systems for the measurement of non-bound fractions or "free" hormone levels of these types of analytes. One strategy that has been successfully applied for the standardization of assays for large molecular weight polypeptide measurands has been to localise the biological activity to a small molecular weight moiety of the meausurand and to establish a reference measurement procedure for this moiety as a surrogate for the total molecule of clinical interest. The standardization or harmonization of assays for heterogeneous polypeptide hormones is also is another area of current research for standardization of clinical immunoassays. The accreditation of medical testing laboratories to ISO15189 standard requires that all testing methods including immunoassays are validated or verified to be fit for purpose including the accuracy of the assay and the estimation of measurement uncertainty as assessed by traceability to certified reference materials through a documented unbroken chain of calibrations.

Keywords: Antibodies, Immunoassays, Standardization.

INTRODUCTION

Immunoassays were first introduced into clinical chemistry laboratories to assist with the diagnosis, prognosis and monitoring of patients particularly in the context of analytes present in biological fluids at what are considered very low concentrations [1]. These are analytes whose concentrations in biological fluids are usually too low for quantification by physical methods such as optical or electrochemical techniques. More often these analytes are present in the nanomolar or femtomolar ranges although some are at micromolar levels. More recently they have been applied to analyses in a variety of laboratories as is discussed later.

The reliability of all laboratory results is dependent on accuracy which has two components, precision and trueness [2]. Trueness describes the comparability of a test result to an accepted reference value for the quantity measured and is of particular importance for the comparability of results between laboratories and clinical centres, which are necessary for the use of internationally-agreed clinical protocols and common reference intervals and decision limits. The concept of trueness has a considerable history in clinical chemistry in general and in immunoassay in particular. The World Health Organisation initiated a program to assist with immunoassays improving trueness through the preparation of International Standards

***Address correspondence to H.A. Morris:** School of Pharmacy and Medical Sciences, University of South Australia, Adelaide, South Australia 5001 and Chemical Pathology, SA Pathology, Adelaide, South Australia 5000 Australia; E-mail: howard.morris@imvs.sa.gov.au particularly for peptide hormone assays [3]. These preparations were Standardized against a biological response using bioassays and their concentration was expressed as a biological activity in International Units (IU). The problem that arose with this strategy was that the quantity of International Standard (IS) in any single preparation was limited and therefore was exhausted at some time. When a second preparation of IS was undertaken the preparative techniques and purity improved and so the mass of peptide per IU was decreased. Bioactivity assays are demanding of technique and time, and therefore unsuitable for routine clinical measurements. Immunoassays however measure mass. Therefore with every new preparation of International Standard the immunoassay measurement was different. Thus traceability of each immunoassay Standardized in this way was dependent on the particular preparation of IS used and such a variation in measurement values is unsuitable for use of internationally-agreed clinical protocols and common reference intervals and decision limits.

Over the last 10 to 15 years considerable advances have been made with technological, theoretical and organisational aspects of this field [4]. Thus we are currently in a period during which much progress is being made with the application of the principles of metrology to achieve traceability and Standardization for immunoassays for specific measurands [5].

THE ROLE OF IMMUNOASSAYS IN THE CLINICAL LABORATORY

Immunoassays were quickly adopted in clinical laboratory testing because they provided a unique technology for assaying a variety of analytes in complex biological fluids with adequate specificity and sensitivity for clinical use [1]. Immunoassays are capable of assaying analytes present in blood serum at levels between 10^{-12} to 10^{-6} molar in the presence of substances to which they share a considerable degree of homology and may be present in concentrations of the order of 10^{-3} molar. For example the steroid hormone cortisol is often measured by immunoassay at levels in blood serum of approximately 10^{-7} molar in the presence of numerous steroid hormones of similar structure and at similar concentrations [6]. Probably most important in this context is the presence of cholesterol, from which all steroid hormones are derived and which forms their backbone structure. Cholesterol is present in human serum at concentrations of 10^{-3} molar which is a 10,000 molar excess compared to cortisol. These properties make immunoassays a most important tool in the clinical laboratory but increase the difficulty to establish their traceability and Standardization.

Immunoassay technology has been amenable to automation with instruments capable of processing some hundreds of patient specimens per hour on a single platform covering a range of 50 or more analytes [1]. These developments have provided clinical laboratories with considerable productivity advantages, the financial benefits of which have been passed onto patients, governments, and insurers *etc.* Such automated technologies have some analytical limitations but these are not so great as to remove them from the clinical laboratory. One such limitation is the necessity to accommodate each assay to a common incubation time and there are considerable advantages to reducing incubation time to the minimum including optimisation of clinical utility and reduction of the time for the result to be issued by the laboratory.

The fundamental principle of immunoassay is the presence of a binding agent, most often an antibody protein. The conditions for the antibody and its specific ligand reaching equilibrium with the antibody-ligand complex are governed by the law of mass action [1]. The ligand may exist as a small molecular weight substance, also known as a hapten, or a large molecular weight substance such as a protein. Consequently any substance present in a biological fluid that can disturb this equilibrium reaction can effect the measurement by immunoassay. These interferences are known as matrix effects and are a major confounding factor for the introduction of traceability and Standardization to this assay strategy. Modification of the assay format to make them suitable for such automated instrumentation includes conditions under which these binding reactions do not reach equilibrium. Such a condition has variable effects on the quality of the assays depending on the properties of the binding agent [7]. Thus it is likely that the quality of many immunoassays has deteriorated when included on such automated platforms particularly through increased interference by matrix effects and the requirement for increased limits of detection which are associated with non-equilibrium immunoassays.

STANDARDIZATION AND TRACEABILITY

Standardization of an assay is achieved through the reliable transfer of measurement values from the highest hierarchical level to those used in the routine analytical laboratory [8]. The key element for such a transfer is a comprehensive measurement system based on metrological principles. The essential components of which are an unequivocally defined analyte, a system of reference materials and reference measurement procedures [5]. A primary reference procedure is used to assign a certified value for a Primary Reference Material. In the case of molecules that can be purified to Analytical Reagent Grade, this procedure could be gravimetry. This primary reference calibrator is used to calibrate a secondary reference procedure which could be a higher-order analytical method such as liquid chromatography-mass spectrometry in some form. The secondary reference procedure is used to calibrate sufficient quantities of secondary reference material that can be distributed to manufacturers of routine assay systems for calibration of their internal higher order reference procedures. These are then used to prepare calibrators for the routine laboratory procedures used to analyse specimens. Through this hierarchical pathway, specimen measurement values are traceable to primary reference materials.

Measurands analysed by immunoassay can vary in molecular weight from some hundreds of Daltons to complex proteins or nucleic acids with molecular weights in the many 100,000's of Daltons [9]. Haptens are substances that because of their relatively small molecular weights of hundreds of Daltons are unable to initiate an immune response unless conjugated to a high molecular weight carrier substance such as a protein. The antibody elicited in the process retains the ability to recognise and bind the small molecular weight substance. These analytes have been incorporated into immunoassay platforms including the steroid and thyroid hormones, therapeutic drugs and other substances [1]. Because of their relatively small molecular weight their structures have been unequivocally identified and identical materials have been prepared using synthetic chemical techniques. Thus they have been defined in the International System of Units (SI, le Systeme internationale d'unites) with highly purified materials available as reference materials. Furthermore these substances have been most amenable to assay by highly specific technologies such as isotope dilution-gas chromatography with mass spectrometry detection. These are the properties required for a reference measurement procedure.

Reference measurement systems for a number of hapten assays used in clinical laboratories have been accomplished including cortisol [10], testosterone [11], estradiol [12] and total thyroid hormones [13]. This work is continuing for other similar measurands [14]. The availability of highly purified material allows gravimetry to be used as the primary reference measurement procedure for assigning the values of the primary calibrator. Many such primary calibrators are available from the National Institute of Standards and Technology (NIST) [15]. As an example the Standard Reference Material (SRM) for cortisol is SRM 921. The Institute for Reference Materials and Measurements (IRMM) is another source of reference materials [16]. These have been catalogued by the Joint Committee for Traceability in Laboratory Medicine and a list is available on their web site (http://www.bipm.org/en/committees/jc/jctlm/). These reference materials are available to calibrate the secondary reference measurement system which for cortisol is isotope dilution-gas chromatography/mass spectrometry (ID-GC/MS). It is recommended that secondary reference procedures be operated in reference laboratories under defined performance conditions linked together through networks. The JCTLM provides a list of these networks and the International Federation of Clinical Chemistry and Laboratory Medicine (IFCC) Committee-Traceability in Laboratory Medicine supervises RELA external quality assessment programmes [17].

Primary reference materials are prepared in a matrix-free format for calibration of a matrix-independent secondary reference procedure. However the clinical utility of all assays depends on their ability to measure these analytes in biological specimens all of which potentially contain substances that interfere with the binding reaction between the binding agent and the analyte. This phenomenon is known as the matrix-effect and defines the commutability of the reference material [8]. Lack of commutability of a primary reference material can also arise from small but significant structural differences from the analyte in biological specimens. For example reference materials prepared from recombinant technology may not exactly duplicate the structure of native analytes. Thus the calibration of a manufacturer's working calibrator must contend with the matrix effects of the manufacturer's standing measurement procedure or routine clinical laboratory measurement procedure as the aim is to provide traceability of the results from the routine procedure on clinical samples to the primary calibrator and primary reference measurement procedure. One method used to account for matrix-effects is to prepare a series of samples in the matrix of the routine method, which in the case of the routine clinical measurement of many analytes is human serum. Thus a series of calibrators made up of serum samples containing the analyte of interest can be assayed by the secondary reference procedure to assign the "true" value and can then be used to calibrate the routine procedure. This method is known as the "split-sample measurement design" [5, 13]. The relationship between the two series of values can be analysed and used to account for the matrix effect of serum in the routine procedure. It must be emphasised that a valid calibration by this method is dependent on a linear relationship between the two sets of values across the whole range using samples from the various specimens submitted for routine measurements. If the routine procedure is imprecise or is subject to different interferences by different types of specimens (for example if male and female samples are interfered to different levels) then this method is unsuitable or must be modified to take such effects into consideration.

TRACEABILITY AND STANDARDIZATION OF THE BIOLOGICALLY ACTIVE FRACTION OF HAPTENS – THE 'FREE' FRACTION

Each of the steroid and thyroid hormones as well as other analytes in plasma exist in at least two forms, a bound form, often bound to protein, and a non-bound or 'free' form [1]. The sum of these fractions is measured as the total plasma level of such substances. There is much evidence to indicate that it is the 'free' form that is biologically active and clinicians in many parts of the world request the 'free' level of such analytes from clinical laboratories. This practice is best exemplified with regard to the thyroid hormones where free thyroxine (fT4) and free liothyronine (fT3) are the requested analytes for many clinicians requiring information on thyroid gland function [1].

The 'free' fraction exists in equilibrium with specific and non-specific binding agents. For example thyroxine binds with high affinity and low binding number to thyroid binding globulin and with low affinity and high binding number to serum albumin [1]. The measurement of 'free' fractions poses a number of significant problems to meet the principles of metrology. Perhaps the most important is the property that any separation of the 'free' fraction from the total amount in serum will disturb the equilibrium between the substance and its binding agents particularly the specific binding agents because of their property of high affinity binding. The IFCC Working Group for Standardization of Thyroid Function Tests (WG-STFT) has proposed a candidate international conventional reference measurement procedure for free thyroxine in serum [18]. This includes an operational definition of the measurand as "thyroxine in the dialysate from equilibrium dialysis of serum prepared under defined conditions". An Isotope Dilution-Mass Spectrometry (ID-MS) reference measurement procedure calibrated with a total thyroxine primary reference material is proposed for the measurement of thyroxine in the dialysate. This strategy breaks new ground for the metrological Standardization of a number of clinically important immunoassays of this kind.

TRACEABILITY AND STANDARDIZATION OF PEPTIDE HORMONE IMMUNOASSAYS

At least two major issues face the application of metrological principles for standardization of immunoassays for the relatively large molecular weight peptide hormones. Firstly their large molecular weight may preclude the intact molecule from assays using the highest levels of analytical technique such as high performance liquid chromatography with mass spectrometry detection. Secondly these hormones very often exist in multiple forms or isotypes for which, with our current knowledge, it is impossible to identify which isotype exerts the biological activity. This means that the assay must measure a family of peptides in order to correctly provide a measure of the biological activity in the form of a measurement of peptide mass, which is the most efficient protocol for routine clinical assays.

A number of approaches have been used to resolve these problems. For peptide hormones of a relatively small molecular weight (less than 10,000 Daltons) isotope dilution-liquid chromatography/tandem mass spectrometry (ID-LC/tandem MS) technology has been used with the measurand being subject to immunoaffinity chromatography-solid phase extraction procedures prior to injection into the liquid chromatographic system. Such a system has been established for insulin [19] and has been used to demonstrate by way of a comparison study that agreement amongst routine clinical methods can be improved by establishing traceability to the ID-LC/tandem MS procedure using a panel of native sera [20].

A commonly used strategy from proteomic strategies is to subject large molecular weight proteins to standardized digestion with trypsin to generate a series of peptides of molecular weight less than 5,000 Daltons molecular weight. Following purification by various techniques including 2-D Fluorescence Difference Gel Electrophoresis (DIGE) the individual peptides can be uniquely identified by LC/tandem MS [21]. This technology has been applied to reference measurement procedures for clinical laboratory measurands such as growth hormone [22]. This method uses ID-LC/tandem MS that is applicable to biological samples containing growth hormone over concentration ranges between 3 to 30 µg/L. Signature peptides, generated by tryptic digestion, are quantified following extraction by two-step liquid chromatography by analysis LC/tandem MS. This method has been used to calibrate a series of human serum pools which are available for calibration of routine clinical laboratory immunoassays. Improvement of the limits of detection of the reference measurement procedure by an order of magnitude is required for it to span all clinical requirements.

Another strategy has been to identify the biologically active element of a large molecular weight measurand thereby reducing it to a substance of low molecular weight that can be prepared by synthetic chemistry technologies to an adequate purity and is available as a primary reference material. Furthermore such a substance is amenable to analysis by the highest level of analytical technology suitable for a primary reference measurement procedure. If these goals can be achieved then the measurand has the necessary components for a reference measurement system suitable to provide traceability for routine clinical assays.

The most successful assay to benefit from this approach has been the work with the glycated hemoglobin (Hb) form HbA_{1c} for the monitoring of diabetes mellitus [23]. The measurement of glycated hemoglobins poses many metrological issues. Firstly glycation can occur at a number of positions including the amino-terminal amino group but also at many of the ε-amino groups of the lysine residues within the α- and β-chains of the globin protein. These analytes are expressed as a percentage of total hemoglobin A_0 and therefore two analytes are required to be defined. The original separation technologies upon which the nomenclature was based were poor such that the composition of the HbA_{1c} fraction varied dependent on the separation technique [24]. The clinical impetus for harmonizing the HbA_{1c} assay heightened following two important clinical trials where its usefulness for monitoring diabetes mellitus and identifying patients at highest risk of developing adverse side-effects was demonstrated. The initial approach involved defining a method which required Standardizing a chromatography system to define the HbA_{1c} fraction. A small network of laboratories was established to provide a service to HbA_{1c} assay manufacturers for standardizing their routine assays marketed to clinical laboratories. In this way routine clinical assays were harmonized by this strategy.

Unfortunately the limitations of this approach quickly became evident over time when the defined chromatography system could not be transferred to other laboratories or even its maintenance could not be guaranteed over the longer term because the technology of the system was outdated. Thus a system based on metrological principles was required that could meet the clinical requirements of traceability and Standardization for HbA1c measurement over the long term such that the measurement was independent of the measurement technology. Such a system can continuously accommodate the further development of measurement technologies.

A Working Group of the IFCC took forward the task of defining both analytes, HbA_{1c} and HbA_0 [24]. These definitions were based on an understanding of the physical chemical properties of the globin peptide chain in which the amino-terminal amine group is the most active with regard to adduct formation such as the glycation reaction. Thus the analytes were defined as the amino-terminal peptide obtained from a tryptic digest of hemoglobin extracted from human blood. For HbA_0 this peptide is a hexapeptide of known sequence while for HbA_{1c} it is this same hexapeptide with the addition of 1-deoxyfructose to the amino-terminal amine group. These analytes can be prepared to sufficient purity such that gravimetry is a suitable primary reference procedure to prepare primary reference materials. Secondary reference measurement procedures have been approved utilising tryptic digestion of whole blood followed by quantification by high performance liquid chromatography with mass spectrometry detection or capillary electrophoresis. An approved reference measurement system is in operation including a network of reference laboratories which has validated the procedure over the mid-term [23]. Thus a full reference measurement system for this analyte was accomplished.

Considerable effort has focussed on standardization of cardiac troponin I (cTnI) measurements through another IFCC Working Group [25]. In blood cTnI exists as a heterogeneous mixture of molecular forms. The Working Group has developed a strategy based on a novel approach. Firstly it has identified a part of the cTnI molecule that is present in each of the various molecular species present in blood. Secondly antibodies against cTnI have been screened for recognition of epitopes within this invariant region. A primary reference material for cTnI is available (NIST Standard Reference Material (SRM) 2921) which utilised mass spectrometry to verify the composition [26] and certified concentration [27]. However the use of SRM 2921 as a common calibrator in various routine clinical cTnI assays did not significantly reduce the variability of measurement values amongst these assays [28]. A number of reasons for this outcome have been proposed including the lack of commutability between the primary reference material and patient serum specimens. Unfortunately spiking of human serum with SRM 2921 has been unsuccessful since such material is highly unstable [25]. Thus the Working Group has proposed the preparation of a series of human serum pools to serve as secondary reference material for cTnI prepared according to the relevant ISO standards.

Such human serum pools of themselves do not provide value assignment for cTnI and the development of a reference measurement procedure is essential. A major limitation of using a well established technology such as mass spectrometry is that it has inadequate sensitivity to measure cTnI levels in serum. Therefore a novel strategy has been proposed to explore the potential of a "higher order" immunoassay using monoclonal antibodies with well-defined epitopes within the invariant region of cTnI. [25]. This "higher order" immunoassay will be required to be calibrated against SRM 2921, provide acceptable assay performance for cTnI in human serum and demonstrate comparable diagnostic power to current routine clinical assays. It is recognised that such developments will take considerable resources including time and that as with any research program there is no guarantee of success.

Immunoassays for heterogeneous antigens or families of closely related isoforms have focussed on a strategy based on the principle of harmonization with a relatively long history beginning in the first half of the 20th Century with International Standards (IS) prepared under the auspices of World Health Organization (WHO). IS were Standardized by bioassays and used to varying levels of success to harmonize immunoassays, which measure mass [4]. An example of success with this strategy is the work conducted on human chorionic gonadotropin (hCG) by the IFCC Working Group [29]. The structure of hCG is complex comprising of a highly heterogeneous family of polypetides which have a high degree of carbohydrate fine structure. The intact molecule comprises of two noncovalently linked polypeptide chains (known as α- and β-chains) with heterogeneous carbohydrate moieties. In biological samples intact hCG is always present along with dissociated (*i.e.* free subunits) or degraded hCG-related polypeptides (nicked forms). The complete elucidation of this structure was not obtained until the 1990's.

Immunoassays for gonadotropins were developed in the 1960's and were standardized against the WHO ARE preparations [3]. It was apparent by the 1980's that the lack of comparability between the routine clinical assays was of clinical significance [4]. It is highly likely that within a heterogeneous family such as hCG some material present in the biological fluid will be immunoreactive without being biologically inactive. Thus as the project developed it became apparent that at least two issues had to be resolved before harmonization of this assay could be achieved. Firstly the structure of each of the members of the hCG family needed to be accurately defined and purified preparations of each be made available. Secondly the cross-reactivity of each of the antibodies used in the routine clinical immunoassays needed to be assessed against each of the members of the family.

Each of these tasks has been completed [30]. Standards of hCG and its most important variants including the β- and α-subunits, the core fragment of hCGβ and two partially cleaved (or nicked) forms are now available from WHO as the 1st Research Reagents (1st RRs). There are some 100 commercial hCG immunoassays available on the market [31]. When these assays were assessed using the 1st RRs as calibrators with a bank of serum samples, the maximum interassay variability of the serum hCG values was reduced to 27% compared to 40 to 60% when the results were calculated on the basis of the standards supplied by the manufacturers. It was clear that the use of impure calibrators is an important contributor to the variation of results between assays. Amongst these commercial assays any of seven antibody combinations can be employed. The variation in the specificity of these antibodies for binding to the different forms comprising the hCG family was found to contribute to greater variation of assay results than the use of impure calibrators.

This work on standardization of hCG assays has lead not only to the characterization and purification of the most common forms of the hCG family of glycoproteins but has developed a nomenclature along with calibration of each preparation in molar terms [30]. These developments have also permitted the mapping of the epitopes for each of the antibodies in commercial use. The WG has recommended that the 1st RRs for hCG and hCGβ be used to recalibrate existing assays for these isoforms and that conversion factors for the reporting of existing assays in mol/L be established.

Major success has been achieved with improving the commutability of serum Prostate Specific Antigen (PSA) assays through the introduction of an international standard comprising purified 90% PSA complexed to α_1-antichymotrypsin (PSA-ACT) and 10% free-PSA [32]. In most instances there was little change in the absolute values achieved for total PSA in serum samples. However the variation between the different assays used in routine clinical laboratories was reduced by approximately 50% [33].

These types of projects provide a very useful outcome of improving comparability between assays through harmonization; however they do not meet the stringent requirements of traceability and standardization of these assays. Currently the only strategy for these types of substances which can meet the metrological principles of a reference measurement system, including a matrix-independent instrumental analytical method such as mass spectrometry, is to identify a surrogate analyte as outlined above for HbA_{1c}. However consideration must be given to the fact that because of the biological complexity of many of these analytes such as the example of the hCG family, will it ever be feasible to define such an analyte? This then raises the question as to the suitability of selecting an immunoassay reference method based on a reference antibody with well-defined epitope specificity. This approach would require the definition of a standard method as has been achieved for enzymes and is being assessed for 'free' hormone assays and cTnI [18, 25, 34].

APPLICATIONS OF IMMUNOASSAYS IN FOOD TECHNOLOGY

Food analysts reviewing the use of immunoassays in analytical laboratories will be aware of the wide variety in chemical structure of measurands to which they can be applied and the suitability of applications for analyses of food samples. In this context immunoassays were originally applied for the testing for species of origin and contamination of food. Legal constraints for the export of meat into many countries require the species of origin to be analytically established and immunoassays are suitable for the assay of species-specific blood proteins, such as albumin with commercial assays for some 14 species currently available, or muscle proteins, such as troponins [35]. The first analytical issues with drug contamination of foods suitable for immunoassay technology arose from presence of antibiotics in food. Microbiological assays are too labour intensive and time consuming and immunoassays were successfully introduced to provide cost-effective assays of adequate accuracy and sensitivity [36]. Requirements for quality control of food products has stimulated the development and use of immunoassays for hormones used as illegal growth promoters [37], drug residues [38], pesticides [39] and other analytes required by the industry. Thus immunoassays are suitable for analyses of source material, including identification of species and more recently whether it is derived from genetically-modified organisms using assays for genetically-modified DNA or products derived from the modified genes [35], contaminants and allergens of commercial interest. This technology has established a considerable niche in the food industry.

ENVIRONMENTAL ANTIGENS AND IMMUNOASSAYS

Identification of environmental contamination is an international issue and often utilises technologies of high analytical performance including various forms of chromatography linked to mass spectrometric detection. However the need for rapid and simple tests performed on site by technicians with limited analytical expertise has lead to the application of immunoassays providing rapid, sensitive analyses for a wide variety of environmental contaminants [40]. Commercial immunoassay kits are available for the assay of dioxins, polychlorinated biphenyls, petroleum hydrocarbons, polyaromatic hydrocarbons, pentachlorophenol amongst others. Such kits are suitable for use during site remediation to detect contaminants and monitor the clean-up process. Currently they are best suited for qualitative rather than quantitative analyses. A limitation for the use of immunoassays is the development of specific antibodies for newly identified contaminants of commercial or health interests. Considerable technological progress is being made in this area with for example the development of phage-display technology yielding a variety of recombinant antibody fragments considerably improving the performance of particular assays and reducing the time for their development [41]. A further area of development is with application of nanoanalytical technology to immunoassays [42]. These systems can accommodate the simultaneous and high throughput measurement of multiple analytes.

ACCREDITATION OF IMMUNOASSAYS

Standards for accreditation of testing laboratories whether they are in the medical, food technology or environmental fields, including the performance of immunoassays are produced by the International Standards Office (ISO). For example the current standard for medical testing is ISO 15189 and ISO 15089 for environmental testing. The accreditation standard or norm relevant to traceability of immunoassays is described in the guidelines for validation and verification of chemical test methods which include immunoassays [2]. Before a test method can be introduced by a testing laboratory, they must demonstrate that it is fit for purpose, either with data supplied by the manufacturer or by the laboratory if it has been developed in-house. Such criteria have been developed and based upon an IUPAC Technical Report [43] and include documentation to define various parameters of the test method. They include traceability to international standards with stated uncertainties and the Measurement Uncertainty which is inexorably linked to traceability [44]. Most countries have legislative requirements that the laboratories providing analytical services in these various fields which are often administered by offices specific for the field. In the USA all human medical laboratory testing is performed under the direction of the Clinical Laboratory Improvements Amendments (CLIA) administered by the Centres for Medicare and Medicaid Services whereas food technology analyses are performed under directives of the US Department of Agriculture while for environmental analyses it is the Environmental Protection Agency which is the responsible government department. In Europe such testing is governed by various Council Regulations of the European Economic Community.

Thus the metrological principles upon which the traceability and standardization of immunoassays are based are now included in the current international standards defining performance of analytical laboratory testing required by either legislation for the operation of or for financial reimbursement of testing laboratories.

CONCLUSIONS

There is still a very large amount of theoretical and practical development work required in this area. It is clear that to apply any of these methods will require considerable laboratory-based fundamental research and therefore expense to identify the structural and biological properties of each of the measurands as well as to develop methods for the large scale preparation of significant amounts of highly purified material required to establish reference measurement systems to establish traceability and standardization of assays. If the standard method strategy is adopted then consideration must be given of the impact that this may have on halting or at least stifling technological development for each assay. The development of the standard method should include consideration that technical developments are likely to occur to improve or even completely change the assay. It cannot be over emphasized that a major benefit of the application of the principles of metrology is to reduce the likelihood that technological developments in routine clinical laboratory assays will require changes in their reference measurement systems.

DISCLOSURE

This chapter was based on the following an article; Morris HA. Traceability and standardization of immunoassays: A major challenge. Clinical Biochemistry 2009; 42: 241-245.

REFERENCES

[1] Wild D. Ed. The Immunoassay Handbook, Third Edition. Amsterdam: Elsevier 2005.

[2] National Association of Testing Authorities, Australia. Guidelines for the validation and verification of chemical test methods. Technical Note 17, April 2009 www.nata.com.au.

[3] Storring PL, Dixon H, Bangham DR. The first international standard for human urinary FSH and for human urinary LH (ICSH) for bioassay. Acta Endocrinol (Copenh) 1976; 83: 700-10.

[4] Sturgeon CM, Ellis AR. Standardization of FSH, LH, and hCG – Current position and future prospects. Mol Cell Endocrinol 2007; 260-262: 301-9.

[5] Thienpont LM, van Uytfanghe K, De Leenheer AP. Reference measurement systems in clinical chemistry. Clin Chim Acta 2002; 323: 73-87.

[6] Lantto O, Bjorkhem I, Blomstrand R, *et al.* Interlaboratory evaluation of 4 RIA kits for determination of plasma cortisol: influence of matrix in calibration standards. Clin Chem 1980; 26: 1899-1902.

[7] Sikaris K, McLachlan RI, Kaslauskas R, *et al.* Reproductive hormone reference intervals in healthy fertile men: evaluation of automated platform assays. J Clin Endocrinol Metab 2005; 90: 5928-36.

[8] Panteghini M. Traceability as a unique tool to improve standardization in laboratory medicine. Clin Biochem 2009; 42: 236-40.

[9] Morris HA. Traceability and standardization of immunoassays: A major challenge. Clin Biochem 2009; 42: 241-45.

[10] Thienpont LM. A reference system for cortisol. Clin Biochem 1998; 31: 483-88.

[11] Thienpont LM, van Uytfanghe K, Blinko CS, *et al.* State-of-the-art of serum testosterone measurement by isotope dilution-liquid chromatography mass spectrometry. Clin Chem 2008; 54: 1290-7.

[12] Vesper HW, Botelho JC, Shacklady C, Smith A, Myers GL. CDC project on standardizing steroid hormone measurements. Steroids 2008; 73: 1286-92.

[13] Thienpont LM, van Uytfanghe K, Marriott J, *et al.* Feasibility of the use of frozen human sera in split-sample comparison of immunoassays with candidate reference measurement procedures for total thyroxine and total triiodothyronine measurements. Clin Chem 2005; 51:2303-11.

[14] http://www.ifcc.org/IFCC Annual Report 2006.

[15] http://ts.nist.gov//measurementservices/referencematerials/index.cfm.

[16] http://irmm.jrc.europa.eu/.

[17] http://www.dgkl-rfb.de links IFCC RELA surveys.

[18] Thienpont LM, Beastall G, Christofides ND, *et al.* Proposal of a candidate international conventional reference measurement procedure for free thyroxine in serum. Clin Chem Lab Med 2007; 45: 934-36.

[19] Rodriguez-Cabaleiro D, van Uytfanghe K, Stove V, Fiers T, Thienpont LM. Pilot study for the standardization of insulin immunoassays with isotope dilution liquid chromatography/mass spectrometry. Clin Chem 2007; 53: 1462-9.

[20] Miller WG, Thienpont LM, van Uytfanghe K, *et al.* Toward standardization of insulin immunoassays. Clin Chem 2009; 55: 1011-8.

[21] McNamara LE, Dalby MJ, Riehle MO, Burchmore R. Fluorescence two-dimensional difference gel electrophoresis for biomaterial applications. J R Soc Interface 2010; 7:S107-18.

[22] Arsene CG, Henrion A, Diekmann N, Manolopoulou J, Bidlingmaier M. Quantification of growth hormone in serum by isotope dilution mass spectrometry. Anal Biochem 2010; March 9 [EPub ahead of print].

[23] Weycamp C, John WG, Mosca A, *et al.* The IFCC Reference Measurement System for HbA1c: A 6-Year Progress Report. Clin Chem 2008; 54: 240-8.

[24] Goodall I. HbA1c Standardization destination-global IFCC Standardization. How, why, where and when--a tortuous pathway from kit manufacturers, *via* inter-laboratory lyophilized and whole blood comparisons to designated national comparison schemes. Clin Biochem Rev 2005; 26: 5-19.

[25] Panteghini M, Bunk DM, Christenson RH *et al.* Standardization of troponin I measurements: an update. Clin Chem Lab Med 2008; 46: 1501-6.

[26] Bunk DM, Dalluge JJ, Welch MJ. Heterogeneity in human cardiac troponin I standards. Anal Biochem 2000; 284: 191-200.

[27] Bunk DM, Welch MJ. Characterization of a new certified reference material for human cardiac troponin I. Clin Chem 2006; 52: 212-19.

[28] Christenson RH, Duh SH, Apple FS, *et al.* Toward standardization of cardiac troponin I measurements Part II : Assessing commutability of candidate reference materials and harmonization of cardiac troponin I assays. Clin Chem 2006; 52: 1685-92.

[29] Stenman UH, Tiitinen A, Alfthan H, Valmu L. The classification, functions and clinical use of different isoforms of HCG. Hum Reprod Update 2006; 12: 769-84.

[30] Stenman UH. Standardization of assays for human chorionic gonadotropin. Clin Chem 2004; 50: 798-800.

[31] Cole LA. Immunoassay of human chorionic gonadotropin, its free subunits and metabolites. Clin Chem 1997; 43: 2233-43.

[32] Stamey TA, Chen Z, Prestigiacomo AF. Reference material for PSA: the IFCC standardization study. Clin Biochem 1998; 31: 473-81.

[33] Sturgeon CM, Ellis AR. Improving the comparability of immunoassays for prostate-specific antigen (PSA): Progress and problems. Clin Chim Acta 2007; 381: 85-92.

[34] Schumann G, Aoki R, Ferrero CA, *et al.* IFCC primary reference procedures for the measurement of catalytic activity concentrations of enzymes at 37 degrees C. Clin Chem Lab Med 2006; 44: 1146-55.

[35] Bonwick GA, Smith CJ. Immunoassays: their history, development and current place in food science and technology. Int J Food Sci Tech 2004; 39: 817-27.

[36] Chesham J, Taylor MJ. The role of immunoassays in monitoring antimicrobial contamination in milk. In (Eds) Morgan MRA, Smith CJ, Williams PA. Food Safety and Quality Assurance: Applications of Immunoassay Techniques. Elsevier, London 1992; pp 159-61.

[37] Johansson MA, Hellenas KE. Immunobiosensor determination of β-agonists in urine using integrated immunofiltration cleanup. Int J Food Sci Tech 2004; 39: 891-8.

[38] Myrtazina MR, Eremin SE, Mozoleva OV, *et al.* Fluorescent polarization immunoassay for sulphadiazine using high specificity antibody. Int J Food Sci Tech 2004; 39: 879-89.

[39] Bonwick CA, Yasmin M, Hancock P, *et al.* Synthetic pyethroids in fish: Analysis by gas chromatography-mass spectrometry operated in negative ion chemical ionisation mode and ELISA. Food Agr Immunol 1996; 8: 185-94.

[40] Plaza G, Ulfig K, Tien AJ. Immunoassays and environmental studies. Pol J Environ Stud 2000; 9: 231-36.

[41] Schneider RJ. Environmental immunoassays. Anal Bioanal Chem 2003; 375: 44-6.

[42] Magliulo M, Michelini M, Simoni P, *et al.* Ultrasensitive and rapid nanodevices for immunoassay. Anal Bioanal Chem 2006; 384: 27-30.

[43] Thompson M, Ellison SLR, Wood R. Harmonised guidelines for single-laboratory validation of methods of analysis (IUPAC Technical Report) Pure Appl Chem 2002; 74: 835-55.

[44] Eurolab - Measurement Uncertainty Revisited: Alternative approaches to uncertainty evaluation, Technical report 1/2007. www.eurolab.org.

CHAPTER 4

Interferences in Immunochemical Methods

Slavica Dodig*

Department of Clinical Laboratory Diagnosis, Srebrnjak Children's Hospital, Srebrnjak 100, 10000 Zagreb, Croatia

Abstract: Immunochemical methods, methods that employ antibodies as analytical reagents, have revolutionized laboratory medicine. Although the noncovalent bound between analyte in biological specimen and complementary antibody in reagent is specific, positive or negative interferences are possible. Interfering substances can be present in both specimen and reagents, respectively. Most interfering substances are inherent in patients' blood under physiological and pathophysiological conditions, especially under diagnostic and therapeutic procedures. Some interferences are similar to those in chemical analyses and some are typical only for immunoassays (hook effect; cross-reactivity with structurally similar or identical epitopes; heterophile antibodies; anti-animal antibodies; autoantibodies; the matrix effect). The main characteristic of all immunoassays is that the reagent which discovers or quantifies the target analyte contains the specific antibody. Results higher than real values are recorded due to a low antibody specificity. Results can also be influenced by pre-analytical factors or assay formulations. One should suspect interferences a) after obtaining an unacceptable result; b) if there is non-linearity during dilution; c) if there is no agreement with other test results or clinical data; d) if different immunoassays in determination of the same analyte provide significantly different results. It is necessary to think about present predictable and always possible unpredictable and unrecognizable interferences. Unawareness and non-recognition of interferences could lead to diagnostic errors, unnecessary laboratory tests, inadequate and unnecessary treatment and therapy. There is no simple and practical way to identify interferences in specimens before analysis. Whenever interference is suspected, there are a few possibilities to solve them, *e.g.* serial dilution, pre-treatment with blocking reagent, use of more specific methods. At the same time a proper information upon pre-analytical diagnostic and therapeutic procedures is needed for accurate interpretation of the results. In this process, consistent communication and compliance between laboratory professionals and clinicians are required.

Keywords: Antibody, Immunoassays, Interferences.

1. INTRODUCTION

Despite the specificity of the noncovalent bond between analyte in biological specimen and complementary antibody in reagent, immunoassays may be compromised by various interferences. Interference is the systematic error in an analysis. It may be defined as the effect of substances that may be present in an analytical system, which causes discrepancy between the measured results and the true values [1]. The interferences may cause false increase (positive interference) or false decrease (negative interference) of measured result [1, 2]. Usually, the magnitude of interference effect depends on the concentration of interfering substance [3]. Interference problems occur in spectra derived from different biological samples (*e.g.* serum or plasma are heterogeneous mixtures of endogenous and sometimes of exogenous antibodies) or from reagent components (reagent contains specific antibodies obtained in different animal species). However, most interferents originate from the biological sample. They can vary from person (patient) to person (patient) and also from time to time in one person (patient) [4]. Analyte-dependent interferences relate to interaction of substances present in biological sample and one [1, 3, 5-9] or more reagent components [10, 11]. The most frequently described interferences are those occurring during determination of hormones [12-15] tumor markers [16], drugs and metabolites [17, 18], troponin [19-21] and during serological analyses [22].

***Address correspondance to Slavica Dodig:** Department of Clinical Laboratory Diagnosis, Srebrnjak Children's Hospital, Srebrnjak 100, 10000 Zagreb, Croatia; Tel: 385-1-6391-128; E-mail: slavica.dodig@zg.t-com.hr

Eline P. Meulenberg (Ed)

Detection of interference is usually very difficult. The best way to detect interferences is during the evaluation and validation of an immunoassay. In these procedures, method comparison studies, usually followed by linearitiy studies, and recovery studies, could be applied [23]. In method comparison studies, both, samples from healthy persons and samples from patients with different diseases (kidney and liver diseases, patients with positive rheumatoid factor, positive anti-nuclear antibodies – ANA, and positive Human Anti-Animal Antibodies (HAAA) should be included. In linearity studies, diluted specimens of samples with a high analyte concentration should be retested. In recovery studies, a small volume of a sample with high analyte concentration is added into samples with known concentration of analyte and than retested.

In routine laboratory practice one should suspect interferences in immunoassays upon receiving an unacceptable result, upon receiving a result that is not coherent with anamnestic and clinical findings, if there is non-linearity during dilution, if different immunoassays in determination of the same analyte provide significantly different results. Lack of specificity and lack of comparability among immunochemical methods may have detrimental effects on clinical outcome.

This chapter gives a review of the most important types of interferences in immunochemical methods: a) the prozone effect, b) cross-reactivity with endogenous and exogenous non antibody-structured substances, c) cross-reactivity with endogenous and exogenous antibody-structured substances, and d) the matrix effect.

2. THE PROZONE EFFECT

Optimal reaction between analyte and specific antibody occur in a zone of equivalence, where the range of reactant ratio is optimal. The prozone effect (or high dose-hook phenomenon) is a common phenomenon in everyday practice of a clinical laboratory. This phenomenon is based on the saturation curve of antibody with analyte (Fig. **1**).

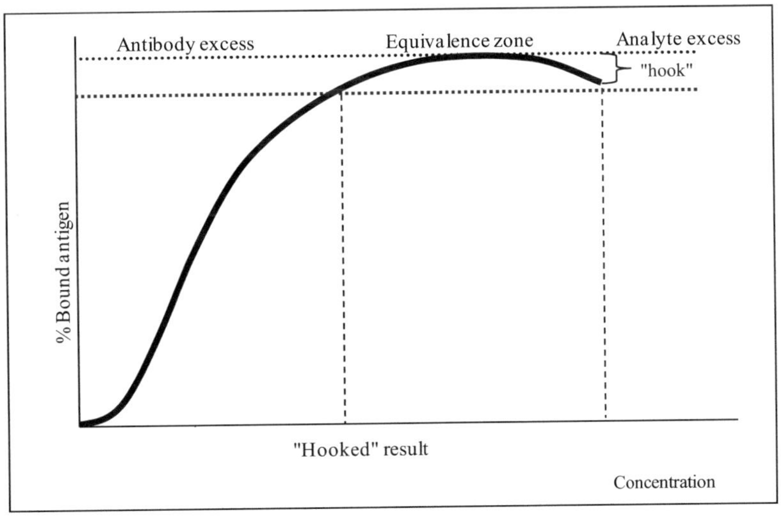

Figure 1: The prozone effect - bell-shaped curve. An excessive amount of analyte overwhelms the binding capacity of the capture antibody. The value of absorbance in the post-zone (down-side of the curve, analyte excess zone) is identical with the absorbance value in the pro-zone (up-side of the curve, antibody excess zone) [24].

It implies the presence of huge excess of analyte which saturates all binding sites on antibody, and a surplus on analytes that did not penetrate to analyte-antibody complex compound. Hence, the prozone effect depends on analyte concentration [24]. Consequence of reactions in the zone of analyte excess is an inappropriately low signal that causes erroneous low or normal result ("hooked" result) for a patient with an excessively elevated serum analyte concentration.

The prozone effect occurs mostly in a single step saturating immunoassays, immuno-turbidimetric and immuno-nephelometric assays, where all components are incubated simultaneously. It exists by analytes known to have a wide range of concentrations, like hormones (at sixfold concentration increase) (human chorionic gonadotrophin – hCG, prolactin, thyroxine – T4, thyroid-stimulating hormone – TSH), tumor markers (especially alpha-fetoprotein – AFP, calcitonin, CA 19-9, CA 125, carcinoembryonic antigen - CEA, prostate specific antigen – PSA), IgE (> thousand fold), ferritin (hundredfold increase), C-reactive protein (hundredfold increase), antistaphylolysin antibodies (tenfold increase) [24, 25]. Tumor marker determination is mostly influenced by possible huge concentration increase (> 10,000 fold) that exists in patients with extreme tumor growth. It can occur if the blood of the patient is tested for the first time. Therefore single step methods are not applicable to determination of these analytes.

2.1. Eliminating Interference

The problem of the prozone effect may be solved by parallel determination, either with diluted samples (dilutions 1 : 10 and 1 : 100) [24] or with altered reagent volume. The sample must be diluted until the results of two different dilutions match (taking into consideration the dilution factor). Most automatic biochemical analysers have a possibility to warn about non-linear reaction what is sufficient to see if the sample needs to be diluted, and in some analysers the sample is being simultaneously diluted. Manufacturers of reagents for immunoturbidimetric assays have reduced the prozone effect by introducing latex particles as carriers on which the reaction between analyte and antibody takes place. In competititve assays the prozone effect was eliminated by introducing a wash step (analysers have programmed this wash step) upon reaction of analyte with the capture antibody and addition of the tracer antibody [26, 27]. Two-step or even three-step methods should be used. Also, manufacturers of reagents reduce the prozone effect by increasing the quantity of the capture and the tracer antibody and by reducing the quantity of samples required for the analysis. There are no cost-effective procedures available for the safe resolution of the prozone effect.

3. CROSS-REACTIVITY

Cross-reactivity is defined as non-specific influence of substances in a sample that structurally resembles analyte (carries similar or identical epitopes like analyte) and competes for the binding site of antibody [24]. It is the most common interference in immunoassays, mostly competitive ones. The interference grade depends upon a few factors: antibody specificity, method and sample preparation [28]. Cross-reactivity presents a problem when the concentration of interferent is at concentration high enough to significantly increase the concentration of the certain analyte. If the concentration of possible interferent is not so significant, variation of final result could be acceptable [23]. Sometimes, in cases when drug metabolites have therapeutic activity, some degree of cross-reactivity could be useful. Cross reaction can be caused by endogenous and exogenous non-antibody-structured substances or antibody-structured substances. The most common examples can be seen during determination of concentrations of hormones (glycoprotein hormones, steroid hormones) [13], drugs [29] and vitamins [24], allergen-specific IgE [30, 31]. The concentration of cross-reactive compounds increase in pathological states, especially in drug immunoassays in patients with liver disease or patients with renal insufficiency.

3.1. Cross-Reactivity with Endogenous and Exogenous Non Antibody-Structured Substances

Well-known example is the similarity in structure of the glycoprotein hormones: Follicle Stimulating Hormone (FSH), hCG, Luteinizing Hormone (LH), TSH, due to their common α-chain. Therefore it is necessary to choose specific antibody which would be able to recognise different epitopes of the certain hormones [32]. Another example are steroid hormones (synthesized from cholesterol) which have identical cyclo-pentano-perhydro-phenanthrene structure [33]. Immunossays may be affected by changes in specific binding proteins, *e.g.* corticotrophin releasing hormone binding protein in corticotrophin releasing hormone measurement or thyroxine binding globulin in the total thyroxine (T4) measurement. Total hormone concentration assays require displacement of the hormone from its binding protein. The use of free hormone assays (free T4 assays) can largely overcome the problem of the effect of binding proteins [13].

Drugs may affect results in two ways: by *in vivo* interactions of the drug with the analyte or by *in vitro* interference in the assay. Cross-reactivity can be caused by metabolite or analyte precursor, *e.g.* conjugated cortisol metabolites by determining the urine cortisol [33] or simultaneous application of medications with similar molecular structure (tricyclic antidepressants). Also, some drugs can interfere with the measurement of thyroid function tests, *e.g.* during heparin therapy in some patients, especially those with increased concentration of free fatty acid [34]. In drug immunoassays, cross-reactive interferences are caused by metabolites of the drug. In the era of organ transplantations it is important to know that immunoassays for determination of immunosuppressant ciclosporin A concentration, can give significantly higher concentration than referent HPLC method [29], due to a large number of its metabolites. Cross-reaction with other drugs can also be a problem, for example during measurement of pentobarbital in the presence of phenobarbital [35]. Digoxin concentration must be interpreted carefully in patients with chronic renal failure undergoing hemodialysis and severe chronic liver disease – caused by digoxin-like factors [36]. Cross-reactivity with other drugs is a problem when screening for drug of abuse (*i.e.* alcohol, amphetamines, benzodiazepines, opioids, marijuana, cocaine, phencyclidine, and tricyclic antidepressants) [37]. Some unexpected cross-reactivity has also been described, *e.g.* a metabolity of cyclamate (synthetic sweetener) in fluorescence-polarization immunoassay [38]. The problem of cross-reactivity by vitamin D[1,25-$(OH)_2D_3$] determination due to possible positive interference of 25-OH D_3 [24] is well known. Cross-reactivity usually causes positive interference, but in some assays negative interference is also possible [39]. The cause of falsely low concentration of analyte can be faster dissociation of an interfering substance than of an analyte during washing or separating free from captured analyte during analysis [40]. Also, cross-reactivity occurs during determination of tumor marker PSA, since PSA exists in several forms (total, PSA; free, fPSA; precursor, proPSA and finally Early Prostate Cancer Antigen, EPCA) [41].

The phenomenon of cross-reactivity has been reported in subjects with allergic diseases. Mostly, cross-reactivity occurs among allergens that are structurally similar or biologically related, such as cow milk allergens [42], mite allergens [43] or seafood allergens [44], and antibiotics [45], but also in biologically unrelated allergens [46]. Recently, cross-reactivity due to glycoepitope-related IgE-activity has been noted [47, 48] by determination of IgE against animal epithelium allergens [30], hymenoptera sting venom allergens [49], peanut allergens [31], and concequently false increased concentration of IgE.

Usually, glycoepitope-related IgE-activity show no symptoms of allergic disease. But, IgE-activity against both, peptide and carbohydrate epitope of the same allergen molecule, could be clinically relevant.

A "component-resolved diagnostics" using recombinant allergens is recommended for the resolution of cross-reactivity between allergens [50].

Cross-reactivity is hard to predict. Therefore, we must be aware of its existence, be up to date with scientific literature and choose the most specific method for analysis.

3.2. Cross-Reactivity with Endogenous and Exogenous Antibody-Structured Substances

Reaction between analyte and antibody in immunoassays can be influenced by antibodies present in biological sample of a patient or antibodies from the reagent [51]. Biological sample can contain exogenous and endogenous antibodies (Fig. **2**). Antibodies for therapeutic and diagnostic imaging belong to the group of exogenous antibodies. Since these antibodies persist in the blood during a certain period of time (depending on half-time) after administration, in some patients they could be a potential source of interference in immunoassays. Endogenous antibodies are presented in about 40% of patients [9] especially after maternal transfer, vaccinations, and intestinal transfer, blood transfusion, infection, immunotherapy with monoclonal antibodies [52]. Heterophylic antibodies [7] are human antibodies that have capability to bind immunoglobulins from other species used in immunoassays, *e.g.* sheep, goat, rabbit, mouse or horse antibodies. These multispecific antibodies have a weak to moderate affinity to various poorly defined antigens, either animal antigens or autoantigens. Antibodies should be called heterophiles when there is no history of medicinal treatment with animal immunoglobulins or other well-defined immunogens [9]. Most of these antibodies can be associated with inflammatory and autoimmune diseases [21, 53], but can also be present in apparently healthy subjects [54]. Around 10% of patients carry heterophilic antibodies [3].

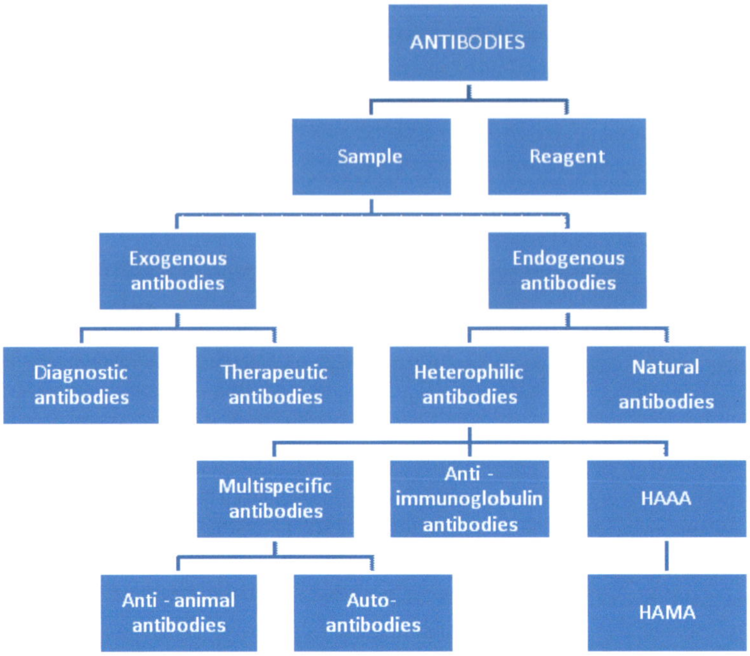

Figure 2: Antibodies which could be present in immunoassay. HAAA - Human Anti-Animal Antibodies; HAMA - human anti-mouse antibodies.

In the general population autoantibody prevalence is between 4% and 27%. Autoantibodies are relatively weak antibodies. However they tend to demonstrate a tight binding to some antigens. So, interference due to autoantibodies, either positive or negative is common in laboratory praxis, *e.g.* anti-thyroglobulin antibodies have the potential to interfere with total thyroglobulin measurement [55], especially in saturating immunoassays [56]. Even newer immunoassays (using blocking agents) are not completely free from interference of anti-thyroid autoantibodies [57] or heterophilic antibodies [54], respectively. Interference in free thyroglobulin measurement is relatively uncommon.

Another category includes anti-immunoglobulin antibodies (*e.g.* rheumatoid factor) that cross-react with animal antibodies. It is present in low concentrations in 5% of the general population and in around 70% of rheumatoid arthritis patients [13].

The most important category consists of antibodies against well-defined animal antigens. These Human Anti Animal Antibodies (HAAA) are high-affinity and high-specificity antibodies [15]. HAAAs are antibodies of high avidity and are synthesised against well defined antigens [8]. HAAAs could be present in subjects with a history of treatment with animal immunoglobulin. Also, antibodies should be considered HAAAs when immunoglobulin from the same species is used in the test [9]. The most common HAAAs are Human Anti-Mouse Antibodies (HAMA) [7, 58-61], but some patients can synthesise HAAAs after exposure to other animal antigens (*e.g.* vaccine produced in chicken or rabbits, in anti-snake venom produced in the horse, pet owners, or in professional exposure animals) [30]. HAMAs are increasingly applied intravenously in diagnostic or therapeutic purposes in oncology [61], autoimmune diseases [62], and allergology [63]. Around 40% of the patients who intravenously received mouse monoclonal antibodies will synthesise HAMAs. Around 39% of patients with IgA deficiency carry anti-goat antibodies and 18% carry HAMAs [14]. HAMA has become a significant problem as many immunoassays now incorporate mouse monoclonal antibodies.

The effect of the interference depend on the type of immunoassay used. It may occur in both competitive and noncompetitive assays, respectively, but in the latter is more common [64]. Interference in immunoassays by antibodies may lead to either falsely elevated [65-67] or decreased results [21, 68-70]. In saturating (sandwich) immunoassay, endo-genous antibodies simultaneously create complexes with capture and tracer antibodies of the reagent (Fig. **3**). False-positive interference of heterophilic antibody in sandwich capture assays occurs because heterophilic antibodies "bridge" the capture and the tracer antibody [71]. False-negative interference occurs due to binding of heterophilic antibodies directly to the capture antibody that disables binding of analytes. Interferences in patients with monoclonal gammopathies [72].

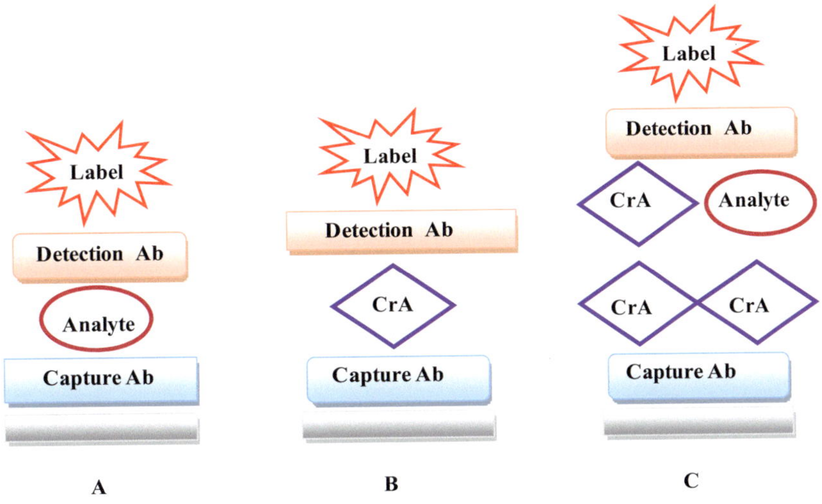

Figure 3: Mechanism of cross-reactive antibodies (CrA) interference in saturating immunoassay: **A** – assay without any interference; **B** – positive interference, "bridge" binding by CrA; **C** – negative interference, masking of the epitope on an analyte surface by CrA of the sample; Ab – antibody.

3.3. Eliminating Interference

A major reason of cross-reactivity and consequent inaccuracy in immunoassays is a lack of specificity of the antibody(s) used. The use of antibodies with weak specificity may result in measuring related molecules and not only the analyte of interest. Since the immunochemical methods have remarkable flexibility and sensitivity as an analytical tool, one of possibilities intended to eliminate interference is to apply the method with more specificity, *i.e.* with more specific antibody. If interference is expected it is useful to have an additional blocking agent that should diminish the nonspecific interference [12, 58, 73, 74]. There is no universal blocking agent for all analytes and all methods. The agent that after validation showed to be the best for reducing the effect of heterophilic antibodies for certain analyte must be applied [58].

4. THE MATRIX EFFECT

Serum or plasma sample is a complex compound of lipids, proteins, carbohydrates, metabolic products, salt and water. The "matrix effect" presents the sum of interferences of all sample components (with exception of analytes) which affect the target analyte to be measured [75]. The matrix effect can be caused by endogenous [76], or exogeonous [77] components of the biological sample. Endogenous elements cause inter-individual [16] and intra-individual variability [78-80] of results. Exogenous components are related to the impact of coagulation activator and separator during serum sampling, or to the impact of anticoagulant during plasma sampling [77]. Gel separator can adsorb analyte what can cause falsely low concentration of some drugs [81]. The drugs can be adsorbed on gel 5-30% and if the sample is kept for longer time (24h) adsorption can be up to 40%. Since there are different types of test tubes with gel of different quality on the market, one should be cautious in choosing them and the need is rising for their validation by determination of certain analytes.

The cause for result variability may be in the matrix of the calibrators or the control samples [10] due to the fact that their matrix is not identical with the biological sample in which some analyte is being determined. Interfering antibodies can affect all types of immunochemical analyses (Table **1**) [82], but they are most frequently present in saturating analyses. That is because in saturating analyses there is an excess of both antibodies (the capture and the tracer one). Their concentration is higher than the usual analyte concentration and the reaction occurs very fast in conditions of high analytic sensitivity. Cross-reactivity is special to competitive immunoassays. Prozone effect and interferences of antibodies are typical mostly for saturating immunoassays.

Table 1: Interferences in particular immunoassays and the ways of possible elimination.

Interference	Methods	Eliminating Interference
Prozone effect	Nephelometric, turbidimetric, saturating	Parallel dilution Use of more specific and more sensitive method
Cross reactivity	All, but mostly competitive	Remove interference from the samples before analysis Use of more specific method
Antibodies	All, but mostly saturating	Use of more specific method
Matrix	All	Choose an appropriate sample

5. CONCLUSIONS

Prevalence of interference is lower in analyses used for longer period of time (manufacturers of reagents and analysers tended to eliminate them) than in those which are in use for shorter period of time. Manufacturers of reagents are obliged to warn about known interferents, and some of them are usually found in instructions for analytic procedures. Information on these issues should necessarily be available in the laboratory handbook. The first step to eliminating interferences from an immunoassay is to recognize them. It is necessary to think about predictable and possible unpredictable and unrecognizable interferences. Unawareness and non-recognition of interferences could lead to diagnostic errors, unnecessary laboratory tests, inadequate and unnecessary treatment and therapy. There is no simple and practical way to identify interferences in specimens before analysis. Whenever interference is suspected, there are a few possibilities to solve them, *e.g.* serial dilution, pre-treatment with blocking reagent, use of more specific method. At the same time a proper information upon pre-analytical diagnostic and therapeutic procedures is needed for accurate interpretation of the results. In this process, consistent communication and compliance between laboratory professionals and clinicians are required.

REFERENCES

[1] Kroll MH, Elin RJ. Interference with clinical laboratory analyses. Clin Chem 1994; 40: 1996-2005.
[2] Preiser W, Brink NS, Hayman A, Waite J, Balfe P, Tedder RS. False-negative HIV antibody test results. J Med Virol 2000; 600: 43-7.
[3] Tate J, Ward G. Interferences in Immunoassay. Clin Biochem Rev 2004; 25: 105-20.
[4] Weber TH, Kapyaho KI, Tanner P. Endogenous interference in immunoassays in clinical chemistry. A review. Scand J Clin Lab Invest 1990; 50: (Suppl. 201): 77-82.
[5] Kricka LJ. Interferences in immunoassays - still a threat. Clin Chem 2000; 46: 1037-8.
[6] Emerson JF, Ngo G, Emerson SS. Screening for interference in immunoassays. Clin Chem 2003; 49: 1163-9.
[7] Kricka LJ. Human anti-animal interferences in immunological assays. Clin Chem 1999; 45: 942-56.
[8] Ismail AAA. A radical approachis needed to eliminate interferences from endogenous antibodies in immunoassays. Clin Chem 2005; 51: 25-6.
[9] Kaplan IV, Levinson SS. When is a heterophile antibody not a heterophile antibody? When it is an antibody against a specific immunogen. Clin Chem 1999; 45: 616-8.
[10] Rigo RB, Panyella MG, Bartolomé LR, Ramos PA, Soria PR, Navarro MA. Variations observed for insulin concentrations in an interlaboratory quality program may be due to interferences between reagents and the matrix of the control materials. Clin Biochem 2007; 40: 1088-91.
[11] Ylander PJ, Bicskei Z, Hänninen P, Soini JT. Theoretical assessments of errors in rapid immunoassays-how critical is the exact timing and reagent concentrations? Biophys Chem 2006; 20: 141-5.
[12] Després N, Grant AM. Antibody interference in thyroid assays: a potential for clinical misinformation. Clin Chem 1998; 44: 440-54.
[13] Jones AM, Honour JW. Unusual results from immunoassays and the role of the clinical endocrinologist. Clin Endocrinol 2006; 64: 234-44.

[14] Knight AK, Bingeman T, Cole L, Cunningham-Rundles C. Frequent false positive beta human chorionic gonadotropin tests in immunoglobuline A deficiency. Clin Exp Immunol 2005; 141: 333-7.

[15] Cavalier E, Carlisi A, Chapelle JP, Delanaye P. False positive PTH results: an easy strategy to test and detect analytical interferences in routine practice. Clin Chim Acta 2008; 387: 150-2.

[16] Berth M, Bosmans E, Everaert J, *et al.* Rheumatodic factor interference in the determination of carbohydrate antigen 19-9 (CA19-9). Clin Chem Lab Med 2006; 44: 1137-9.

[17] Melanson SE, Lee- Lewandrowski E, Griggs Da, Long WH, Flood JG. Reduced interference by phenothiazines in amphetamine drug of abuse immunoassays. Arch Pathol Lab Med 2006; 130: 1834-8.

[18] Dasgupta A. Endogenous and exogenous digoxin-like immunoreactive substances: impact on therapeutic drug monitoring of digoxin. Am J Clin Pathol 2002; 118: 132-40.

[19] Panteghini M. Selection of antibodies and epitopes for cardiac troponin immunoassays: Should we revise our evidence-based beliefs? Clin Chem 2005; 51: 803-4.

[20] Lum G, Solarz DE, Farney L. False positive cardiac troponin results in patients without acute myocardial infarction. Labmedicine 2006; 37: 546-50.

[21] Eriksson S, Halenius H, Pulkki K, Hellman J, Pettersson K. Negative interference in cardiac troponin I immunoassays by circulating troponin autoantibodies. Clin Chem 2005; 51: 839-47.

[22] Duverlie G, Driencourt M, Roussel C, Orfila J. Heterophile IgM, IgA, and IgE antibodies in infectious mononucleosis. J Allergy Clin Immunol 2007; 119: 640-5.

[23] Miller JJ, Levinson SS. Interferences in immunoassays. In Immunoassay, Diamandis EP and Christopoulos TK ed. Academic Press. San Diego 2007, pp. 165-190.

[24] Wu JT. Quantitative immunoassay: A practical guide for assay establishment, troubleshooting, and clinical application. AACC Press, Washington 2000.

[25] Butch AW. Dilution Protocols for Detection of Hook Effects/Prozone Phenomenon . Clin Chem 2000; 46: 1719-20.

[26] Van Lente F. Light scattering immunoassays. Rose NR de Macario EC Folds JD Lane HC Nakamura RM eds. Manual of clinical laboratory immunology, 5th ed 1997: 13-19 ASM Press Washington.

[27] Charrie A, Charriere G, Guerrier A. Hook effect in immunometric assays for prostate-specific antigen. Clin Chem 1995; 41: 480-1.

[28] Gosling JP. Immunoassays. A practical approach. Oxford: Oxford University Press, 2000.

[29] Steimer W. Performance and specificity of monoclonal immunoassays for cyclosporine monitoring: how specific is specific? Clin Chem 1999; 45: 371-81.

[30] Adédoyin J, Johansson SGO, Grönlund H, van Hage M. Interference in immunoassays by human IgM with specificity for the carbohydrate moiety of animal proteins. J Immunol Methods 2006; 310: 117-25.

[31] ItoK, Morishita M, Ohshima M, Sakamoto T, Tanaka A. Cross-reactive carbohydrate determinant contributes to the false positive IgE antibody to peanut. Allergol International 2005; 54: 387-92.

[32] Nilsson C, Seppälä, Pettersson K. Immunological sharacterization of human luteinizing hormone with special regard to a common genetic variant. J Endocrinol 2001; 168: 107-16.

[33] Lee C, Goeger DE. Interference of 6 β-hydroxycortisol in the quantitation of urinary free cortisol by immunoassay and its elimination by solid phase extraction. Clin Biochem 1998; 31: 229-33.

[34] Laji K, Rhidha B, John R, Lazarus J, Davies JS. (2001) Abnormal serum free thyroid hormone levels due to heparin administration. Q J Med 2001; 94: 471-3.

[35] Earl R, Sobeski L, Timko D, Markin R. Pentobarbital quantification in the presence of phenobarbital by fluorescence polarization immunoassay. Clin Chem 1991; 37: 1774-7.

[36] Avendaño C, Alvarez JS, Sacristan JA, Adin J, Alsar MJ. Interference of digoxin-like immunoreactive substances with TDx digoxin II assay in different patients. Ther Drug Monit 1991; 13: 523-7.

[37] Moeller KE. Urine drug screening: practical guide for clinicians. Mayo Clin Pros 2008; 83: 66-76.

[38] Martz W, Schütz HW. Synthetic sweetener cyclamate as a potential source od false-positive amphetamine results in the TDx system. Clin Chem 1991; 37: 2016-7.

[39] Cao Z, Swift TA, West CA, Rosano TG, Rej R. Immunoassay of Estradiol: unanticipated suppression by unconjugated estriol. Clin Chem 2004; 50: 160-5.

[40] Valdes R Jr, Jortani SA. Unexpected supression of immunoassay results by cross reactivity; now a demonstrated cause for concern. Clin Chem 2002; 48: 405-6.

[41] Wright JL, Lange PH. Newer potential biomarkers in prostate cancer. Urology 2007; 9: 207-13.

[42] Cantisani A, Giuffrida, Fabris C, *et al.* Detection of specific IgE to human milk proteins in sera of atopic infants. FEBS Lett 1997; 412: 515-7.

[43] Aalberse RC. Allergens from mites: implications of cross-reactivity between invertebrate antigens. Allergy 1998; 53: 47-8.

[44] Chou MC, Yuo CY, Lan WS, Huang SP. Seral IgE of atopic individuals exhibit the reactivity to multiple allergens. J Biomed Lab Sci 2001; 13: 1-5.

[45] Furmin J, Gallagher JC. Allergic cross-sensitivity between penicillin, carbapenem, and monobactam antibiotics: what are the chances? Ann Pharmacother 2009; 43: 304-15.

[46] Fuchs T, Spitzauer S, Vente C, *et al.* Natural latex, grass pollen, and weed pollen share IgE epitopes. J Allergy Clin Immunol 1997; 100: 356-64.

[47] Mari A, Iacovacci P, Afferni C, *et al.* Specific IgE to cross-reactive carbohydrate determinants strongly affect the *in vitro* diagnosis of allergic diseases. J Allergy Clin Immunol 1999; 103: 1005-11.

[48] Malandain E. IgE reactive carbohydrate epitopes - Classification, cross-reactivity and clinical impact. Eur Ann Allergy Clin Immunol 2005; 37: 122-8.

[49] Hemmer W, Focke M, Kolarich D, *et al.* Antibody binding to venom carbohydrates is a frequent cause for double positivity to honeybee and yellow jacket venom in patients with stinging-insect allergy. J Allergy Clin Immunol 2001; 108: 1045-52.

[50] Valenta R, Lidholm J, Hayek B, Niederberger V, Kraft D, Grönlund H. The recombinant allergen-based concept of component-resolved diagnostics and immunotherapy (CRD and CRIT). Clin Exp Allergy 1999; 29: 896-904.

[51] Emerson JF, Ellis MJ, LiveseyJH. Techniques for identifying heterophile antibody interference are assay specific: study of seven analytes on two automated immunoassay analyzers. Clin Chem 2005; 51: 639-41.

[52] Choy EH, Schantz A, Pitzalis C, Kingsley GH, Panayi GS. The pharmacokinetics and human anti-mouse antibody response in rheumatoid arthritis patients treated with a chimeric anti-CD4 monoclonal antibody. Rheumatol 1998; 37: 801-2.

[53] Zouwail SA, O'Toole AM, Clark PMS, Begley JP. Influence of thyroid hormone autoantibodies on 7 thyroid hormone assays. Clin Chem 2008; 54: 927-8.

[54] Levinson SS. Antibody multispecificity in immunoassay interference. Clin Biochem 1992; 25: 77-87.

[55] Madureira D, Prazeres S, Pedro MS, Pereira T, Font AP, Bugalho MJ. In vitro assays to test the interference of anti-thyroglobulin antibodies on thyroglobulin measurement. Endocrine 2008; 33: 40-4.

[56] Spencer CA, Bergoglio LM, Kazarosyan M, Fatemi S, LoPresti JS. Clinical impact of thyroglobulin (Tg) and Tg autoantibody method differences on the management of patients with differentiated thyroid carcinomas. J Clin Endocrinol Metab 2005; 90: 5566-75.

[57] Dai J, Dent W, Atkinson JW, Cox JG, Dembinski TC. Comparison of three immunoassay kits for serum thyroglobulin in patients with thyroid cancer. Clin Biochem 1996; 29, 461-5.

[58] Ellis MJ, LiveseyJH. Techniques for identifying heterophile antibody interference are assay specific: study of seven analytes on two automated immunoassay analyzers. Clin Chem 2005; 51: 639-41.

[59] Oei Al, Sweep FC, Massuger LF, Olthaar AJ, Thomas CM. Transient human anti-mouse antibodies (HAMA) interference in CA 125 measurements during monitoring of ovarian cancer patients treated with murine monoclonal antibody. Gynecol Oncol 2008; 109: 199-202.

[60] Bertholf RL, Johannsen L, Benrubi G. False elevation of serum CA-125 level caused by human anti-mouse antibodies. Ann Clin Lab Sci 2002; 32: 414-8.

[61] Oldham RK. Monoclonal Antibodies in Cancer Therapy: 25 Years of Progress. J Clin Oncol 2008; 26: 1774-7.

[62] Schulze-Koops H, Lipsky PE. Anti-CD4 Monoclonal Antibody Therapy in Human Autoimmune Diseases. In: Fathman C.G. (ed): Biologic and Gene Therapy of Autoimmune Disease.Curr Dir Autoimmun. Basel, Karger, 2000, vol 2, pp 24-49.

[63] Dodig S, Richter D, Čepelak I, Benko B. Anti-IgE therapy with omalizumab in asthma and allergic rhynitis. Acta Pharm 2005; 55: 123-38.

[64] Selby, C. Interference in immunoassay. Ann Clin Biochem 1999; 36: 704-21.

[65] Levinson SS, Miller JJ. Towards a better understanding of heterophile (and the like) antibody interference with modern immunoassays. Clin Chim Acta 2002; 325: 1-15.

[66] Jeremias A, Gibson CM. Narrative review: Alternative causes for elevated cardiac troponin levels when acute coronary syndromes are excluded. Ann Int Med 2005; 142: 786-92.

[67] Preissner CM, O'Kane DJ, Singh RJ, Morris JC, Grebe SK. Phantoms in the assay tube: heterophile antibody interferences in serum thyroglobulin assays. J Clin Endocrinol Metab 2003; 88: 3069-74.

[68] Giovanella L, Ghelfo A. Undetectable serum thyroglobulin due to negative interference of heterophile antibodies in relapsing thyroid carcinoma. Clin Chem 2007; 53:1871-2.

[69] Luzzi VI, Scott MG, Gronowski AM. Negative thyrotropin assay interference associated with an IgG{kappa} paraprotein. Clin Chem 2003; 49: 709-10.

[70] Eriksson S, Junikka M, Laitinen P, Majamaa-Voltti K, Alfthan H, Pettersson K. Negative interference in cardiac troponin I immunoassays from a frequently occurring serum and plasma component. Clin Chem 2003; 49: 1095-104.

[71] Martins TB, Pasi BM, Litwin CM, Hill HR. Heterophile antibody interference in a multiplexed fluorescent microsphere immunoassay for quantitation of cytokines in human serum. Clin Diagn Lab Immunol 2004; 11: 325-9.

[72] Halsall DJ, Mangi M, Soos M, et al. Hypoglycemia due to an insulin binding antibody in a patient with an IgA-{kappa} myeloma. J Clin Endocrinol Metab 2007; 92: 2013-6.

[73] Bjerner J, Bormer OP, Nustad K. The war on heterophilic antibody interference. Clin Chem 2005; 51: 9-11.

[74] Warren J, Bjerner J, Paus E, Bormer OP, Nustad K. Use of an in vivo biotinylated single-chain antibody as capture reagent in an immunometric assay to decrease the incidence of interference from heterophilic antibodies. Clin Chem 2005; 51: 830-8.

[75] Wood GW. «Matrix effect» in immunoassay. Scand J Clin Lab Invest 1991; 51: 105-12.

[76] Feng-Bo Wu, You-Feng He and Shi-Quan Han. Matrix interference in serum total thyroxin (T4) time-resolved fluorescence immunoassay (TRFIA) and its elimination with the use of streptavidin-biotin separation technique. Clin Chim Acta 2001; 308: 117-26.

[77] Wu AHB, Fen YJ, Moore R, *et al*. Characterization of cardiac troponin subunit release into serum after acute myocardial infarction and comparison of assays for troponin T and I. Clin Chem 1998; 44: 1198-208.

[78] Gerhardt W, Nordin G, Herbert AK, *et al*. Troponin T and I assays show decreased concentrations in heparin plasma compared with serum: lower recoveries in early than in late phases of myocardial injury. Clin Chem 2000; 46: 817-21.

[79] Katrukha AG, Bereznikova AV, Esakova TV, et al. Troponin I is released in bloodstream of patients with myocardial infarction not in free form but as a complex. Clin Chem 1997; 43: 1379-85.

[80] Hirsh J, Raschke R, Warkentin TE, Dalen JE, Deykin D, Foller L. Heparin: mechanism of action, pharmacokinetics, dosing, considerations, monitoring, efficacy, and safety. Chest 1995; 108 (Suppl 4): 258-75.

[81] Karppi J, Akerman KK, Parviainen M. Suitability of collection tubes with separator gels for collecting and storing blood samples for therapeutic drug monitoring (TDM).Clin Chem Lab Med 2000; 38: 313-20.

[82] Dodig S. Interferences in quantitative immunochemical methods. Biochemia medica 2009; 19: 50-62.

CHAPTER 5

Antibodies as Bioanalytical Tools in Food Analysis

Georg Mahlknecht*

Weizmann Institute of Science, Department of Immunology, 76100 Rehovot, Israel

Abstract: With new developments in agriculture and food production in the past two decades, bioanalytical detection of toxins and allergens in foods became a challenging task. In addition, efficient validation and labelling of food products demand reliable technical approaches. Complex, heterogeneous matrices and low amounts of specific analytes complicate detection and characterization of harmful substances in food. A highly relevant tool to achieve this goal is represented by several immunochemical approaches, based on antibody technology. Different types of antibodies have been developed, which are characterized by high affinity and specificity. Although, alternative methods have been introduced into food analysis (*e.g.*, mass-spectrometry and PCR), antibodies still play a key role, especially in detection and characterization of allergens. In this chapter, I discuss basic immunochemical methods of food analysis based on antibody technologies. The increasing importance of establishing suitable detection schemes for several allergens (*e.g.*, allergens from peanut and soy) in an immunoanalytical approach, will be particularly emphasized.

Keywords: Antibodies, Immunoassays, Food Allergens.

INTRODUCTION

Food allergy is a major health problem in westernized countries, affecting both children and adults. Between 5 and 8% of children and up to 2% of adults show typical symptoms after exposure to specific allergens in foods [1-3]. Nevertheless, recent population studies indicate that beside careful evaluation, estimates have to consider prevalence estimates which show in fact a vast heterogeneity, as demonstrated in a Canadian population-based study on peanut, tree nut, fish, shellfish and sesame allergy [4]. This heterogeneity has, for example, also been shown in an earlier study, where prevalence estimates of sensitization or perceived allergic reactions to plant food were evaluated [5].

Food allergy is basically an adverse immune reaction to substances present in foods [6]. The term "adverse" implicates a reaction which doesn't necessariliy refer to an immunologic response. Especially, enzyme deficiencies (*e.g.* lactose intolerance) and pharmacological responses are common causes of pathological symptoms [3]. Allergic responses can be attributed to food allergens that provoke reactions with IgE antibodies, induce allergic reactions and allergic sensitization. So called "complete allergens" instigate all three mentioned reactions, some will only induce IgE-mediated responses and are termed "non elicitors". "Non sensitizing elicitors" are unable to induce sensitization at all [7]. Clinical symptoms instigated by food allergens can include gastrointestinal, cutaneous and respiratory disorders [8].

Food allergens from plants comprise a relatively small group of protein families and show considerable similarity and comparable bio- and physicochemical features, which include thermal stability and resistance to proteolysis [9]. The cupin and prolamin superfamilies, as well as proteins making part of the plant defense system represent the most common source of proteins with allergenic properties [10]. Beside structural features, functional characteristics (*e.g.*, enzymatic activity) may play an important role in allergic processes [11]. Many allergens are glycoproteins that interact with IgE *via* N-glycan moieties [12]. These glycosylated sites increase the structural stability of proteins and improve their resistance [13].

***Address correspondence to Georg Mahlknecht:** Weizmann Institute of Science, Department of Immunology, 76100 Rehovot, Israel; E-mail: georgmahlknecht@gmx.at

Nevertheless, the importance and significance of carbohydrate determinants, which are the major targets for IgE epitopes, is restricted and has only a low clinical impact [14]. But still, indications that there might exist an involvement of such glycosylated areas have been reported [15]. The identification of allergenic epitopes is rather complex and database searches based on sequence similarity are currently one of the most accepted tools of such approaches. The characterization of specific motifs may play an even bigger role than overall similarity [16]. The involvement of linear and conformational epitopes seems to influence specific IgE binding in allergic reactions. Such allergenic areas can be compared with databases which enable now also similarity searches, based on physicochemical properties and not only the primary sequence [17]. In a lot of cases, allergens do not only contain conformational or linear epitopes, but display combinations of such epitopes. A recent characterization of tree nut allergens revealed, for example, presence of both variants on the respective protein [18, 19]. Furthermore, structural homology modelling can reveal structural features that may represent indications of allergenicity of a specific protein [20]. The detection and quantification of food allergens has become a major issue with rising numbers of people, affected by allergic reactions to foods.

The development of suitable technological approaches is of high importance, in order to prevent contact of allergens with patients suffering from diverse immunological responses to specific compounds. The reliability and robustness of selected test systems has to be validated in terms of sensitivity, specificity and reproducibility. The complexity of food matrices represents a major obstacle in the development of these test systems [21]. Different allergens present in a specific food product could lead to unexpected cross-reactivities, and therefore to false positive results. Hence, higly specific antibodies are needed in immunochemical approaches to guarantee reliable measurements of allergens. Elaborated extraction methods have to be established to ensure, that allergens are available in adequate amounts and in the original biochemical conformation. Analysis of specific proteins can be facilitated in a significant way, if the right methodological extraction-tools are applied as shown by Natarajan *et al.* for low abundant soy proteins and Hildebrandt *et al.* for allergens in hen's egg [22, 23]. Purification and characterization of the soy allergen profilin (Gly m 3) represents an example where a combination of affinity chromatography, dialysis and ultrafiltration resulted in a purified allergen [24]. The fact that most food products are processed during industrial production, which leads to denatured proteins, complicates bioanalytical approaches. Detection of conformational epitopes can be highly influenced by such treatments. Therefore, the specificity of antibodies for specific allergens (epitopes) has to be evaluated before test systems are incorporated into evaluation processes. The traditional strategies to detect allergens are characterized by immunochemical and PCR methods. But new developments in the field of proteomics, mainly based on progresses made in mass-spectrometry, represent a valuable alternative [25]. In this chapter, different methods based on immunochemical, molecular interactions between allergens and antibodies will be presented and discussed.

METHODS FOR DETECTION AND CHARACTERIZATION OF ALLERGENS

In a vast number of publications several technical approaches to detect and characterize allergens have been described. Among immunochemical test systems, the RAST/EAST inhibition, immunoblotting, rocket immuno-electrophoresis, ELISA, dipsticks and biosensors can be enumerated [26]. Cell based methods like the basophile histamine release assay and the hexosaminidase release assay are additional immunochemical tools [25]. In most assays, monoclonal or polyclonal antibodies are in use. Antibodies represent a suitable tool for analytical purposes in food and environmental research as well as in clinical approaches [27]. Monoclonal antibodies recognize a singular, specific epitope, whereas polyclonal sera are able to characterize multiple epitopes with high sensitivity. They have shown impressive efficacy and reliability even as therapeutic antibodies in clinical approaches. The humanized, monoclonal antibody Omalizumab confirms this claim in various clinical settings of allergic diseases [28, 29]. Polyclonal antibodies are produced with lower costs and play an important role in several ELISA test kits [30]. In addition, characterization of allergens can also be achieved with human IgE serum from sensitized and allergic individuals. Such sera are especially applied in RAST/EAST inhibition approaches and as primary antibodies in immunoblotting [31].

RAST INHIBITION

The RAST (RadioAllergoSorbentTest) test is a common methodology to titrate IgE in serum. The test was first proposed in the late '60s and became soon a very helpful tool in clinical diagnosis of allergic reactions [32, 33]. A well characterized antigen is bound to a solid phase and competes with a non further characterized sample for free binding sites on radiolabelled serum-IgE. The specific interaction of IgE with antigen coated to a solid phase is therefore, more or less inhibited. Known antigen and labelled IgE are inversely proportional to each other. Several variations of the test system are known, available as test kits and comprise enzyme catalyzed reactions (EAST inhibition, EnzymeAllergoSorbentTest), fluorescence and chemiluminometric labels [34].

ELISA

The ELISA (Enzyme Linked Immunosorbent Assay) is the most common used assay for diagnostical purposes in the detection and analysis of toxins and allergens in food. In an ELISA test system a specific analyte is detected and in most cases quantified with enzymatic labelled antibodies. Horse radish peroxidase and alcalic phosphatase are the most frequently applied labels. Depending on the immunochemical assembly of assays, homogenic or heterogenic ELISAs can be distinguished. Furthermore, competitive and non-competitive variations can be applied. In the analysis of food products, competitive and Sandwich ELISAs are methods of choice and play a dominant role among all immunochemical options [26]. The competitive approach is in most settings characterized by the presence of an antigen bound to a solid phase. A pre-incubation of antibodies with a specific sample precedes an incubation of the antibody-sample complex. The binding of antibodies to immobilized antigen can therefore be inhibited by the presence of a specific sample. The intensity of the absorbance measured in a photometer, depends on the amount of labelled antibody binding to the immobilized antigen and is inversely proportional to antigen amounts present in the sample. In Sandwich ELISAs an antibody coated to a solid phase (*e.g.*, microtiter plate) serves as primary capture antibody for specific allergens. A secondary, labelled antibody enables a proper colorimetric reaction. It is important to mention, that in order to avoid cross-reactivity, primary and secondary antibodies should derive from different species. The developed colorimetric signal is proportional to the amount of antigen in a specific sample.

Several ELISA test kits have been developed for allergens in different plant and animal species [35]. These assays include, for example, the detection of allergens from peanut, almond, soy and several other allergens from animals, like casein and egg like protein. The detection limits range from 0,05 to 10 mg kg^{-1} [35]. In addition, several publications describe attempts to detect allergens in food products with a plethora of technological innovations which paved the way for the development of industrial utilization. ELISAs described (see Table **1**), characterize, for example, allergens in hazelnut, peanut, Brazil nut and hen's egg [36-41].

Table 1: Overview of ELISAs to several target compounds with detection limits as indicated by the authors.

Methodology	Target Compounds	Matrix	Detection Limit (as Indicated by the Authors)	Reference
ELISA	hazelnut protein	extracts from hazelnut and several food products	5 ng/ml	36
	hazelnut protein	extracts from hazelnut and several food products	10 µg/l	37
	hazelnut protein	extracts from hazelnut and several food products	0,1 mg/kg	38
	Brazil nut	extracts from Brazil nut and several food products	1 ppm	39
	Peanut (Ara h1, Ara h2, total protein)	peanut extracts	comparison of extraction methods	40
	Hen's egg	ovalbumin	comparison of extraction methods	41

The development of an ELISA protocol requires sufficient amounts of target molecules. These targets are in many cases purified from raw extracts (*e.g.* plant extracts) or can be expressed as recombinant molecules in suitable hosts (*e.g. E. coli*). The selection of the right test format has to be oriented on availability of reagents, sensitivity, and specificity requirements (*e.g.* Sandwich ELISAs for highly sensitive measurements). Once test-conditions are established, specific characterization of target molecules and detecting antibodies can be carried out. The determination of cross-reactivity and specific epitopes recognized by antibodies plays thereby a major role. The basic step in the development of an ELISA - protocol are illustrated in Fig. **1**.

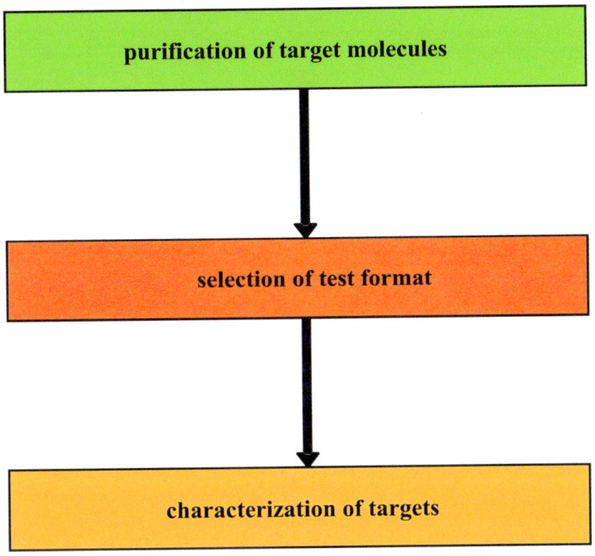

Figure 1: Basic steps in the development of ELISA protocols.

ELISAs have proven reliability in qualitative and quantitative assessments of food authenticity and are together with DNA-based methods suitable tools for successful regulatory food controls [42].

IMMUNOBLOTTING

Immunoblotting enables the detection of specific allergens in a mixture of proteins. The protein mixture is separated into singular proteins in a SDS-Page which are blotted to a membrane (*e.g.* nitrocellulose, polyvinyldenfluoride). Comparable to an ELISA assay, blotted proteins (*e.g.* allergens) are detected with specific monoclonal, polyclonal antibodies or IgE sera. Secondary, labelled antibodies recognize bound primary antibodies and a colorimetric reaction can be detected. This approach is also known as Western blotting. The Dot-blot represents a faster version of the described Western blot. Protein mixtures are directly blotted to a membrane. The detection of a specific analyte follows the same principle as described for the Western-Blot. This methodology has shown also proven reliability if simultaneous detection of multiple allergens was requested [43]. Immunoblots were used in several occasions for characterizing antigens (see Table **2**) from selected species and proofed to be a reliable qualitative test method [44-46].

ROCKET IMMUNO-ELECTROPHORESIS

Rocket immuno-electrophoresis is only a rarely used methodology for allergen detection and characterization [31]. Antibodies which are supposed to form antibody-antigen immunocomplexes are introduced into a gel. A specific sample migrates through such a gel in an electrophoretic run and antibody-antibody complexes with typical shapes (rocket) are formed. The antigen/antibody ratio has to be constant and determines the height of the rocket which is proportional to the antigen present in a sample [26]. The methodology is less described and applied in recent publications, but good examples which have their scientific relevance can be mentioned [47, 48].

Table 2: Overview of cited Immunoblots to several target compounds with detection limits as indicated by the authors.

Methodology	Target Compounds	Matrix	Detection Limit (as indicated by the authors)	Ref.
Immunoblotting	Hazelnut protein, Brazil nut protein, peanut protein	extracts from Hazelnut, Brazil nut, peanut and several food products	0,01-0,03 µg/ml	[43]
	Birch pollen proteins (Bet v I, Bet v II)	Recombinant protein extracts from E. coli and native protein extracts	5 µg / strip of nitrocellulose	[44]
	Birch pollen proteins (Bet v I, Bet v II)	Recombinant protein extracts from E. coli and native protein extracts	5 µg/1ml serum dilution for each recombinat protein in IgE inhibition immunoblot experiments	[45]
	HPLC purified peptides from Avocado allergen (Prs a 1)	Avocado extract	50 % IgE binding inhibition	[46]

BIOSENSORS

Biosensors represent a valuable analytical tool in clinical analysis, biochemistry and recently also in environmental sciences [49-51]. Biosensors are at a crossrad where biology, physics and electronics meet [52]. Biosensors allow in contrast to ELISA-approaches real time measurements, which means, that they show also an improved time efficacy. In experimental settings with Biosensors, an antibody or a single stranded DNA molecule with specificity and affinity to allergenic proteins or the capability to hybridize with allergenic DNA fragments from food samples are immobilized on a specific transducer element (*e.g.* amperometric electrodes, piezoelectric crystals). Changes in the refractive index lead to a qualitative and quantitative characterization of samples [26]. Several attempts to involve Biosensors into food processing chains have been carried out. A recent example is the SPREETA™ evaluation kit which can be applied during food production, but has limited reliability on processed samples. Nevertheless, a detection limit of 0.7 µg/ml, real time measurements and robust quantitative results turn this biochip into a useful analytical tool [53].

DIPSTICKS

Considering the necessity to detect allergens in very short time frames, dipsticks (lateral flow immunochromatographic assays) represent a suitable and efficient bioanalytical tool. They make part of those techniques, which use immunochemical interactions to detect specific antigens (*e.g.* allergens). A specific allergen present in a sample is incubated with labelled antibodies and runs along a test strip that contains an area with allergen-specific antibodies. Once the allergen-antibody (labelled antibodies) complex is captured by immobilized, allergen-specific antibodies, a colour reaction can be detected that enables a clear and specific qualitative characterization of the analyte. Mills *et al.* for example described already in the '90s the development of a rapid dipstick to detect peanut-allergen conarachin contaminations in food [54]. They were able to identify protein concentrations in a range from 0.01 to 0.1 % (w/w). Dipsticks are reliable in qualitative measurements, but lack the ability to perform well in quantitative approaches. Nevertheless, their easy handling and the fast generation of results without sophisticated lab instrumentations, justifies their use also in analytical approaches in the future.

BASOPHILE HISTAMINE RELEASE ASSAY AND HEXOSAMINIDASE ASSAY RELEASE ASSAY

In this type of immunochemical assay the release of histamine and ß-hexosaminidase after binding of specific allergens to basophil and mast cells is measured. With augmented amounts of allergen an increasing direct proportional signal is detected and thus, a quantitative output can be obtained. This methodology represents a useful tool in order to test the antigenicity of allergens (native and recombinant) as exemplified by Lüttkopf *et al.* and Bauermeister *et al.* [55, 56].

CONCLUSIONS

Despite new, innovative technologies applied in the field of food analysis, immunochemical methods remain a major player on the market. They are highly reliable, robust and easy to handle. Their sensitivity and specificity enables qualitative and (semi-)quantitative detection of allergens in food.

Complex matrices are still a big obstacle in immunochemical detection systems and new approaches (*e.g.* CREATE Project) for international standardization of allergy diagnostics and vaccines are established [57]. It is necessary to standardize natural and recombinant allergens for calibration, and develop certified immunoassays [57]. In addition, the introduction of new genes into crops by means of genetical engineering and correlating potential allergenicity pose new challenges in evaluation of food quality [58-60].

In order to avoid major health threats by contact with specific allergens for people suffering from diverse types of allergies, a clear labelling of food products is of demanding importance. Criteria to define the potential risks of specific allergens have to be assessed and allergen lists have to be established [61]. Advisory labellings on food products demonstrate in many cases ambiguities that lead to misinterpretations by consumers of food products which could be avoided by using a more sophisticated terminology which has to be based on efficient evaluation methods [62]. Clear and efficient evaluation on the other hand, has to be based on technical guidelines for specific test methods, as exemplified by Abbott *et al.* for ELISAs [63]. In summary, the quality of food risk management has to be improved in terms of augmented research to gain better evaluation criteria and well defined alternative perspectives [64, 65].

REFERENCES

[1] Bock S. Prospective appraisal of complaints of adverse reactions to foods in children during the first 3 years of life. Pediatrics 1987; 79: 683-688.

[2] Niestijl J, Kardinall A, Huijbers G, *et al.* Prevalence of food allergy and intolerance in the adult Dutch population. J Allergy Clin Immunol 1994; 93: 446-456.

[3] Kagan RS. Food allergy: An overview. Environmental Health Perspectives 2003; 111: 223-225.

[4] Ben-Shoshan M, Harrington DW, Soller L, *et al.* A population-based study on peanut, tree nut, fish, shellfish, and sesame allergy prevalence in Canada. J Allergy Clin Immunol 2010; in press.

[5] Zuidmeer L, Goldhahn K, Rona RJ, *et al.* The prevalence of plant food allergies: A systematic review. J Allergy Clin Immunol 2010; 121: 1210-1218.e4.

[6] Sicherer SH, Sampson HA. Food allergy. J Allergy Clin Immunol 2010; 125: S116-S125.

[7] Aalberse RC. Food allergens. Environ Toxicol Pharmacol 1997; 4:55-60.

[8] Sampson HA. Update on food allergy. J Allergy Clin Immunol 2004; 113: 805-819.

[9] Breiteneder H, Mills ENC. Molecular properties of food allergens. J Allergy Clin Immunol 2010; 115: 14-23.

[10] Breiteneder H, Radauer C. A classification of plant food allergens. J Allergy Clin Immunol 2004; 113: 821-830.

[11] Bredehorst R, David K. What establishes a protein as an allergen? J Chromatogr B Biomed Sci Appl 2001; 756:33-40.

[12] Van Ree R. Carbohydrate epitopes and their relevance for the diagnosis and treatment of allergic diseases. Int Arch Allergy Immunol 2002; 129: 189-197.

[13] Wormald MR, Dwek RA. Glycoproteins: glycan presentation and protein-fold stability Structure 1999; 7:R155-160.

[14] Chunsheng J, Hantusch B, Hemmer W, *et al.* Affinity of IgE and IgG against cross-reactive carbohydrate determinants on plant and insect glycoproteins. J Allergy Clin Immunol 2008; 121:185-190.e2.

[15] Amigo-Benavent M, Athanasopoulos VI, Ferranti P, *et al.* Carbohydrate moieties on the *in vitro* immunoreactivity of soy ß-conglycinin. Food Res Int 2009; 42: 819-825.

[16] Ivanciuc O, Garcia T, Torres M, *et al.* Characteristic motifs for families of allergenic proteins. Mol Immunol 2009; 46:559-568.

[17] Ivanciuc O, Schein CH, Garcia T, *et al.* Structural analysis of linear and conformational epitopes of allergens. Regul Toxicol Pharmacol 2009; 54: S11-S19.

[18] Robotham JM, Xia L, Willison LN, *et al.* Characterization of a cashew allergen, 11S globulin (Ana o 2), conformational epitope. Mol Immunol 2010; 47: 1830-1838.

[19] Xia L, Willison LN, Porter L, *et al.* Mapping of a conformational epitope on the cashew allergen Ana o 2: A discontinuous large subunit epitope dependent upon homologous or heterologous small subunit association. Mol Immunol 2010; 47: 1808-1816.

[20] Robotham JM, Hoffman GG, Teuber SS, *et al.* Linear IgE-epitope mapping and comparative structural homology modelling of hazelnut and English walnut 11S globulins. Mol Immunol 2009; 46: 2975-2984.

[21] Ge B, Meng J. Advanced technologies for pathogen and toxin detection in foods: current applications and future directions. JALA 2009; 14: 235-241.

[22] Natarajan SS, Krishnan HB, Lakshman S, Garrett WM. An efficient extraction method to enhance analysis of low abundant proteins from soybean seed. Anal Biochem 2009; 394: 259-268.

[23] Hildebrandt S, Steinhart H, Paschke A. Comparison of different extraction solutions for the analysis of allergens in hen's egg. Food Chem 2008; 108: 1088-1093.

[24] Amnuaycheewa P, Gonzalez de Mejia E. Purification, characterization, and quantification of the soy allergen profilin (Gly m3) in soy products. Food Chem 2010; 119: 1671-1680.

[25] Kirsch S, Fourdrilis S, Dobson R, Scippo ML, Maghuin-Rogister G, De Pauw E. Quantitative methods for food allergens: a review. Anal Bioanal Chem 2009; 395(1):57-67.

[26] Van Hengel AJ, Anklama E, Taylor SL, Hefle SL. Analysis of food allergens. Practical applications. In: Pico Y, Eds. Food Toxicants Analysis. Amsterdam, Elsevier, 2007; pp. 189-229.

[27] Franek M, Hruska K. Antibody based methods for environmental and food analysis: a review. Vet Med-Czech 2005; 50: 1:1-10.

[28] Hsu CL, Shiung YY, Lin BL, *et al.* Accumulated immune complexes of IgE and omalizumab trap allergens in an vitro model. Int Immunopharmacol 2010; 10: 533-539.

[29] Chang TW. The pharmacological basis of anti-IgE therapy. Nat Biotechnol 2000; 18: 157-162.

[30] Monaci L, Visconti A. Immunochemical and DNA-based methods in food allergen analysis and quality assurance perspectives. Trends in Food Science & Technology 2010; In Press: xx:1-12.

[31] Besler M. Determination of allergens in foods. Trends Anal chem 2001; 20: 662-672.

[32] Wide L, Bennich H, Johansson SGO. Diagnosis of allergy by an *in vitro* test for allergen antibodies. The Lancet 1967; 290: 1105-1107.

[33] Ceska M, Eriksson R, Varga JM. Radioimmunosorbent assay of allergens. J Allergy Clin Immunol 1972; 49: 1-9.

[34] Poulsen LK. *In vivo* and *in vitro* techniques to determine the biological activity of food allergens. J Chromatogr B Biomed Sci Appl 2001; 756: 41-55.

[35] Schubert-Ullrich P, Rudolf J, Ansari P, *et al.* Commercialized rapid immunoanalytical tests for determination of allergenic food proteins: an overview. Anal Bioanal Chem 2009; 395: 69-81.

[36] Koppelman SJ, Knulst AC, Koers WJ, *et al.* Comparison of different immunochemical methods for the detection and quantification of hazelnut proteins in food products. J Allergy Clin Immunol 1999; 229: 107-120.

[37] Baumgartner ES, Bremer M, Kemmers-Voncken A, *et al.* Detection of hidden hazelnut protein in food by IgY-based indirect competitive enzyme immunoassay. Analytica Chimica Acta 2004; 520: 223-228.

[38] Faeste CK, Holden L, Plassen C, Almli B. Sensitive time-resolved fluoroimmunoassay for the detection of hazelnut (Corylus avellana) protein traces in food matrices. J Immunol Methods 2006; 314: 114-122.

[39] Clemente A, Chambers SJ, Lodi F, *et al.* Use of the indirect competitive ELISA for the detection of Brazil nut in food products. Food Control 2004; 15: 65-69.

[40] Chassaigne H, Brohée M, Nørgaard JV, van Hengel AJ. Investigation on sequential extraction of peanut allergens for subsequent analysis by ELISA and 2D gel electrophoresis. Food Chem 2007; 105: 1671-1681.

[41] Watanabe Y, Aburatani K, Mizumura T, *et al.* Novel ELISA for the detection of raw and processed egg using extraction buffer containing a surfactant and a reducing agent. J Immunol Methods 2005; 300: 115-123.

[42] Asensio L, González I, García T, Martín R. Determination of food authenticity by enzyme-linked immunosorbent assay (ELISA). Food Control 2008; 19: 1-8.

[43] Blais BW, Gaudreault M, Phillippe LM. Multiplex enzyme immunoassay system for the simultaneous detection of multiple allergens in foods. Food Control 2003; 14: 43-47.

[44] Valenta R, Duchene M, Vrtala S, *et al.* Recombinant allergens for immunoblot diagnosis of tree pollen allergy. J Allergy Clin Immunol 1991; 88: 889-894.

[45] Kazemi-Shirazi L, Pauli G, Purohit A, *et al.* Quantitative IgE inhibition experiments with purified recombinant allergens indicate pollen-derived allergens as the sensitizing agents responsible for many forms of plant food allergy. J Allergy Clin Immunol 2000; 105: 116-125.

[46] Díaz-Perales A, Blanco C, Sánchez-Monge R, *et al.* Analysis of avocado allergen (Prs a 1) IgE-binding peptides generated by simulated gastric fluid digestion. J Allergy Clin Immunol 2003; 112: 1002-1007.

[47] Lind P, Norman PS, Newton M, *et al.* The prevalence of indoor allergens in the Baltimore area: House dust-mite and animal-dander antigens measured by immunochemical techniques. J Allergy Clin Immunol 1987; 80: 541-547.

[48] Mäkinen-Kiljunen S, Turjanmaa K, Palosuo T, Reunala T. Characterization of latex antigens and allergens in surgical gloves and natural rubber by immunoelectrophoretic methods. J Allergy Clin Immunol 1992; 90: 230-235.

[49] Hock B, Seifert M, Kramer K. Engineering receptors and antibodies for biosensors. Biosens Bioelectron 2002; 17: 239-249.

[50] Scheller F, Schubert F. Biosensoren. Berlin: Akademie-Verlag, 1989.

[51] Spichiger-Keller UE. Chemical Sensors and Biosensors for Medical and Biological applications. Weinheim: Wiley-VCH, 1998.

[52] Luong JHT, Groom CM, Male KB. The potential role of biosensors in the food and drink industries. Biosens Bioelectron 1991; 6: 547-554.

[53] van Hengel AJ. Food allergen detection methods and the challenge to protect food-allergic consumers. Anal Bioanal Chem 2007; 389: 111-118.

[54] Mohammed I, Mullett WM, Lai EPC, Yeung JM. Is biosensor a viable method for food allergen detection? Analytica Chimica Acta 2001; 444: 97-102.

[55] Mills ENC, Potts A, Plumb GW, Lambert N, Morgan MRA. Development of a rapid dipstick immunoassay for the detection of peanut contamination of food. Food Agric Immunol 1997; 9: 37 - 50.

[56] Lüttkopf D, Müller U, Skov PS, *et al.* Comparison of four variants of a major allergen in hazelnut (Corylus avellana) Cor a 1.04 with the major hazel pollen allergen Cor a 1.01. Mol Immunol 2002; 38: 515-525.

[57] Bauermeister K, Ballmer-Weber BK, Bublin M, *et al.* Assessment of component-resolved *in vitro* diagnosis of celeriac allergy. J Allergy Clin Immunol 2009; 124: 1273-1281.e2.

[58] Chapman MD, Ferreira F, Villalba M, *et al.* The European Union CREATE Project: A model for international standardization of allergy, diagnostics and vaccines. J Allergy Clin Immunol 2008; 122: 882-889.e2.

[59] Ladics GS, Selgrade MJK. Identifying food proteins with allergenic potential: Evolution of approaches to safety assessment and research to provide additional tools. Regula Toxicol Pharmacol 2009; 54: S2-S6.

[60] Gallo M, Sayre R. Removing allergens and reducing toxins from food crops. Curr Opin Biotechnol 2009; 20: 191-196.

[61] Goodman RE. Performing IgE serum testing due to bioinformatics matches in the allergenicity assessment of GM crops. Food Chem Toxicol 2008; 46: S24-S34.

[62] Björkstén B, Crevel R, Hischenhuber C, *et al.* Criteria for identifying allergenic foods of public health importance. Regul Toxicol Pharmacol 2008; 51: 42-52.

[63] Abbott M, Hayward S, Ross W, *et al.* Validation procedures for quantitative food allergen ELISA methods: community guidance and best practices. J AOAC Int 2010; 93: 442-450.

[64] Pieretti MM, Chung D, Pacenza R, Slotkin T, Sicherer SH. Audit of manufactured products: Use of allergen advisory labels and identification of labelling ambiguities. J Allergy Clin Immunol 2009; 124: 337-341.

[65] Houghton JR, Rowe G, Frewer LJ, *et al.* The quality of food risk management in Europe: Perspectives and priorities. Food Policy 2008; 33: 13-26.

CHAPTER 6

Immunoassays for Antibiotics in the Food Chain

Willem Haasnoot*

RIKILT-Institute of Food Safety, Wageningen UR, Wageningen, The Netherlands

Abstract: The food chain is threatened by various hazards and the presence of residues of antibiotics, used during cattle-breeding, is one of the serious risks for consumers. In food and feed analysis for antibiotics, screening technologies are powerful tools that provide a rapid screen of large numbers of samples when conventional analytical methods are too cumbersome. Due to their simplicity and/or high-throughput capacity, immunoassays are applicable for screening at critical control points in the food chain and in control laboratories. However, in general, they are very specific, and only suitable for the detection of one or two antibiotics, which seriously limits their application. New antibodies and new assay formats with multiplex capacity might give new possibilities for control agencies and food industries for increased and more efficient controls on antibiotics and other food contaminants. Multiplex applications and future perspectives of poly- and monoclonal as well as recombinant antibodies for the compound- or group-specific detection of antibiotics, using different immunoassay formats (*e.g.* ELISAs, dip sticks, biosensors and flow cytometers), are described and discussed.

Keywords: Antibodies, Immunoassays, Antibiotics, Food.

ANTIBIOTICS IN THE FOOD CHAIN

Antibiotic means "against life" and antibiotics are medicines that kill or cause growth retardation of micro-organisms. In the original definition, an antibiotic was described as any substance produced by a micro-organism that is antagonistic to the growth of other micro-organisms. This excluded synthetic compounds such as the sulfonamides and quinolones. In modern usage, an antibiotic is any chemotherapeutic agent with activity against micro-organisms such as bacteria, fungi or protozoa [1]. The variety of antibiotics is enormous and there are hardly any processes in the living cell that are not sensitive to one of these antibiotics. Some antibiotics are still produced and isolated from living organisms, such as the aminoglycosides. Many others are produced *via* purely synthetic means, such as the quinolones and sulfonamides.

Veterinary drugs are used to treat disease and improve health in animals, analogous to pharmaceuticals in human beings. The use of antibiotics as feed additives is one of the most effective management tools available to meat cattle producers [2]. Added in low doses to the feed of farm animals, they improve growth performance. Therefore, antibiotics have extensively been used in animal production worldwide for decades. The serious problems caused by the emergence and spread of antimicrobial resistance was the reason for an EU-wide ban on the use of antibiotics as growth promoters in animal feed which has been effective since 2006 [3]. This ban was the final step in the phasing out of antibiotics used for non-medicinal purposes. Antibiotics are now only allowed to be added to animal feed for veterinary medicine. However, so far, this EU regulation did not result in a major decrease in the use of veterinary medicines. The Dutch Organization of Manufacturers and Importers of Veterinary Medicines reported a total use of 543 tons of antibiotics in 2006, which implies a 7% increase compared with 2005 with a comparable number of farm animals [4]. In 2007, the total use of veterinary drugs increased again with 9% to 590 tons with the same number of farm animals [5] and finally in 2008, a 12% decrease to 521 tons was observed with a small increase of farm animals [6]. However, the still massive use of antibiotics in food-producing animals, may result in residues in food (*e.g.* milk, eggs or meat). This is especially the case when products from animals have been sent for processing within the withdrawal periods - ranging from a few days to a few weeks - of approved therapeutic antibiotics, or when animals have had access to excreted residues in their environment [7].

***Address correspondence to Willem Haasnoot:** RIKILT-Institute of Food Safety, Wageningen UR, Wageningen, The Netherlands; E-mail: willem.haasnoot@wur.nl

To guarantee a high level of consumer protection, European Community legislation [8] requires that the toxicity of potential residues is evaluated before the use of a medicinal substance in food-producing animals is authorized. If considered necessary, Maximum Residue Limits (MRLs) are established and in some cases the use of the relevant substance is prohibited. All pharmacologically active substances are divided into two groups: (i) Group A compounds, which comprise prohibited substances (listed in the Directive 96/22/EC [9] and in Annex IV of the Council Regulation (EC, 1990) [8]); (ii) Group B compounds, which comprise substances with final and provisional MRLs (listed in Annex I and III of the regulation [8]). Veterinary medicinal products can only be authorized or used in food-producing animals if pharmacologically active substances contained therein have been assessed as safe according to this MRL regulation and rules concerning the documentation of use, prescription and distribution have been established [10].

Within the EU, residue monitoring plans for antibiotics and other groups of compounds are established from 1996 [11]. They include the frequencies and level of sampling, investigation procedures and requirements on the documentation of use. The plans give indications for sanctions in case of non-compliance, requirements for targeted investigations and for the establishment, reporting and the groups of substances to be controlled for each food commodity. Another Commission Decision [12] lays down additional rules for milk, eggs, honey, rabbits and game. A summary report for 2006 [13] on the results of the national residue monitoring plans in food of animal origin in all EU member states described that the percentage of non-compliant results for antibacterials (exceeding the MRL levels) increased from 0.20% in 2005 to 0.30% in 2006 and that antibacterials remain the main problem for meat (bovine, pigs, sheep, goats, poultry, and rabbits), milk and honey.

DETECTION OF ANTIBIOTICS IN FOOD

For the detection of antibiotics in food and related products (*e.g.* blood, urine, renal pelvis fluid, *etc.*), three techniques are mainly applied: (i) microbial inhibition screening tests; (ii) chromatography-based screening and confirmation methods; and (iii) immuno- or receptor-based screening assays.

Because of their high cost-effectiveness and broad spectrum characteristics, microbial inhibition methods are preferred for large scale surveillance programs on veterinary drug residues. The methods usually use a medium inoculated with a susceptible bacterium and rely on diffusion of the antimicrobial residue. Inhibition of growth indicates the presence of antimicrobial compounds. Many test systems have been developed based on this principle, and methods using one to seven agar plates have been reported. The Fast Antimicrobial Screening Test (FAST) is a one-plate microbial method with *Bacillus megaterium* that requires a minimum of 6 h for development [14]. The Premi® test uses a vial containing spores of the thermophile *B. stearothermophilis* in agar, and acts similarly to a single-plate method [15]. This test is more rapid, with development times typically from 3 to 4 h. A similar test, the kidney inhibition swab (KIS™) test of Charm Sciences uses a differently configured vial of *B. stearothermophilis* spores in agar, and also allows results within 3-4 h. These three fast tests were compared for screening antibiotic residues in beef kidney juice and serum [16] and one of the conclusions was that there is not one rapid screening microbial inhibition assay for antibiotics that is ideal for all analytes. To cover all possibilities, one would have to run a number of different assays or separate plates. Such a five-plates test has been described [17], and comprises various microbes for the group-specific identification of antimicrobial residues in slaughter animals, the so-called Nouws Antibiotic Test (NAT screening). The NAT screening combines a simple and efficient sampling and sample processing strategy with a high detection capability because it detects the great majority of antibiotics used in veterinary medicine at or below their maximum residue levels in kidney. However, it requires a rather lengthy incubation time of 16-18 h.

A faster alternative for the microbial inhibition assay is a whole-cell-based bioassay, also named whole-cell biosensor, which has been described for the detection of tetracyclines [18]. They constructed a genetically engineered luminescent bacterial strain that contained the regulation unit of tetracycline resistance factor (tetracycline-responsive element) to control the expression of the luciferase operon. This resulted in a tetracycline-dependent light production. The time needed for optimal induction of light emission was 90 min. They found that this kind of sensor cell can be freeze-dried without any loss of sensitivity or overall performance which simplifies the applicability of the assay system. This tetracycline group-specific bioassay was sensitized to meet the EU MRL for tetracycline residues in poultry tissue (100 ng g^{-1}) by adding membrane-permeabilizing and chelating agents and sensitivities of 5 ng g^{-1} for doxycycline, 7.5 ng g^{-1} for chlortetracycline and 25 ng g^{-1} of tetracycline were reached [19]. The assay was performed in 96-well flat bottom microtiter plates within 4 h with little preparation, as lyophilized cells are always ready, and a multitude of samples can be assayed easily in this format. Being at least as sensitive and better suited for high-throughput analysis, whole-cell biosensors have the potential to displace growth inhibition assays as the favored method for tetracycline residue screening. However, such bioassays are not yet described for other antibiotics although the use of the multidrug-binding repressor protein (QacR) from *Staphylococcus aureus* [20] might offer an interesting approach for the future development of a multi-drug biosensor. Currently, cellular biosensors - based on various microbial species containing reporters that are specifically induced *via* selected promotors - are widely used in pharmaceutical drug discovery and in environmental biology [21] and for monitoring environmental chemical contaminants [22]. This will also further influence the development of new bioassays for the detection of antibiotics in food.

Of the chromatographic techniques, High-Performance Thin-Layer Chromato-Graphy (HPTLC) has been applied successfully for the qualitative and quantitative detection of multi-residues in food samples even though its use has rapidly decreased during the last decade [23]. The use of High-Performance Liquid Chromatography (HPLC) expanded during the 1990s and the availability of automation facilitated its use as a screening technique. The choice of the detection system is very important to obtain both sufficient selectivity and sensitivity. UV-diode array detection in combination with reversed-phase HPLC has been applied for the detection of many antibiotics in a lot of different food matrices. Nowadays, more than 80% of the analytical techniques for the determination of veterinary drugs use HPLC in combination with Mass Spectrometry (MS) [24]. Chromatographic methods are mainly used for the simultaneous detection and quantification of closely related compounds belonging to a single drug class. In combination with an MS/MS technique they fulfill the established criteria [25] for confirmation of identity of drugs [26-28]. Recently, Ultra-Performance Liquid Chromatography Combined With Time-Of-Flight Mass Spectrometry (UPLC-Tof-MS) was used for the screening and quantification of more than 100 veterinary drugs in milk [29] and in muscle, kidney and liver [30]. This technique combines high resolution for both LC and MS with high mass accuracy, and as such is very powerful for the multi-compound analysis of veterinary drugs. However, in general, chromatography-based methods are laborious and require trained personnel with high expertise and expensive equipment which make them only suitable for specialized laboratories and less suitable for measurements in the food chain. According to the General Food Law [31], the food and feed industries are responsible for the safety of their products and their demand for simplified and rapid test methods at critical control points in the entire chain has never been greater. These methods must be able to detect an analyte or class of analytes at the level of interest. Some false positives (false non-compliants) are acceptable, as they will be further submitted for confirmatory analysis. However, the test must avoid or reduce to a minimum the number of false negative results (false compliants), because they will not be further analyzed.

IMMUNOASSAYS FOR ANTIBIOTICS

In immunoassays for antibiotics, polyclonal (Pabs), monoclonal (Mabs) and occasionally recombinant antibodies (Rabs) are used. Pabs are applied most frequently. The main problem with polyclonal antisera is the batch quantity and the batch-to-batch variation. Therefore the amount of tests is limited. However, with for instance a batch of 25 ml of a polyclonal antiserum and a usually optimum dilution of 40,000 times (total volume = 1,000,000 ml of which 2.5 ml is used per microtiter plate), 400,000 microtiter plate tests kits can be prepared. For most of the drug residue test kits, this is much more than the world-wide market needs for 50 or more years. In special circumstances, *e.g.* for high volume (on-line) testing, test strips, immunoaffinity chromatography (IAC) and for "best-sellers", more antibodies are necessary. Increased volumes of Pabs can be obtained by mixing different batches of (rabbit) antisera obtained after different boosters or from different rabbits. However, in most cases, the quality of antisera improves after several boosters (antibody maturation) and mixing with lower-quality batches might reduce the test performance. Other possibilities are the immunization of larger animals (goat, sheep, donkey, *etc.*) or the use of chicken eggs. The usefulness of Mabs stems from three characteristics: their specificity of binding, their homogeneity, and their ability to be produced in unlimited quantities. The production of Mabs allows the isolation of reagents with a unique, chosen specificity. Because all of the antibodies produced by descendants of one hybridoma cell are identical, Mabs are powerful reagents for testing for the presence of a desired epitope. In addition, one unique advantage of hybridoma production is that impure antigens can be used to produce specific antibodies. The limitations of hybridoma technology include the extensive commitment of time, labor and expense, the requirement for animal use and specialized cell culture facilities, and the expertise needed to prepare and screen large number of hybridomas to select the best ones [32]. Until the late 1980s, the production of antibodies relied primarily on animal immunization. From then, the development of molecular methods for the expression of recombinant antibody fragment in bacteria and techniques for production and screening of combinatorial libraries has opened a wide range of opportunities for the selection of recombinant antibodies and their engineering [33]. Several *in vitro* methods have been developed for the production of antibodies [34], but the most commonly used technology is phage display [35]. Phage display refers to the display of functional foreign peptides, proteins or antibody fragments on the surface of a bacteriophage. This is accomplished by fusion of the DNA coding sequences of the protein to be displayed into the phage genome to the gene encoding one of the phage surface proteins. Surface display of the antibodies allows affinity selection of antibodies by exposing the phage library to immobilized antigen molecules. The captured phage particles are eluted from the antigen, amplified by infecting *Escherichia coli* host cells and used in a subsequent round of affinity selection. After the final round of affinity selection, phage particles are amplified in order to prepare and characterize their displayed antibodies individually and the monoclonal phage population with the desired binding specificities can be isolated.

With regard to antigenic specificity, different types of phage libraries are used for selection of specific recombinant antibodies: (1) a specific library sourced from immunized animals, (2) a single-pot (general) library created with no specificity against a particular analyte which avoids the use of laboratory animals [36]. The most popular recombinant antibody format is the single-chain variable fragment (scFv), containing the variable domains of the heavy and light chain (Fig. **1**) linked to a single protein by a polypeptide linker. It contains a complete binding site and it is the smallest effective antibody fragment (26-27 kDa). Spinks *et al.* [37] used this technique to study the development of broad-specificity (generic) antibodies to beta-lactams and aminoglycosides. Other Rab applications are described for sulfonamides by Korpimäki *et al.* [38-41], for pesticides [42, 43] and potato glycoalkaloids [44]. In comparison to Pabs and Mabs, Rabs, using the phage display technique, can be prepared faster, in a more automatic process and with reduced consumption of laboratory animals [35].

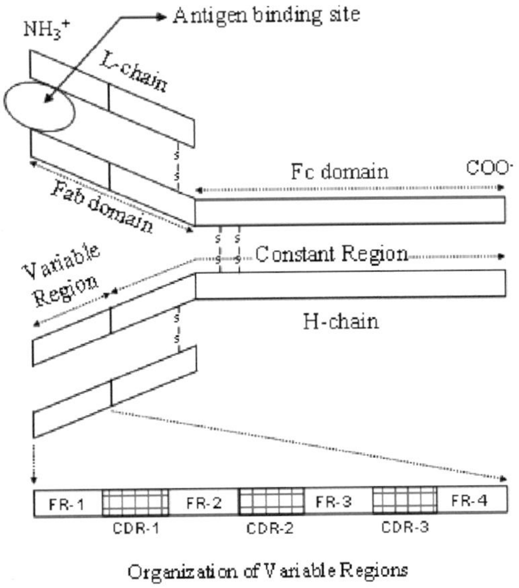

Figure 1: Schematic representation of a typical immunoglobulin-G molecule. The organization of the variable portions of the heavy and light-chains depicting the Framework Regions (FR) and the Complementarity Determining Regions (CDRs) is shown in the lower portion of the figure.

Of the immunochemical methods, the 96-wells microtiter plate Enzyme-Linked Immunosorbent Assay (ELISA) is most frequently used and many test kits to detect specific compounds or groups of compounds are commercially available. In general, they are sensitive and easy to use, have a high specificity, require minimal sample preparations, and are therefore suitable for the screening of a large number of samples in a short time (about 2-3 h). These tests can be used within food-producing facilities. For instance, antibiotic-ELISAs are described for the detection of sulfamethazine in swine urine and plasma [45] and meat [46], aminoglycosides in milk and kidney [47], chloramphenicol in urine, tissue, milk and eggs [46-49], nitroimidazoles in eggs and chicken muscle [50], gentamicin in milk [51] and tetracyclines in goat and sheep meat [46]. Font *et al.* [52] used antibody-coated magnetic nanoparticles for target capture/enrichment in the assay for sulfonamides in milk and hair. A multianalyte ELISA for the immunochemical screening of sulfonamides, fluoroquinolones and ss-lactams antibiotics in milk, using three class-selective bioreceptors in a planar microarray configuration, was described recently [53].

Immunochromatographic or lateral flow tests or dip sticks are much faster antibody-based assays, which can be performed in minutes. In these tests, all ingredients are already present in the test device, and the sample (extract) is needed only to perform an assay. Therefore, this format is ideal for some food-producing facilities and field applications. Such fast tests are described for the detection of sulfadimidine in calf serum [54], sulfonamides in eggs and chicken muscles [55], (dihydro) streptomycine [56] and cephems [57] in milk. Based on this technology, Unisensor (Angleur, Belgium) developed a receptor-based assay dipstick format (Twin sensor^{BT}) for the rapid detection of β-lactams and tetracyclines molecules in raw milk. Other examples of commercially available products are the Rapid One Step Assay (ROSA$^{®}$) tests for β-lactams, tetracyclines, enrofloxacin and sulfadimethoxine/sulfamethazine of Charm Sciences Inc. (Lawrence, MA, USA). The commercial availability of these rapid tests is still limited to a few antibiotics.

Another more recent approach to screen animal products for veterinary drugs consists of the application of biomolecule-based biosensors. While bioassays or cellular biosensors utilize the response of whole cells to detect biologically active agents, these biosensor instruments use a biological recognition element (*e.g.* antibodies, enzymes, lectins, receptors and nucleic acids) in close contact with a signal transduction element (*e.g.* optical, acoustic, and electrochemical) connected to data acquisition and processing systems [22]. Thus, the signal from the biological element is converted to a quantifiable signal, *e.g.*, electrical. Enzymatic biosensors utilize specific enzymes for the capture and catalytic generation of the product, which is then directly determined using a range of transducers (*e.g.* electrochemical, optical, photothermal, amperometric, and acoustic). In contaminant analysis, enzyme biosensors have largely been used for organophosphorus and carbamate pesticide and herbicide analysis, with fewer applications being reported for antibiotics, *e.g.* for the detection of penicillins using penicillinase [58].

Antibody-based immunosensors are frequently described with transduction elements based on piezoelectric, electrochemical, and optical components. A piezoelectric immunosensor is a device based on materials such as quartz crystals, which resonate on application of an external alternating electric field. The frequency of the resulting oscillation is a function of the mass of the crystal. This mass increases during interactions of *e.g.* antibodies to immobilized antigens, and thus yields a directly measurable decrease in the frequency. Such a fast (5 min) inhibition piezoelectric immunosensor is described for the detection of the mycotoxin ochratoxin A in liquid food samples [59].

For the detection of antibiotics, electrochemical and optical immunosensors are most frequently applied. Electrochemical biosensors include potentiometric and amperometric immunosensors. The potentiometric immunosensors are based on the change in potential that occurs when an antigen in a sample reacts with the corresponding antibody previously immobilized to an electrode. The potential difference between an antibody-immobilized electrode and a reference electrode is a function of the analyte in the sample. Amperometric immunosensors rely on the measurement of current generated when an electroactive species is either oxidized or reduced at an antibody- (or antigen-) coated electrode to which an analyte (or antibody) binds specifically. Zacco *et al.* [60] developed a novel electrochemical immunosensing strategy for the detection of sulfonamide antibiotics in milk based on magnetic beads coated with class-specific anti-sulfonamide antibodies and a sulfonamide-peroxidase as tracer.

The interest in optical biosensors for food analysis, with fluorescent, bioluminescent or chemiluminescent labels for detection, as well as the direct (label-free) detection, is increasing. Label-free biosensors do not require the use of reporter elements to generate a signal, which is convenient during assay development and during application by saving washing steps and time [61]. One of the most popular label-free technologies for performing rapid analysis is based on commercially available automated multi-channel Surface Plasmon Resonance (SPR)-based biosensors (Fig. **2**).

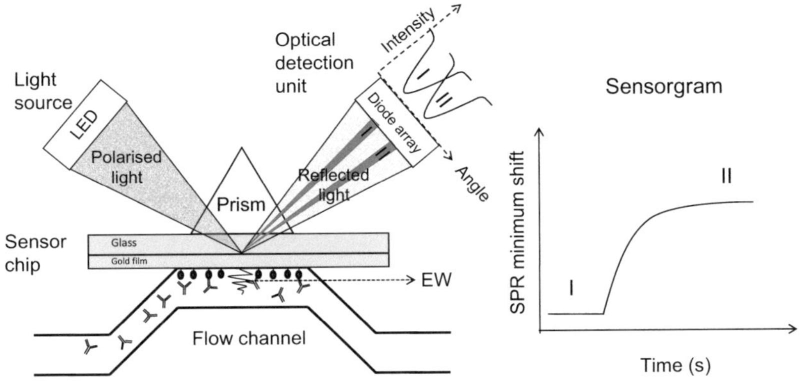

Figure 2: Schematic view of the optical and flow channel setup of a Biacore system (reproduced from www.biacore.com).

With such a biosensor, direct biosensor immunoassays (BIAs), using Mab-coated biosensor chips, were developed which detected gentamicin [62] and (dihydro)streptomycin [63] in milk far below the Maximum Residue Limits (MRLs). However, with milk, interferences were observed which were probably due to the nonspecific binding of milk proteins to the protein-coated sensor chips. Better results, less matrix interferences and more stable chips, were obtained in the inhibition BIA in which four aminoglycosides (gentamicin, neomycin, kanamycin and a streptomycin derivative) were directly immobilized (without coupling to proteins) onto the sensor surface in the four flow channels of the Biacore 3000 that were serially connected [64]. These flow channels were used in combination with a mixture of four specific antibodies. Milk samples were diluted ten times in the antibodies-containing buffer and the Limits Of Detection (LODs) in milk were far below the MRLs (varying from 100 to 1500 ng ml^{-1}) and the total run time between samples was 7 min.

Another approach of a multiplex immunoassay is the development of group-specific antibodies which were described for fluoroquinolones [65] and sulfonamides [66, 67] in which generic structures were used for the development of antibodies. In the case of sulfonamides, a sulfathiazole derivative (Fig. **3**) was synthesized and linked to carrier proteins in such a way that the aromatic amino group, common to all sulfonamides, was distal to the proteins. Mice were immunized and Mabs were obtained of which the best one (Mab 27G3) recognized in an ELISA eight structurally different sulfonamides at concentrations less than 100 ng ml^{-1}, however, they were less sensitive for other sulfonamides [66]. The use of mutated Rabs, after the modification of the single chain variable fragment (scFv) molecules of the wild-type Mab 27G3, resulted in improved immunoassays [38-41]. The applications of two genetically modifications (mutants A.3.5 and M.3.4) and the wild-type Mab 27G3 were evaluated in the biosensor using a CM5 sensor chip coated with the sulfonamide-derivative (TS, Fig. **3**) and chicken serum as sample material [68].

TS

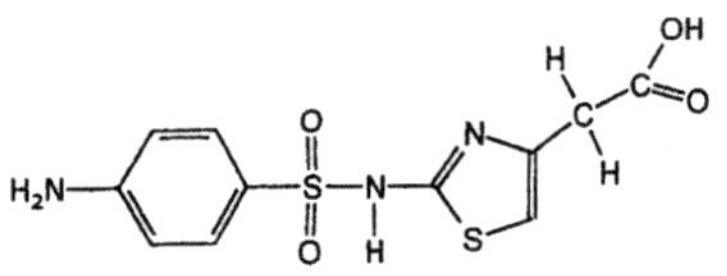

Figure 3: Molecular structure of N1-[4-(carboxymethyl)-2-thiazolyl]sulfanilamide (TS), the immunogen used for the development of generic Pabs and Mabs.

The improvements in inhibition, due to the presence of different sulfonamides added to chicken serum at the 100 ng ml^{-1} level, are shown in Fig. **4** for the three antibodies. With the wild-type Mab 27G3 and mutants A.3.5 and M.3.4, the number of sulfonamides showing significant inhibitions of the response (>20%) were 7, 12 and 17, respectively. The performance of the best mutant was compared in a biosensor immunoassay (BIA) format with other multi-sulfonamide antibodies and it was found to be the most sensitive towards most of the sulfonamides [69]. The Rab-based BIAs were successfully applied to the detection of sulfonamides in serum and levels were higher and correlated well with levels in tissue as measured with LC-MS/MS [70]. Serum and milk were found to be suitable sample materials for the biosensor detection of antibiotics in the food chain. Such assays are fast, robust, automated, easy to handle, and require simple sample preparations (dilutions in antibody-containing buffer). However, the applied four-channel biosensor systems are expensive, too limited in multiplexing and antibodies are too specific for the simultaneous detection of antibiotics from different groups and the systems are therefore less suitable for control agencies and food industries to provide an increased and more efficient control on food contaminants (such as antibiotics) in the food chain. Cheaper alternatives and more extended multiplex systems need to be explored.

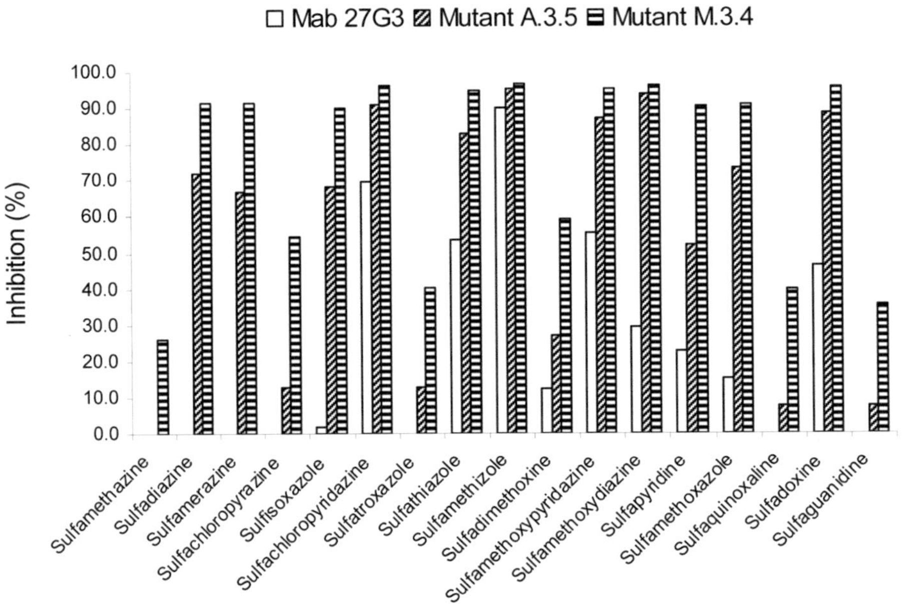

Figure 4: Inhibition (%) of the maximum responses obtained with a BIA, due to the presence of different sulfonamides added to a blank chicken serum at 100 ng ml^{-1}, using the wild-type Mab 27G3 and mutants A.3.5 and M.3.4. Chicken serum (20 µl) was diluted with 100 µl of the antibody-containing buffer of which 50 µl was injected at a flow rate of 20 µl min^{-1} [68].

FUTURE PERSPECTIVES FOR ANTIBIOTIC DETECTION

Biosensors. The application of a low-cost SPR-based prototype biosensor system (Spreeta™) has been described previously [71] in which the sensitivities with inhibition assays for endocrine disruptors were comparable to those obtained with a Biacore 3000. However, this system was less robust and built with a single flow-channel only. Alternative eight-channel SPR sensor instruments were developed and used for the detection of low molecular weight endocrine-disrupting compounds [72] and an environmental contaminant in a miniaturized and portable format [73], which are interesting approaches for future research. Beyond that, an SPR system with the possibility for the simultaneous detection of 20 spots in 4 flow-channels (Biacore A100) is available (GE Healthcare). However, the imaging SPR (iSPR) technology takes multiplex SPR analysis a step further [74]. With iSPR, broad-beam monochromatic polarized light from a laser diode (at a specific wavelength) illuminates the whole functionalized area of the biosensor chip surface. The high resolution CCD video camera provides real-time difference images across the array format with up to hundreds of active spots and it captures all of the local changes at the surface of the biochip (Fig. **5**).

There are several commercial iSPR instruments available, *e.g.* Biacore Flexchip (GE Healthcare), SPRi-Plex™ (Genoptics Bio interactions), ProteOn™ XPR 36 (Bio-Rad laboratories), SPRimager®II ARRAY system (GWC Technologies) and IBIS iSPR (IBIS Technologies B.V.). The instruments differ in optics, fluidics, sample handling and surface preparation. Rebe Raz *et al.* [75] used the IBIS iSPR for the simultaneous detection of eight model antibiotics from four major antibiotic families (aminoglycosides, sulfonamides, fenicols, and fluoroquinolones) in milk. By multiplexing seven immunoassays in a competitive format, they were able to measure all the target compounds at parts per billion (ppb) levels.

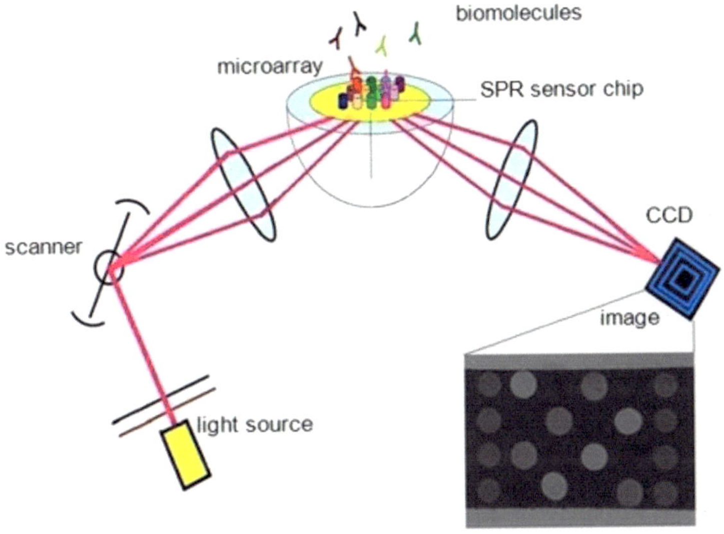

Figure 5: Schematic representation of an iSPR assembly.

Another interesting automated multiplex biochip array technology (Evidence®) is marketed by Randox (www.randox.com) in which 25 immunoassays can be measured simultaneously using chemiluminescent signals and spots are measured with a CCD camera. They supply arrays for growth-promoters and antimicrobials but a major disadvantage is that it is a closed system which is not suitable for assay development. The different immunoanalytical microarray systems based on fluorescence, chemiluminescence, electrochemical, and label-free microarray readout systems have recently been reviewed [76].

Flow cytometry. Seidel & Niessner [76] also included in their review an interesting and commercially available suspension microarray in a flow cytometer. This promising and evolving suspension microarray is the Multi Analyte Profiling (xMAP®) technology of Luminex Corporation, which is an open system suitable for assay development. This technology uses small carboxylated polystyrene microspheres (5.6 μm beads), which are internally dyed with a red and an infrared fluorophore. By varying the ratio of the two fluorophores, up to 100 different color-coded bead sets can be distinguished (Fig. **6**), and each bead set can be coupled to a different biological probe. In combination with flow cytometry, it is possible to simultaneously measure up to 100 different biomolecular interactions in a single well. The carboxylated bead surface allows simple chemical coupling of capture reagents such as antibodies or drug-protein conjugates. This technology was already applied for the detection of sulfonamides in milk [77] and in blood serum, meat drip and eggs [78] using the Rab M.3.4 and for the simultaneous detection of aminoglycosides and sulfonamides in milk and blood serum [79]. These experiments demonstrate that this technology is suitable for multiplexing of antibiotic assays in food materials and it is a serious option for future multiplex applications.

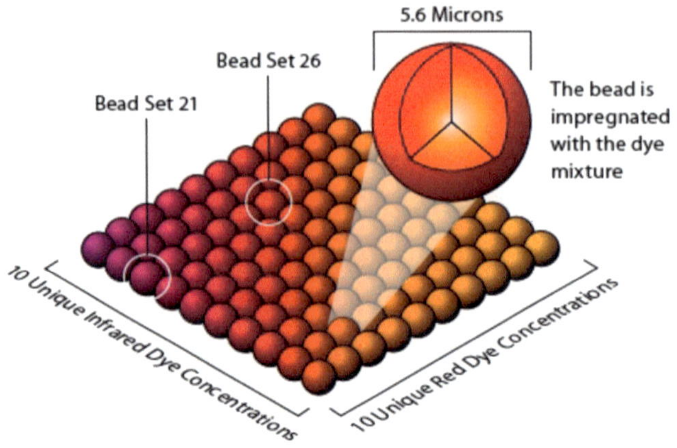

Figure 6: The 100 different bead sets of the xMAP® technology prepared by mixing a red and an infrared dye each in 10 different unique concentration.

A five-fold increase in multiplexing capabilities can be obtained with the FlexMAP 3D™ platform of Luminex, using a third fluorophor, which offers 500-plex capability and runs three times faster compared with the Luminex100 or -200 systems. More relevant to food diagnostics is the development of the new Luminex multiplex platform called MagPix™ which is a lower-cost, compact, rugged, diagnostic and environmental testing xMAP analyzer which moves away from a flow cytometry-based system to an instrument based on their already existing magnetic bead array (MagPlex™) analyzed on a magnet in a 2D readout with inexpensive Light Emitting Diodes (LEDs) and a CCD imager. It is expected to be launched in 2010 and this development will make future multiplexing faster, cheaper and more robust and applicable in the food chain.

Nanoparticles. The former described particles used in flow cytometry are on a microscale and nanoparticle research is currently an area of intense scientific investigations, due to a wide variety of potential applications in biomedical, optical, and electronic fields. Nanoparticles (NPs) are defined as particles having one or more dimensions in the sub-100 nanometer range. In analytical biochemistry, they are used as biosensor response enhancers [80] and as labels in clinical and food diagnostics due to their unique characteristics as the high surface-to-volume ratio and the size-dependent optical or magnetical properties. Yuan *et al.* [81] reported about the use of larger gold NPs (40 nm) for signal enhancement on a mixed self-assembled monolayer (mSAM) sensor surface which resulted in a twenty-fold increase in signal and, due to a large reduction in antibody concentration, in a thirty times more sensitive assay for chloramphenicol. The use of gold NPs and other new nanodiagnostic tools (*e.g.* Quantum Dots (QDs)) for diagnostic applications promise increased sensitivity, multiplexing capabilities, and reduced costs [82]. The nanometer sized colloidal gold particles are frequently used as labels in lateral flow tests [55] because of their ability to adhere proteins (*e.g.* antibodies) and their intense red color which is due to localized SPR (LSPR) a common phenomenon for nanometer-sized metallic structures [83]. Localized Surface Plasmons (LSPs) are charge density oscillations confined to metallic NPs. Excitation of LSPs by an electric field (light) at an incident wavelength where resonance occurs results in strong light scattering, in the appearance of intense Surface Plasmon (SP) absorption bands, and an enhancement of the local electromagnetic fields. The frequency (*i.e.* absorption maxima or color) and intensity of the SP absorption bands are characteristic of the type of material (gold, silver or platinum), and highly sensitive to the size, size distribution, and shape of the nanostructures, as well as to the environments which surround them. The fact that the color of metallic NPs depends markedly on the refractive index of the surrounding medium has been exploited for sensing applications. LSPR sensing is based on a simple optical extinction measurement, is not temperature sensitive, and requires only common laboratory equipment. Molecular interaction analysis of gold NPs on a solid transparent substrate (glass), to avoid the possibility of aggregation, have been reported by several groups. Such an LSPR-based immunosensor was developed for the detection of casein in milk [84] in which anti-casein antibodies were immobilized to gold-capped silica NPs on a glass slide substrate and the binding of casein could be monitored by the peak absorbance intensity increments at around 520 nm using a UV-Vis spectrophotometer. Kreuzer *et al.* [85] developed an LSPR-based biosensor for the detection of stanozolol using gold colloids (100 nm), coated with a stanozolol-protein conjugate, chemically sized on an activated glass substrate. Binding of anti-stanozolol antibodies was observed by a shift of the resonance wavelength (with a maximum of 13 nm) and the detection limit of the system was calculated as 2.4 nM or 0.7 ng ml^{-1}. Gold-silica core nanoshells, spherical silica core surrounded by a gold shell of a few nanometers in thickness, with different core/shell ratios result in different optical resonances and can be used for multiplexing [86]. Advantages of the LSPR devices were described as the simplicity of the optical configuration, easy fabrication, the great potential for miniaturization, simple handling, low-cost, short assay times, and high sensitivity.

Advances in nanomaterials have produced a new class of fluorescent labels which is more suitable for multiplex detection by conjugating semiconductor nanocrystals, also known as Quantum Dots (QDs), with biorecognition molecules [87]. These QDs (2-8 nm) are atom clusters comprising a core, shell, and coating. The core is made up of a few hundred to a few thousand atoms of a semiconductor material often composed of atoms from group II-VI (*e.g.* CdSe, CdTe, CdS, and ZnSe) or group III-V elements (*e.g.* InP and InAs) in the periodic table. A semiconductor shell (typically zinc sulfide) surrounds and stabilizes the core, improving both the optical and physical properties of the material. An amphiphilic polymer coating then encases the core and shell, providing a water-soluble surface that can be modified. For some of these QDs, this amphiphilic inner coating is covalently modified with a functionalized polyethylene glycol (PEG) outer coating to reduce nonspecific binding. By varying the size and composition of QDs, the emission wavelength can be tuned and the broad absorption spectra, useful for the simultaneous excitation of different-sized QDs, and narrow symmetric emission spectra make QDs very well suited to optical multiplexing [88]. More multicolor optical coding for biological assays has been achieved by embedding different-sized QDs into polymeric microbeads at precisely controlled ratios [89]. Other advantages of QDs are excellent brightness, negligible photobleaching, fairly high quantum yields, and photostability. These extraordinary fluorescence properties can be attributed to the unique fluorescence mechanism of semiconductor materials which fluoresce through the formation of excitons, or Coulomb-correlated electron-hole pairs, upon absorption of a photon of light. Compared with the excited state of a fluorophore, this exciton typically exhibits a much longer lifetime (up to about 200 nanoseconds). For diagnostic multiplex applications, a set of seven amine-, or carboxyl-derivatized or streptavidin-labeled Qdot® nanocristals with a broad excitation and narrow symmetric emission properties (maxima at: 525, 565, 585, 605, 655, 705 and 800 nm) is commercially available (www.invitrogen.com). Although QDs have proven to be suitable labels in bioanalysis, their application in quantitative immunoassays is still limited. Ding *et al.* [90] developed a competitive Fluorescence-Linked Immunosorbent Assay (cFLISA) in a microtiter plate for the detection of sulfamethazine in chicken muscle tissue extracts using a commercially available QD (QD 655 (Quantum Dot Corp, Hayward, CA, USA) as the fluorescent label coupled to the secondary antibody. The same QD was used for the detection of enrofloxacin in chicken muscle tissue [91] and the high emission amplitude of the QD (655 nm) led to significant improvements in the signal to noise ratios of the final detected signals. Nichkova *et al.* [92] described the application of two commercially available QDs as labels in an immunoassay microarray for the simultaneous microscopic detection of two biomarkers of exposure to two major classes of compounds: pyrethroid insecticides and triazine herbicides. Goldman *et al.* [93] prepared bioinorganic conjugates of highly luminescent nanocrystals (CdSe-ZnS core-shell QDs) and antibodies to develop a fourplex immunoassay in a microtiter plate for the simultaneous detection of four toxins (cholera toxin, ricin, shiga-like toxin 1 and staphylococcal enterotoxin B) in a single well using QDs with emission maximums of 510, 555, 590 and 610 nm.

Artificial "Antibodies". The most critical and time-consuming reagent in an immunoassay is the antibody and artificial "antibodies" such as Molecularly Imprinted Polymers (MIPs) and aptamers are described as potential alternatives. These alternatives can be prepared *in vitro*, avoiding the need for animals, and against non-immunogenic and toxic targets.

MIPs have been demonstrated to be a promising class of synthetic receptors that can be tailored to meet specific end-use recognition requirements. MIP technology is a general strategy of synthesis that allows preparation of polymeric materials with "memory" of a particular molecule (analyte). Most modern imprinting is performed through a process called non-covalent imprinting in which a template molecule interacts with a functional monomer to form a pre-polymerization complex in the presence of a solvent (Fig. **7**). The solvent is known as the porogen because of its role in pore forming during polymerization. A cross-linking monomer is added to the pre-polymerization complex to form a scaffold around the binding site during polymer synthesis. The template is removed from the polymer and the result is a highly cross-linked polymer with exposed imprinted cavities capable of analyte binding. The serious problem of interferences in analysis by bleeding of residual template (analyte) was successfully solved by the use of analogs as templates [94]. For antibiotics, HPLC, as for sulfadimethoxine [95], and Molecularly Imprinted Solid-Phase Extraction (MISPE), as for fluoroquinolones [96], are the analytical techniques where MIPS have found most applications [97]. They are usually synthesized in bulk, ground, sieved, sedimented to remove fine particles and packed in columns. MIP-based SPE columns for the selective pre-concentration of the antibiotics chloramphenicol and fluoroquinolones (with high recoveries for sarafloxacin, norfloxacin, enrofloxacin, ciprofloxacin, lomefloxacin and ofloxacin) are commercially available *via* the company MIP Technologies (Lund, Sweden).

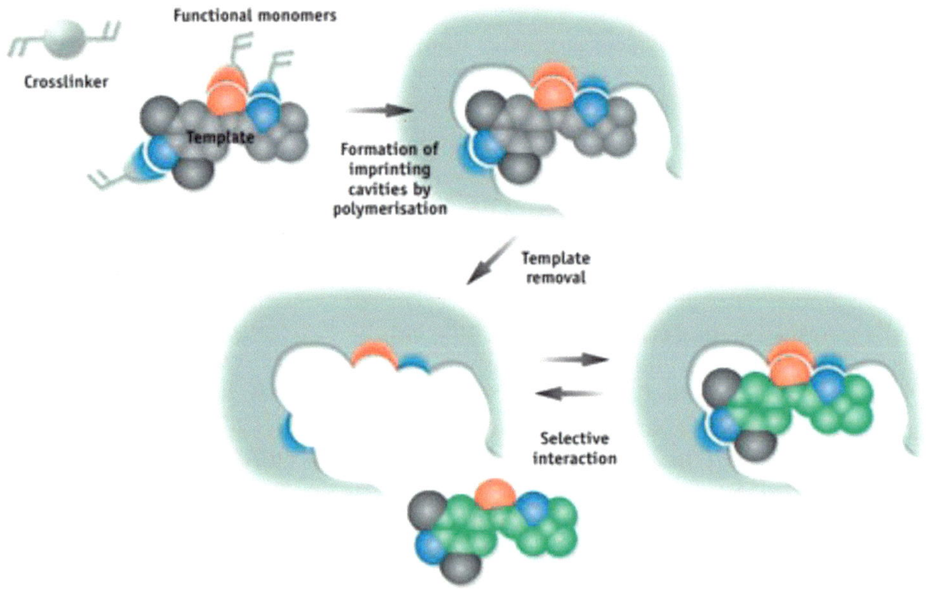

Figure 7: Production scheme of MIPs (*http://www.miptechnologies.com*).

While the selectivity, high capacity, robustness, low costs, and easy handling and synthesis of MIPs make them an ideal choice for the development of sensing devices, their use for antibiotic sensing is an unexplored field that deserves further research. In residue analysis, MIPs are most frequently described for mycotoxin detection [94, 98]. Yu and Lai [99] described an SPR sensor (Spreeta) chip surface which was covered with a thin molecularly imprinted polypyrrole (MIPPy) film by electrochemical polymerization. The same procedure was followed be Choi *et al.* [100] for the preparation of a MIPPy film with zearalenone on bare gold biosensor chips. These chips were successfully applied for the direct detection of ochratoxin A in wheat and wine extracts and zearalenone in corn extracts, which are interesting examples for future research with MIPs in optical biosensors.

Aptamers are oligonucleotides (DNA or RNA) with the ability to bind to non-nucleic acid target molecules such as peptides, proteins and antibiotics with high affinity and specificity. They are isolated from combinatorial libraries of synthetic single-stranded nucleic acids of 10^{14}-10^{15} DNA or RNA molecules containing a random region flanked on both sides with fixed primer sequences for amplification. This isolation by exponential enrichment, *via* an *in vitro* iterative process of adsorption, recovery and reamplification is known as systematic evolution of ligands by exponential enrichment (SELEX). The enriched library is cloned and sequenced, and individual sequences are chosen for their best affinity and specificity. The final selected aptamer(s) can now be produced in sizeable quantities by chemical syntheses. The high affinity of aptamers for their targets is given by their capability of folding upon binding their target molecule. They can incorporate small molecules into their nucleic acid structure or integrate into the structure of larger molecules such as proteins. Thanks to their unique characteristics and chemical structure, aptamers offer themselves as ideal candidates for use in analytical devices and techniques. The mainly clinical applications are reviewed [101-103]. Aptamers have been selected for binding to several antibiotics (tetracyclines, aminoglycosides, chloramphenicol and viomycin [104] however, they were used to study the mode of interaction of these antibiotics with RNA and not in a screening assay. Stead *et al.* [105] described the first aptamer-based and food control-related screening assay for the detection of malachite green in salmon tissue extracts. The assay uses an RNA-based aptamer with an affinity for malachite green of which the complex showed a circa 2000 times increase in fluorescence signal and this detection principle was used for the spectrofluorimetric detection. They described a rapid complex formation (within 10 min) and the complex was found to be stable for circa 18 hours. It should be mentioned that malachite green was known to bind to RNA and DNA at forehand since it has been used as an interacting dye for many years. A further broadening of aptamers into an area as food control will have to address the new challenge of complex matrices. However, just as with antibodies, MIPs and aptamers are relatively target specific.

Bio-effect related assays. For the broader detection of compounds or bio-effect related detections, the application of whole cells or other biomolecules (transport proteins or receptors) might be more interesting for future applications in food diagnostics. For the detection of tetracyclines in poultry tissue, such a whole-cell-based bioassay in a 96-well microtiter plate format, based on a genetically engineered luminescent bacterial strain containing the regulation unit of tetracycline resistance factor, has been applied [19]. This assay is better suited for high-throughput analysis and has the potential to displace growth inhibition assays. However, such bioassays are not yet described for other antibiotics although the use of the multidrug-binding repressor protein (QacR) from *Staphylococcus aureus* [20] might be an interesting approach for the future development of a multi-drug biosensor. Currently, cellular biosensors, based on various microbial species containing reporters which are specifically induced *via* selected promoters, are more widely used in pharmaceutical drug discovery and in environmental biology [21] and for monitoring environmental chemical contaminants [22] and this will also influence the development of new bioassays for the detection of antibiotics in food.

Whole cell-based assays need incubation times of a few hours and by the use of their functional ingredients (*e.g.* receptors) in multiplex diagnostic platforms, faster functional binding assays can be developed. Such fast receptor-based lateral flow tests are already commercially available for the detection of beta-lactams in combination with tetracyclines (*e.g.* Twin sensor^{TM} of Unisensor (Angleur, Belgium)). The combination of a receptor assay for β-lactams antibiotics with antibody-based assays for groups of sulfonamides and fluoroquinolones in an ELISA format has also been described as an interesting option for multi-analyte detection [53].

CONCLUSIONS

According to an EU definition (2002/657/EC), screening methods are used to detect the presence of a substance or class of substances at the level of interest with the capability for a high sample throughput. They are used to sift large numbers of samples for potential non-compliant results and they are specifically designed to avoid false compliant results. Of the multiplex technologies described above, only two of the flow cytometers have high-throughput capacities (see Table **1**).

Different potential end-users (*e.g.* farmers, inspectors, food industries, or control laboratories), require different strategies for screening (from low- to high-throughput, handheld to automated on-line devices and from single analyte to multiplex systems) and the suitability of the different technologies for the different end-users are presented in Table **1**. The dip sticks or lateral flow tests are most suitable for farmers and inspectors, because of the lack of investment in equipment, easy format and performance and speed (minutes per sample), but they are most limited in multiplex capacity and qualitative results (compliant or suspected non-compliant) are obtained. All other suggested technologies are quantitative when calibrations curves are used for the calculations of concentrations. Multiplex capacities of more than 100 (like the FlexMap 3D and iSPR) are not very useful and realistic in food control. Future multiplexing will probably consist of combinations of 5 to 25 assays and most technologies are capable of handling that. The nanoparticle-based assays are limited in multiplex capacity (<10) but some (*e.g.* LSPR) require less investment in equipment compared with the other technologies of which the cost-prices of the flow cytometers are estimated as <25 and 50 k€ for the MagPix and Luminex 200, respectively. The multiplex developments described above bring great promise for future custom-made and cost-effective screening assays in the different areas of the control of the food chain.

Table 1: The possible multiplex capacity (MC: the estimated theoretically maximum number of assays in the multiplex format), sample throughput (TP: high (H), medium (M) or low (L)), costs of investment in equipment (Inv:. high (H) >100 k€, medium (M) 25-50k€, low (L) <25 k€, or no costs (N)), application format (AF: handheld (H), automated with on-site possibility (A), or not automated (N)) and end-users of the multiplex technologies described in the future perspectives.

Technology	MC	TP	Inv.	AF	End-User		
					Farmer/ Inspector	Food Industry	Control Labs
Biosensors							
- Multichannel	20	M	H	A	-	+	+
- iSPR	>100	M	H	A	-	+	+
- Evidence	25	M	H	A	-	+	+
Flow cytometry							
- Luminex 200	100	H	M	A	-	+	+
- FlexMAP 3D	500	H	H	A	-	-	+
- MagPix	50	M	M	A	-	+	+
Nanoparticles							
- LSPR	<10	M	L	N	-	+	+
- QDs	<10	M	M	N	-	+	+
Dip sticks	4	L	N	H	+	+	-

- not or less suitable, + suitable.

REFERENCES

[1] Davey PG. Antimicrobial chemotherapy. In Ledingham JGG, Warrell DA, Eds. Concise Oxford Textbook of Medicine. Oxford, Oxford University Press, 2000; p. 1475.

[2] Gillespie JR, Ed. Modern Livestock & Poultry Production. Florence, KY, USA: Cengage Delmar Learning 2004; p. 15.

[3] EC Regulation (EC) No. 1831/2003 of the European Parliament and of the Council of 22 September 2003, on additives for use in animal nutrition. Off J Eur Union 2003; L268: 29-43.

[4] FIDIN Working Group Antibiotic policy. Antibiotic report 2006, The Hague, The Netherlands, FIDIN June 2007.

[5] FIDIN Working Group Antibiotic policy. Antibiotic report 2008, The Hague, The Netherlands, FIDIN September 2008.

[6] FIDIN Working Group Antibiotic policy, Antibiotic report 2009, The Hague, The Netherlands, FIDIN September 2009.

[7] Kümmerer K. Significance of antibiotics in the environment. J Antimicr Chemoth 2003; 52: 5-7.

[8] Council Regulation (EEC) No. 2377/90 of 26 June 1990, laying down a community procedure for the establishment of maximum residue limits of veterinary medicinal in foodstuffs of animal origin. Off J Eur Commun 1990; L224: 1-8.

[9] Council Directive 96/22/EC of 29 April 1996 concerning the prohibition on the use in stock farming of certain substances having a hormonal or thyrostatic action and of β-agonists, and repealing Directives 81/602/EEC, 88/146/EEC and 88/229/EEC. Off J Eur Commun 1996; L125: 3-10.

[10] Directive 2001/82/EC of the European Parliament and of the Council of 6 November 2001 on the Community Code relating to veterinary medicinal products. Off J Eur Commun 2001; L311: 1-66.
[11] Council Directive 96/23/EC of 29 April 1996 on measures to monitor certain substances and residues thereof in live animals and animal products repealing Directives 85/358/EEC and 86/469/EEC and Decisions 89/187/EEC and 91/664/EEC. Off J Eur Commun 1996; L125: 10-32.
[12] Commission Decision 97/747/EC of 27 October 1997, fixing the levels and frequencies of sampling provided for by Council Directive 96/23/EC for the monitoring of certain substances and residues thereof in certain animal products. Off J Eur Commun 1997; L303: 12-15.
[13] SANCO/1313/2008, Report for 2006 on the results of residue monitoring in food of animal origin in the Member States. European Commission, Health & Consumer Directorate-General, Brussels.
[14] Dey BP, Thaker NH, Bright SA, Thaler AM. Fast antimicrobial screen test (FAST): Improved screen test for detecting antimicrobial residues in meat tissue. J AOAC Int 2005; 8(2): 447-54.
[15] Cantwell H, O'Keeffe M. Evaluation of the Premi® Test and comparison with the One-Plate Test for the detection of antimicrobials in kidney. Food Add Cont 2006; 23(2): 120-25.
[16] Schneider MJ, Lehotay SJ. A comparison of the FAST, Premi® and KIS™ tests for screening antibiotic residues in beef kidney juice and serum. Anal Bioanal Chem 2008; 390: 1775-79.
[17] Pikkemaat MG, Oostra-van Dijk S, Schouten J, *et al.* A new microbial screening method for the detection of antimicrobial residues in slaughter animals: The Nouws antibiotic test (NAT-screening). Food Control 2008; 19: 781-89.
[18] Korpela MT, Kurittu JS, Karvinen JT, Karp MT. A recombinant *Escherichia coli* sensor strain for the detection of tetracyclines. Anal Chem 1998; 70: 4457-62.
[19] Virolainen NE, Pikkemaat MG, Elferink JWA, Karp MT. Rapid detection of tetracyclines and their 4-epimer derivatives from poultry meat with bioluminescent biosensor bacteria. J Agric Food Chem 2008; 56: 11065-70.
[20] Schumacher MA, Miller MC, Grkovic S, *et al.* Structural mechanisms of QacR induction and multidrug recognition. Science 2001; 294: 2158-63.
[21] Urban A, Eckermann S, Fast B, *et al.* Novel whole-cell antibiotic biosensors for compound discovery. Appl Environ Microbiol 2007; 73 (20): 6436-43.
[22] Patel PD. Overview of affinity biosensors in food analysis. J AOAC Int. 2006; 89 (3): 805-18.
[23] Toldrá F, Reig M, Methods for rapid detection of chemical and veterinary drug residues in animal Foods. Trends Food Sci Techn 2006; 17: 482-89.
[24] Gentili A. (2008) Drug residues in animal-food products. http://topics.scirus.com/Drug_residues_in_animal_food-products.html, approached on 2009-03-30.
[25] Commission Decision 2002/657/EEC of 12 August 2002, implementing Council directive 96/23/EC concerning the performance of analytical methods and the interpretation of results. Off J Eur Commun 2002; L221: 8-36.
[26] Danaher M, De Ruyck H, Crooks SRH, *et al.* Review of methodology for the determination of benzimidazole residues in biological matrices. J Chromatogr B 2007; 845: 1-37.
[27] Yuan Y, Xu C, Peng C, *et al.* Analytical methods for the detection of corticosteroids-residues in animal-derived foodstuffs. Crit Rev Anal Chem 2008; 227-41.
[28] Nielen MWF, Lasaroms JJP, Essers ML, *et al.* Multiresidue analysis of beta-agonists in bovine and porcine urine, feed and hair using liquid chromatography electrospray ionization tandem mass spectrometry. Anal Bioanal Chem 2008; 391: 199-10.
[29] Stolker AAM, Rutgers P, Oosterink E, *et al.* Comprehensive screening and quantification of veterinary drugs in milk using UPLC-ToF-MS. Anal Bioanal Chem 2008; 391: 2309-22.
[30] Kaufmann A, Butcher P, Maden K, Widmer M. Quantitative UPLC-TOF multiresidue method for 100 different veterinary drugs. Proceedings EuroResidue VI Conference 2008, Egmond aan Zee, the Netherlands, 19-21 May 2008, pp. 87-91.
[31] EC Regulation No. 178/2002 of the European Parliament and of the Council of 28 January 2002 laying down the general principles and requirements of food law, establishing the European Food Safety Authority and laying down procedures in matters of food safety. Off J Eur Commun 2002; L31:1-24.
[32] Lipman NS, Jackson LR, Trudel LJ, Weis-Garcia F. Monoclonal versus polyclonal antibodies: Distinguishing characteristics, applications, and information resources. ILAR J 2005; 46: 258-68.
[33] Maynard J, Georgiou G. Antibody engineering. Ann Review Biom Engin 2000; 2: 339-76.
[34] Bradbury A, Velappan N, Verzillo V, *et al.* Antibody in proteomics I. Trends Biotechn 2003; 21: 275-81.

[35] Brichta J, Hnilova M, Viskovic T. Generation of hapten-specific recombinant antibodies. Antibody phage display technology. A review Vet Med Czech 2005; 50: 231-52.

[36] Willats WG. Phage display: practicalities and prospects. Plant Mol. Biol 2002; 50: 837-54.

[37] Spinks CA, Bull VJ, Chambers SJ, *et al.* The veterinary drug detection puzzle: Getting the pieces to fit. Proceedings EuroResidue III Conference 1996, Rijksuniversiteit Utrecht, Faculteit Diergeneeskunde, Utrecht, the Netherlands, pp. 879-84.

[38] Korpimäki T, Rosenberg J, Virtanen P, *et al.* Improving broad specificity hapten recognition with protein engineering. J Agric Food Chem 2002; 50: 4194-01.

[39] Korpimäki T, Rosenberg J, Virtanen P, *et al.* Further improvement of broad specificity hapten recognition with protein engineering. Prot Eng 2003; 16: 37-46.

[40] Korpimäki T, Brockmann E-V, Kuronen O, *et al.* Engineering of a broad specificity antibody for simultaneous detection of 13 sulfonamides at the maximum residue level. J Agric Food Chem 2004; 52: 40-47.

[41] Korpimäki T, Hagren V, Brockmann E-V, Tuomola M. Generic lanthanide fluoroimmunoassay for the simultaneous screening of 18 sulfonamides using an engineered antibody. Anal Chem 2004; 76: 3091-98.

[42] Kramer K, Hock B. Recombinant antibodies for pesticide immunoanalysis. In Beier RC, Stanker LH, Eds. Immunoassays for Residue Analysis- Food Safety, ACS Symposium Series 621; 1996: pp. 471-84.

[43] Kramer K, Hock B. Recombinant antibodies for environmental analysis. Anal Bioanal Chem 2003; 377: 417-26.

[44] Kamps-Holtzapple C, Stanker LH. Development of recombinant single-chain variable portion of recognizing potato glycoalkaloids. In Beier RC, Stanker LH, Eds. Immunoassays for Residue Analysis- Food Safety, ACS Symposium Series 621; 1996: pp. 485-99.

[45] Haasnoot W, Korsrud GO, Cazemier G, *et al.* Application of an enzyme immunoassay for the determination of sulphamethazine (sulphadimidine) residues in swine urine and plasma and their use as predictors of the level in edible tissue. Food Addit Contam 1996; 13 (7): 811-822.

[46] Mahgoub O, Kadim IT, Mothershaw A, *et al.* Use of enzyme linked immunosorbent (ELISA) for detection of antibiotic and anabolic residues in goat and sheep meat. World J Agric Sc 2006; 2 (3): 298-302.

[47] Haasnoot W, Stouten P, Cazemier G, *et al.* Immunochemical detection of aminoglycosides in milk and kidney. Analyst 1999; 124: 301-05.

[48] Cazemier G, Haasnoot W, Stouten P. Screening of chloramphenicol in urine, tissue, milk and eggs in consequence of the prohibitive regulation. Proceedings EuroResidue III Conference, 6-8 May, 1996, Veldhoven, the Netherlands, pp. 315-19.

[49] Gaudin V, Cadieu N, Maris P. Inter-laboratory studies for the evaluation of ELISA kits for the detection of chloramphenicol residues in milk and muscle. Food Agric Immunol 2003; 15: 143-57.

[50] Huet AC, Mortier L, Daeseleire E, *et al.* Development of an ELISA screening test for nitroimidazoles in egg and chicken muscle. Anal Chim Acta 2005; 534: 157-62.

[51] Jin Y, Jang JW, Han CH, Lee MH. Development of ELISA and immunochromatographic assay for the detection of gentamicin. J Agric Food Chem 2005; 53: 7639-43.

[52] Font H, Adrian J, Galve R, *et al.* Immunochemical assays for direct sulphonamide antibiotic detection in milk and hair samples using antibody derivatized magnetic nanoparticles. J Agric Food Chem 2008; 56: 736-43.

[53] Adrian J, Pinacho DG, Granier B, *et al.* A multianalyte ELISA for immunochemical screening of sulphonamide, fluoroquinolone and β-lactam antibiotics in milk samples using class-selective bioreceptors. Anal Bioanal Chem 2008; 391 (5): 1703-12.

[54] Verheijen R, Stouten P, Cazemier G, Haasnoot W. Development of a one step strip test for the detection of sulfadimidine residues. Analyst 1998; 123: 2437-41.

[55] Wang X, Li K, Shi D, *et al.* Development of an immunochromatographic lateral-flow test strip for rapid detection of sulfonamides in eggs and chicken muscles. J Agric Food Chem 2007; 55 (6): 2072-78.

[56] Verheijen R, Osswald IK, Dietrich R, Haasnoot W. Development of a one step strip test for the detection of (dihydro) streptomycin residues in raw milk. Food Agric Immunol 2000; 12: 31-40.

[57] Xie H, Ma W, Liu L, *et al.* Development and validation of an immunochromatographic assay for rapid multi-residues detection of cephems in milk. Anal Chim Acta 2009; 634: 129-33.

[58] Kiran BR, Kale KU. Transformed E. Coli JM 109 as a biosensor for penicillin. Indian J Pharm Sci 2002; 83 (3): 205-08.

[59] Hauck S, Kosslinger C, Drost S, Wolf H. Biosensor system for the determination of ochratoxin A. In Proceedings of the 12th European Conference on Solid-State Transducers and the 9th UK Conference on Sensors and their Applications, Southampton, UK, 13-16 September 1998, EUROSENSOR XII, Ed. by N. M. White, Institute of Physics Publishing Bristol and Philadelphia, Sensors Series, volume 1, pp. 515-518.

[60] Zacco E, Adrian J, Galve R, *et al.* Electrochemical magneto immunosensing of antibiotic residues in milk. Biosens Bioelectr 2007; 22: 2184-91.

[61] Morrow KJ. Label-free biosensors show early promise; optical and nonoptical platforms are on the heel of conventional ELISA. Gen Engin Biotechn News 2007; Vol. 27, No. 4.

[62] Haasnoot W, Verheijen R. A direct (non-competitve) immunoassay for gentamicin residues with an optical biosensor. Food Agric Immunol 2001; 13: 131-34.

[63] Haasnoot W, Loomans EEMG, Cazemier G, *et al.* Direct versus competitive biosensor immunoassays for the detection of (dihydro)streptomycin residues in milk. Food Agric Immunol 2002; 14: 15-27.

[64] Haasnoot W, Cazemier G, Koets, M, Amerongen van A. Single biosensor immunoassay for the detection of five aminoglycosides in reconstituted skimmed milk. Anal Chim Acta 2003; 488: 53-60.

[65] Huet AC, Charlier C, Tittlemier SA, *et al.* Simultaneous determination of (fluoro)quinolone antibiotics in kidney, marine products, eggs and muscle by ELISA. J Agric Food Chem 2006; 54: 2822-27.

[66] Haasnoot W, Du Pré J, Cazemier G, *et al.* Monoclonal antibodies against a sulfathiazole derivative for the immunochemical detection of sulfonamides. Food Agric Immunol 2000; 12: 127-38.

[67] Haasnoot W, Cazemier G, Du Pré J, *et al.* Sulfonamide antibodies: from specific polyclonals to generic monoclonals. Food Agric Immunol 2000; 12: 15-30.

[68] Haasnoot W, Bienenmann-Ploum M, Korpimäki T, *et al.* Biosensor detection of sulfonamides: from specific to multi-sulfonamide assays. In: Amerongen van A, Barug D, Lauwaars M, Eds. Rapid Methods for biological and chemical contaminants in food and feed. Wageningen Academic Publishers 2005, pp. 321-37.

[69] Bienenmann-Ploum M, Korpimäki T, Haasnoot W, Kohen F. Comparison of multi-sulfonamide biosensor immunoassays. Anal Chim Acta 2005; 529: 115-22.

[70] Haasnoot W, Bienenmann-Ploum M, Lamminmäki U, *et al.* Application of a multi-sulfonamide biosensor immunoassay for the detection of sulfadiazine and sulfamethoxazole residues in broiler serum and its use as predictor of the levels in edible tissue. Anal Chim Acta 2005; 552: 87-95.

[71] Marchesini GR, Koopal K, Meulenberg E, *et al.* Spreeta-based biosensor assays for endocrine disruptors. Biosens Bioelectron 2007; 22: 1908-15.

[72] Dostálek J, Přibyl J, Homola J, Skládal P. Multichannel SPR biosensor for detection of endocrine-disrupting compounds. Anal Bioanal Chem 2007; 389: 1841-47.

[73] Kim SJ, Gobi V, Iwasaka H, *et al.* Novel miniature SPR immunosensor equipped with all-in-one-microchannel sensor chip for detecting low-molecular-weight analytes. Biosens Bioelectron 2007; 23: 701-07.

[74] Steiner G. Surface plasmon resonance imaging. Anal Bioanal Chem 2004; 379; 328-31.

[75] Rebe-Raz S, Bremer MGEG, Haasnoot W, Norde W. Label-free and multiplex detection of antibiotic residues in milk using surface Plasmon resonance-based immunosensor. Anal Chem 2009; 81: 7743-49.

[76] Seider M, Niessner R. Automated analytical microarrays: a critical review. Anal Bioanal Chem 2008; 391: 1521-44.

[77] Keizer de W, Bienenmann-Ploum ME, Bergwerff AA, Haasnoot W. Flow cytometric immunoassay for sulfonamides in raw milk. Anal Chim Acta 2008; 620: 142-49.

[78] Bienenmann-Ploum ME, Keizer de W, Eekelen van HDLM, *et al.* Flow cytometric immunoassay for sulfonamides in milk, blood serum, meat drip and eggs. Proceedings of the EuroResidue VI conference, 19-21 May, 2008, Egmond aan Zee, the Netherlands, pp. 425-30.

[79] Haasnoot W, Eekelen van HDLM, Bienenmann-Ploum ME, *et al.* Multiplex flow cytometric immunoassay for drug residues using the xMAP technology. Proceedings of the EuroResidue VI conference, 19-21 May, 2008, Egmond aan Zee, the Netherlands, pp. 431-36.

[80] Guo S, Dong S. Biomolecule-nanoparticle hybrids for electrochemical biosensors. Trends in Anal Chem 2009; 28 (1): 96-09.

[81] Yuan J, Oliver R, Aquilar M-I, Wu Y. Surface plasmon resonance assay for chloramphenicol. Anal Chem 2008; 80 (21): 8329-33.

[82] Azzazy HME, Mansour MMH, Kazmierczak SC. Nanodiagnostics: A new frontier for clinical laboratory medicine. Clin Chem 2006; 52 (7): 1238-46.

[83] Hutter E, Fendler JH. Exploitation of localized surface Plasmon resonance. Adv Mater 2004; 16 (19): 1685- 06.

[84] Hiep HM, Endo T, Kerman K, *et al.* A localized surface Plasmon resonance based immunosensor for the detection of casein in milk. Sci Technol Advanc Mater 2007; 8: 331-38.

[85] Kreuzer MP, Quidant R, Salvador J-P, *et al.* Colloidal-based localized surface Plasmon resonance (LSPR) biosensor for the quantitative determination of stanozolol. Anal Bioanal Chem 2008; 391: 1813-20.

[86] Prodan E, Nordlander P, Halas NJ. Electronic structure and optical properties of gold nanoshells. Nano Letters 2003; 3 (10): 1411-15.

[87] Chan WCW, Maxwell DJ, Gao XH, *et al.* Luminescent quantum dots for multiplexed biological detection and imaging. Curr Opin Biotechnol 2002; 13 (1): 40-46.

[88] Algar WR, Massey M, Krull UJ. The application of quantum dots, gold nanoparticles and molecular switches to optical nucleic-acid diagnostics. Trends Anal Chem 2009; 28 (3): 292-06.

[89] Han M, Gao, X, Su JZ, Nie S. Quantum-dot-tagged microbead for multiplexed optical coding of biomolecules. Nature Biotechn 2001; 19: 631-35.

[90] Ding S, Chen J, Jiang H, *et al.* Application of quantum dot-antibody conjugates for detection of sulfamethazine residue in chicken muscle tissue. J Agric Food Chem 2006; 54 (17): 6139-42.

[91] Chen J, Xu F, Jiang H, *et al.* A novel quantum dot-based fluoroimmunoassay method for detection of Enrofloxacin residue in chicken muscle tissue. Food Chem 2009; 113: 1197-01.

[92] Nichkova M, Dosev D, Davies AE, *et al.* Quantum dots as reporters in multiplexed immunoassays for biomarkers of exposure to agrochemicals. Anal Lett 2007; 40: 1423-33.

[93] Goldman ER, Clapp AR, Anderson GP, *et al.* Multiplexed toxin analysis using four colors of quantum dot fluororeagents. Anal Chem 2004; 76: 684-88.

[94] Urraca JL, Marazuela MD, Moreno-Bondi MC. Molecularly imprinted polymers applied to the clean-up of zearalenone and α-zearalenol from cereal and swine feed sample extracts. Anal Bioanal Chem 2006; 385: 1155-61.

[95] Hung CH, Huang YT, Hwang CC. Molecular recognition and identification of sulfapyridine and sulfadimethoxine by high performance liquid chromatography with molecular imprinted polymer as the stationary phase. J Food Drug Anal 2008; 16 (4): 8-14.

[96] Turiel E, Martín-Esteban A, Tadeo JL. Molecular imprinting-based separation methods for selective analysis of fluoroquinolones in soils. J Chromatogr A 2007; 117: 97-04.

[97] Fernández-González A, Guarida L, Badía-Laíño R, Díaz-García ME. Mimicking molecular receptors for antibiotics – analytical implications. Trends Anal Chem 2006; 25 (10): 949-57.

[98] Appell M, Maragos CM, Kendra DF. Molecularly imprinted polymers for mycotoxins in Food contaminants: In: Siantar DP, Truckness MW, Scott PM, Eds. Mycotoxins and Food Allergens, ACS Symposium Series 1001, 2008, Washington, DC., pp 152-69.

[99] Yu JCC, Lai EPC. Interaction of ochratoxin A with molecularly imprinted polypyrrole film on surface plasmon resonance sensor. React Funct Polym 2005; 63: 171-76.

[100] Choi S-W, Chang H-J, Lee N, *et al.* Detection of mycoestrogen zearalenone by a molecularly imprinted polypyrrole-based surface plasmon resonance (SPR) sensor. J Agric Food Chem 2009; 57: 1113-18.

[101] Tombelli S, Minunni M, Mascini M. Analytical applications of aptamers. Biosens Bioelectron 2005; 20: 2424-34.

[102] Hamula CLA, Guthrie JW, Zhang H, *et al.* Selection and analytical applications of aptamers. Trends Anal Chem 2006; 25 (7): 681-91.

[103] Mairal T, Özalp VC, Sánchez PL, *et al.* Aptamers: molecular tools for analytical applications. Anal Bioanal Chem 2008; 390: 989-07.

[104] Lorenz C, Schroeder R. Aptamers to antibiotics. In: Klussmann S, Ed. The Aptamer Handbook, Wiley-VCH Verlag GmbH & Co 2006, Weinheim, Germany, pp. 116-30.

[105] Stead S, Tarbin JA, Sharman M, *et al.* A novel aptamer-based procedure for the rapid detection of malachite green in fish tissue. Proceedings of the EuroResidue VI conference, 19-21 May, 2008, Egmond aan Zee, the Netherlands, pp. 71-75.

CHAPTER 7

Immunoassays for Detecting Prohibited Growth Promoters in the Food Chain

Ph. Delahaut*

CER Groupe, Rue du point du jour, 8 – B-6900 Marloie

Abstract: The use of growth promoters to fatten cattle, once widespread, is now banned or strictly regulated worldwide, with a view to protecting consumer health. The European Union, in particular, has issued directives, regulations, and guidelines for controlling such substances. Immunoassays (radioimmunoassays, ELISAs, biosensor assays) provide quick, sensitive, low-cost, and high-throughput screening tools for detecting steroids, corticosteroids, and β-agonists in live animals and meat. Their development has led, for instance, to eradication of the use of the dangerous compound diethylstilbestrol. Current challenges include the growing number of growth-promoting "black market" substances and the emergence of "cocktails" containing low levels of several mutually potentiating compounds. New analytical approaches, such as immunochemical multiplexing or the development of receptor-based assays, may contribute to meet these challenges.

Keywords: Antibodies, Immunoassays, Growth Hormones.

1. INTRODUCTION

The objective of modern agriculture is to produce a maximum of food at minimal cost in order to feed the ever-increasing world population. This is made possible by mechanization and by progress in zootechnics, as rational feeding and modern selection methods have yielded animals characterized by remarkable production. In parallel, trade globalization has considerably changed people's dietary habits.

Meat producers want to increase the amount of muscle protein while reducing the proportion of fat. The use of anabolic agents makes it possible to reach this goal more quickly by improving the conversion yield of the nitrogen ingested by the animal. The economic impact of hormones on meat production has long been known in ruminants, which are poor transformers of dietary nitrogen. The estimated weight gain is 10 to 20%. Before hormones were banned in Europe, 50 to 60% of all meat livestock in England was receiving implants while in France, 70% of calves and 50% of bulls were being treated in this manner. In the US, an estimated 90% of all meat animals receive anabolic agents.

In 1938, diethylstilbestrol (DES) became the first synthetic hormone to be used in poultry and bovines, remaining popular until the mid-1970s. Later many estrogens and androgens endowed with anabolic properties were developed by the pharmaceutical industry, the same molecules being used to increase the athletic performance of both humans and racehorses.

Under its Directive 96/22/EC [1] and 96/23/EC [2], the European Union requires its Member States to monitor certain substances and residues thereof in live animals and animal products. The directives cover two groups of substances. Group A comprises substances having a hormonal or thyreostatic action, β-agonists used in stock farming, and veterinary drugs that are now banned (Annex IV of Council Directive EC. 2377/90 [3]). Group B comprises other veterinary drugs and a list of contaminants.

Currently the fight against fraud relies essentially on control methods based on physico-chemical analysis (GCMS, LCMS, HPLC). The drawback of such methods is the limited number of samples that can be analyzed, because they are expensive and hard to implement.

***Address correspondence to Ph. Delahaut:** CER Groupe, Rue du point du jour, 8 – B-6900 Marloie; E-mail: p.delahaut@cergroupe.be

Eline P. Meulenberg (Ed)

The present chapter describes, on the one hand, the main developments and applications of classical immunological methods (radioimmunoassays, ELISAs, biosensor assays). Additionally, the aim is to present current prospects for detecting hormones and other prohibited substances such as corticosteroids and β agonists, particularly in the light of novel approaches such as multiplexing or the use of receptors, making it possible to assay many molecules simultaneously.

2. TIMELINE

It was Pasteur who, in 1880, really laid down the principles of preventive immunization against infectious disease by injection of attenuated germs. The English physician Jenner had previously applied the concept in 1798, after observing that people in contact with animals suffering from cowpox never contracted smallpox. He imagined a smallpox prevention strategy based on inoculating humans with material derived from blisters appearing on cows with cowpox.

It wasn't until 1960 that Yalow and Berson [4] proposed, for the first time, a radioimmunoassay (RIA) for a polypeptide hormone: insulin. Immunochemical methods were subsequently to undergo remarkable development, especially in endocrinology. This technique was the first to reach µg/kg-level (ppb-level) sensitivity.

Unfortunately, the penetration of such methods into the agro-food sector, which requires obtaining results quickly and near the production site, was limited by the use of radioisotopes.

In 1971, Engvall and Perlman [5] on the one hand and Van Weemen and Schuurs [6] on the other discovered the possibility of introducing an enzyme instead of a radioisotope to visualize the competition reaction. The term « ELISA» (enzyme-linked immunosorbent assay) was initially coined to describe an excess-reagent enzyme immunoassay of specific antibodies or antigens. Nowadays, the terms ELISA and EIA (enzyme immunoassay) are often used interchangeably. This type of assay is currently the most frequently used format. Later developments, emerging around the 1990s, include the Fluorescence Polarization Immunoassay (FPIA), the Time-Resolved FluoroImmunoAssay (TR-FIA), and the Dissociation Enhanced Lanthanide FluoroImmunoAssay (Delfia). These techniques enjoy limited popularity.

A new technological advance, in the early 2000s, was the development of biosensors. The main advantage of biosensor technology is the possibility of measuring a signal linked to a change in concentration of a molecule bound to the surface of a detector. Furthermore, it is not necessary to produce a tracer or a conjugate to visualize the antibody-antigen reaction. Biosensors currently have a wide range of applications requiring, unfortunately, a well-equipped laboratory.

The main problem with traditional immunoassays is that they can determine only one compound or group of compounds at a time. With the appearance of flow cytometry and the possibility of detecting microspheres of different sizes and colors, multiplexing has become possible. Microspheres coated with different antigens are detected and sorted by size and color. The other steps of the assay resemble those of an ELISA.

In parallel with these advances, many developments reflect attempts to create field-use assays (*i.e.* assays for use on the farm or in the slaughterhouse or factory). The lateral flow device is currently the most popular format for this type of development.

3. ANALYTICAL METHODS

3.1. General Considerations

To ensure product quality and protect the consumer, it is essential to have quick, reliable, low-cost, high-throughput analytical methods for monitoring foods. Immunological methods, which use antibodies and other biological reagents, have features that make them well suited for this purpose.

Such methods are called screening methods because they currently constitute ideal tools for quickly identifying a problem in the food production chain. A screening method must indicate whether a target analyte is present above or below a threshold. Generally, screening methods are qualitative rather than quantitative, but inasmuch as they yield an estimate of the analyte concentration, they are considered semi-quantitative. The percentage of false positives should be low to avoid the costs and delays linked to confirmatory testing, but it is above all imperative to avoid any risk of obtaining a false negative.

Sample screening and the identification of positive samples must be a very rapid process. This requires minimizing the extraction and purification steps as well as the cost and response time of the analysis. For positive samples it is recommended to confirm the result by means of a standard physico-chemical method (typically LC/MS or GC/MS).

In the early 1970s, the effort to detect anabolic agents focused mainly on stilbenes. One method used was the histological examination of the Bartolin glands in female animals and of the prostate in males [7]. Another was thin-layer chromatography[8]. These methods were adequate for animals receiving high doses.

Since 1975, authorities have used immunoassays reaching ppb-level sensitivity. Another advantage of this technology is its specificity for a single molecule or for a group of molecules sharing a similar structure.

There are many problems to be solved in the effort to control anabolic agents and other prohibited substances. The need to screen for a growing number of molecules increases the number of tests that have to be developed and validated. The range of molecules administered by injection, orally, or subcutaneously includes over thirty anabolic agents, as many β-agonists, and about ten corticosteroids. To tackle this problem, the ideal is to have multiresidue screening methods that can detect several molecules of the same family. Specific methods are justified when the aim is to fight the widescale use of toxic substances. In addition to the parent compound, it is often necessary to identify and detect, also at ppb level, its major metabolites. One problem is that xenobiotic metabolization may differ from one species to another. Another issue concerns the stability of the residues in their biological matrices during food transformation and conservation.

As animals can naturally produce molecules such as estradiol, progesterone, testosterone, nortestosterone [9], and boldenone [10, 11], this physiological reality must be taken into account to avoid unwarranted sanctions against well-meaning farmers.

Today most immunochemical methods for determining anabolic agents are enzymatic (of the ELISA type). Some development of biosensors has also occurred in this field. In contrast, techniques of the « dipstick » type are not frequently applied because of poor sensitivity.

3.2. Key Aspects of Immunoassays

3.2.1. Antibodies

Antibodies are the key element of any immunoassay. Hormones and veterinary medicines are haptens, *i.e.* non-immunogenic molecules with a molecular mass below 5,000. It is thus indispensable to couple them chemically to a protein, such as Bovine Serum Albumin (BSA) or Keyhole Limpet Hemocyanin (KLH), having a higher molecular mass and the ability to induce antibody production in an animal. Doses of 50 to 1,000 μg are generally used for immunizing rabbits. High doses allow a rapid response, whereas lower doses tend to favor antibody affinity [12]. The specificity of an antibody is determined by the choice of the position on the hormone at which the carrier molecule is coupled. Usually the part of the molecule that lies opposite the coupling site confers the specificity of antigen-antibody recognition. This synthesis step is crucial in the development of an immunoassay. Examples are presented later on.

Most immunoassays developed for the food sector use polyclonal antibodies, because they afford higher sensitivity than monoclonal antibodies. The amount of antiserum available for method development is seldom a problem.

Polyclonal antibodies are obtained by hyperimmunization of animals, particularly rabbits. The standard protocol involves once-monthly multisite subcutaneous injection of the immunogen, followed by blood collection about 10 days after the third injection. To increase the immune response, adjuvants are regularly associated with the immunogen. The antibodies produced during immunization result from the activity of several cell clones, hence the name "polyclonal". They thus constitute a mixture of B-lymphocyte-secreted antibodies directed against different epitopes and displaying different specificities and affinities [13].

Monoclonal antibodies [14], used increasingly since the 1970s, derive from a single cell clone. As a result, they have the same epitope specificity and binding affinity. After mouse immunization, antibody-producing lymphocytes are fused *in vitro* with myeloma cells, *i.e.* tumor cells capable of multiplying indefinitely. After various culture steps on selective media, the chosen clone will be able to produce antibodies either « *in vivo* » or « *in vitro* ».

Most immunoassays have been developed to measure individual contaminants, but it is now more advantageous to use them to identify two or more targets simultaneously. To achieve this, it is possible to raise numerous antibodies recognizing individual targets and to include all the antibodies in a single test. This approach is not cheap and there can be problems with antibody affinity. This is why it is desirable to produce a single antibody that can identify several analytes in a single test. Hapten design and assay optimization have played an important role in producing assays with appropriate specificity and sensitivity.

Recently, new techniques have emerged for modifying *in vitro* the specificity or affinity of a given antibody. Protein engineering of existing antibodies could produce a recombinant antibody capable of detecting a large number of compounds in one assay [15]. To date, however, there exist few applications in the field of anabolic steroid or β-agonist detection.

Since the 1980s, new approaches have been envisaged with a view to producing antibodies that bind whole groups or families of compounds. The alternative use of receptors has the advantage of identifying a wide range of compounds having receptor-binding activity without necessarily requiring knowledge of a substance's chemical properties. As early as 1989, Arts *et al.* [16] routinely used a receptor isolated from the calf uterus as a ligand for detecting estrogens in bovine urine samples. Similar developments have focused on β-agonists [17]. In both cases, the receptors were taken from tissues collected from animals at the slaughterhouse. Currently this technique is seldom applied because of the difficulty of adapting it for routine laboratory use, and also because biological receptors do not always recognize the whole range compounds in a target group with sufficient sensitivity [18].

To avoid these problems, the production of recombinant receptors by genetic engineering may be a good solution. As an additional advantage, this approach should offer an inexhaustible, homogeneous source of receptors. Also envisaged is plasmid-based production of recombinant proteins sharing sequence similarity with natural receptors. This technique has been used successfully to detect glucocorticoids, β-agonists, and endogenous steroids (progesterone, estrogens, and androgens) [19].

Another approach in the same line involves using steroid hormones to create cells that are sensitive to the hormones to be detected. The cells are genetically engineered to produce, in the presence of hormones, the enzyme luciferase, which catalyses the production of light through the transformation of luciferin. The cells are thus equipped with a luciferin-encoding gene (a reporter gene) under the control of a steroid response element acting as a promoter of the reporter gene when the steroid binds to its receptor. Hence, when steroids are present in a sample, the cells produce luciferase, whose activity can be measured. Cell lines have been developed for the detection of andogens, estrogens, progesterones, and glucocorticoids [20]. The best-known cell-based tests, whose principle is the same, are used to detect dioxins and related compounds (CALUX – **C**hemically **A**ctivated **LU**cifèrase gene e**X**pression).

3.2.2. Assay Formats

For detecting low-molecular-mass compounds, competitive immunoassays are generally used. The response is inversely proportional to the amount of antibody-linked substance.

Radioimmunoassays were developed in the 1970s to measure levels of anabolic steroids in animal tissues. As one cannot incorporate an ^{125}I atom directly into such molecules, the preferred approach was to replace a hydrogen atom with tritium (^{3}H), which emits β radiation. The major advantage of this technique is that the labeled molecule is immunologically identical to the antigen to be assayed [21].

In the 1980s, this technique was used to screen for DES, trenbolone, zeranol, and natural hormones. The main drawback of the tritium radiolabel is the need for specific installations for radioisotope use and waste management. RIAs are still used today to determine natural hormones in animal plasma [22].

Currently, ELISA-type immuno-enzymatic methods are more frequently used. In a competitive ELISA, the antigen is chemically coupled to an enzyme catalyzing a reaction that generates a change in optical density that depends on the amount of analyte in the sample. For detecting small molecules, there are two competitive ELISA formats. Most often, the anti-hapten antibodies are immobilized on a support. Alternatively, the immobilized antibody is an antibody directed against immunoglobulins of the species in which the anti-hapten antibodies are raised (for example, anti-rabbit immunoglobulins if the anti-hapten antibodies are raised in a rabbit). The bound antibodies can then capture the antibodies recognizing the hapten to be assayed. This procedure, which better respects the binding capacity of the anti-hapten antibody, improves the reproducibility of the assay.

In the competitive indirect ELISA, the analyte, usually coupled to a carrier protein such as bovine serum albumin, is immobilized on the solid phase. In this case, the amount of bound analyte-specific antibodies is quantified by addition of an enzyme-conjugated second antibody that specifically binds the first antibody. The competitive indirect format is not often used for the detection of prohibited growth promoters in the food chain.

There currently exist commercial ELISA kits for detecting the main anabolic agents, β-agonists, and corticosteroids in animals.

In parallel with the emergence of classical microplate ELISAs, many types of immunosensors have been described. Their aim is to solve problems related to the use of plates, such as the long incubation time required. There exist various types of immunosensors classified according to the mode of detection and type of label used.

A biosensor is an analytical device combining the specificity of a biological interaction with a transducer producing a signal proportional to the target analyte concentration [23]. The biological recognition element (an antibody, a receptor, an enzyme…) is in close contact with a signal transducer (*e.g.* optical, amperometric, potentiometric, or acoustic) coupled to a data acquisition system.

The system currently embodied in the greatest number of substance control applications in the agro-food sector is the Surface Plasmon Resonance (SPR) immunosensor. In principle, this sensor measures the mass concentration change caused by binding of an antibody (or analyte) to the corresponding analyte (or antibody) on the sensor surface [24]. The SPR phenomenon occurs when plane polarized light is reflected from a gold film deposited on a glass support. Photons react with the free electron cloud in the metal film at a specific angle, the SPR angle, and cause a drop in the reflected light. Refractive index changes near the surface give rise to a shift in the resonance angle. The shift is directly proportional to the mass increase, and mass concentration can thus be measured [25]. This analysis principle is summarized in Fig. **1**. An additional advantage of this technique is that it does not require synthesizing labeled antigens or antibodies in order to detect a signal, as in other immunoassays.

Recently, the development of a microsphere-based competitive fluorescence immunoassay had been described for the determination of low-molecular-weight compounds in food [26]. It relies on the use of microspheres of different sizes and different fluorescence intensities, to which the molecules of interest (antigens) are covalently bound. Specific antibodies bind to these antigens. Detection of the microspheres is done by multiparametric flow cytometry. Quantitation is based on the intensity of the reporter signal emitted by the primary or secondary antibody according to whether the fluorochrome is coupled to the

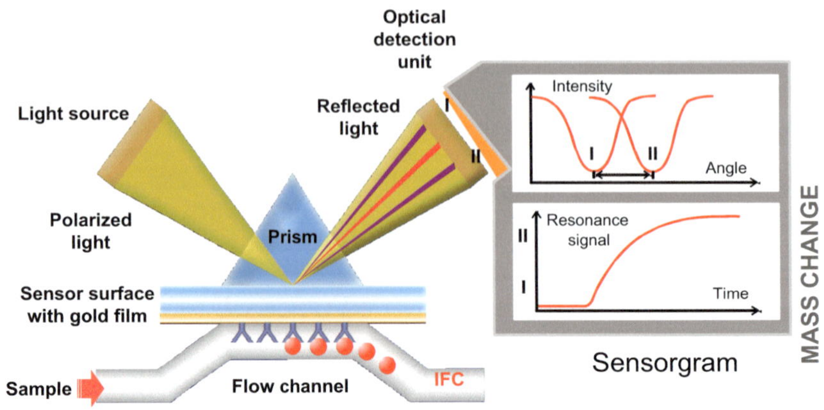

Figure 1: Principle of the Surface Plasmon Resonance (SPR) biosensor. Binding of biomolecules to the surface increases the refractive index, which induces a shift in the SPR angle. The shift is directly proportional to the mass increase.

former or the latter (Fig. **2**). This technique analyzes samples particle by particle, making it possible to sort the particles and divide them into different subpopulations. Each microsphere has a unique character in terms of size and fluorescence intensity. These different combinations make it possible to multiplex by analyzing several molecules simultaneously. To prepare a multiplexed assay, individual sets of microspheres are conjugated with the target molecules required for each reaction. In this case, the target molecules are antigens. A fluorescent reporter may be coupled directly to the specific antibody or to a secondary antibody, depending on whether the immunoassay is direct or indirect (Fig. **2**). After optimizing the parameters of each assay separately in a non–multiplexed format, the assays can be multiplexed by simply mixing the different sets of microspheres with a mixture of analytes, followed by the cocktail of antibodies. After a short incubation period, the mixture of microspheres is washed and then incubated with the fluorescent reporter. The mixture of microspheres, now containing various amounts of fluorescent reporters on their surfaces, is analyzed with a flow cytometer. Data acquisition, analysis, and reporting are done in real time on all microsphere sets included in the multiplex assay. As each individual microsphere is analyzed by the flow cytometer, all of them are classified into distinct sets on the basis of both the internal and external fluorescence values, which are recorded.

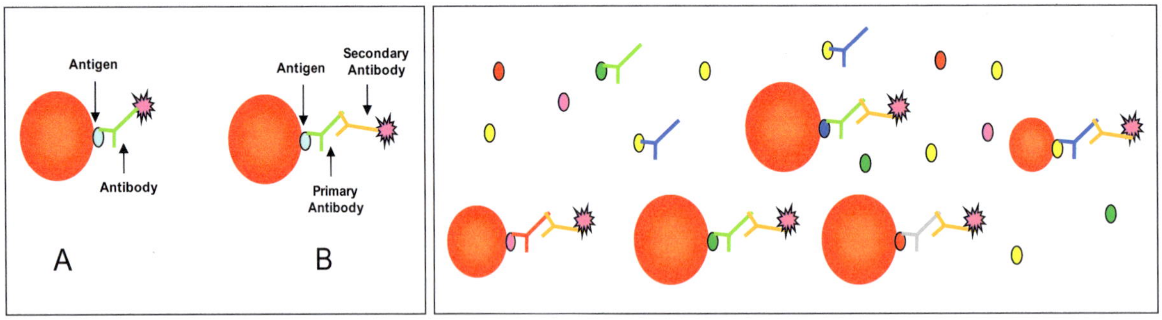

Figure 2: General principle of the direct and indirect immunoassays in which the antigen to be assayed is bound to a microsphere; Principle of multiplexing in an assay using 3 microspheres of different sizes and four different antibodies.

The main advantages of this technique are that it requires a small sample volume and offers a better surface of contact with the various reagents (due to the fact that the microspheres are in suspension). This allows higher sensitivity and a shorter incubation time.

Flow-through techniques and lateral-flow test strip assays based on an antibody-antigen reaction have few applications, to date, in prohibited substance detection, although they are used routinely for molecules such as antibiotics in milk or mycotoxins in cereals. The first tests were made for the detection of human chorionic gonadotrophin (hCG) [27]. Many format variants are possible, but they all have in common the formation of a complex between a detector particle that is free in the sample and a capture reagent bound to the membrane at the test line.

Such tests are applicable directly on the farm or in the slaughterhouse, so that animals passing the screening test can be placed rapidly on the market.

3.2.3. Validation

In the European Union, a group of experts has defined the criteria that routine and confirmation methods must meet. These criteria are laid down in EC Council Directive 2002/657 [28]. In this text, here is no mention of immunological methods; the emphasis is on physico-chemical (confirmation) methods. More recently, a working group has been elaborating *guidelines for initial validation and transfer of screening methods*, but to date these guidelines are not binding and they are subject to much discussion, especially as regards their applicability in real-life situations. It is requested, however, that the values of the following parameters be specified for newly developed immunoassays:

The decision limit (CCα): the limit at and above which it can be concluded with an error probability of α that a sample is positive. For the prohibited substances of EC Council Directive 96/23/EC [2], the error α (percentage of false negatives) must be below 1%. To determine this criterion it is necessary to analyze at least 20 different biological « blanks » per type of matrix. The decision limit is calculated from the mean of the value obtained plus three standard deviations.

The detection capacity (CCβ): the smallest quantity of substance that can be detected in a sample with an error probability of β. For prohibited substances (tolerance level zero), the detection capacity is the lowest concentration at which a method can identify samples that are really contaminated with a statistical certainty of 1-β. For all substances of Directive 96/23/EC, the error β (percentage of false positives) must be below 5%. For this, one can analyze 20 blanks spiked with a concentration of analyte near the decision limit. To the value obtained one adds the standard deviation multiplied by1.64 to obtain the detection capacity.

Recovery: the percentage of the real concentration of a substance recovered in the analysis. To estimate the recovery rate, samples are spiked at different concentrations and the quantity recovered is measured for each sample.

Specificity: the capacity of the method to generate signals related to the presence of the analyte, to the exclusion of all other compounds. In immunoassays it is important to use appropriate extraction and purification procedures to avoid matrix effects as much as possible. The specificity of immunoassays is measured above all by calculating the cross-reactivity of the antiserum with related molecules and metabolites.

The standard curve can yield an estimate of the amount of analyte present in a sample. Five different concentrations are required to establish a standard curve. In some cases it may be necessary to prepare a standard curve in the biological matrix so as to avoid errors due to potential interferences.

Robustness: the sensitivity of a method to variations of certain experimental parameters. These factors may be numerous and hard to identify.

The stability must be determined by testing the main reagents at different temperatures.

Common control strategies integrate a combination of immunological methods for screening and physico-chemical methods for confirmation of positive results.

4. MOLECULES IN CURRENT USE

Anabolic agents are molecules that are very active in muscle cell formation in both humans and animals. It is hard to classify them in a manner that is relevant to all uses. They can be classified according to their structure (steroid or non-steroid), their origin (endogenous or exogenous), or their pharmacological activity.

The classes generally distinguished in the steroid group include androgens, estrogens, and progestagens; their basic structure is the sterane nucleus, whose backbone resembles that of cholesterol. This backbone includes four rings: three hexagonal rings called A, B, and C and one pentagonal ring (D). The carbon atoms are numbered as in Fig. **3**.

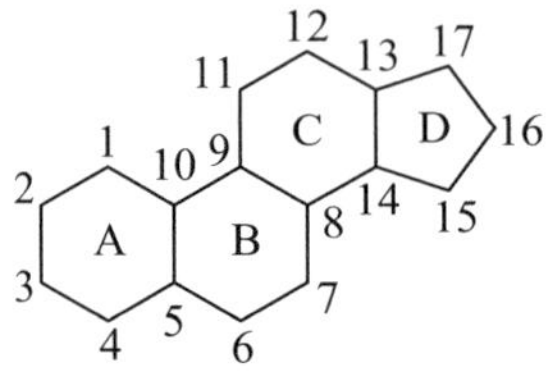

Figure 3: Basic structure of steroids : the sterane nucleus.

Only the stilbenes and the lactones like zeranol derived from resorcylic acid do not share this basic structure.

Other groups used fraudulently to fatten cattle are the corticosteroids and β-agonists.

4.1. Estrogens (Fig. 4)

Natural estrogens (17β-estradiol, estrone, and estriol) are essentially synthesized in the ovaries and placenta. These hormones participate in the regulation of many physiological processes of the reproductive system, such as ovulation, fertilization, implantation of the embryo, and lactation. Natural and synthetic estrogens ensure the sexual development of females. They are little used in veterinary therapeutics.

Alongside these endogenous molecules there exist synthetic molecules with similar activity. Ethinylestratiol is frequently used in association with progestagens in contraceptive pills.

The stilbenes (diethylstilbestrol, hexestrol, and dienestrol), whose chemical structure is different, display strong estrogenic activity. Their use is formally prohibited in all countries because of carcinogenic effects observed in women and their descent.

Zeranol, originally extracted from molds of the type « *Giberella Zea* », displays rather low estrogenic activity but a real anabolic effect. This molecule is used in the US as an implant placed at the base of the ear in bovines.

Immunoassays are available for all molecules of this group. Details of their development are presented later in this chapter.

4.2. Androgens (Fig. 5)

This family includes many synthetic molecules in addition to natural testosterone. The development of synthetic testosterone analogs has led to the appearance of new molecules with anabolic effects. Because these derivatives have short half-lives, they are most often administered as esters offering prolonged action through release of the active principle.

Indications for the use of androgens in veterinary therapeutics are very limited, but to increase spectacularly the musculature of athletes and animals, trenbolone and stanozolol are very effective.

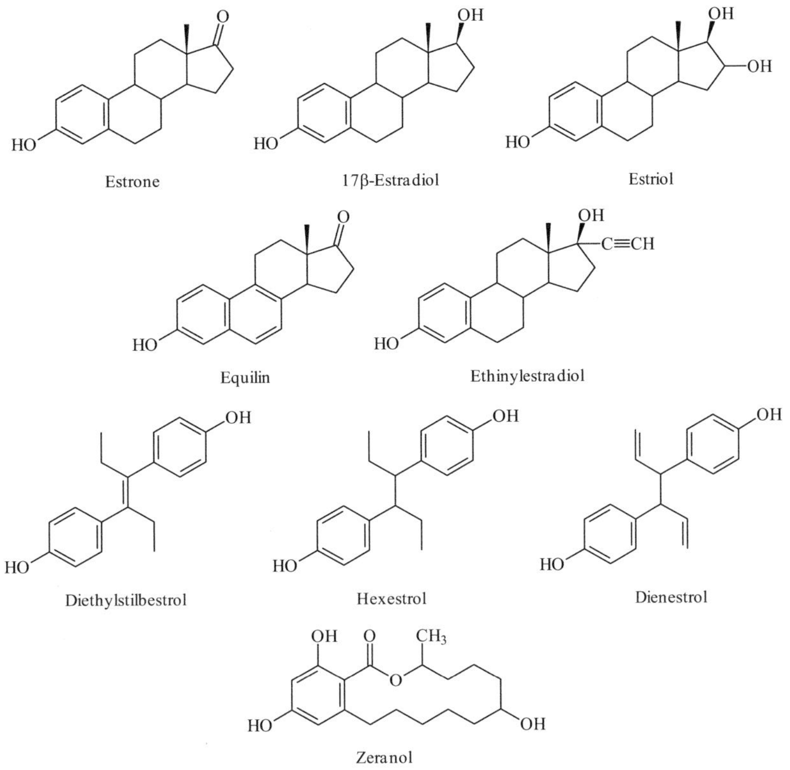

Figure 4: Chemical structures of the main estrogens.

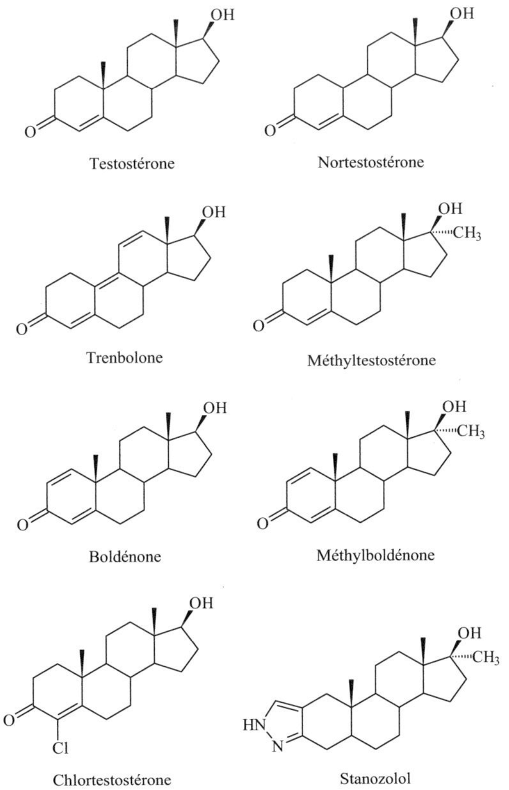

Figure 5: Chemical structures of testosterone and of the main synthetic androgens.

4.3. Progestagens (Fig. 6)

There exist both natural (progesterone) and synthetic molecules with progestative activity. Progesterone is produced by the corpus luteus and placenta. Its role is to prepare for and maintain pregnancy.

In the cocktails used to "anabolize" animals, progestagens are often associated with estrogens and androgens to avoid the disturbances of sexual behavior often caused by these molecules (agitation, untimely mounting…).

Screening for these compounds is done on samples of perirenal fat, where high concentrations can accumulate. Several immunoassays are currently available for this group of molecules.

Progesterone, an endogenous hormone, has been analyzed for years by RIA for early diagnosis of gestation [29].

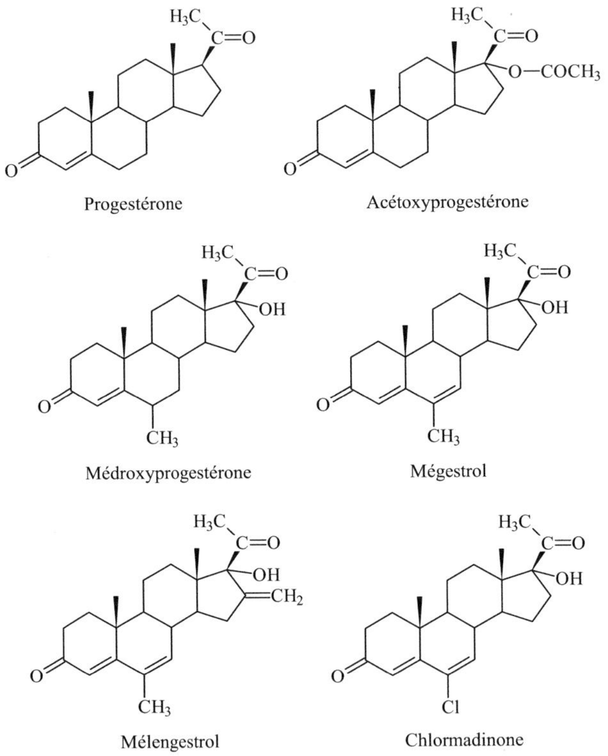

Figure 6: Chemical structures of progesterone and of the main synthetic progestagens.

4.4. β-Agonists (Fig. 7)

In response to the prohibition of anabolic agents and to the development of sensitive methods for detecting their residues in animal tissues, new substances capable of increasing animal body mass have emerged: the β-agonists. Initially, clenbuterol was prescribed for the treatment of respiratory deficiencies in horses and bovines. Various studies have shown that the products belonging to this family also have the ability to decrease the proportion of fat and increase the amount of muscle. They have been called fat-distributing agents. Their chemical structure resembles that of natural catecholamines like adrenalin. The use of clenbuterol is strictly regulated in Europe [28]. In pig production in the US, only ractopamine is authorized, and the same applies to zilpaterol in Mexico.

Several cases of poisoning due to clenbuterol misdosing in animal feed have been reported in people having consumed contaminated livers. Symptoms include muscle twitching, tachycardia, palpitations, and nervousness.

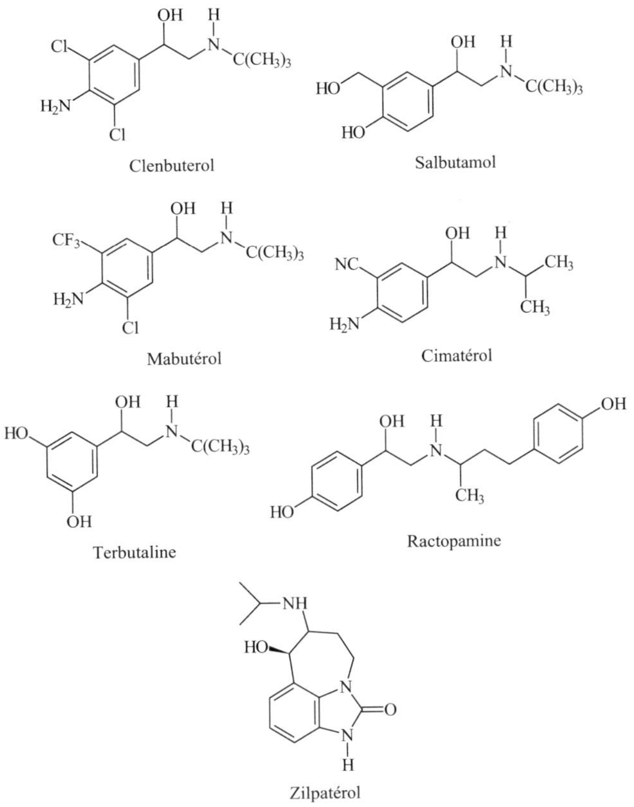

Figure 7: Chemical structures of several β-agonists.

4.5. Glucocorticosteroids (Fig. 8)

The only features distinguishing different glucocorticosteroids from one another are their levels of anti-inflammatory activity and mineralocorticoid activity and the duration of their action. These molecules are indicated in veterinary therapeutics for all pathologies involving an acute or chronic immune or inflammatory process. They induce a catabolic effect and favor neoglucogenesis. These substances are not anabolic agents. Livestock farmers use them because they favor water retention and meat tenderness.

Dexamethasone and its isomer betamethasone, along with triamcinolone acetophenide, are the molecules most often found in controls carried out in various countries.

5. IMMUNOLOGICAL METHODS FOR THE DIFFERENT GROUPS

5.1. Natural Hormones

Controlling the use of natural hormones in animals is difficult, because exogenous and endogenous molecules are chemically highly similar. A quantitative method is required to distinguish animals that have been treated with estradiol, testosterone, or progesterone from ones that have not. Immunochemical assays (RIAs or ELISAs) are recommended because they afford ppb- or even ppt-level sensitivity [30].

Physiological levels vary in animals according to sex, age, and season. Some pathological conditions are associated with abnormal levels.

The plasma level of *testosterone* varies between 1 and 4 µg/l in male bovines aged 4 to 7 months, reaching about 10 µg/l in adult bulls. Testosterone secretion is pulsatile, and in the same animal, major nyctemeral variations occur. Furthermore, lower plasma levels of this hormone are observed in bulls treated with testosterone esters than in untreated animals. This is due to the fact that pituitary stimulation mechanisms are altered by this exogenous input. For control purposes, the recommended threshold for testosterone is 10 μg/l in males less than six months old and 30 μg/l in older males. In non-gestating females, the threshold is around 0.5 μg/l.

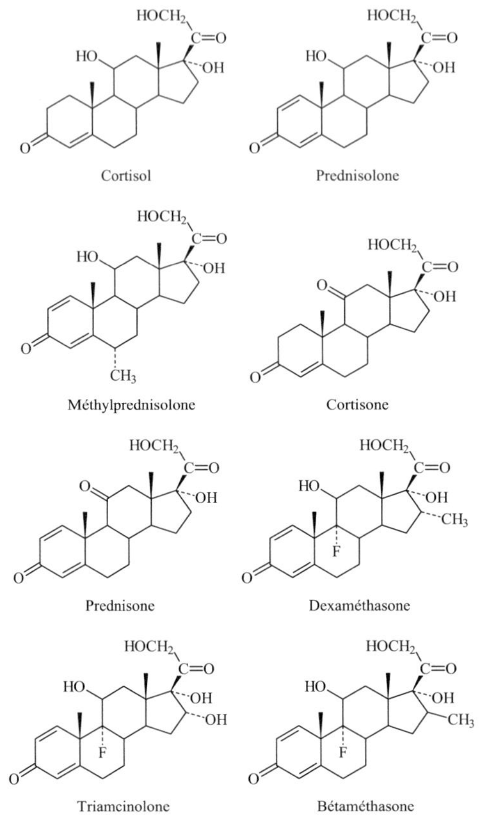

Figure 8: Chemical structures of the main glucocorticosteroids.

Plasma levels of *17β–estradiol* are about 0.01 to 0.02 μg/l in cows during the estral phase. The compound can be free or conjugated. Most authors refer to the free titer measured by means of an RIA. A preliminary purification step is recommended in order to reduce potential matrix interferences. An animal is considered treated with an estradiol preparation if the measured titer is above 0.04 μg/l.

The RIA for *progesterone* has been used since the 1970s for early diagnosis of gestation in cows, between day 21 and 24 post-insemination. In pubescent females, plasma levels range between 0 and 10 μg/l.

Tissue concentrations of these three steroids are low, and increase very little in treated animals.

Table **1** shows the main characteristics of the RIAs used in our laboratory to monitor endogenous steroids. The tritium-labeled tracers are commercially available, and the various polyclonal antibodies are produced from the immunogens indicated in the table [31]. The progesterone and estradiol assays are relatively specific, but interferences are greater for exogenous and endogenous molecules in the RIA for testosterone.

Several ELISA-type assays have been described for these steroids and are used extensively in clinical chemistry.

Development and validation of a biosensor-based immunoassay for progesterone in milk is described in [32]. Its detection limit was 3.56 ng/ml, as opposed to 1 ppb for RIAs and ELISAs.

Table 1: Main characteristics of RIAs for natural hormones.

Hormone	Radioactive Tracer	Antibody	Concentration at 50 % B/B0 (ng/ml)	Main cross-Reactions (%)	
Testosterone	[1α, 2α-^{3}H (N)]-Testosterone	Testosterone-3-CMO-BSA	0.13	Testosterone	100
				Boldenone	50
				Dihydrotestosterone	32
				Nortestosterone	19
17β-Estradiol	[2,4,6,7,16,17-^{3}H]-Estradiol	17β-Estradiol-6-CMO-BSA	0.06	17β-Estradiol	100
				Estrone	1.40
				17α-Estradiol	0.47
				Estriol	0.12
Progesterone	[1 α, 2α-^{3}H (N)]-Progesterone	Progesterone-3-CMO-BSA	0.20	Progesterone	100
				21α-Hydroxyprogesterone	3.16
				17α-Hydroxyprogesterone	1.90
				Pregnenolone	1

In the late 1980s, a dipstick for determining progesterone in milk appeared on the market, for quick on-farm diagnosis of pregnancy by farmers and veterinarians. Applied to a milk sample 21 to 24 days post-insemination, this test shows whether the animal is pregnant or not. In a non-pregnant animal the progesterone level remains at its base level in milk, but in a gestating animal the level in milk exceeds 10 ng/ml. The test is an enzymatic test in which the antibody is bound to the solid phase. Its low popularity is due to the difficulty of interpreting quantitative progesterone levels. It is more suitable as a semi-quantitative assay.

5.2. Stilbenes

The various scandals linked to the use of these substances in the early 1980s made necessary the early development of immunochemical methods for effective control.

A determining step turned out to be organic synthesis of the various derivatives, the antibody used being produced from an ether formed with one of the hydroxyl groups of DES (preferably an ether very sensitive to hydrolysis) [33]. The mixed anhydride process was used for hapten binding to free amino groups on BSA (Fig. **9**).

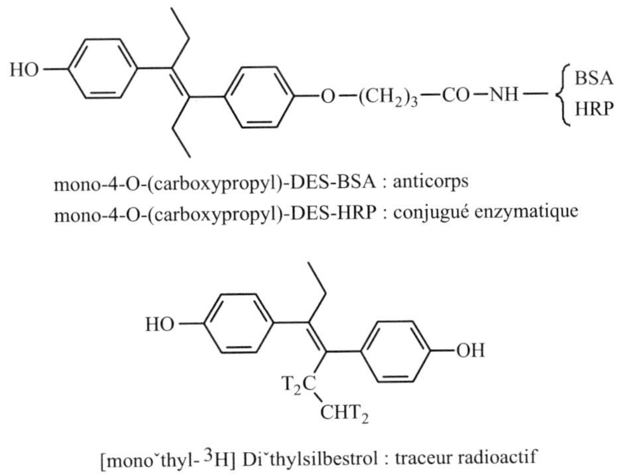

Figure 9: Chemical structures of the immunogen, the radioactive tracer, and the enzyme conjugate in the DES assay.

The radioactive tracer ([monoethyl-^{3}H] diethylstilbestrol) was produced by introducing a tritium atom on one of the ethyl groups of DES [33]. Since the 1990s this reagent has no longer been commercially available, making it necessary to prepare an enzymatic conjugate by binding an enzyme (horseradish peroxidase, HRP) to a mono-4-O-(carboxypropyl)-diethylstilbestrol derivative [34]. The pathway of synthesis is the same as for preparing the immunogen, except that an enzyme is used instead of bovine serum albumin (Fig. **9**).

The concentration at 50% binding in the RIA is 0.3 ng/ml and the cross-reactions with dienestrol and hexestrol yield respectively about 3 and 1%. In the ELISA, 50% binding is observed at 0.8 ng/ml, but the cross-reactions with dienestrol and hexestrol yield 10%. The positive impact of these immunologogical methods is demonstrated by the fact that DES is no longer used in animal production.

5.3. Synthetic Androgens, Estrogens, and Progestagens

In the identified black-market cocktails, androgens are often associated with estrogens and progestagens, so that each compounds is present only at low dosage. Product effects are additive and the concentration levels to be determined are low.

The multiplicity of molecules and the similarity of their structures to those of testosterone and some of its metabolites, which may be produced in large quantities in animals, have complicated the task of developing a multiresidue test for *synthetic androgens* (Fig. **5**). The only assays of interest are those for nortestosterone and stanozolol.

Trenbolone (Fig. **5**), a potent anabolic agent developed by Roussel-Uclaf, is authorized in the United States for fattening bovines. Its principle metabolite 17α-trenbolone is found in the liver, kidneys, urine, and feces, whereas its unaltered form (17β-trenbolone) is found in muscle and fat.

The first RIA for trenbolone residues could detect them down to 0.1-µg/l concentration [27]. Later on, ELISAs with equivalent performance levels were developed [35]. Depending on whether the aim is to detect one form specifically (17α- or la 17β-trenbolone) or both molecules simultaneously in the same assay, immunogen synthesis is different. Assay specificity is determined by the choice of the site on the hapten to which the BSA molecule is coupled. By coupling the albumin or the enzyme to trenbolone-17β-hémisuccinate, one obtains an aspecific system in which the antibody shows strong cross-reactivity towards trenbolone, its epimer, and its metabolites (Table **2**). To assay α-trenbolone or β-trenbolone specifically, it is necessary to start with a carboxymethyloxime of the molecule to be assayed (Table **2**) [31]. This example is a perfect illustration of the analytical performance level attainable with an immunological test by varying the chemical structure of some of its elements.

Table 2: Main characteristics of ELISAs developed to assay trenbolone.

ELISA	Antibody	Conjugate	Cross-Reactions (%)			Concentration at 50 % of B/Bo (ng/ml)
			17β-Trenbolone	17α-Trenbolone	Triendione	
Generic	17β-Trenbolone-17-hemisuccinate-BSA	17β-Trenbolone-17-hemisuccinate-HRP	100	54	100	0.30
α-Trenbolone	17α-Trenbolone-3-carboxymethyloxime-BSA	17α-Trenbolone-3-carboxymethyloxime-HRP	0.03	100	0.10	0.20
β-Trenbolone	17β-Trenbolone-3-carboxymethyloxime-BSA	17β-Trenbolone-3-carboxymethyloxime-HRP	100	< 0.02	0.10	0.30

Stanozolol is another potent synthetic androgen used regularly by high-level athletes and in meat animals. Its chemical structure is close to that of methyltestosterone, except for a pyrazole ring attached to cycle A (Fig. **10**). It is not possible to use the same ELISA to detect the use of stanozolol in humans and bovines, because animals and humans metabolize this compound differently (Fig. **10**). In man, stanozolol is metabolized to 3'-hydroxystanozolol and 4β-hydroxystanozolol, whereas in bovines, 16β-hydroxystanozolol appears as the preponderating metabolite (Fig. **10**) [36].

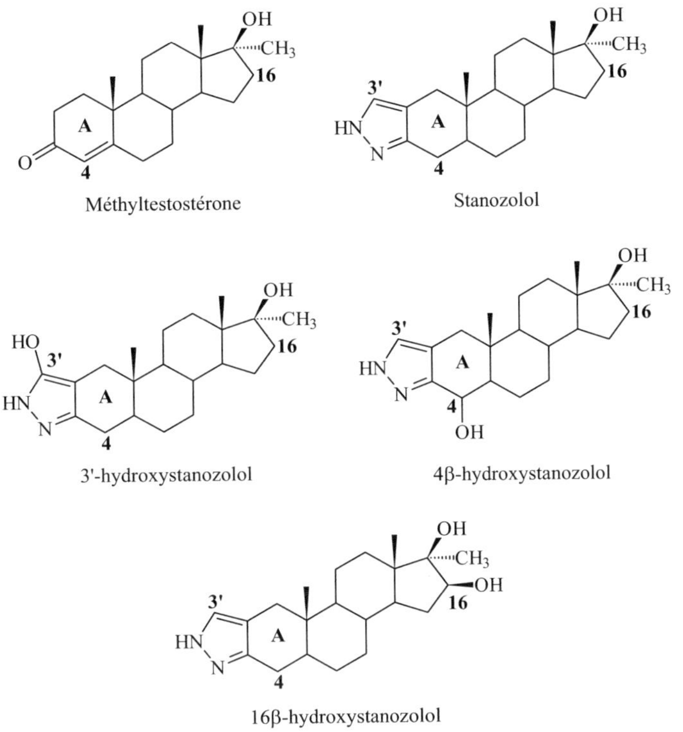

Figure 10: Chemical structures of methyltestosterone, stanozolol, and the metabolites of stanozolol.

Interferences due to the presence of large quantities of testosterone metabolites in human urine prevent the development of an immunoassay for detecting stanozolol. For bovines, on the contrary, we have successfully raised an adequate antibody with a stanozolol-17-carboxymethyloxime hapten coupled to KLH. We then coupled this antibody to the enzyme HRP to produce the conjugate. This test displays 100% cross-reactivity between stanozolol and 16β-hydroxystanozolol, but only 0.01% and 0.3% cross-reactivity with 3'-hydroxystanozolol and 4β-hydroxystanozolol respectively. The concentration allowing 50% binding (B/Bo) is about 0.3 ng/ml [36]. This example illustrates the importance of species-specific metabolism of the products administered. Among the other assays developed for androgens, the test for *nortestosterone* has proved quite useful in eradicating large-scale use of this compound.

In the *estrogen* family (Fig. **4**), assays for ethinylestradiol and zeranol have been validated for detection of residues in animal production. The main difficulty encountered in attempts to develop and RIA for *ethinylestradiol* was the necessity of producing an antiserum insensitive to the endogenous estrogens secreted by cows, particularly when they are in heat or gestating. To this end we hyperimmunized rabbits with the derivative 17α-ethinylestradiol-6-carboxyméthyloxime coupled to albumin [37]. In this way, positions C3 and C17 of the sterane nucleus (features of 17β-estradiol and of its main metabolites) were left free.

Zeranol is sold in the US as an implant to be placed at the base of the ear in bovines. Many immunoassays (RIAs and ELISAs) exist on the market [38]. One should remain cautious when interpreting the results, however, because ingestion of mycotoxin-contaminated feed (yielding zeranol or its metabolites) may lead to false positives.

Synthetic progestagens are sought in samples of perirenal fat, where they accumulate in unchanged form to high concentrations. The usual way to detect them is thin-layer chromatography followed by LC/MS. Currently, there exists on the market only one generic ELISA for the molecules of this group [39].

5.4. β-Agonists

In the late 1980s a « black market » for β-agonists (particularly clenbuterol) developed in Europe. These molecules are active when administered orally and they are quickly eliminated in the urine and feces without being metabolized. An immunoassay was needed because of several cases of severe poisoning observed in humans having consumed contaminated beef.

In 1991, a specific RIA for detecting clenbuterol in bovine plasma, urine, and feces was validated [40].

To obtain a generic test detecting all compounds of the group, it was necessary to use a succinyl derivative of salbutamol to raise the antibody [41]. The only molecules not recognized by this antibody were those possessing a second aromatic cycle (*e.g.* fenoterol and ractopamine). The sensitivity of β-agonist detection can be significantly increased by using a heterologous system (a clenbuterol tracer and an anti-salbutamol antibody).

Many ELISAs have appeared on the market since the development of this first immunoassay. To obtain an enzyme conjugate, the enzyme is bound to clenbuterol by diazotization. Table **3** shows the main features of the tests developed for molecules of this group [31].

Table 3: Main characteristics of RIAs and ELISAs for detecting β-agonists.

Tests	A	B	C	D	E	F
Concentration at 50 % of B/B0 (ng/ml)	0.40	0.13	1.05	1.13	0.43	0.32
Cross-reactions (%)						
- Clenbuterol	100	100	100	100	60	115
- Salbutamol	8	100	18	82	100	100
- Mabuterol	100	60	143	40	44	65
- Cimbuterol	100	100	96	99	18	-
- Terbutaline	9	30	8	34	20	31
- Clenpenterol	-	62	41	31	50	-
- Mapenterol	-	30	61	8	32	-
- Cimaterol	3	15	9	8	9	13

A – RIA : antibody anti-clenbuterol – tracer ^{3}H clenbuterol.

B – RIA : antibody anti-salbutamol – tracer ^{3}H clenbuterol.

C – ELISA : antibody anti-clenbuterol – conjugate clenbuterol-HRP.

D – ELISA : antibody anti-salbutamol – conjugate clenbuterol-HRP.

E – ELISA : antibody anti-clenbuterol and anti-salbutamol – conjugate clenbuterol-HRP.

F – ELISA : antibody anti-salbutamol – conjugate salbutamol-HRP.

Manufacturers aim to cover as many molecules as possible at µg/l-level sensitivity. For this it is necessary to introduce a preliminary extraction-purification step.

A comprehensive evaluation of existing tests was carried out in 1996 by the β-agonist reference laboratory [42]. Control laboratories use these tests routinely to detect β-agonists in various matrices such as urine, feces, hair, and eyes.

Detection of most $ß_2$ agonist residues by use of a surface plasma resonance biosensor was validated by Traynor and coworkers in 2003 [43]. In 2001, Johansson [44] published a description of a sensor chip for simultaneous detection of $ß_2$ agonists and synthetic hormones such as ethinylestradiol, trenbolone, and hexestrol.

A bioassay based on a solubilized $ß_2$ adrenoreceptor as a group-specific binding protein has been validated for detecting a wide range of $ß_2$ agonists. The assay is specific and its sensitivity is closely related to the biological activity of the different substances [45].

To date, intense monitoring has practically led to the eradication of the use of these molecules in Europe.

5.5. Glucocorticosteroids

Dexamethasone is the glucocorticosteroid on which efforts to develop immunochemical tests have focused most intensely, the main reason being large-scale misuse of drugs intended for treating inflammation in animals.

To produce the immunogen, coupling to the protein can be done at position C3 or C6 on the sterane nucleus or at C21 on the side chain carried by C17 (Fig. **8**). The results obtained to date with different systems do not allow total elimination of interferences due to endogenous substances (notably cortisol). This problem can be solved by including a step of purification by High Performance Liquid Chromatography (HPLC), with collection of the dexamethasone fraction.

6. CONCLUSIONS

There is an increasing consumer demand for quality food. To meet this demand, adapted legislation and high-performance analytical techniques are needed. Several European directives produced in recent years address these issues.

A problem arising in this field is the growing number of new substances on the « black market ». Each year new substances with anabolic properties and used as growth promoters are detected. This phenomenon is also well known in high-level sports. Another problem is the generalized use of cocktails where each substance is present in small amount and thus more difficult to detect, but whose various constituents act synergistically to produce an effect similar to that obtained with a single substance at higher dosage. For analysis, control laboratories have immunological screening methods and physico-chemical techniques for confirming initial positive results.

Screening methods must be quick, sensitive, and easy to implement. Around the 1970s, emphasis was on developing RIAs for detecting specific single compounds, but the disadvantages of using radioactive tracers later led laboratories to develop ELISAs. This approach led in turn to stopping the use of DES, whereas the physico-chemical methods of the time couldn't cope with the large numbers of samples to be analyzed. This success led some fatteners to use cocktails associating several molecules potentiating each other's effects.

From this time onward it became necessary to develop multiresidue tests for detecting molecules of a same family. Unfortunately this approach has not always been possible, notably for the many synthetic androgens. Methods based on mass spectrometry have made it possible to bridge this gap.

Progress in the development of new immunoassays always depends on the availability of antibodies having the desired specificity and affinity. The current trend is to produce antibodies capable of detecting several analytes in a single test. To reach this goal, innovative immunochemical and recombinant approaches should be favored.

New developments are oriented towards producing tests for use directly on the farm or in the slaughterhouse. Immunosensors may constitute an advantageous alternative to standard ELISAs.

Because they are easy to use and sensitive, immunochemical techniques are and always will be an ideal means of detecting anabolic agents. Since the 1970s, they have amply proven their efficacy.

REFERENCES

[1] EC Council Directive 96/22, Off J Eur Commun 1996; L 125: 3.

[2] EC Council Directive 96/23, Off J Eur Commun 1996; L 125: 10.

[3] EC Council Directive 2377/90, Off J Eur Commun 1990; L 224: 1-8.

[4] Yalow, R. Remembrance project: origins of RIA. Endocrinology 1991; 129(Pt 4): 35-6.

[5] Engvall E, Perlmann P. Enzyme-linked immunosorbent assay (ELISA), quantitative assay of immunoglobulin G. Immunochemistry 1971; 8: 871-4.

[6] Van Weemen B, Schuurs A. Immunoassay using antigen-enzyme conjugates. FEBS Lett 1971; 15: 232-6.

[7] Schilt R, Groot MJ, Berende, PLM *et al.* Pour on application of growth promoters in veal calves: analytical and histological results. Analyst 1998; 123: 2665-70.

[8] Verbeke R. Sensitive multi-residue method for detection of anabolics in urine and in tissues of slaughtered animals. J Chromatogr 1979; 177: 69-84.

[9] Scarth J, Akre C, van Ginkel L *et al.* Presence and metabolism of endogenous androgenic-anabolic steroid hormones in meat-producing animals: a review. Food Addit Contam Part A 2009; 26 (5): 640-71.

[10] Arts C, van Baak M, Haenen G, van der Greef J. Œstrogen radioreceptor assay for the screening of bovine urine for œstrogenic anabolic compounds. Food Addit Contam 1993; 6: 103-16.

[11] Arioli F, Gavinelli M, Fraccchiolla M *et al.* Evaluation of boldenone formation and related steroids transformations in veal faeces by liquid chromatography/tandem mass spectrometry. Rapid Commun Mass Spectrom 2008; 22: 217-23.

[12] Fodey T, Gree N, Crooks S. Antibody production: Low dose immunogen vs. low incorporation hapten using salmeterol as a model. Anal Chim Acta 2009; 637: 328-32.

[13] Leenaars P, Hendriksen C, Deleuw W *et al.* The production of polyclonal antibodies in laboratories in laboratory animals report and recommendations of ECVAM workshop. Atla 1999; 27: 79-102.

[14] Köhler G, Milstein C. Continuous culture of fused cells secreting antibody of predefined specificity. Nature 1975; 256: 495-7.

[15] Korpimäki T, Hagren V, Brockmann E-V. Tumola M. Generic lanthanide fluoroimmunoassay for the simultaneous screening of 18 sulfonamides using an engineered antibody. Anal Chem 2004; 76: 3091-8.

[16] Arts C, Van Den Berg H. Multi-residue screening of bovine urine on xenobiotic oestrogens with an oestrogen radioreceptor assay. J Chromatogr 1989; 489: 225-34.

[17] Helbo V, Vandenbroeck M, Maghuin-Rogister G. Development of a radioreceptor assay for the β2 adrenergic agonists. Arch Lebensmittelhyg 1994; 45: 57-61.

[18] Hasnoot W, Schilt R. Immunochemical and receptor technologies. In: O'Keeffe M, Ed. Residue Analysis in Food. Priniciples and Application. Amsterdam, Harwood Academic Publishers, 1999; pp. 107-44.

[19] Scippo M.-L, Willemsen, S, Danyi, S *et al.* Receptor-based screening assays: new perspectives in anti-doping control. Chromatographia 2004; 59: 1-5.

[20] Willemsen P, Scippo, M-L, Maghuin-Rogister G *et al.* Use of specific bioluminescent cell lines for the detection of steroid hormone (ant)agonists in meat producing animals. Anal Chimica Acta 2002; 473: 119-26.

[21] Franchimont P. Les principes généraux des dosages radio-immunologiques. Ann Biol Clin 1970; 28: 3-14.

[22] Scippo M-L, Gaspar P, Degand G. *et al.* Control of the illegal administration of natural steroid hormones in urine and tissues of veal calves and in plasma of bulls. Anal Chim Acta 1993; 275: 57-74.

[23] Mulchandani A, Bassi AS. Principles and applications of biosensors for bioprocess monitoring and control. Crit Rev Biotechnol 1995; 15: 105-24.

[24] Patel PD. (Bio)sensors for measurements of analytes implicated in food safety: a review. Trends in Analytical chemistry 2002; 21: 96-115.

[25] Stenberg E, Persson B, Roos H, Urbaniczky C. Quantitative determination of surface concentration of protein with surface plasmon resonance by using radiolabelled protein. J Colloid Inter Sci 1991; 143: 513-26.

[26] Zou M, Gao H, Li J *et al.* Rapid determination of hazardous coumpounds in food based on a competitive fluorescence microsphere immunoassay. Anal Biochem 2008; 374: 318-24.

[27] David GS, Greene HE, Immunometric assays using monoclonal antibodies. US 4376110. 1983.

[28] EC Council Directive 2002/657, Off. J Eur Commun. 2002; L 221: 8-36.

[29] Delahaut P, Beckers JF, Ectors F. Diagnostic de gestation chez les différentes espèces animales. Ann Méd Vét 1978; 122: 205-8.

[30] Scippo M-L, Maghuin-Rogister G. Methods of detection and surveillance of natural sex steroid hormones. In: Scientific Conference on Growth Promotion in Meat Production; 1995; Brussels, Belgium: European Commission, Directorate-General VI Agriculture; 1996. pp 541-66.

[31] Delahaut P. In: Méthodes d'analyses immunochimiques pour le contrôle de qualité dans les IAA. Arbault P, Daussant J, Eds. Paris, Lavoisier Tec et Doc, 2005; pp 197-220.

[32] Gillis E, Gosling J, Sreenan J, Kane M. Development and validation of a biosensor-based immmunoassay for progesterone in bovine milk. J Immunological Methods 2002; 267: 131-38.

[33] Rombauts P, Pierdet A, Jouquey A. Préparation et propriétés d'immunsérums anti-diéthylstilbestrol. C R Acad Sc Paris 1973; 277(D): 1921-24.

[34] Degand G, Schmitz P, Maghuin-Rogister G. Enzyme immunoassay screening procedure for the synthetic anabolic estrogens and androgens, diethylstilbestrol, nortestosterone and trenbolone in bovine urine. J Chromatogr 1989; 489: 235-43.

[35] Jouquey A, Mouren M, Salmon J. Méthodes de dosage de la trenbolone. In: Meissonnier E, Ed. OIE Symposium Anabolisants en production animale; 1983; Paris, France: OIE; 1984. pp 447-65.

[36] Delahaut P, Tailleu X, Dubois M *et al.* Detection of stanozolol metabolites in bovine urine after intramuscular injection. Arch Lebensmittlhyg 1998; 49: 3-7.

[37] Delahaut P, Bodson P, Dubois, M *et al.* Mise au point du dosage radioimmunologique de l'éthynylœstradiol: application à des bovins traités. Ann Med Vét 1990; 134: 155-60.

[38] Wang S, Wang XH. Analytical methods for the determination of zeranol in animal products: a review. Food Addit Contam 2007; 24(6): 573-82.

[39] Hageleit M, Daxenberger A, Meyer H. A sensitive enzyme immunoassay (EIA) for the determination of melengestrol acetate (MGA) in adipose and muscle tissues. Food Addit Contam 2001; 18(4): 285-95.

[40] Delahaut P, Dubois M, Pri-Bar I *et al.* Development of a specific radioimmunoassay for the detection of clenbuterol residues in treated cattle. Food Addit Contam 1991; 8: 43-53.

[41] Degand G, Bernes-Duyckaerts A, Delahaut P, Maghuin-Rogister G. Determination of β-agonists in urine by an anti-salbutamol antiserum. Anal Chim Acta 1993; 275: 241-7.

[42] Hahnau S, Jülicher B. Evaluation of commercially available ELISA test kits for the detection of clenbuterol and other β2-agonists. Food Addit Contam 1996; 13: 259-74.

[43] Traynor I, Crooks S, Bowers J, Elliott C. Detection of multi-β-agonist residues in a liver matrix by use of a surface plasma resonance biosensor. Anal Chim Acta 2003; 483: 187-91.

[44] Johansson A, Hellenäs K.-E. Sensor chip preparation and assay construction for immunobiosensor determination of beta-agonists and hormones. Analyst 2001; 126: 1721-27.

[45] Boyd S, Heskamp H; Bovee T *et al.* Development, validation and implementation of a receptor based bioassay capable of detecting a broad range of ß-agonists drugs in animal feedingstuffs. Anal Chim Acta, 2009; 637: 24-32.

CHAPTER 8

Application of Antibodies in the Field of Environmental Analysis – An Overview

Eline P. Meulenberg*

ELTI Support VOF, Ambachtsweg 5, 6581 AX Malden, The Netherlands

Abstract: The application of antibodies for environmental analysis has a long history. In the first few years there have been developed several immunoassays, predominantly EIAs/ELISAs, for the detection of pesticides in water, which have been reviewed by many authors. Subsequently, the formats of the immunoassays were changed from enzyme immunoassays to fluorescent, (chemi/bio) luminescent, polarization fluorescent and other assays and from tube or microtiter plate to flow injection, lateral flow strips, dipstick, immune biosensor assays, *etc.* The goal was always to design faster and more sensitive assays. In addition, the range of target compounds was substantially extended. Initially, the more polar pesticides were chosen as target compounds for analysis because of their simple couplings chemistry for the synthesis of tracers and coating conjugates. However, more apolar pesticides followed as well as various industrial pollutants and even toxins and microorganisms. In the last few years, the attention was focused on other unwanted compounds present in the environment, such as Endocrine Disrupting compounds (EDC) and pharmaceuticals. Given the development in other fields of investigation, such as analytical chemistry, toxicology and bioassays, the list of emerging target compounds is increasing.

In this chapter, an overview is given of the development of immunoassays in various formats from the earlier days until now. In addition, attention will be given to various target compounds and organisms as well as the basis of selection.

Keywords: Antibodies, Immunoassays, Immunosensors, Environmental Application, Pollutants, EDC, Obesogens.

1. INTRODUCTION

The first real immunoassay, a radioimmunoassay (RIA), was developed by Yalow & Berson [1, 2] for the measurement of insulin in blood. The usefulness of immunoassays was soon recognized in the field of environmental analysis. The same problems of a complex matrix and low concentrations of target compounds made the immunoassay highly suitable to detect, quantify and monitor *e.g.* pesticides in the water environment. Because radioisotopes were not appropriate in the scope of environmental analysis due to their disposal and health problems, the introduction of enzyme tracers in the enzyme immunoassay (EIA) or the Enzyme Linked-Immunosorbent Assay (ELISA) was a great step forward in the safety and applicability of such immunoassays [3]. Initially, they were used in environmental analysis for the detection and monitoring of water pollution, the presence of pesticides on crops and for natural toxins. To this end, immunoassays were developed either in-house or purchased commercially.

From the nineties of last century there was published a logarithmically increasing number of articles and reviews with regard to the development of immunoassays formats for all kinds of matrices, such as surface water, drinking water, effluents, rain, snow, sediments, soil, food, blood, *etc.* In addition, there were great advances at the field of antibody production (polyclonal, monoclonal, recombinant, phage antibodies, antibody fragments), the synthesis of immunogens in the case of small compounds, and tracer conjugates. In particular, target compounds lacking active groups for coupling of proteins for the synthesis of immunogens, coating conjugates or tracers appeared to be a challenge. Some haptens had to be resynthesized such that they contained a coupling site. Another challenge comprised the production of

***Address correspondence to Eline P. Meulenberg:** Ambachtsweg 5, 6581 AX Malden, The Netherlands; E-mail: E.Meulenberg@eltisupport.nl highly, single-compound specific or broad-spectrum antibodies. In this case, the site of coupling is crucial for the specificity or cross-reactivity of the antibodies.

With the increase in immunoassays and applications there also was a need for protocols, validation procedures and norms. When established, immunoassays could be used as validated analytical methods comparable with standard analytical methods such as GC and HPLC.

In the course of time, many new target compounds were found based on contaminants detected with conventional analysis, new findings in toxicology and exposure data.

All of the above subjects will be discussed in this chapter, with a short view on the newest and future applications. Biosensors or immunosensors will only form a minor part because they are subject of other parts of this book.

2. IMMUNOCHEMICAL METHODS

Methods using antibodies as main component are called immunochemical methods. They include immunoassays, immunoaffinity chromatography, lateral flow immunotests, dipsticks, immunosensors (see *e.g.* [4]). In all of these systems antibodies are used to bind their target, followed by detection of this binding event and optionally calculation of the concentration of the target; except in immunoaffinity chromatography, where antibody on a solid phase is used to isolate, purify and/or concentrate the target compound. Various formats of the above systems have been described, as well as the application of the different antibody forms and fragments. For the interested reader I refer to some text books and reviews about the different types of antibodies and their characteristics [5, 6] the production of antibodies including recombinant antibodies and fragments [7-9], the design of immunogens derived from haptens [10-13], labels used [14-20], the principle and design of immunoassays [13, 21-23], the advantages and disadvantages of immunoassays for environmental assays [24], standardization, validation, interpretation/calculation, norms, guidelines and user's guides [25-32]. And of course the various chapters in this book provide excellent descriptions of the different fields. In this chapter the main focus will be on the application of antibodies and immunochemical methods for environmental analysis and target compounds will be extensively described.

3. TARGET COMPOUNDS IN IMMUNOASSAYS

Pesticides

In order to protect crops against all kinds of infestations and to prevent weed growth pesticides have been used for many years in high amounts. Soil, water and sediment have been polluted and crops contaminated. Due to their inherent toxicity their presence is unwanted, especially in drinking water and food. The first immunoassays to be used for environmental detection and monitoring comprised those for pesticides, industrial pollutants and some of their metabolites. Reviews listing in-house and/or commercially available assays, ideally including some parameters such as detection limit, working range, cross-reactivities, precision and matrix effects, were published by several authors [12-14, 20, 21, 33-47]. Table **1** summarizes the different target pesticides and the immunoassay formats for environmental analysis. Other matrices such as fruit, food, feed, biological fluids *etc.* are excluded.

Table 1: Pesticides as targets in immunoassays (compiled from reviews of 1988-2003).

Target	***Format***	***Kit***
2,4-D	RIA/ELISA/	
EIA/FIA/FFIA		+
2,4,5-T	RIA/ELISA	+
Alachlor	ELISA/EIA	+

Table 1: cont…

Aldicarb	ELISA/EIA	+
Aldrin	ELISA	+
Allethrin	ELISA	
Atrazine	ELISA/EIA/	
FIA/FFIA		+
Benomyl/Carbendazim	ELISA/EIA/RIA	+
Bentazon	ELISA	
s-Bioallethrin	ELISA	
Bioresmethrin	ELISA	+
Blasticidine S	ELISA	
Bromacil	ELISA	
Captan	ELISA/EIA	+
Carbaryl	ELISA/EIA	+
Carbofuran	ELISA/EIA	+
Clomazone	ELISA	
Chlordane	ELISA	+
Chloropyrophosmethyl	ELISA	
Chlorotoluron	ELISA	+
Chlorpyrifos	ELISA/EIA	+
Chlorsulfuron	ELISA	+
Chlorthalonil	EIA	+
Chlorpyrifos	ELISA/EIA	+
Clomazone	ELISA	
Cyanazine	EIA	+
Cyclodiene	ELISA	+
Cypermethrin	ELISA	
Cyclopiazonic acid	ELISA	
DDE	ELISA	+
DDT	ELISA	+
Diazinon	ELISA	
Dichlorprop	FIA	
Dieldrin	ELISA	+
Dichlfop-methyl	EIA	
Dichlorprop	RIA	
De-ethylatrazine	ELISA	
Diflubenzuron	ELISA	
Diuron	ELISA/FFIA	+
Endosulfan	ELISA	+
Endrin	ELISA	+
Fenitrothion	ELISA	+
Fenoxycarb	ELISA	+
Fenpropimorph	ELISA	

Table 1: cont...

Heptachlor	ELISA	+
Hydroxyatrazine	ELISA	
Imazapyr	ELISA	+
Imazaquin	ELISA	+
Imazethapyr	FFIA	
Imazmethabenz	EIA	
Ioprodione	ELISA	
Irgarol	FFIA	
Isoproturon	ELISA	+
Lindane	ELISA	+
Linuron	ELISA	+
Malathion	ELISA	
MATP	ELISA	
Mecoprop	ELISA	
Metalochlor	ELISA	+
Metazachlor	ELISA	
Methabenzthiazuron	ELISA	
Metalaxyl	ELISA	+
Methomyl	ELISA	+
Methoprene	ELISA	+
Metolachlor	EIA	+
Metribuzin	EIA	+
Metsulfuron	ELISA	+
Molinate	ELISA	
Monolinuron	ELISA	
Norflurazon	ELISA	
Paraquat	ELISA/EIA	+
Paraoxon	ELISA	
Parathion	ELISA	+
PCP	ELISA	+
Permethrin	ELISA	
Picloram	RIA/EIA	
Procymidone	ELISA/EIA	+
Propazine	ELISA/FIA	+
Pirimiphos	ELISA	+
Simazine	ELISA/FIA	
Soman	ELISA	
Sulfathiazole	ELISA	
Sylvex	EIA	+
Triadimefon	ELISA	
Trichlorpyridinol	EIA	+
Terbutylazine	ELISA	

Table 1: cont…

Terbutryn	ELISA	
Thiobencarb	ELISA	
Trifluralin	ELISA	+
Triasulfuron	ELISA	+
Triclopyr	ELISA	+
Terbutryn	ELISA	+

Legend: RIA, radioimmunoassay; EIA, enzyme immunoassay (tube assay); ELISA, enzyme-linked immunosorbent assay; FIA, fluorescent immunoassay; FFIA, flow-injection fluorescent immunoassay; +, kit available. Specifications of the immunoassays are to be found in the respective reviews and kit inserts.

The above immunoassays developed were based on the need to detect the presence of pesticides in several environmental matrices, in particular surface and ground water and soil. They were selected as target compounds on the basis of several criteria: 1. their use for crop protection; 2. persistence; 3. toxicity; 4. occurrence in (drinking) water or food; 5. conventional analytical methods. Results of the analyses can be used to trace sources, lower the used amounts to prevent human exposure or for remediation purposes. At the field of drinking water production, especially from surface water, it is particularly important to screen and monitor the presence of polar pesticides that may pass purification devices. Examples are chlorophenoxy acetic acid pesticides that are used as herbicides on crop fields and for weed control in urban areas in spring time and that are present in run-off water and enter surface water, especially after rain periods. Due to their highly polar nature they have been found in drinking water in certain periods. At levels above a certain limit the intake of surface water for the production of drinking water is stopped, a situation that has occurred several times in the Netherlands.

In addition to the immunoassays for pesticides as listed above from reviews for the period 1988-2003, many more immunoassays for pesticides have been published after that time. These included newly developed pesticides, those resulting from advanced analytical techniques, immunoassays with improved sensitivity or specificity, immunoassays with broad-spectrum versus single-compound specificity, assays adapted for alternative matrices, and immunoassays in alternative format. For example, the RIA/ELISA/EIA formats as listed in Table **1** are heterogeneous assays requiring a step of separating bound and free fraction after the immunochemical reaction. To avoid this separation step the fluorescence polarization immunoassay has been developed, which is based on the increase in fluorescence polarization of fluorescent-labeled small antigens when bound by specific antibody. An overview of target compounds has been given by Smith & Eremin (2008) [48]. Further developments include immunosensors that represent label-free, real-time immunoassays. Such devices have the advantage of very short assay times and high sensitivity; however, the equipment is often quite expensive. Several reviews about principles, types and application fields have been published [49-57]. Immunosensors for specifically for pesticides and other environmental pollutants have also been reviewed. [58-62]; pathogens as targets for immunosensors are discussed by Wark *et al.* (2010) [63].

Toxins

Many microorganisms produce and secrete toxins, often as metabolites, that are harmful for humans and animals upon exposure. Such microorganisms include fungi/molds, algae, dinoflagellates, diatoms, bacteria and cyanobacteria both in the terrestrial and aqueous environment. The need to detect such toxins in order to avoid health problems after consumption of contaminated food and feed was recognized already in the 70-ies of last century. Fungal mycotoxins present on/in food and feed present a worldwide problem. For example, one group consists of fumonisins and contamination of harvested crops, food and feed has been extensively reviewed by Weidenbörner (2001) and Binder (2007), respectively [64, 65]. Although the analysis of marine toxins is predominantly performed in food, these target compounds are not strictly environmental, but given their origin and efforts to protect consumers, immunoassays developed for such toxins are worth mentioning. For an overview of natural toxins occurring in food, see Dolan *et al.* (2010) and Gerssen *et al.* (2010) [66, 67]. Marine toxins are divided in shell fish toxins according to their effect: amnesic shellfish poisoning (ASP, *e.g.* domoic acid), diarrheic shell fish poisoning (DSP, *e.g.* okadaic acid, dinophysis toxins, pectenotoxins), Neurotoxic

Shellfish Poisoning (NSP, *e.g.* brevetoxins), paralytic shellfish poisoning (PSP, *e.g.* saxitoxin); ciguatera fish poisoning. In some cases, analysis of sea water has also been performed. Bacterial toxins can cause diseases worldwide, especially in disaster areas and bad hygienic circumstances. The development of antibodies against toxins by the immunization of laboratory animals poses some serious problems in that on the one hand pure toxins are not easily available or very expensive, and on the other hand immunization procedures have to be performed very carefully due to the toxicity of the compounds. Initially, toxins were detected by mouse bioassays, but it will be clear that immunoassays and immunosensors offer many advantages in terms of animal use, costs and time. Reviews about mycotoxin assays using biosensor technology have been given by Pohanka *et al.* (2007) [68] and Prieto-Simón *et al.* (2007) [69]. A further use of antibodies against mycotoxins is in immunoaffinity chromatograpy (IAC), wherein the particular antibody is coupled to column solid support and used to isolate, purify, concentrate and even quantify mycotoxins. For most of the mycotoxins IAC columns are commercially available. Mycotoxins as targets for immunoassays are listed in Table **2**, marine toxins in Table **3**, and bacterial toxins in Table **4**.

Reviews regarding immunochemical detection methods for toxins have been given by Pestka *et al.* 1995, Tseng 1995, Trucksess 2001, Urusov *et al.* 2010 (mycotoxins) [21, 70-72] Märtlbauer & Becker 1996, van Emon & Lopez-Avila 1992, Pimbley & Patel 1998 (bacterial toxins) [73, 35, 74], Vilarino *et al.* 2009, 2010, Camacho *et al.* 2007, Taitt *et al.* 2008, Wang & Wang 2008, Posthuma-Trumpie *et al.* 2009, Fremy *et al.* 2006 (mycotoxins, bacterial toxins, microcystins) [75-80], and marine toxins by Fremy *et al.* 1999 and Humpage *et al.* 2010 [81, 82]. In addition, further ELISAs for brevetoxins, domoic acid, okadoic acid and saxitoxin were developed [83-88]. Palytoxin, a very potent marine toxin, was the target compound for the development of an ELISA using phage display technology [89]. Recent advances comprise the development of antibody-based biosensors for toxin detection, including a multi-analyte array biosensor, reviewed by several authors [75, 78, 79] and applied already in 1999 for the detection of fumonisins in maize [90]. Marine toxins have also been subject of several recent international cooperation projects. Additional data about RIAs, ELISAs and fluorescence polarization immunoassay for mycotoxins in feed can be found in a report of Yu *et al.* (1999) [91].

Table 2: Mycotoxins as targets for immunoassays.

Target	***Format***	***Kit***
Aflatoxins	RIA/ELISA/IS/IA	+
Citrinine	ELISA	n.a.
Cyclopropiazonid acid	ELISA	+
Deoxynivalenol	ELISA/IS/IAC	+
Diacetoxyscirpenol	ELISA	n.a.
Ergot alkaloids	ELISA	+
Fumonisin	ELISA/FFIA/IS/IAC/	
	FPIA	+
Fusachromanone	ELISA	+
Fusarenone	ELISA	n.a.
Ochratoxin	ELISA/IS/IAC	+
Patulin	ELISA	n.a.
PR toxin	RIA	+
Rubratoxin	RIA	+
Sterigmatocystins	ELISA	+
T-2 toxin	ELISA/IS/IAC	+
Trichothecenes	RIA/ELISA	+
Zearalenone	ELISA/IS/IAC	+

Legend: See Table 1; IS = immunosensor; IAC = immunoaffinity chromatograph; n.a. = not available.

A large survey of the presence of mycotoxins and derivatives produced by *Fusarium, Aspergillus* and *Penicillium* in wheat and maize samples using ELISA kits and compared to HPLC was described in 1998 by Curtui *et al.* [92]. Various other food, feed and liquid matrices were subject of the development of methods for analysis of mycotoxins with immunochemistry [93-101]. The chemical structure of *e.g.* aflatoxin is given in Fig. **1**.

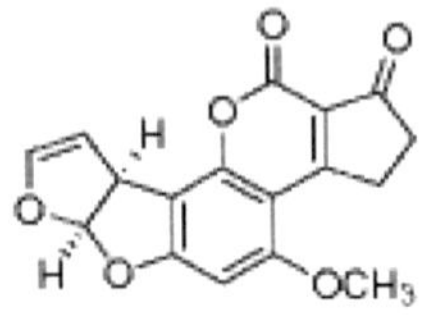

Figure 1: Chemical structure of aflatoxin.

Table 3: Marine toxins as targets for immunoassays.

Target	***Format***	***Kit***
ASP toxins	ELISA	+
Azaspiracid	ELISA	+
Brevetoxin	RIA/ELISA/IS	n.a.
Calyculin	n.a.	
Ciguatoxins	RIA/ELISA/SIA	+
Cyclic imines	n.a.	
Domoic acid	ELISA/IS	+
Dinophysistoxins	IS	n.a.
DSP toxins	ELISA	+
Gempylotoxin	n.a.	
Gonyautoxin	ELISA	n.a.
Okadaic acid	RIA/ELISA/IS	+
Palytoxin	ELISA	n.a.
Pectenotoxin	n.a.	
PSP toxins	ELISA	+
Saxitoxins	ELISA/IS	+
Tetrodotoxin	ELISA/IS	n.a.
Yessotoxin	ELISA	+

Legend: See Table **1** and **2**.

Individual antibodies and immunoassays developed for toxins include those for domoic acid [102], okadaic acid [84], ciguatoxin [103], saxitoxin [86]. A stick test for ciguatoxin was patented [104]. The possibility of using a battery of ELISAs for screening of marine toxins in shellfish extracts was described by Garthwaite *et al.* (2001) [105]. An example of the chemical structure of a marine toxin, saxitoxin, is given in Fig. **2**.

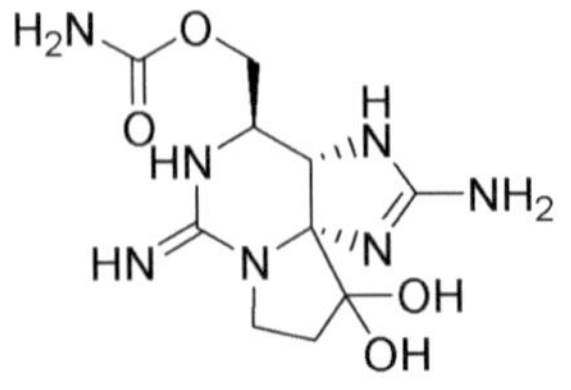

Figure 2: Chemical structure of saxitoxin.

Table 4: Bacterial toxins as targets for immunoassays.

Target	*Format*	*References*
Anthrax	EIA	[106]
Botulinum toxins	FIIA/IS	[107-111]
Cholera toxin	ELISA/IS	[112-116]
Clostridium toxins	ELISA	[117, 118]
Diphtheria toxin	ELISA	[119, 120]
Staphylococcus toxins	ELISA/FIA/SIA	
	IS/ELIFA/IAC	[111, 121-142]
Tetanus toxin	ELISA	[143,144]
Verotoxin	ELISA	[145-150]

Legend: See Tables **1** and **2**; FIIA = flow injection immunoassay; ELIFA = Enzyme-linked immunoflow assay.

Toxins of cyanobacteria, *i.e.* microcystins, cyanotoxins, nodularins, anatoxins, cylindrospermopsin, constitute a distinct problem as they occur worldwide in fresh water used for recreational purposes. Contact of humans or animals with microcystins causes skin and lung problems, but they are also hepatotoxic, neurotoxic and carcinogenic [151-154]. In periods with high temperatures and low wind the cyanobacteria may lead to algal blooms with levels of up to 6000 μg/l, whereas surface water samples may contain also very high concentrations of microcystins (see Fig. **3**). The EU has set a limit of 10-20 μg/L for recreational waters, in which case either a warning is given or water recreation is prohibited. Microcystins have even caused incidents in wild animals in Africa [155-158]. An overview of members of the family of cyanobacterial toxins and physicochemical and biochemical detection methods is given by Codd *et al.* (2001) and Sangolkar *et al.* (2006) [159,160]. There are commercial immunoassays kits available for quantitative screening [161]. However, as the appearance of algal blooms can be quite sudden and the ELISA takes at least two days from sampling to result, there is a need for on-site detection of microcystins. Various in-house immunoassays for the detection of microcystins and application in water have been described in several publications [162-170]. The development of immunosensors was also reported, including an SPR-based biosensor for detection of microcystins in drinking water [171-175]. Recently, cyanobacterial toxins have also been detected by immunoassay in brackish water and the marine environment [176,177].

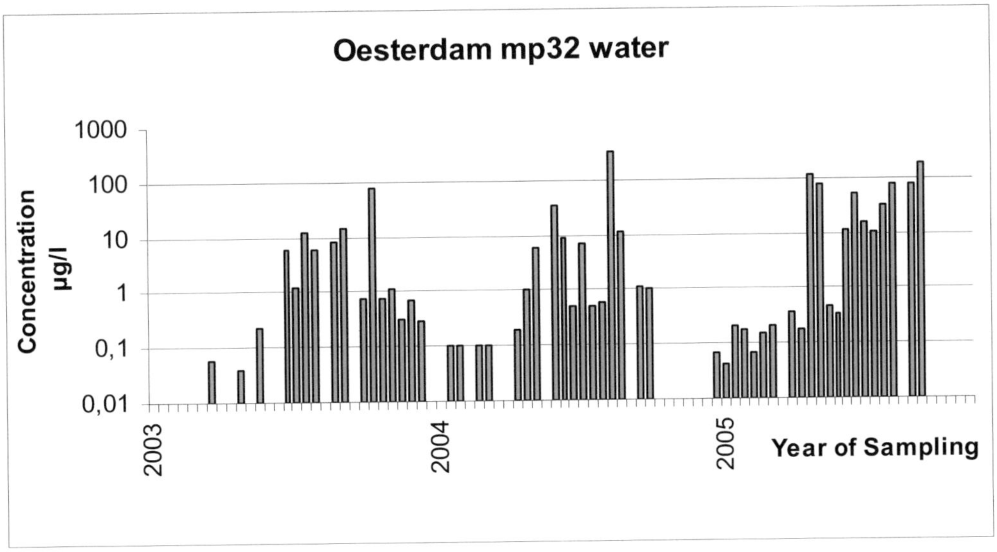

Figure 3: Concentrations of microcystins in recreational surface water in the province of Zeeland (the Netherlands) measured with an ELISA kit over 3 years.

Industrial Pollutants

Among anthropogenic pollutants that may be toxic and a threat for human health are industrial pollutants and residues of combustion and fuel spills, such as PAH, PCBs, dioxins, flame retardants, BTEX, phenolics, organic solvents and explosives. Some of these are highly toxic and they are ubiquitous in the environment, especially in soils. The need to localize and quantify such compounds was recognized in the 80-ies and various immunoassays and kits have been developed and applied for environmental analysis to locate polluted sites and for remediation purposes. Epidemiologic studies have revealed that the human population is continuously exposed to such compounds as they can be detected in body fluids and tissues. Table **5** summarizes immunoassays and kits developed or applied for industrial pollutants. Data were retrieved from reviews and published articles [21, 35, 37, 44, 178-181].

Table 5: Industrial pollutants as targets for immunoassays.

Target	*Format*	*Kit*	*References*
Benzpyrene(adducts)	RIA/ELISA/IS	+	[181-187]
BTEX	ELISA	+	[188, 189]
Dibutylphthalate	FIA	n.a.	[190]
Dioxins	EIA/ELISA	+	[191]
Nitrated PAHs	ELISA	n.a.	[180]
PAH	EIA/ELISA/FPIA	+	[192]
PCBs	RIA/ELISA/SIA	+	[193]
PCDDs/PCDFs	ELISA	+	[194]
PCP	ELISA/EIA	+	[195]
2,3,7,8-TCDD/F	RIA/EIA	+	[196, 197]
Phenolics	ELISA	+	[198]
Phthalate esters	FIA	n.a.	[199]
Phthalic acid esters	ELISA	n.a.	[200]
Pyrene	ELISA/IAC	n.a.	[201]
TNT	ELISA/IS	+	[202, 203]
Triton X-100	ELISA	n.a.	[204]

Legend: See Tables **1** and **2**; FPIA = Fluorescence polarization immunoassay; SIA = Strip immunoassay.

The advantage of using an antibody-coated tube kit for PCBs in soil screening for remediation has been described by Baek (1993) [205]. The kit has also been evaluated by Waters *et al.* 1994 [178] with regard to soil matrices, cross-reactivity and sensitivity (1 ppm). The performance of a antibody-coated tube kit for PAHs was similarly evaluated by McDonald *et al.* (1994) [177]. Both groups of contaminants consist of various compounds which makes it difficult to design an immunoassay that detects the most important representatives. For example, in the PAH kit the standard chosen is phenanthrene and it appeared that at least anthracene, benzo(a)anthracene and fluoranthene showed more than 50 % cross-reactivity. The advantages of using such kits for the screening of large areas of contaminated soils are their low price per sample and the rapidity of analysis (less than 1 hour including extraction) [206]. A homogeneous fluorescence polarization immunoassay for PAH was described by Goryacheva *et al.* (2007) [201]. Monoclonal and polyclonal antibodies were compared as well as different fluorescein-labeled PAH-derivatives. It was assessed that the structure of the derivative used to synthesize the tracer greatly influenced the performance of the assay. Detection limits for benzo[a]pyrene, naphthalene and anthracene of 0.9, 1.1 and 3.4 ng/ml, respectively, were found using spiked river water. In Fig.**4** is shown a comparison of the chemical structure of these compounds.

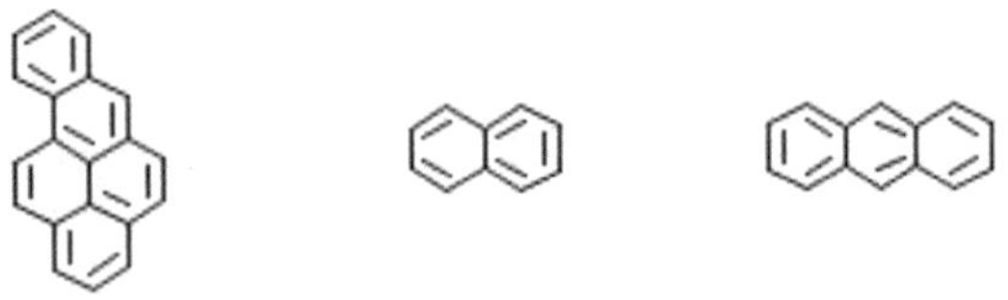

Figure 4: Chemical structure of benz[a]pyrene, naphthalene and anthracene.

A single-compound specific field test kit, for PCP (used as wood preservative) was evaluated by Mapes *et al.* (1992) [207]. The kit detected PCP at levels above 0.5 ppm and immunoassay results compared very well with GC-MS. A more recent study into the development of an ELISA for PCP involved the investigation of hapten design for the production of polyclonal sheep antibodies with high specificity and a comparison of heterologous and homologous ELISA by Abuknesha & Griffith (2004) [195]. In river water a detection limit of 0.2 ng/ml could be reached.

Another field-test for PCBs in two formats was designed by Roberts & Durst (1995) [193]. This assay is a type of lateral flow immunoassay using dye-encapsulated PCB-tagged liposomes and nitrocellulose strips coated with anti-PCB antibody. Aroclors were used for testing on specificity and real samples were compared with GC-MS.

Microorganisms

Among the numerous microorganisms there are some that are present in water and pose a threat for human beings. From time to time there are reported outbreaks of diseases such as enterogastitis, diarrhea, vomiting, dehydration, caused by microorganisms. In particular, E. coli, Campylobacter, Cryptosporidium, Giardia, Mycobacterium, Yersinia, Vibrio, Aeromonas, Legionella and Salmonella are bacteria that have been found in several water types; Hepatitis A, Astroviruses, Enteroviruses, Rotaviruses, Flaviviruses, Caliciviruses, Norwalk virus, and Norwalk-like virus are pathogenic viruses found in water. Some microorganisms, called indicator organisms, are regarded as indicators of water quality: E. coli, Shigella, Vibrio cholerae, Salmonella typhi, Campylobacter, Aeromonas, Yersinia, Giardia, Entamoeba, Cryptosporidium, Streptococcus, Enterococcus [208]. Additional reviews about the occurrence of harmful microorganisms in environment and food have been published [209-212]. Although nowadays PCR methods are the method of choice to detect and identify microorganisms, there have been developed antibodies and immunoassays for screening purposes as well as several kits for quantitative analysis, often after enrichment (Table **6**). Advances in the development of biosensors to detect viruses in food and environment are reviewed by Yadav *et al.* (2010) [213].

Table 6: Microorganisms as targets for immunoassays.

Target	***Format***	***Kit***	***References***
Bacteria/Protozoa			
Aeromonas	dot-blot	n.a.	[214]
Bacillus anthracis (spores)	IS	n.a.	[215-217]
Campylobacter	ELISA/EIA	+	[218, 219]
Clostridium	ELISA	+	[220]
Cryptosporidium	ELISA, FIA	+	[221-224]
E. coli	ELISA	+	[225, 226]
Enterococcus	dot-blot	n.a.	[227]
Giardia	ELISA	n.a.	[221]
Helicobacter pylori	ELISA	+	[219, 228, 229]

Legionella	ELISA	+	[230]
Steptococcus	ELISA/IS	+	[231]
Staphylococcus	ELISA/IS	+	[232, 233]
Vibrio	FIIA/dot-blot	n.a.	[234, 235]
Viruses			
Adenovirus	ELISA	+	[236, 237]
SRSV	EIA	n.a.	[238]
Caliciviruses	EIA	n.a.	[239]
Norovirus	ELISA	n.a.	[240, 241]
Norwalk(-like) virus	ELISA	n.a.	[238]
Hepatitis A/E	ELISA/EIA/IS	n.a.	[236, 242, 243]
Polyoma virus	ELISA	n.a.	[236]

Legend: See Tables **1** and **2**; SRSV = small round structured viruses.

In addition, for those molds producing mycotoxins, *Aspergillus/Penicillium/Fusarium*, a sandwich ELISA was developed and described employing mixed monoclonal antibodies for simultaneous detection in food or agricultural commodies [244].

Antibiotics/Pharmaceuticals

In veterinary and human medical practice antibiotics and medicines are used for the treatment of various diseases and disorders. Their occurrence in the environment, especially in water due to spills, faeces and urine, has raised much concern with respect to the emergence of resistance and subsequent exposure of humans to these resistant organisms as well as unwanted effects of substances. Further, allergic reactions may occur in humans at undesired exposure, especially to antibiotics. As a results of surveys all over the world there have been listed many compounds and metabolites found in various water bodies, even some in drinking water. A summary of compounds found in various types of water bodies, including WWTPs and influents/effluents, is given in Table **7**, compiled from reports and publications [245-263]. Additional references for pharmaceuticals and immunoassays, when available, are given in the table below under 'References'. Characteristics and further information of commercially available immunoassays and thus the antibody contained therein can be found in the kit inserts. Some of the immunoassays for pharmaceuticals have been developed for clinical application, but they can also be adopted for environmental analysis. It should be taken into account that as a consequence of additive or synergistic effects the health hazard of pharmaceuticals in water may be even higher than expected.

Table 7: Antibiotics and pharmaceuticals found in water.

Compound	***Class***	***Immunoassay***	***Kit***	***References***
Acetaminophen	antipyretic	RIA/ELISA	+	
Acetylsalicylic acid	anti-inflammatory	-	n.a.	
Amidotrizoinic acid	contrast chemical	-	n.a.	
Aminopyrine	analgesic	-	n.a.	
Amitriptyline	antidepressant	ELISA	+	[264]
Ampicillin	antibiotic	ELISA	+	
Atenolol	beta-blocker	ELISA	n.a.	[265]
Betaxolol	beta-blocker	-	n.a.	
Bezafibrate	lipid-regulator	ELISA	n.a.	
Biphenylol	antiseptic	-	n.a.	
Bisopropol	beta-blocker	ELISA	n.a.	[265]

Table 7: cont…

Bleomycin	antibiotic	ELISA	+	
Caffeine	stimulant	ELISA	+	[266]
Carazolol	beta-blocker	ELISA	+	
Carbamazepine	anti-epileptic	ELISA/EMIT/	n.a.	[267-270]
CMIA				
Citalopram	drug	ELISA	+	
Clarithromycine	antibiotic	-	n.a.	
Chloramfenicol	antibiotic	ELISA	+	
Chlorophene	antiseptic	-	n.a.	
Chloroxylenol	antiseptic	-	n.a.	
Chlortetracyclin	antibiotic	ELISA	n.a.	[271]
Cimetidine	antacid	-	n.a.	
Ciprofloxacin	antibiotic	ELISA	+	[272]
Chloramphenicol	antibiotic	ELISA	+	
Clenbuterol	antibiotic	ELISA	+	
Clindamycine	antibiotic	-	n.a.	
Clofibric acid	lipid regulator	ELISA	n.a.	[273, 274]
Codeine	analgesic	ELISA	+	
Coprostanol	biomarker	ELISA	n.a.	
Cotinine	metabolite	ELISA	+	
Cyclophoshamide	cytostatica	ELISA	+	
Dehydronifendipine	anti-anginal	-	n.a.	
Dextropropoxyphene	analgesic	-	n.a.	
Diatrizoate	contrast chemical	-	n.a.	
Diazepam	antidepressant	ELISA	+	
Diclofenac	anti-inflammatory	ELISA	n.a.	[275, 276]
Diltiazem	antihypertensive	-	n.a.	
Dimethylxanthine	bronchodilator	FPIA/EMIT	n.a.	
Enalapril(at)	antihypertensive	ELISA/EIA	n.a.	[277, 278]
Erythromycine	antibiotic	ELISA	+	[279]
Ethinylestradiol	oral contraceptive	RIA/ELISA	+	
Etofibrate	lipid regulator	-	n.a.	
Fenacetine	analgesic	-	n.a.	
Fenazon	analgesic	-	n.a.	
Fenfluramine	anorexic	ELISA	+	
Fenofibrate	lipid regulator	-	n.a.	
Fenofibric acid	metabolite	-	n.a.	
Fenoprofen	analgesic	-	n.a.	
Fenoterol	bronchodilator	-	n.a.	
Fluoroquinolones	antibiotics	ELISA	+	[280, 281]
Fluoxetine	antidepressant	ELISA	+	
Fluvoxamine	antidepressant	-	n.a.	

Table 7: cont…

Gemfibrozil	antihyperlipidemic	-	n.a.	
Gentisic acid	metabolite	-	n.a.	
Ibuprofen	anti-inflammatory	ELISA	+	[282, 283]
Ifosfamide	antineoplastic	-	n.a.	
Indometacin	antibiotic	-	n.a.	
Ivermectine	antiparasitic	ELISA	+	
Ketoprofen	analgesic	ELISA	+	
Levonorgestrel	oral contraceptive	ELISA	n.a.	[284]
Lidocaine	analgesic	ELISA	+	
Lincomycin	antibiotic	ELISA	+	
Meclofenamic acid	analgesic	-	n.a.	
Metaxalone	relaxant	-	n.a.	
Methaqualone	hypnotic	-	n.a.	
Metformin	antidiabetic	-	n.a.	
Metoprolol	beta-blocker	ELISA	n.a.	[265]
Methotrexate	cytostatica	ELISA	+	
Metronidazole	antibiotic	-	n.a.	
Nadolol	beta-blocker	-	n.a.	
Naproxen	anti-inflammatory	ELISA	n.a.	[282]
Nebivolol	beta-blocker	-	n.a.	
Norethisterone	hormone	RIA/ELISA	n.a.	
Norfloxacin	antibiotic	ELISA	+	
Omeprazole	antiacid	-	n.a.	
Oxycodone	drug	ELISA	+	[285]
Oxytetracycline	antibiotic	ELISA	+	
Pantoprazole	antiacid	-	n.a.	
Paroxetine	antidepressant	ELISA	+	
Pentoxifylline	lipid regulator	ELISA	+	
Phenazone	analgesic	-	n.a.	
Phenytoin	anticonvulsant	ELISA/EMIT	+	[267]
Pindolol	beta-blocker	RIA/ELISA	n.a.	[265]
Primidone	anti/epileptic	EMIT/EIA	+	[267]
Propanolol	beta-blocker	-	n.a.	
Propyfenazone	analgesic	-	n.a.	
Propoxyphene	analgesic	ELISA	+	
Propylphenazon	analgesic	-	n.a.	
Ranitidine	antacid	-	n.a.	
Roxythromycin	antibiotic	-	n.a.	
Salbutamol	bronchodilator	-	n.a.	
Salicylic acid	metabolite	-	n.a.	
Sotalol	beta-blocker	ELISA	+	[286]
Sulfadimethoxine	antibiotic	ELISA	n.a.	

Table 7: cont...

Sulfamethazine	antibiotic	ELISA	+	
Sulfamethizol	antibiotic	-	n.a.	
Sulfamethoxazole	antibiotic	ELISA	+	
Sulfonamide	antibiotic	ELISA	+	
Terbutaline	bronchodilator	-	n.a.	
Tetrabromo-*o*-cresol	antiseptic	-	n.a.	
Tetracycline	antibiotic/IS	ELISA/IS	+	[287-290]
Theophylline	anti-epileptic	FIA/EIA/	n.a.	[267, 291, 292]
EMIT/FFIA				
Timolol	beta-blocker	-	n.a.	
Tolfenamic acid	analgesic	-	n.a.	
Triclosan	antiseptic	EIA/ELISA	+	[293]
Trimethoprim	antibiotic	-	n.a.	
Tylosin	antibiotic	ELISA	n.a.	[289]
Venlafaxine	antidepressant	-	n.a.	
Verapamil	antihypertensive	-	n.a.	

Legend: See Tables **1** and **2**; CMIA = carbonyl metallo-immunoassay; - = not yet developed; n.a. = not available.

Although the health hazard of pharmaceuticals in water bodies is recognized and they have been detected by conventional methods, for some of them no immunoassay exists. These can be regarded as interesting target compounds for the development of antibodies and/or immunochemical detection methods depending on the occurrence rate and the optional health hazard. A further special group of pharmaceuticals found in surface water comprise contrast chemicals. These iodinated compounds comprise iodipamide iohexol, iomeprol, iopamidol, iopanoic acid, iopromid, iotalaminic acid, ioxaglinic acid, ioxitalaminic acid and ioxynil [261]. Since they are used in relatively high amounts in hospitals and occur in river water and no immunoassays are available, they also form an interesting group to develop antibodies and immunoassays for.

Although most of the pharmaceutical compounds listed above are prescribed drugs, some over-the-counter drugs are taken in large amounts; for example, the analgesics/anti-inflammatory drugs ibuprofen, naproxen and diclofenac. Their occurrence and environmental behavior in rivers and wastewater was subject of studies by Buser *et al.* (1999) [276, 283]. Although there are similarities between pesticides and pharmaceuticals with regard to undesired pollution of the environment, the difference is that some metabolites of pesticides are more toxic than their parent compound, whereas this does not apply for pharmaceuticals. In addition, combination effects of pharmaceuticals on humans may pose a higher threat due to the sometimes low effective dose. The European norm is set at 0.01 µg/l, a factor 10 lower than the norm for individual pesticides of 0.1 µg/l. To predict health hazards for humans and animals, it is important to determine the fate of pharmaceutical chemicals in the environment [294, 295] and to extend ecologic and toxic effects studies [296, 297].

4. EDC

EDC means endocrine disruptive compounds. Since the observation of sex conversion in wild life there has been much investigation into the presence of anthropogenic and natural substances in the environment that may have an endocrine disruptive activity. The group of EDC is very diverse and their effects may influence one or more of the hormonal systems in the animal or human body. They may be grouped into compounds showing (anti)estrogenic, (anti)androgenic, (anti)progestagenic, (anti)thyroidal, (anti)glucocorticosteroidal activity. Effects have been determined using whole organisms with regard to development, organ size, sex reversal, reproductive effects, protein synthesis (*e.g.* vitellogenin in male fish liver as indicator for estrogenicity); much used are receptor-based assays; bioassays based on tissue-specific cell lines; but they may also influence enzymes involved in the synthesis, degradation, interconversion and other components of endocrine pathways as well as their transport in blood by the binding globulins Corticosteroid Binding Globulin (CBG), Sex Hormone Binding Globulin (SHBG), Thyroid Binding Globulin (TBG). In the sixties and seventies of the last century SHBG and CBG have been used in the first binding assays to assess an estrogenic, progestagenic or androgenic activity of pharmaceuticals such as oral contraceptives [298-302]. The background for such binding assays was that those steroids that bind to their cognate transport globulins in blood show a very delicate equilibrium between the bound fraction and the relatively very low free, biological active fraction. Any disturbance of this equilibrium may lead to hormonal disorders. Similarly, TBG determines for the greater part the free fraction of thyroid hormones in blood. While binding proteins transport hormones from the glands to their target cells, receptors on and in these cells are required for their biological activity. Receptor-based assays may use isolated receptors such as the 96-well plate AR assay [303] or the Enzyme-Linked Receptor Assay (ELRA) [304, 305], but more often receptor genes are isolated and transferred into yeast, mammalian or microbial cells, often simultaneously with a reporter gene, yielding cell lines that respond to EDC. Examples are the E-screen, the YES-assay, the Rikilt Yeast Assay, the Calux ER/PR/AR/GR assays [306]. In addition, several mammalian cell lines have been used for the assessment of the endocrine activity of chemicals, such as the MCF-7 breast cancer cell line for estrogenic activity, which is also used in the E-screen; effects are related to growth stimulation or inhibition during culture of the cells. The difference between competitive receptor assays and receptor-based bioassays is that in the former yields information about the binding/affinity of a particular compound to the receptor, whereas in the latter a biological effect on the cells is determined, either positive or negative. Cell bioassays using the Aryl hydrocarbon (AhR) and Estrogen Receptor (ER) to detect activity in environmental samples was reviewed by Hilscherova *et al.* (2000) [307] giving a list of chemicals and their endocrine disrupting activity in the respective bioassay. Thyroid-disrupting environmental chemicals are discussed by Kashiwagi *et al.* 2009 and Zoeller 2010 [308, 309]. A general review of EDC and their effect on the brain and behavior with effects on sexual differentiation as well as transgenerational effects was published by Gore & Crews (2009) [310]. Further, several classes of pesticides may influence pregnancy outcomes, length of gestation and sexual development [311]. Exposure to pesticides and health risks, in particular for the fetus, is discussed by Gilden *et al.* 2010, Latini *et al.* 2010 [312, 313]. Pesticides and their endocrine disrupting effects have been summarized by several authors [314-317].

The importance of the knowledge of levels of EDC in the environment and exposure risks for humans is based on the fact that even the slightest disturbance of one or more hormonal pathways may have profound health effects, such as disorders, hormone-related cancers, developmental and reproductive disturbances, because exposure may be for a long term. In particular the fetus and newborns may be very vulnerable, because many EDC pass the feto-placental unit and also mother milk may contain apolar persistent contaminants. It has been shown in animal studies that exposure in the antenatal and early postnatal period may have unwanted effects in adult life. Some effects are even epigenetic, which means that traits are inherited by descendants [317]. A recent review regarding EDC and water quality and answers to many questions in this matter is given by Burkhardt-Holm (2010) [318]. Exposure to xeno-estrogenic compounds can even occur through precipitation according to Peters *et al.* (2008) [319], who analyzed BPA, alkylphenols, alkylphenol ethoxylates, phthalates, flame retardants and synthetic musk compounds in rain samples. Additional data were retrieved from [320-325].

Once characterized as EDC, immunoassays for the respective compounds have been developed or adopted from clinical chemistry or developed in order to detect such compounds in the environment. A selection of EDC assessed using bioassays and targeted conventional methods such as LC-MS, and immunoassays developed for these compounds, if available, are listed in Table **8**. Characteristics of antibodies/immunoassays can be found in the respective kit inserts and some relevant literature is given under 'References'.

Table 8: EDC as targets for immunoassays.

Compound	***Type***	***Immunoassay***	***Kit***	***References***
2,4-D	A	ELISA	+	
17OH-progesteron	P	RIA/ELISA	+	
19-Norethisterone	A	ELISA	+	
6α-Methylprednisone	G	ELISA	+	
Androstanedione	A	RIA/ELISA	+	[326]
APEs	E	ELISA	n.a.	
Atrazine	E	ELISA/EIA/IS	+	
Benomyl	A-E/E	EIA	+	
BDEs	Th	ELISA	n.a.	[327]
Bisphenol A	E/Th/N	ELISA/IS/IAC	+	[328, 329]
BFR	Th	ELISA	n.a.	[330]
Br-PCBs	Th	ELISA	n.a.	
Chlordane	E	ELISA	n.a.	
Chlorophenols	A-E	ELISA	n.a.	
Cortisol	G	RIA/ELISA	+	
Cortisone	G	RIA/ELISA	+	
DDE	A/A-A/Th	ELISA/EIA	+	
DDT	E	ELISA/EIA	+	
DES	E	RIA/ELISA	+	
Dexamethasone	G	ELISA	+	
Dieldrin	A-E	EIA	+	
Dihydrotesterone	A	RIA/ELISA	+	
Dioxins	E	ELISA	+	
Endosulfan	E	ELISA	+	
Estradiol	E	RIA/ELISA/FIIA	+	[331, 332]
Estriol	E	ELISA	+	
Estrone	E	ELISA	+	
Ethynylestradiol	E	ELISA	+	
Flame retardants	T	-	n.a.	
Ketoconazole	A-G	-	n.a.	
Linuron	A-A	ELISA	n.a.	
Mecoprop	Th	ELISA	n.a.	
Mestranol	E	ELISA	+	
Methoxychlor	E/Th	ELISA	n.a.	
Nonylphenol	E/Th	ELISA	n.a.	[333]
Norgesterel	P	ELISA	+	
Octylphenol	E	ELISA	n.a.	[333]
OH-PCBs	Th	-	n.a.	
PAHs	G	EIA	+	
PBDE	T/A-Th/E	ELISA	+	[334, 335]
PCB	A-E/A-A/Th/N	EIA/ELISA	+	

Table 8: cont…

Perchlorate	Th	-	n.a.	
Phthalates	E/Th	ELISA	n.a.	
Phthalate esters	E	EIA/ELISA	n.a.	[336]
Procimidone	A-A	EIA/ELISA	+	
Prednisolone	G	ELISA	n.a.	
Prednisone	G	ELISA	n.a.	
Progesterone	P	RIA/ELISA	+	
Simazine	E	ELISA	+	
Tamoxifen	E	ELISA	+	
Testosterone	A	ELISA	+	[326]
Toxaphene	E	ELISA	n.a.	
UV filters	Th	-	n.a.	[337]
Vinclozolin	E/A-A	-	n.a.	[338]

Legend: E = estrogenic; A-E = anti-estrogenic; A = androgenic; A-A = anti-androgenic; Th = thyroidal; G = glucocorticoidal; P = progestagenic; A-G = anti-glucocorticoidal; N = neurosteroidal;- = not yet developed; += kit available.

A particularly interesting group of compounds in this respect are the so-called obesogens. These comprise a very diverse group of compounds and exposure may explain the enormous increase in obesity worldwide. A hypothesis to explain the global obesity epidemic is posed by Baillie-Hamilton (2002) [339] and Drahl (2009) [340], also reviewed by Newbold (2008, 2010) [341, 344]. The association between EDC and obesity concluded from epidemiologic studies is described by Hatch *et al.* [345]. Nowadays, obesity is regarded as a debilitating disease and prevention has a high focus. It has long been known that steroid and thyroid hormones are involved in metabolism and adiposity. For example, women show an increase in body fat in the postmenopausal period, whereas administration of testosterone has the opposite effect. Castrated men (eunuchs) are characterized by high fat deposits. From clinical chemistry it is known the disorders Cushing's syndrome and Addison's disease are characterized by abdominal fat and very low fat reserves, respectively. The same applies for hypo- and hyperthyroidism. This implies that estrogens, androgens, glucocorticoids and thyroids are involved in adiposity. However, obesity is strongly related to the metabolic syndrome, that is regulated by complex hormonal interactions, several receptors, enzymes and signaling pathways. Apart from the well-known causes of obesity, excessive food intake and no exercise, endocrine disruption may also be effective. Exposure during the fetal and early postnatal period to obesogens may lead to metabolic diseases and obesity in adult life. Even epigenetic modification can occur and these may lead to inherited disorders. Environmental compounds related to obesity and the metabolic syndrome, including diabetes type 2, as well as mechanisms involved, are retrieved from literature [343-358] and listed in Table **9**. Details about specific obesogens can be found in the respective reference. Antibodies and immunochemical assays to monitor exposure routes and presence in body fluids of obesogens is a very promising field. The availability of antibodies and/or immunochemical detection methods can be found in the tables above.

Table 9: Obesogens as targets for immunoassays.

Compound	**References**
Alachlor	[346]
Aldrin	[346]
BFR	[353]
BPA	[341- 344, 359-363]
Carbamates	[348]
Chlordane	[346]

Table 9: cont…

Cyanazine	[346]
DDT/DDE	[346]
DEHP	[364]
DES	[341-344]
Diazenon	[351]
Dichlorfos	[346]
Dimethoate	[351]
Dithiocarbamates	[351]
Endosulfan	[349]
Fibrates	[356]
Heptachlor	[344]
Mancozeb	[351]
Lindane	[351]
Nonylphenol	[355]
Octylphenol	[355]
Organotins	[344, 365-369]
PCB/PCDD	[356]
PFOA	[370]
Phthalates	[345, 349, 371]
TCDD/PCDD	[356]
Trichlorfos	[346]

A notorious environmental and food contaminant is bisphenol A that is used extensively in the plastic and resins industry. Potential health effects of BPA (and phthalates) are updated at http://vitalhealthzone.com/health/articles/bisphenol_A_BPA_and_phthalates.html. According to numerous studies, BPA has estrogenic, thyroidal and obesogenic activities and it is associated with disruptive effects on reproductive function in fertile men and rat offspring [359, 360] and on glucose homeostasis [348].

5. EMERGING COMPOUNDS/NEW TARGET COMPOUNDS

Due to advancements in analytical techniques, new regulations (*e.g.* REACH), but also the detection of increasingly more and different pollutants in biological fluids make various compounds very interesting for monitoring and thus for the development of new antibodies and immunochemical assay methods. For example, it has been found that human milk may contain environmental chemicals such as pharmaceuticals, organochlorine pesticides, PCBs, dioxins, and PBDEs [372-374]. That means that neonates, that are particularly vulnerable, are exposed to this chemicals and can develop disorders and diseases in their later life. The ratio of plasma/milk for several drugs and environmental pollutants has been described by Abraham *et al.* (2009) and this parameter may be used to predict an exposure risk for children [375]. A review with regard to EDC transferred from the mother to the offspring and possible effects has been given by Cummings *et al.* (2010) [376]. Another interesting tissue for investigations into effects of exposure to environmental contaminants is adipose tissue. In particular apolar compounds are accumulated into fat, such as flame retardants and personal care products [377]. In the course of a lifetime concentrations may increase and affect behavior and wellbeing, especially if neurotoxic compounds accumulating in neurons and brain cells are involved. Maybe early and ongoing exposure to such contaminants could explain the increasing incidence of neurological, motorical, mental, social and behavior deficits in children and young adults, such as aggression and ADHD. Maybe even Alzheimer has an origin in exposure to pollutans. Exposure to industrial chemicals during pregnancy and neurodevelopmental toxicity risks has been reviewed by Julvez & Grandjean (2009) [378].

The range of drugs found in the environment will be extended due to the application of advanced techniques in analysis. An example is the development of an analytical method for the detection of the presence of antiviral drugs (acyclovir, abacavir, lamivudine, nevirapine, oseltamivir, penciclovir, ribavirin, stavudine, zidovudine). Some of these drugs have been found in German river water and raw wastewater [379]. Another group of new compounds found includes antidepressants and metabolites such as Viagra due to increased use [380]. These also form an interesting group of target compounds for monitoring studies using immunochemical assays.

Thus, with regard to antibodies and immunochemical methods there is a need for the development and applications of existing and new ones. In addition, in the tables above many immunoassays are missing and have not been developed yet. There have been published several epidemiologic reports about the occurrence of pollutants in blood and mother milk that are somehow related to the development of diseases and disorders . For both epidemiologic and monitoring studies existing immunoassays can be adapted to measurements in biological fluids. Otherwise it may be advantageously to develop new antibodies and immunochemical methods. For environmental studies it is important to keep track of new pesticides and antibiotics developed and applied and new toxins detected. Another aspect of pollutants comprises biotransformation of chemicals. A recent publication describes the biotransformation of permethrin to estrogenic metabolites in fish [381]. The same may occur in humans with regard to ingested pesticides and other organic pollutants.

The advantage of antibodies and immunochemical methods is the ease to develop them. Techniques have been described and reviewed. In addition, such methods are rapid, cost-effective and especially suited for the analysis of large series of samples of any origin. In addition, chemical or synthetic antibodies, such as aptamers and MIP (molecular imprinted polymers constitute useful substitutes for conventional antibodies due to their similarities in specificity and binding affinity. However, although some applications have been described, environmental studies are awaited for.

6. SUMMARY

This chapter summarizes antibodies and immunochemical methods applied in environmental studies. It will be clear that this overview is not comprehensive and that, besides those methods listed, many more have been published. For example, a group of compounds called phytoestrogens has not been discussed. Compounds such as genistein and daidzein, are secondary plant metabolites and they are present in certain types of food and feed. It is known that they can have estrogenic activities like the estrogenic EDC. There have been developed immunoassays for the detection and quantification of such compounds, but it is beyond the scope of this overview to discuss them. In addition, plant pathogens may also be interesting from an economical view. However, the same applies for immunochemical methods for such microorganisms in the scope of this overview. Also heavy metals, some of which can have an endocrine effect have been subject of the development of immunoassays. Further, the field of research into chemicals with hormonal activity is expanding. Although discussed above, there certainly will be found many more compounds showing such activities. For example, in addition to bioassays to assess estrogenic activity there is a need for the development and application of more bioassays to detect androgenic, progestagenic, thyroidal and glucocorticoidal activity. Here an interdisciplinary approach between chemical, biological, clinical and epidemiological investigators may be promising.

In some cases antibodies are commercially available, but not a commercial immunoassay kit. In such cases immunoassays, IAC columns or immunosensors may be designed and developed using available antibodies. In this regard a database containing all antibodies raised and/or available should be very helpful for future research.

The advanced as well as new reader in this field may take use of the information about immuochemical methods as applied in environmental investigations. With regard to commercially available immunoassay kits and immunoaffinity chromatography columns, additional information about their performance may be requested from the suppliers or producers.

REFERENCES

[1] Berson SA, Yalow RS. Quantitative aspects of the reaction between insulin and insuling-binding antibody. J Clin Invest 1959; 38: 1996-2016.

[2] Yalow RS, Berson SA. Immunoassay of endogenous plasma insulin in man. J Clin Invest 1960; 39: 1157-75.

[3] Engvall E, Perlmann P. Enzyme-linked immunosorbent assay, Elisa. J Immunol 1972; 109: 129-135.

[4] Shetty, N. Immunology: Introductory Textbook, 2nd ed.; New Age International Publishers, 2005.

[5] Coico R, Sunshine G. Immunology: A short course, 6th ed.; Wiley-Blackwell, 2009.

[6] Hefle SL. Immunoassays fundamentals. Food Technol 1995; 49: 102-7.

[7] Konterman R, Dübel S. Antibody Engineering, 2nd ed.; Springer, 2010.

[8] Marasco WA. Intrabodies: turning the humoral immune system outside in for intracellular immunization 1997; 4: 11-5.

[9] Lo BKC. Antibody Engineering: Methods and Protocols. Humana Press, 2004.

[10] Brandon DL, Binder RG, Bates AH, Montague WC. In: Kurtz DA, Skerrit JH, Stanker L, Ed. New Frontiers in Agrochemical Immunoassay. Arlington, AOAC Int. 1995; pp. 77-89.

[11] Lawruk TS, Hottenstein CS, Flekker JR, Rubio FM, Herzog DP. Factors influencing the specificity and sensitivity of triazine immunoassays. In: Meyer MT, Thurman EM, Ed.ACS Symposium Series 630, Herbicide metabolites in surface water and groundwater. 1996; pp. 43-52.

[12] Surdoki F, Jaeger L, Harris A, Kido , Wengatz I, Goodrow MH, Szekacs A. Wortberg M. Zheng J. Stoutamire DW, Sanborn JR, Gilman SD, Jones AD, Gee SJ, Choudary PV, Hammock BD. Rapid assays for environmental and biological monitoring. J Environ Sci Health 1995; B31: 451-458.

[13] Hennion M-C, Barcelo D. Strenghts and limitations of immunoassays for effective and efficient use for pesticide analysis in water samples: a review. Anal Chim Acta 1998; 362: 3-34.

[14] Ahern H. Immunoassay techniques proven to be outstanding in several fields. The Scientist 1995; Oct.:18-19.

[15] Brecht A, Abuknesha R. Multi-analyte immunoassays application to environmental analysis. Trends Anal Chem 1995; 14: 361-371.

[16] Kricka LJ, Stanley PE. Bioluminescence and chemiluminescence literature. J Biolumin Chemilumin. 1995; 10: 301-22.

[17] Gosling JP. Enzyme immunoassay. In: Meyer MT, Thurman EM, Ed.ACS Symposium Series 630, Herbicide metabolites in surface water and groundwater. 1996; pp. 287-307.

[18] Kricka LJ. Chemiluminescence immunoassay. In: Meyer MT, Thurman EM, Ed. ACS Symposium Series 630, Herbicide metabolites in surface water and groundwater. 1996; pp. 337-353.

[19] Sammes PG, Yahioglu G. Modern bioassays using metal chelates as luminescent probes. Nat Prod Rep 1996; 13: 1-28.

[20] Schobel U, Barzen C, Gauglitz G. Immunoanalytical techniques for pesticide monitoring based in fluorescence detection. Fres J Anal Chem 2000; 366: 646-658.

[21] Tseng T-C. Immunochemical methods for detection of toxins and pesticides. In: Singh RP, Singh US, Ed. Molecular methods in plant pathology. Boca Raton: Lewis Publishers 1995; pp. 445-460.

[22] Chernesky MA, Mahony JB. In: Mahy BWJ, Kangro HO, Ed. Virol Meth Manual 1996; pp. 123-141.

[23] Puchades R, Maquiera A. Recent developments in flow injection immunoanalysis. Crit Rev Anal Chem 1996; 26: 195-218.

[24] Plaza G, Ulfig K, Tien AJ. Immunoassays and environmental studies. Pol J Environ Studies 2000; 9: 231-236.

[25] Brady JF. In: Nelson JO, Karu AE, Wong RB, Ed. Immunoanalysis of agrochemicals. Washington, ACS Symposium Series 586. 1995; pp. 266-87.

[26] Krotzky AJ, Zeeh B. Immunoassays for residue analysis of agrochemicals: proposed guidelines for precision, standardization and quality control. Pure Appl Chem 1995; 67: 2065-88.

[27] Mihaliak CA, Berberich SA. In: Nelson JO, Karu AE, Wong RB, Ed. Immunoanalysis of agrochemicals. Washington, ACS Symposium Series 586. 1995; pp. 288-300.

[28] Rocke DM. In: Kurtz DA, Skerrit JH, Stanker L, Ed. New Frontiers in Agrochemical Immunoassay. Arlington, AOAC Int. 1995; pp. 251-259.

[29] Hock B, Hansen P-D, Krotzky A, Meitzel L, Meulenberg E, Müller G, Obst U, Spener F, Strotmann U, Weil L, Wittman C. In: Meyer MT, Thurman EM, Ed. ACS Symposium Series 630, Herbicide metabolites in surface water and groundwater. 1996; pp. 53-62.

[30] Hill ARC, Reynolds SL. Guidelines for in-house validation of analytical methods for pesticide residues in food and animal feed. Analyst 1999; 124: 953-8.

[31] ISO norm 15089; 1998

[32] Gee SJ, Hammock BD, Van Emon JM. A user's guide to environmental immunochemical analysis: www.epa.gov/heasd/edrb/chemistry/immunochem/user-guide.html
[33] VanderLaan M, Watkins BE, Stanker B. Environmental monitoring by immunoassay. Environ Sci Technol 1988; 22: 247-54.
[34] Knopp D, Dobberkau H-J, Degenkolb H. Immunoassays. Leistungsfähige Analysenmethoden für die Umwelttoxikologische Forschung und Praxis. Z gesamte Hyg 1989; 35: 122-124.
[35] Van Emon JM, Lopez-Avilla V. Immunochemical methods for environmental analysis. Anal Chem 1992; 64: 79A-87A.
[36] Hock B. Immunochemisch Verfahren in der Umweltanalytik und ihre Perspektiven. Z. Umweltchem Ökotox 1993; 5: 309-19.
[37] Niessner R. Immunoassays in environmental analytical chemistry: Some thoughts on trends and status. Anal Meth Instrum 1993; 1: 134-44.
[38] Jordon JR. Immunoassay kits for environmental analysis. The Referee 1995; 19: 2-12.
[39] Meulenberg EP, Mulder WH, Stoks PG. Immunoassays for pesticides. Environ Sci Technol 1995; 29: 553-61.
[40] Sherry JP. Immunodetection of ecosystem contaminants. In: Comstock MJ, Ed. Immunoanalysis of Agrochemicals, ACS 1995; pp. 335-53.
[41] Van Emon JM, Gerlach CL. A status report on field-portable immunoassay. Environ Sci Techonol 1995; 29:312A-317A.
[42] Watts CD, Hagerty B. Use of immunoassays for the analysis of pesticides and some other organics in water samples. Pure Appl Chem 1995; 67: 1533-48.
[43] Yang SS, Goldsmith AI, Smetena I. Recent advances in the residue analysis of N-methylcarbamate pesticides. J Chromat A 1996; 754: 3-16.
[44] Dankwardt A. In: Meyers RA, Ed. Encyclopedia of analytical chemistry. Chichester, John Wiley & Sons. 1998; pp. 1-27.
[45] Nunes GV, Toscano IA, Barcelo D. Trends Anal Chem 1998; 17: 79-87.
[46] Gabaldon JA, Maquieira A, Puchades R. Current trends in immunoassay-based kits for pesticide analysis. Crit Rev Food Sci Nutr. 1999; 39: 519-38.
[47] Eremin SA, Smith DS. Fluorescent polarization immunoassays for pesticides. Combinat Chem High Throughput Screening 2003; 6: 79-99.
[48] Smith DS, Eremin SA. Fluorescence polarization immunoassays and related methods for simple, high-throughput screening of small molecules. Anal Bioanal Chem 2008; 391: 1499-1507.
[49] Skadal P. Advances in electrochemical immunosensors. Electroanal 1997; 9: 737-45.
[50] Hock B. Antibodies for immunosensors. A review. Anal Chim Acta 1997; 347: 177-86.
[51] Marty J-L, Leca B, Noguer T. Biosensors for the detection of pesticides. Analusis Magazine 1998; 26: M144-M149.
[52] Rogers KR. Principles of affinity-based biosensors. Mol Biotechnol 2000; 14: 109-29.
[53] Wolfbeis OS. Fiber-optic chemical sensors and biosensors. Anal Chem 2000; 72: 81R-89R.
[54] Baird CL, Myszka DG. Current and emerging commercial optical biosensors. J Mol Recog 2001; 14: 261-268.
[55] Luppa PB, Sokoll LJ, Chan DW. Immunosensors – principles and applications to clinical chemistry. Clin Chim Acta 2001; 314: 1-26.
[56] Marazuela MD, Moreno-Bondi MC. Fiber-optic biosensors – an overview. Anal Bioanal Chem 2002; 372: 664-82.
[57] Conroy PJ, Hearty S, Leonard P, O'Kennedy RJ. Antibody production, design and use for biosensor-based applications. Seminars Cell Develop Biol 2009; 20: 10-26.
[58] Rekha K, Thakur MS, Karanth NG. Biosensors for the detection of organophosphorus pesticides. Crit Rev Biotechnol 2000; 20: 213-35.
[59] Suri CR, Raje M, Varshney GC. Immunosensors for pesticide analysis: Antibody production and sensor development. Crit Rev Biotechnol 2002; 22: 15-32.
[60] Ives JT, Doss HM, Sullivan BJ, Stires JC, Bechtel JH. In: Lieberman RA, Ed. Chemical, and Environmental Fiber Sensors X. Proceedings 3540. Bellingham. 1999; pp. 36-44.
[61] Laschi S, Palchetti I, Marrazza G, Mascini M. Disposable electrochemical sensors and biosensors for environmental and food analysis. Indian J Chem 2003; 42A: 2968-73.
[62] Badihi-Mossberg M, Buchner V, Rishpon J. Electrochemical biosensors for pollutants in the environment. Electroanalysis 2007; 19: 2015-28.
[63] Wark AW, Lee J, Kim S, Faisal SN, Lee HJ. Bioaffinity detction of pathogens on surfaces. J Ind Engn Chem 2010; 16: 169-77.
[64] Weidenbörner M. Foods and fumonisins. Eur Food Res Technol 2001; 212: 262-73.

[65] Binder EM. Managing the risk of mycotoxins in modern feed production. Anim Feed Sci Technol 2007; 133: 149-66.
[66] Dolan LC, Matulka RA, Burdock GA. Naturally occurring food toxins. Toxins 2010; 2: 2289-2332.
[67] Gerssen A, Pol-Hofstad IE, Poelman M, Mulder PPJ, van den Top HJ, de Boer J. Marine toxins: Chemistry, toxicity, occurrence and detection, with special reference to the Dutch situation. Toxins 2010; 2: 878-904.
[68] Pohanka M, Jun DM Kuca K. Mycotoxin assays using biosensor technology: A review. Drug Chem Toxicol 2007; 30:1-9.
[69] Prieto-Simón B, Noguer T, Campas M. Emerging biotools for assessment of mycotoxins in the past decade. Trends Anal Chem 2007; 26: 689-702.
[70] Pestka JJ, Abouzied MN, Sutikno. Immunological assays for mycotoxin detection. Food Technol 1995; 2: 120-8.
[71] Trucksess MW. Mycotoxins. J AOAC Int. 2001; 84: 202-11.
[72] Urusov AE, Zherdev AV, Dzantiev BB. Immunochemical methods of mycotoxin analysis (Review). Appl Biochem Microbiol 2010; 46: 253-66.
[73] Märtlbauer, E, Becker H. Immunological determination of microorganisms and toxins in food : application and prospects. Fleischwirtschaft 1996; 76: 54-7.
[74] Pimbley DW, Patel PD. A review of analytical methods for the detection of bacterial toxins. J Appl Microbiol Symp Suppl 1998; 84: 98S-109S.
[75] Vilarino N, Fonfría ES, Louzao MC, Botana LM. Use of biosensors as alternative to current regulatory methods for marine biotoxins. Sensors 2009; 9: 9414-43.
[76] Virarino N, Lourzao MC, Vieytes MR, Botana LM. Biological methods for marine toxin detection. Anal Bioanal Chem 2010; 397: 1673-81.
[77] Camacho GF, Rodríguez JG, Mirón AS, García MCC, Belarbi EH, Chisti Y, Grima EM. Biotechnological significance of toxic marine dinoflagellates. Biotechnol Adv 2007; 25: 176-94.
[78] Taitt CR, Shriver-Lake LC, Ngundi MM, Ligler FS. Array biosensor for toxin detection: Continued advances. Sensors 2008; 8: 8361-77.
[79] Wang X-H, Wang S. Sensors and biosensors for the determination of small molecule biological toxins. Sensors 2008; 8: 6045-54.
[80] Posthuma-Trumpie GA, Korf J., van Amerongen A. Lateral flow (immuno)assay: its strengths, weaknesses, opportunities and threats. A literature survey. Anal Bioanal Chem 2009; 393: 569-82.
[81] Fremy JM, Puech L, Krys S, Dragacci S. Recent advances in analytical procedures for the detection of diarrhetic phycotoxins: a review. J Appl Phycol 1999; 11: 377-84.
[82] Humpage AR, Magalhaes VF, Froscio SM. Comparison of analytical tools and biological assays for detection of paralytic shellfish poisoning toxins. Anal Bioanal Chem 2010; 397: 1655-71.
[83] Trainer VL, Baden DG. An enzyme immunoassay for the detection of Florida red tide brevetoxins. Toxicon 1991; 29: 1387-94.
[84] Shestowsky WS, Quilliam, Sikorska HM. An idiotypic-anti-idiotypic competitive immunoassay for quantitation of okadaic acid. Toxicon 1992; 30: 1441-48.
[85] Smith DS, Kitta DD. Enzyme immunoassay for the determination of domoic acid in mussel extracts. J Agric Food Chem 1995; 43: 367-71.
[86] Micheli L, Di Stefano S, Moscone D, *et al.* Production of antibodies and development of highly sensitive formats of enzyme immunoassay for saxitoxin analysis. Anal Bioanal Chem 2002; 373: 678-84.
[87] Dubois M, Demoulin M, Charlier C, *et al.* Development of ELISAs for detecting domoic acid, okadaic acid, and saxitoxin and their applicability for the detection of marine toxins in samples collected in Belgium. Food Addit Contam Part A Chem Anal Control Expo Risk Assess 2010; 27: 859-68.
[88] Renyan L, Daoyan X, Yubo L. Preparation of monoclonal antibody against okadaic acid and development of a sensitive ELISA for detection diarrhetic shellfish poisoning in shellfish.Environ Sci Inform Appl Technol 2009; 2: 550-5.
[89] Garet E, Cabado AG, Vieites JM, González-Fernández A. Rapid isolation of single-chain antibodies by phage display technology directed against one of the most potent marine toxins: Palytoxin. Toxicon 2010a; 55: 1519-26.
[90] Maragos CM, Thompson VS. Fiber-optic immunosensor for mycotoxins. Nat Toxins 1999; 7: 371-376.
[91] Yu W, Yu F-Y, Undersander DJ, Chu FS. Immunoassays of selected mycotoxins in hay, silage and mixed feed. Food Agric Immunol 1999; 11: 307-19.
[92] Curtui V, Usleber E, Dietrich R, Lepschy J, Märtlbauer E. A survey on the occurrence of mycotoxins in wheat and maize from western Romania. Mycopathol 1998; 143: 97-103.
[93] Barna-Vetró, I, Balázs E, Solty L. Immunodiagnostics for food and feed safety. Circle Reader Service 2000a; 91:64-6.

[94] Barna-Vetró, I, Szabó E, Fazekas B, Solti L. Development of a sensitive ELISA for the determination of fumonisin B1 in cereals. J Agric Food Chem 2000b; 48: 2821-25.

[95] Castellari M, Fabbri S, Fabiani A, Amati A, Galassi S. Comparison of different immunoaffinity clean-up procedures for high-performance liquid chromatographic analysis of ochratoxin A in wines. J Chromat A 2000; 888: 129-36.

[96] Ho J, Durst RA. Preparation of reagents for the determination of fumonisin B1 by flow-injection immunoanalysis. Anal Chim Acta 2000; 414: 51-60.

[97] Thirumala-Devi K, Mayo MA, Reddy G, Reddy SV, Delfosse P, Reddy DVR. J Agric Food Chem 2000; 48: 5079-82.

[98] Visconti A, Pascale M, Centonze. Determination of ochratoxin A in domestic and imported beers in Italy by immunoaffinity clean-up and liquid chromatography. J Chromat A 2000; 888: 321-26.

[99] Maragos CM, Jolley ME, Plattner RD, Nasir MS. Fluorescence polarization as a means for determination of fumonisins in maize. J Agric Food Chem 2001; 49: 596-602.

[100] Solfrizzo M, De Girolamo A, Visconti A. Determination of fumonisins B1 and B2 in cornflakes by high performance liquid chromatography and immunoaffinity clean-up. Food Addit Contam 2001; 18: 227-35.

[101] Dall'Asta C, De Dea Lindner J, Galaverna G, Dossena A, Neviani E, Marchelli R. The occurrence of ochratoxin A in blue cheese. Food Chem 2008; 106: 729-34.

[102] Smith DS, Kitta DD. Enzyme immunoassay for the determination of domoic acid in mussel extracts. J Agric Food Chem 1995; 43: 367-71.

[103] Campora CE, Dierking J, Tamaru CS, Hokama Y, Vincent D. Detection of ciguatoxin in fish tissue using sandwich ELISA and neuroblastoma cell bioassay. J Clin Lab Anal 2008; 22: 246-53.

[104] Yoshitsugi H. Rapid stick test for detection of ciguatoxin and other polyether toxins from tissues. US 07/056130; 1987.

[105] Garthwaite I, Ross KM, Miles GO, *et al.* Integrated enzyme-linked immunosorbent assay screening system for amnesic, neurotoxic, diarrhetic, and paralytic shellfish poisoning toxins found in New Zealand. J AOAC Int 2001; 84: 1643-48.

[106] Tang S, Moayeri M, Chen, Z, Harma H, Zhao J, Hu H, Purcell RH, Leppla SH, Hewlett IK. Detection of anthrax toxin by an ultrasensitive immunoassay using europium nanoparticles. Clin Vaccine Immunol 2009; 16: 408-13.

[107] Kwon Y, Hara CA, Knize MG, *et al.* Magnetic bead based immunoassay for autonomous detection of toxins.Anal Chem 2008; 80: 8416-23.

[108] Stanker LH, Merrill P, Scotcher MC, Cheng LW. Development and partial characterization of high-affinity monoclonal antibodies for botulinum toxin type A and their use in analysis of milk by sandwich ELISA. J Immunol Meth 2008; 336: 1-8.

[109] Volland H, Lamourette P, Nevers M-C, *et al.* A sensitive sandwich enzyme immunoassay for free or complexed *Clostridium botulinum* neurotoxin type A. J Immunol Meth 2008; 330: 120-9.

[110] Ekong TAN, McLellan K, Seardic D. Immunological detection of Clostridium botulinum toxin type A in therapeutic preparations. J Immunol Meth 1995; 180: 181-91.

[111] Gatto-Menking DL, Yu H, Bruno JG, Goode MT, Miller M, Zulich AW. Sensitive detection of biotoxoids and bacterial spores using an immunomagnetic electrocheminescence sensor. Biosensors Bioelectr 1995; 10: 501-7.

[112] Alfonta L, Willner I. Electrochemical and quartz crystal microbalance detection of the cholera toxin employing horseradish peroxidase and GM1-functionalized liposomes. Anal Chem 2001; 73: 5287-95.

[113] Ahn-Yoon S, DeCory TR, Baeumner A, Durst RA. Ganglioside-liposome immunoassay for the ultrasensitive detection of cholera toxin. Anal Chem 2003; 75: 2256-61.

[114] Ahn S, Durst RA. Detection of cholera toxin in seafood using a ganglioside-liposome immunoassay. Anal Bioanal Chem 2008; 391: 473-8.

[115] Li Y, Wang Y, Yu H, Jiang J, Kong R, Shen G, Yu R. A simple and sensitive piezoelectric immunosensor for cholera toxin based on GM1-incorporated liposome agglutination. Chin J Chem 2010; 28: 1678-84.

[116] Chiriaco MS, Primiceri E, D'Amone E, Ionescu RE, Rinaldi R, Maruccio G. EIS microfluidic chips for flow immunoassay and ultrasensitive cholera toxin detection. Lab Chip 2011; in press.

[117] Anderson M, Songer JG. Evaluation of two enzyme immunoassays for detection of Clostridium difficile toxins A and B in swine. Vet Microbiol 2008; 128: 204-6.

[118] Herrera-Cáceres JO, Camacho-Ortiz A, Galindo-Fraga A, *et al.* Concordance between two enzyme immunoassays for the detection of Clostridium difficile toxins. Arch Med Res 2010; 41: 92-6.

[119] Hallas G, Harrison TG, Samuel D, Colman G. Detection of diphtheria toxin in culture supernatants of Corynebacterium diphtheria and C. ulcerans by immunoassay with monoclonal antibody. J Med Microbiol 1990; 32: 247-53.

[120] Valyakina TI, Lakhtina OE, Komaleva RL, *et al.* Production and characteristics of monoclonal antibodies to the diphtheria toxin. Russ J Bioorg Chem 2009; 35: 556-65.

[121] Dupont H, Therasse J, Pinon JM, Binder P. Detection of staphylococcal enterotoxin B: A comparative study of ELISA and ELIFA systems. J Immunol Meth 1990; 128: 287-91.

[122] Goyache J, Orden JA, Blanco JL, *et al.* Murine monoclonal antibodies against staphylococcal enterotoxin B: production and characterization. FEMS Microbiol Lett 1992; 89: 247-254.

[123] Bhatti AR, Siddiqui YM, Micusan VV. Highly sensitive fluorogenic enzyme-linked immunosorbent assay: detection of staphylococcal enterotoxin B. J Microbiol Meth 1994; 19: 179-87.

[124] Bradstreet CM, Digherd MW, Gilbert RJ, Wieneke AA. Raising antibodies to staphylococcal enterotoxins A and B. J Appl Bacteriol 1977; 42: 117-22.

[125] Spero L, Morlock BA, Metzger JF. On the cross-reactivity of staphylococcal enterotoxins A, B, and C. J Immunol 1978; 120: 86-89.

[126] Lee AC-M, Robbins RN, Reiser RF, Bergdoll MS. Isolation of specific and common antibodies to staphylococcal enterotoxins B, C1 and C2. Infect Immun 1980; 27: 431-34.

[127] de Oliveira TC, Hirooka EY. Low cost production and purification of polyclonal antibodies to staphylococcal enterotoxin A. Rev Microbiol 1999; 30: 120-4.

[128] King KD, Anderson GP, Bullock KE, Regina MJ, Saaski EW, Ligler FS. Detecting staphylococcal enterotoxin B using an automated fiber optic biosensor. Biosensors Bioelectr 1999; 14: 163-70.

[129] Wadkins RM, Golden JP, Pritisolas LM, Ligler FS. Detection of multiple toxic agents using a planar array immunosensor. Biosensors Bioelectr 1998; 13: 407-15.

[130] Harteveld JLN, Nieuwenhuizen MS, Wils ERJ. Detection of staphylococcal enterotoxin B employing a piezoelectric crystal immunosensor. Biosensors Bioelectr 1997; 12: 661-67.

[131] Homola J, Dostálek J, Chen S, Rasooly A, Jiang S, Yee SS. Spectral surface Plasmon resonance biosensor for detection of staphylococcal enterotoxin B in milk. Int J Food Microbiol 2002; 75: 61-9.

[132] Lam MT, Boulet CA, Le XC. Development of a tetramethylrhodamine-labeled probe for a capillary electrophoresis-based competitive immunoassay of staphylococcal enterotoxin B. Anal Chim Acta 2002; 457: 21-8.

[133] Slavik R, Homola J, Brynda E. A miniature fiber optic surface Plasmon resonance sensor for fast detection of staphylococcal enterotoxin B. Biosensors Bioelectr 2002; 17: 591-5.

[134] Khan AS, Cao CJ, Thompson RG, Valdes JJ. A simple and rapid fluorescence-based immunoassay for the detection of staphylococcal enterotoxin B. Mol Cell Probes 2003; 17: 125-6.

[135] Lin H-C, Tsai W-C. Piezoelectric crystal immunosensor for the detection of staphylococcal enterotoxin B. Biosensors Bioelectr 2003; 18: 1479-83.

[136] Alefantis T, Grewal P, Ashton J, Khan AS, Valdes JJ, Del Vecchio VG. A rapid and sensitive magnetic bead-based immunoassay for the detection of staphylococcal enterotoxin B for high-through put screening. Mol Cell Probes 2004; 18: 379-82.

[137] Ruan C, Zeng K, Varghese O, Grimes CA. A staphylococcal enterotoxin B magnetoelastic immunosensor. Biosensors Bioelectr 2004; 20: 585-91.

[138] Chatrathi MP, Wang J, Collins GE. Sandwich electrochemical immunoassay for the detection of staphylococcal enterotoxin B based on immobilized thiolated antibodies. Biosensors Bioelectr 2007; 22: 2932-2938.

[139] Yang M, Kostov Y, Rasooly A. Carbon nanotubes based optical immunodetection of staphylococcal enterotoxin B (SEB) in food. Int J Food Microbiol 2008; 127: 78-83.

[140] Rong-Hwa S, Shiao-Shek T, Der-Jiang C, Yao-Wen H. Gold nanoparticles-based lateral flow assay for detection of staphylococcal enterotoxin B. Food Chem 2009; 118: 462-6.

[141] Yang M, Kostov Y, Bruck HA, Rasooly A. Gold nanoparticle-based enhanced chemiluminescence immunosensor for detection of staphylococcal enterotoxin B (SEB) in food. Int J Food Microbiol 2009; 133: 265-71.

[142] Kull S, Pauly D, Stormann B, *et al.* Multiplex detection of microbial and plant toxins by immunoaffinity enrichment and matrix-assisted laser desorption/ionization mass spectrometry. Anal Chem 2010; 82: 2916-24.

[143] Kiessig ST, Hentschel C, Jahn S, Mehl M, Starke R, Porstmann T. A solid-phase enzyme immunoassay for the detection of tetanus toxin using human and murine monoclonal antibodies. J Basic Microbiol 1991; 31: 135-40.

[144] Burkin MA, Sviridov VV, Perelygina OV. Determination of tetanus toxin and toxoid by ELISA using monoclonal antibodies. Appl Biochem Microbiol 2004; 40: 409-14.

[145] Ball HJ, Finlay D, Burns L, Mackie DP. Application of monoclonal antibody-based sandwich ELISAs to detect verotoxins in cattle faeces. Res Vet Sci 1994; 57: 225-32.

[146] Yutsudo T, Nakabayashi N, Hirayama T, Takeda Y. Pyurification and some properties of a Vero toxin from Escherichia coli O157:H7 that is immunologically unrelated to Shiga toxin. Microb Pathog 1987; 3: 21-30.

[147] Padhye VV, Zhao T, Doyle MP. Production and characterisation of monoclonal antibodies to Verotoxins 1 and 2 from Escherichia coli of serotype O157:H7. J Med Microbiol 1989; 30: 219-6.
[148] Weeratna RD, Doyle MP. Detection and production of verotoxin 1 of Escherichia coli O157:H7 in food. Appl Environ Microbiol 1991; 57: 2951-55.
[149] Williams JA, Byrne LM, Pugh CSG. Methods for producing avian verotoxin antitoxin. US patent 6.652.857 B2; 2003.
[150] Capps KL, McLaughlin EM, Murray AW, *et al.* Validation of three rapid screening methods for detection of verotoxin-producing Escherichia coli in foods: interlaboratory study. J AOAC Int 2004; 87: 68-77.
[151] Duy TN, Lam PKS, Shaw GR, Connell DW. Toxicology and risk assessment of freshwater cyanobacterial (blue-green algal) toxins in water. Rev Environ Contam Toxicol 2000; 163: 113-86.
[152] Svrcek C, Smith DW. Cyanobacteria toxins and the current state of knowlegde on water treatment options: a review. J Environ Eng Sci 2004; 3: 155-85.
[153] Dittman E, Wiegand C. Cyanobacterial toxins – occurence, biosynthesis and impact on human affairs. Mol Nutr Food Res 2006; 50: 7-17.
[154] van Apeldoorn ME, van Egmond HP, Speijers GJA, Bakker GJI. Toxins of cyanobacteria. Mol Nutr Food Res 2007; 51: 7-60.
[155] Oberholster PJ, Botha A-M, Myburgh JG. Linking climate change and progressive eutrophication to incidents of clustered animal mortalities in different geographical regions of South Africa. Afr J Biotechnol 2009a; 8: 5825-32.
[156] Oberholster PJ, Mthethwa BLS, Botha AM. Development of a rapid and sensitive battery of bioassays for risk assessment of cyanobacterial microcystin-LR in drinking water of rural water treatment plants, South Africa. Afr J Biotechnol 2009b; 8: 4562-71.
[157] Oberholster PJ, Myburgh JG, Govender D, Bengis R, Botha A-M. Identification of toxigenic Microcystis strains after incidents of wild animal mortalities in the Kruger National Park, South Africa. Ecotoxicol Environ Safety 2009; 72: 1177-82.
[158] Masango MG, Myburgh JG, Labuschage L, Govender D, Bengis RG, Naicker D. Assessment of Microcystis bloom toxicity associated with wildlife mortality in the Kruger National Park, South Africa. J Wildlife Dis. 2010; 46: 95-102.
[159] Codd GA, Metcalf JS, Ward CJ, *et al.* Analysis of cyanobacterial toxins by physicochemical and biochemical methods. J AOAC Int 2001; 84: 1626-35.
[160] Sangolkar LN, Maske SS, Chakrabarti T. Methods for determining microcystins (peptide hepatotoxins) and microcystin-producing cyanobacteria. Water Res 2006; 40: 3485-96.
[161] Bruno M, Melchiorre S, Messineo V, *et al.* Microcystin detection in contaminated fish from Italian lakes using Elisa immunoassays and Lc-Ms/Ms analysis. In: Gault PM, Marler HJ, Ed. Nova Sci Pub 2009; pp. 191-210.
[162] McDermott CM, Feola R, Plude J. Detection of cyanobacterial toxins (microcystins) in waters of northeastern Wisconsin by a new immunoassay. Toxicon 1995; 33: 1433-42.
[163] Ueno Y, Nagata S, Tsutsumi T, *et al.* Detection of microcystins, a blue-green algal hepatotoxin, in drinking water sampled in Haimen and Fusui, endemic areas of primary liver cancer in China, by highly sensitive immunoassay. Carcinogenesis 1996; 17: 1317-21.
[164] Ueno Y, Nagata S, Tsutsumi T, Hasegawa, A, Yoshida F, Suttajit M, Mebs D, Pütsch M, Vasconselos V. Survey of microcystins in environmental water by a highly sensitive immunoassay based on monoclonal antibody. Nat Tox 1996; 4: 271-6.
[165] Nagata S, Tsutsumi T, Hasegawa A, Yoshida F, Ueno Y. Enzyme immunoassay for direct determination of microcystins in environmental water. J AOAC Int 1997; 80: 408-17.
[166] Nagata S, Tsutsumi T, Yoshida F, Ueno Y. A new type sandwich immunoassay for microcystin: production of monoclonal antibodies specific to the immune complex formed by microcystin and an anti-microcystin monoclonal antibody. Nat Tox 1999; 7: 1-7.
[167] Tsutsumi T, Nagata S, Yoshida F, Ueno Y. Development of sandwich immunoassays for microcystins, a natural contaminant in environmental water: an assay based on anti-immune complex antibodies. Jpn J Toxicol Hlth 1998;44: P-25.
[168] Weller MG, Zeck A, Eikenberg A, Nagata S, Ueno Y, Niessner R. Development of a direct competitive microcystin immunoassay of broad specificity. Anal Sci 2001; 17: 1445-48.
[169] Zeck A, Eikenberg A, Weller MG, Niessner R. Highly sensitive immunoassay based on monoclonal antibody specific for [4-arginine]microcystins. Anal Chim Acta 2001; 441: 1-13.
[170] Young FM, Metcalf JS, Meriluoto JAO, Spoof L, Morrison LF, Codd GA. Production of antibodies against microcystin-RR for the assessment of purified microcystins and cyanobacterial environmental samples. Toxicon 2006; 48: 295-306.

[171] Campas M, Marty J-L. Highly sensitive amperometric immunosensors for microcystin detection in algae. Biosensors Bioelectr 2007; 22: 1034-40.

[172] Loyprasert S, Thavarunkul P, Asawatreratanakul P, Wongkittisuksa B, Limsakul C, Kanatharana P. Label-free capacitive immunosensor for microcystin-LR using self-assembled thiourea monolayer incorporated with Ag nanoparticles on gold electrode. Biosensors Bioelectr 2008; 24: 78-86.

[173] Yu H-W, Lee J, Kim S, Nguyen GH, Kim IS. Electrochemical immunoassay using quantum dot/antibody probe for identification of cyanobacterial hepatotoxin microcystin-LR. Anal Bioanal Chem 2009; 394: 2173-81.

[174] Long F, Zhu J-W, He M, Shi H-C. Matrix effects on the microcystin-LR fluorescent immunoassay based on optical biosensor. Sensors 2009; 9: 3000-10.

[175] Herranz S, Bocková M, Marazuela MD, Homola J, Moreno-Bondi MC. An SPR biosensor for the detection of microcystins in drinking water. Anal Bioanal Chem 2010; 398: 2625-34.

[176] Carmichael WW, Li RH. Cyanobacterial toxins in the Salton Sea. Saline Systems 2006; 2: 1-13.

[177] Lopes VR, Fernández N, Martins RF, Vasconcelos V. Primary screening of the bioactivity of brackishwater cyanobacteria: Toxicity of crude extracts to Artemia salina larvae and Paracentrotus lividus embryos. Mar Drugs 2010; 8: 471-82.

[178] Waters LC, Smith RR, Stewart JH, Jenkins RA, Counts RW. Evaluation of two field screening test kits for the detection of PCBs in soil by immunoassay. J AOAC Int 1994; 77: 1664-71.

[179] McDonald PP, Almond RE, Mapes JP, Friedman SB. PAH RIS® soil test – A rapid, on-site screening test for polynuclear aromatic hydrocarbons in soil. J AOAC Int 1994; 77: 466-72.

[180] Harrison RO, Eduljee GH. Immunochemical analysis for dioxins – progress and prospects. Sci Total Environ 1999; 239: 1-18.

[181] Zielinska B, Samy S. Analysis of nitrated polycyclic aromatic hydrocarbons. Anal Bioanal Chem 2006; 386: 883-90.

[182] Kado NY, Wei ET, Radioimmunoassay for benzo[a]pyrene. J Natl Cancer Inst 1978; 61: 221-5.

[183] Poirier MC, Stanley JR, Beckwith JB, Weinstein IB, Yuspa SH. Indirect immuonofluorescent localization of benzo[a]pyrene adducted to nucleic acids in cultured mouse keratinocyte nuclei. Carcinogenesis 1982; 3: 345-48.

[184] Vo-Dinh T, Tromberg BJ, Griffin GD, Ambrose KR, Sepaniak MJ, Gardenhire EM. Antibody-based fiberoptics biosensor for the carcinogen benzo[a]pyrene. Appl Spectr 1987; 41: 735-38.

[185] Ius A, Bacigalupo MA, Roda A, Vaccari C. Development of a time-resolved fluoroimmunoassay of benzo(a)pyrene in water. Fres J Anal Chem 1992; 343: 55-6.

[186] Borrebaeck CA, Glad C, Mattiasson B, Jergil B. Enzyme immunoassay of benzo[a]pyrene conjugated to DNA, RNA and microsomal proteins using a monoclonal antibody. Cancer Lett 1984; 22: 163-70.

[187] Roda A, Bacigalup MA, Ius A, Minutello A. Development and applications of an ultrasensitive quantitative enzyme immune-assay for benzo(a)pyrene in environmental samples. Environ Toxicol 1991; 12: 1027-35.

[188] Geloglazova NV, Goryacheva IY, Mikhirev DA, De Saeger S, Niessner R, Knopp D. New immunochemically-based field test for monitoring benzo[a]pyrene in aquous samples. Anal Sci 2008; 24: 1613-17.

[189] Allen RL, Manning WB, McKenzie KD, Withers TA, Mapes JP, Friedman SB. A rapid and sensitive immunoassay for the detection of gasoline and diesel fuel in contaminated soil. J Soil Contam 1992; 1: 227-37.

[190] Maiolini E, Knopp D, Niessner R, Eremin S, Bolelli L, Ferri EN, Girotti S. Chemiluminescent ELISA for the BTEX determination in water. Anal Sci 2010; 26: 773-7.

[191] Zhang M-C, Wang Q-E, Zhuang H-S. A novel competitive fluorescence immunoassay for the determination of dibutyl phthalate. Anal Bioanal Chem 2006; 386: 1401-6.

[192] Nording M, Nichkova M, Spinnel E, Persson Y, Gee S, Hammock B, Haglund P. Anal Bioanal Chem 2006; 385: 357-66.

[193] Goryacheva IY, Eremin SA, Shutaleva EA, Suchanek M, Niessner R, Knopp D. Development of a fluorescence polarization immunoassay for polycyclic aromatic hydrocarbons. Anal Lett 2007; 40: 1445-60.

[194] Roberts MA, Durst RA. Investigation of liposome-based immunomigration sensors for the detection of polychlorinated biphenyls. Anal Chem 1995; 67: 482-91.

[195] Nording M, Denison MS, Baston D, Persson Y, Spinnel E, Haglund P. Analysis of dioxins in contaminated soils with the CALUX and CAFLUX bioassays, an immunoassay, and gas chromatography/high-resolution mass spectrometry. Environ Toxicol Chem 2007; 26: 1122-29.

[196] Abuknesha RA, Griffith HM. Evaluation of a polyclonal antiserum to pentachlorophenol-acetic acid-KLH immunogen: binding properties and use with heterologous PCP derivatives in ELISA for pentachlorophenol. Anal Bioanal Chem 2004; 379: 411-6.

[197] Sherry J, ApSimon J, Collier L, Wilkinson R, Albro P, Afghan B. The use of radioimmunoassay for the detection of polychlorinated dibenzo-p-dioxins in fish samples. Chemosphere 1989; 19: 255-61.

[198] Luster MI, Albro PW, Chae K, Lawson LD, Corbett JT, McKinney JD. Radioimmunoassay for quantitation of 2,3,7,8-tetrachlorodibenzofuran. Anal Chem 1980; 52: 1497-1500.

[199] Puig D, Barcelo D. Determination of phenolic compounds in water and waste water. TRAC 1995; 15: 362-75.

[200] Ius A, Bacigalupo A, Meroni G, Pistillo A, Roda A. Development of a time-resolved fluoroimmunoassay for phthalate esters in water. Fres J Anal Chem 1993; 345: 589-91.

[201] Yanaihara N, Kato I, Nagasawa S, Kodaira T. Immunoassay for phthalic acid esters. US patent 6.399.318; 2002.

[202] Goryacheva IY, Beloglazova NV, Eremin SA, Mikhirev DA, Niessner R, Knopp D. Gel-based immunoassay for non-instrumental detection of pyrene in water. Talanta 2008; 75: 517-22.

[203] Shankaran DR, Matsumoto K, Toko K, Miura N. Development and comparison of two immunoassays for the detection of 2,4,6-trinitrotoluene (TNT) based on surface Plasmon resonance. Sensors Actuators B 2006; 114: 71-9.

[204] Charles PT, Adams AA, Howell PB, Trammell SA, Deschamps JR, Kusterbeck AW. Fluorescence-based sensing of 2,4,6-trinitrotoluene (TNT) using a multichanneled poly(methyl methacrylate) (PMMA) microimmunosensor. Sensors 2010; 10: 876-89.

[205] Wie SI, Hammock BD. The use of enzyme-linked immunosorbent assays (ELISA) for the determination of Triton X nonionic detergents. Anal Biochem 1982; 125: 168-76.

[206] Baek NH. Evaluation of immunoassay tests in screening soil contaminated with polychlorinated biphenyls. Bull Environ Contam Toxicol 1993; 51: 844-51.

[207] Mapes JP, McKenzie KD, McClelland LR, Movassaghi S, Reddy RA, Allen RL, Friedman SB. Penta RISc™ - A rapid, on-site screening test for pentachlorphenol in soil. Bull Environ Contam Toxicol 1992; 49: 334-41.

[208] Stedtfeld RD, Yurtsever D, Duran M, Alm EW, Hashsham SA. Detection and occurrence of indicator organisms and pathogens. Water Environ Res 2006; 78: 1054-77.

[209] Gantzer C, Maul A, Audic JM, Schwartzbrod L. Detection of infectious enteroviruses, enterovirus genomes, somatic coliphages and Bacteroides fragilis phages in treated wastewater. Appl Environ Microbiol 1998; 64: 4307-12.

[210] Abbaszadegan M, Stewart P, LeChevallier M. A strategy for detection of viruses in groundwater by PCR. Appl Environ Microbiol 1999; 65: 444-9.

[211] Gasanov U, Hughes D, Hansbro PM. Methods for the isolation and identification of Listeria spp. and Listeria monocytogenes: a review. FEMS Microbiol Rev 2005; 29: 851-75.

[212] Giangaspero A, Berrill F, Brandonisio O. Giardia and Cryptosporidium and public health: the epidemiological scenario from the Italian perspective. Parasitol Rev 2007; 101: 1169-82.

[213] Yadav R, Dwivedi S, Kumar S, Chaudhury A. Trends and perspectives of biosensors for food and environmental virology. Food Environ Virol 2010; 2: 53-63.

[214] Hang J, Sundaram AK, Zhu P, *et al*. Development of a rapid and sensitive immunoassay for detection and subsequent recovery of Bacillus anthracis spores in environmental samples. J Microbiol Meth 2008; 242-246.

[215] Longyant S, Chaiyasittrakul K, Rukpratanporn S, Chaivisuthangkura P, Sithigorngul P. Simple and direct detection of Aeromonas hydrophila infection in the goldfish, Carassium auratus (L.), by dot blotting using specific monoclonal antibodies. J Fish Dis 2010; 33: 973-984.

[216] Longchamp P, Leighton T. Molecular recognition specificity of Bacillus anthracis spore antibodies. J Appl Microbiol 1999; 87: 246-9.

[217] Gatto-Menking DL, Yu H, Bruno JG, Goode MT, Miller M, Zulich AW. Sensitive detection of biotoxoids and bacterial spores using an immunomagnetic electrochemiluminescence sensor. Biosensors Bioelectr 1995; 10: 501-7.

[218] Hochel I, Slavíckova D, Viochna D, Skvor J, Steinhauserová I. Detection of Campylobacter species in foods by indirect competitive ELISA using hen and rabbit antibodies. Food Agric Immunol 2007; 18: 151-67.

[219] Sack DA, Lastovica AJ, Chang SH, Pazzaglia G. Microtiter assay for detecting Campylobacter spp. And Helicobacter pylori with surface gangliosides which bind cholera toxin. J Clin Microbiol 1998; 36: 2043-5.

[220] McCourt MT, Finlay DA, Laird C, Smyth JA, Bell C, Ball HJ. Sandwich ELISA detection of Clostridium perfringens cells and α-toxin from field cases of necrotic enteritis of poultry. Vet Microbiol 2005; 106: 259-264.

[221] Rimhanan-Finne R, Enemark HL, Kolehmainen J, Toropainen P, Hänninen ML. Evaluation of immunofluorescence microscopy and enzyme-linked immunosorbent assay in detection of Cryptosporidium and Giardia infections in asymptomatic dogs. Vet Parasitol 2007;145: 345-348.

[222] Kramer MF, Vesey G, Look NL, Herbert BR, Simpson-Stroot JM, Lim DV. Development of a Cryptosporidium oocyst assay using an automated fiber-optic-based biosensor. J Biol Eng 2007; 1: 3-9.

[223] Inpankaew T, Jittapalapong S, Phasuk J, Pinyopanuwut N, Chimnoi W, Kengradomkit C, Sunanta C, Zhang G, Aboge GO, Nishikawa Y, Igarashi I, Xuan X. Seroprevalence of Cryptosporidium parvum infection of dairy cows in three northern provinces of Thailand determined by enzyme-linked immunosorbent assay using recombinant antigen CpP23. J Vet Res 2009; 76: 161-5.

[224] Wang C, He H, Duan M. Development and evaluation of a recombinant CP23 antigen-based ELISA for serodiagnosis of Cryptosporidium parvum. Exp Parasitol 2009; 121: 157-62.

[225] Kamma S, Tang L, Leung K, Ashton E, Newman N, Suresh MR. A rapid two dot filter assay for detection of E. coli O157 in water samples. J Immunol Meth 2008; 336: 159-65.

[226] Jurkevica A, Halsall HB, Seliskar CJ, Heineman WR. Effect of some physico-chemical conditions on an immunoassay for viable Escherichia coli. Anal Bioanal Chem 2010; 397: 3133-36.

[227] Caruso G, Monticelli LS, Caruso R, Bergamasco A. Development of a fluorescent antibody method for the detection of Enterococcus faecium and its potential for coastal aquatic environment monitoring. Marine Poll Bull 2008; 56: 318-24.

[228] Erzin Y, Altun S, Dobrucali A, Aslan M, Erdamar S, Dirican A, Kocazeybek B. Evaluation of two enzyme immunoassays for detecting Helicobacter pylori in stool specimens of dyspeptic patients after eradication therapy. J Med Microbiol 2005; 54: 863-6.

[229] Blanco S, Forné M, Lacoma A, Prat C, Cuesta MA, Latorre I, Viver JA, Fernández G, Molinos S, Domínguez J. Comparison of stool antigen immunoassay methods for detecting Helicobacter pylori infection before and after eradication treatment. Diag Microbiol Inf Dis 2008; 61: 150-5.

[230] Blanco S, Prat C, Sánchez MD, Ferrer D, Pellicer T, Haba L, Latorre I, Vilaplana C, Ausina V, Domínguez J. Evaluation of a Legionella urinary antigen enzyme immunoassay for rapid detection of Legionella pneumophila in water samples. Int J Hyg Environ Health 2008; 211: 168-71.

[231] Leskinen S, Lim DV. Rapid ultrafiltration concentration and biosensor detection of enterococci from large volumes of Florida recreational water. Appl Environ Microbiol 2008; 74: 4792-98.

[232] Shi-Hui S, Jin-Hua C, Fen-Jiao H, Li-Hua N, Shou-Zhuo Y. Electrochemically modified piezoelectric crystal biosensor for detection of Staphylococcus aureus. Chin J Chem 1996; 14: 222-7.

[233] Jianming Y, Pivarnik PE, Senecal AG, Rand AG. Rapid detection of Staphylococcus aureus using a membrane fiber optic biosensor. SPIE Proceeding Series 1999; 3544: 2-9.

[234] Manti A, Falcioni T, Campana R, Sisti D, Rocchi M, Medina V, Dominici S, Papa S, Baffone W. Detection of environmental Vibrio parahaemolyticus using a polyclonal antibody by flow cytometry. Environ Microbiol Rep 2010; 2: 158-65.

[235] Pengsuk C, Longyant S, Rukpratanporn S, Chaivisuthangkura P, Sriduylyakul P, Sithigorngul P. Development of monoclonal antibodies for simple detection and differentiation of Vibrio mimicus from V. cholerae and Vibrio spp. by dot blotting. Aquaculture 2010; 300: 17-24.

[236] Richardson SD. Water analysis: emerging contaminants and current issues. Anal Chem 2007; 79: 4295-324.

[237] Valanne A, Huopalahti S, Soukka T, Vainionpää R, Lövgren T, Härmä H. A sensitive adenovirus immunoassay as a model for using nanoparticle label technology in virus diagnostics. J Clin Virol 2004; 33: 217-23.

[238] Vipond IB, Pelosi E, Williams J, *et al.* A diagnostic EIA for detection of the prevalent SRSV strain in United Kingdom outbreaks of gastroenteritis. J Med Virol 2000; 61: 132-37.

[239] Atmar RL, Estes MK. Diagnosis of noncultivatable gastroenteritis viruses, the human caliciviruses. Clin Microbiol Rev 2001; 14: 15-37.

[240] Kamata K, Shinozake K, Okada M, *et al.* Expession and antigenicity of virus-like particles of norovirus and their application for detection of noroviruses in stool samples. J Med Virol 2005; 76: 129-36.

[241] Maunula L. Waterborne norovirus outbreaks. Future Virol 2007; 2: 101-12.

[242] Liu YS, Green A. A monoclonal-antibody enzyme immunoassay for detection of hepatitis B surface antigen with use of a biotin-avidin system. Clin Chem 1985; 31: 202-5.

[243] König B, Grätzel M. A piezoelectric immunosensor for hepatitis viruses. Anal Chim Acta 1995; 309: 19-25.

[244] Kwak B-Y, Kwon B-J, Kweon C-H, Shon D-H. Detection of Aspergillus, Penicillium, and Fusarium species by sandwich enzyme-linked immunosorbent assay using mixed monoclonal antibodies. J Microbiol Biotechnol 2004; 14: 385-9.

[245] Stumpf M, Ternes TA, Haberer K, Seel P, Baumann W. Nachweis von Arzneimittelrückständen in Kläranlangen und Fließgewässern. Vom Wasser1; 86: 291-303. 1996

[246] Halling-Sorensen B, Nielsen SN, Lanzky PF, Ingerslev LF, Holten Lützhoft HC, Jorgensen SE. Occurrence, fate and effects of pharmaceutical substances in the environment – A review. Chemosphere 1998; 36: 357-93.

[247] Ternes TA. Occurrence of drugs in German sewage treatment plants and rivers. Wat Res 1998; 32: 3245-60.

[248] Daughton CG, Ternes TA. Pharmaceuticals and personal care products in the environment: Agents of subtle change? Environ Health Persp 1999; 107: 907-38.

[249] Heberer T. Tracking persistent pharmaceutical residues from municipal sewage to drinking water. J Hydrol 2001; 266: 175-89.

[250] Heberer T. Occurrence, fate, and removal of pharmaceutical residues in the aquatic environment: a review of recent research data. Toxicol Lett 2002; 131: 5-17.

[251] Derksen JGM, Eijnatten GM, Lahr J, van der Linde P, Kroon AGM. Environmental effects of human pharmaceuticals. RIWA Report 2000.052, 2001; pp 1-226.

[252] Ternes T, Bonerz M, Schmidt T. Determination of neutral pharmaceuticals in wastewater and rivers by liquid chromatography-electrospray tandem mass spectrometry. J Chromat A 2001; 938: 175-85.

[253] Jux U, Baginski RM, Arnold H-G, Krönke M, Seng PN. Detection of pharmaceutical contaminations of river, pond, and tap water from Cologne (Germany) and surroundings. Int J Hyg Environ Health 2002; 205: 393-8.

[254] Kolpin DW, Furlong ET, Meyer MT, Thurman EM, Zaugg SD, Barber LB, Buxton HT. Pharmaceuticals, hormones, and other organic wastewater contaminants in U.S. streams, 1999-2000: A national reconnaissance. Environ Sci Technol 2002; 36: 1202-11.

[255] McQuillan D, Hopkins S, Chapman TH, Sherrell K, Mills D. Drug residues in ambient water: initial survey in New Mexico, USA. Abstract. 7th Annual New Mexico Environmental Health Conference, New Mexico, 2002; 1-9.

[256] Webb S, Ternes T, Gibert M, Ol K. Indirect human exposure to pharmaceuticals *via* drinking water. Toxicol Lett 2003; 142: 157-67.

[257] Nikolaou A, Meric S, Fatta D. Occurrence patterns of pharmaceuticals in water and wastewater environments. Anal Bioanal Chem 2007; 387: 1225-34.

[258] Kuster M, López de Alda MJ, Hernando MD, Petrovic M, Martín-Alonso J, Barceló D. Analysis and occurrence of pharmaceuticals, estrogens, progestogens and polar pesticides in sewage treatment plant effluents, river water and drinking water in the Llobregat river basin (Barcelona, Spain). J Hydrol 2008; 358: 112-23.

[259] Halford B. Side effects. Chem Eng News 2008; 86: 13-7.

[260] Peng X, Tan J, Tang C, Yu Y, Wang Z. Multiresidue determination of fluoroquinolone, sulfonamide, trimethoprim, and chloramphenicol antibiotics in urban waters in China. Environ Toxicol Chem 2008; 27: 73-9.

[261] ter Laak TL, van der Aa, Houtman CJ, Stoks PG, van Wezel AP. Relating environmental concentrations of pharmaceuticals to consumption: A mass balance approach for the river Rhine. Environ Int 2010; 36: 403-9.,

[262] van Nuijs ALN, Tarconicu I, Simons W, Bervoets L, Blust R, Jorens PG, Neels H, Covaci A. Optimization and validation of a hydrophilic interaction liquid chromatography-tandem mass spectrometry method for the determination of 13 top-prescribed pharmaceuticals in influent wastewater. Anal Bioanal Chem. 2010; 398: 2211-22.

[263] Kessler R. Pharmaceutical factories as a source of drugs in water. Environ Health Persp 2010; 118: A383.

[264] Denis H, Marullo S, Hoebeke J, Strosberg AD. Enzyme-linked immunosorbent assay for amitriptyline and other antidepressants using a monoclonal antibody. Clin Chim Acta 1986; 159: 257-67.

[265] Yu L. Antibodies specific to multiple beta blockers and methods for their use. US Patent 7.229.782.

[266] Carvalho JJ, Weller MG, Panne U, Schneider RJ. A highly sensitive caffeine immunoassay base don a monoclonal antibody. Anal Bioanal Chem 2010; 396: 2617-28.

[267] Knight D. Enzyme immunoassay of phenobarbital, phenytoin, primidone, carbamazepine and theophylline with the abbott VP bichromatic analyzer. Clin Chem 1981; 14: 14-15.

[268] Varenne A, Vessières A, Salmain M, Brossier P, Jaouen G. Production of specific antibodies and development of a non-isotopic immunoassay for carbamazepine by the carbonyl metallo-immunoassay (CMIA) method. J Immunol Meth 1995; 186: 195-204.

[269] Brummond BA, Saini MS, Ponticello IS. Immunoassays with novel labeled carbamazepine hapten analogues. US patent 5.578.457, 1980.

[270] Bahlman A, Weller MG, Panne U, Schneider RJ. Monitoring carbamazepine in surface and wastewaters by an immunoassay based on a monoclonal antibody. Anal Bioanal Chem 2009; 395: 1809-20.

[271] Sheedy C. Development of an immunoassay and antibodies for the veterinary antibiotic chlortetracycline. WCTOW Canada, presentation, 2007.

[272] Gomes FB, Riedstra S, Ferreira JP. Development of an immunoassay for ciprofloxacin based on phage-displayed antibody fragments. J Immunol Meth 2010; 358: 17-22.

[273] Buser H-R, Müller MD, Theobald N. Occurrence of the pharmaceutical drug clofibric acid and the herbicide mecoprop in various Swiss lakes and in the North Sea. Environ Sci Technol 1998; 32: 188-92.

[274] Stan H-J, Heberer T, Linkerhägner M. Vorkommen von Clofibrinsäure im aquatischen System – Führt die therapeutisch Anwendung zu einer Belastung von Oberflächen-, Grund- und Trinkwasser? Vom Wasser 1994; 83: 57-68.

[275] Deng A, Himmelsback M, Zhu Q-Z, Frey S, Seng M, Buchberger W, Niessner R, Knopp D. Residue analysis of the pharmaceutical diclofenac in different water types using ELISA and GC-MS. Environ Sci Technol 2003; 37: 3422-29.

[276] Buser H-R, Poiger T, Müller MD. Occurrence and fate of the pharmaceutical drug diclofenac in surface water: rapid photodegradation. Environ Sci Technol 1998; 32: 3449-56.

[277] Arafat T, Awad R, Hamad M, Azzam R, Al-Nasan A, Jehanil A, Matalka K. Pharmacokinetics and pharmacodynamics profiles of enalapril maleate in healthy volunteers following determination of enalapril and enalaprilat by two specific enzyme immunoassays. J Clin Pharmacol Ther 2005; 30: 319-28.

[278] Metalka K, Arafat T, Hamad M, Jehani A. Determination of enalapril and enalaprilat by enzyme immunosorbent assays: application to pharmacokinetic and pharmacodynamic analysis. Fund Clin Pharmacol 2002; 16: 237-44.

[279] Albrecht U, Walte H, Hammer P. Detection of erythromycin in raw milk by an antibody-capture-iimunoassay. Kieler Milchwissenschaftliche Forschungsberichte 1998; 50: 163-70.

[280] Golet EM, Alder AC, Hartmann A, Ternes TA, Giger W. Trace determination of fluoroquinolone antibacterial agents in urban wastewater by solid-phase extraction and liquid chromatography with fluorescence detection. Anal Chem 2001; 73: 3632-38.

[281] Golet EM, Alder AC, Giger W. Environmental exporsure and risk assessment of fluoroquinolone antibacterial agents in wastewater and river water of the Glatt Valley watershed, Switserland. Environ Sci Technol 2002; 36: 5455-62.

[282] Meulenberg EP, Peelen GOH, Lukkien E, Koopal K. Immunochemical detection methods for bioactive pollutants. Int J Environ Anal Chem 2005; 85: 861-70.

[283] Buser H-R, Poiger T, Müller MD. Occurrence and environmental behavior of the chiral pharmaceutical drug ibuprofen in surface waters and in wastewater. Environ Sci Technol 1999 ; 33: 2529-35.

[284] Pu C, Wy Y-F, Yang H, Deng A-P. Trace analysis of contraceptive drug levonorgestrel in wastewater samples by a newly developed indirect competitive enzyme-linked immunosorbent assay (ELISA) coupled with solid phase extraction. Anal Chim Acta 2008; 628: 73-79.

[285] Le NL, Reiter A, Tomlinson K, Jones J, Moore C. The detection of oxycodone in meconium specimens. J Anal Toxicol 2005; 29: 54-57.

[286] Pujos E, Cren-Olivé C, Plaise O, Flament-Waton MM, Grenier-Loustalot MF. Comparison of the analysis of ß-blockers by different techniques. J Chromat B 2009; 877: 4007-14.

[287] Andree U, Mueller-Seitz E, Usai I, Loeber S, Gmeiner P, Wimmer C, Hillen W, Petz M. Tetracycline sensing using novel doxycycline derivatives immobilized on different surface Plasmon resonance biosensor surfaces. Bioanal 2010; 2: 217-27.

[288] Zhang Y, Lu S, Liu W, Zhao C, Xi R. Preparation of anti-tetracycline antibodies and development of an indirect heterologous competitive enzyme-linked immunosorbent assay to detect residues of tetracycline in milk. J Agric Food Chem 2007; 55: 211-8.

[289] Kumar K, Thompson A, Singh AK, Chander Y, Gupta SC. Enzyme-linked immunosorbent assay for ultratrace determination of antibiotics in aqueous samples. J Environ Qual 2004; 33: 250-6.

[290] Pastor-Navarro N, Morais S, Maquieira A, Puchades. Synthesis of haptens and development of a sensitive immunoassay for tetracycline residues: Application to honey samples. Anal Chim Acta 2007; 594: 211-8.

[291] Locasio-Brown L, Plant AL, Horvath V. Liposome flow injection immunoassay: implication for sensitivity, dynamic range, and antibody regeneration. Anal Chem 1990; 62: 2587-2593.

[292] Danilova ND, Vasilov RG. Production and characterization of anti-theophylline monoclonal antibodies suitable for immunoassay. Immunol Lett 1991; 28: 79-83.

[293] Kantiani L, Farré M, Asperger D, Rubio F, González S, López de Alda MJ, Petrovic M, Shelver WL, Barceló D. Triclosan and methyl-triclosan monitoring study in the northeast of Spain using a magnetic particle enzyme immunoassay and confirmatory analysis by gas chromatographyt-mass spectrometry. J Hydrol 2008; 361: 1-9.

[294] Richardson M, Bowron J. The fate of pharmaceutical chemicals in the aquatic environment. J Pharm Pharmacol 1985; 37: 1-12.

[295] Boreen AL, Arnold WA, McNeill K. Photodegradation of pharmaceuticals in the aquatic environment: a review. Aquat Sci 2003; 65: 320-41.

[296] Rönnefart I, Koschorreck J, Kolossa-Gehring M. Arzneimittel in der Umwelt. Mitteilungsblatt Fachgruppe Umweltchemie Ökoltoxikol. 2002; 8: 1-6.

[297] Halling-Sorensen B, Nielsen SN, Lanzky PF, Ingerslev F, Holten Lützhoft HC, Jorgensen SE. Occurrence, fate and effects of pharmaceutical substances in the environment – A review. Chemosphere 1998; 36: 357-93.

[298] Murphy BEP. Binding of testosterone and estradiol in plasma. Can J Biochem 1968; 46: 299-302.
[299] Bruning PF, Bonfrèr, Hart AA. Non-protein bound oestradiol, sex hormone binding globulin, breast cancer and breast cancer riskt. Br J Cancer 1985; 51: 479-84.
[300] Bonfrer JMG, Bruning PF, Nooijen WJ. A simple method for the measurement of the steroid fraction bound to sex hormone binding globulin in serum. J Steroid Biochem 1989; 33: 227-31.
[301] Dunn JF, Nisula BC, Rodbard D. Transport of steroid hormones: Binding of 21 endogenous steroids bound to both testosterone-binding globulin and corticosteroid-binding globulin in human plasma. J Clin Endocrinol Metab 1985; 53: 58-68.
[302] Pugeat MM, Dunn JF, Nisula BC. Transport of steroid hormones: Interaction of 70 drugs with testosterone-binding globulin and corticosteroid-binding globulin in human plasma. J Clin Endocrinol Metab 1981; 53: 69-75.
[303] Hartig PC, Cardon MC, Blystone CR, Gray LE, Wilson VS. High throughput adjustable 96-well plate assay for androgen receptor binding: A practical approach for EDC screening using the chimpanzee AR. Toxicol Lett 2008; 181: 126-131.
[304] Seifert M, Haindl S, Hock B. Development of an enzyme linked receptor assay (ELRA) for estrogens and xenoestrogens. Anal Chim Acta 1999; 398: 191-9.
[305] Hock B, Kramer K, Seifert M. Environmental analysis using antibody and receptor based techniques. Intern J Environ Anal Chem 2000; 78: 289-303.
[306] Campbell CG, Borglin SE, Green FB, Grayson A, Wozei E, Stringfellow WT. Biologically directed environmental monitoring, fate, and transport of estrogenic endocrine disrupting compounds in water: A review. Chemosphere 2006; 65: 1265-80.
[307] Hilscherova K, Machala M, Kannan K, Blankenship A, Giesy JP. Cell bioassays for detection of aryl hydrocarbon (AhR) and estrogen receptor (ER) mediated activity in environmental samples. Environ Sci Pollut Res 2000; 7: 159-71.
[308] Kashiwagi K, Furuno N, Kitamura S, Ohta S, Sugihara K, Utsumi K, Hanada H, Taniguchi K, Suzuki K, Kashiwagi A. Disruption of thyroid hormone function by environmental pollutants. J Health Sci 2009; 55: 147-160.
[309] Zoeller TR. Environmental chemicals targeting thyroid. Hormones 2010; 9: 28-40.
[310] Gore AC, Crews D. Environmental endocrine disruption of brain and behavior. Hormones, Brain and Behavior 2009; 3: 1789-1816.
[311] Colborn T, Carroll LE. Pesticidees, sexual development, reproduction, and fertility: Current perspective and future direction. Human Ecol Risk Assessm 2007; 13: 1078-110.
[312] Gilden RC, Huffling K, Sattler B. Pesticides and health risks. J Obstet Gynecol Neonat Nursing 2010; 39: 103-10
[313] Latini G, Knipp G, Mantovani A, Marcovecchio ML, Chiarelli F, Soder O. Endocrine disruptors and human health. Mini Rev Med Chem 2010; 10: 846-55.
[314] Sonneveld E, Riteco JAC, Jansen HJm Pieterse B, Brouwer A, Schoonen WG, van der Burg B. Comparison of *in vitro* and *in vivo* screening models for androgenic and estrogenic activities. Toxicol Sci 2006; 89: 173-187.
[315] Yamada H, Ishii Y, Yamamoto M, Oguri K. Induction of the hepatic cytochrome P450 2B subfamily by xenobiotics: Research history, evolutionary aspect, and relation to tumorigenesis, and mechanism. Curr Drug Metab 2006; 7: 397-409.
[316] Janosek J, Hilscherová K, Bláha L, Holoubek I. Environmental xenobiotics and nuclear receptors – Interactions, effects and *in vitro* assessment. Toxicol *In Vitro* 2006; 20: 18-37.
[317] McKinlay R, Plant JA, Bell JNB, Voulvoulis N. Endocrine disrupting pesticides: Implications for risk assessment. Environ Int 2007; 34: 168-83.
[318] Anway MD, Cupp AS, Uzumcu M, Skinner MK. Epigenetic transgenerational actions of endocrine disruptors and male fertility. Science 2005; 308: 1466-69.
[319] Burkhardt-Holm P. Endocrine disruptors and water quality: A state-of-the-art review. Water Resources Develop 2010; 26: 477-93.
[320] Peters RJB, Beeltje H, van Delft RJ. Xeno-estrogenic compounds in precipitation. J Environ Monit 2008; 10: 760-9.
[321] Richardson SJ. Cell and molecular biology of transthyretin and thyroid hormones. Int Rev Cytol 2007; 258: 137-93.
[322] Quednow K, Püttmann W. Organophosphates and synthetic musk fragrances in freshwater streams in Hessen/Germany. Clean – Soil, Air, Water 2008; 36: 70-8.
[323] Streck G. Chemical and biological analysis of estrogenic, progestagenic and androgenic steroids in the environment. Trends Anal Chem 2009; 28: 635-52.
[324] Chang H, Hu J, Shao B. Occurrence of natural and synthetic glucocorticoids in sewage treatment plants and receiving river waters. Environ Sci Technol 2007; 41: 3462-68.

[325] Höhne C, Püttmann W. Occurrence and temporal variations of the xenoestrogens bisphenol A, 4-tert-octylphenol, and tech. 4-nonylphenol in two German wastewater treatment plants. Environ Sci Pollut Res 2008; 15: 405-16.

[326] Chang H, Wu S, Hu J, Asami M, Kunikane S. Trace analysis of androgens and progestogens in environmental waers by ultra-performance liquied chromatography-electrospray tandem mass spectrometry. J Chromat A 208; 1195: 44-51.

[327] Ahn KC, Gee SJ, Tsai H-J, Bennett D, Nishioka MG, Blum A, Fishman E, Hammock BD. Immunoassay for monitoring environmental and human exposure to the polybrominated diphenyl ether BDE-47. Environ Sci Technol 2009; 43: 7784-90.

[328] Marchesini GR, Koopal K, Meulenberg E, Haasnoot W, Irth H. Spreeta-based biosensor assays for endocrine disruptors. Biosensors Bioelectr 2007; 22: 1908-15.

[329] Li L, Wang J, Zhou S, Zhao M. Development and characterization of an immunoaffinity monolith for selective on-line extraction of bisphenol A from environmental water samples. Anal Chim Acta 2008; 620: 1-7.

[330] Shelver WL, Keum YS, Kim HJ, Rutherford D, Hakk HH, Bergman A, Li QX. Hapten synthesis and antibody generation for the development of a polybrominated flame retardant ELISA. J Agric Food Chem 2005; 53: 3840-7.

[331] Huang C-H, Sedlak DL. Analysis of estrogenic hormones in municipal wastewater effluent and surface water using enzyme-linked immunosorbent assay and gas chromatography/tandem mass spectrometry. Environ Toxicol Chem 2001; 20: 133-9.

[332] Tschmelak J, Proll G, Gauglitz G. Improved strategy for biosensor-based monitoring of water bodies with diverse organic carbon levels. Biosensors Bioelectr 2005; 21: 979-83.

[333] Meulenberg EP, Koopal K, Rhemrev R. Immunoassays for alkylphenolic pollutants with endocrine disrupting activity. Intern J Environ Anal Chem 2005; 85: 871-83.

[334] Chevrier J, Harley KG, Bradman A, Gharbi M, Sjödin A, Eskenazi B. Polybrominated diphenyl ether (PBDE) flame retardants and thyroid hormone during pregnancy. Environ Health Persp 2010; 118: 1444-49.

[335] Pacyniak EK, Cheng X, Cunningham ML, Crofton K, Klaassen CD, Guo GL. The flame retardants, polybrominated diphenyl ethers, are pregnane X receptor activators. Toxicol Sci 2007; 97: 94-102.

[336] Parveen M, Inoue A, Ise R, Tanji M, Kiyama R. Evaluation of estrogenic activity of phthalate esters by gene expression profiling using a focused microarray (estrarray®). Environ Toxicol 2008; 27: 1416-25.

[337] Schmutzler C, Bacinski A, Gotthardt I, *et al.* The ultraviolet filter benzophenone 2 interferes with the thyroid hormone axis in rats and is a potent *in vitro* inhibitor of human recombinant thyroid peroxidase. Endocrinol 2007; 148: 2835-44.

[338] Nilsson EE, Anway MD, Stanfield J, Skinner M. Transgenerational epigenetic effects of the endocrine disruptor vinclozolin on pregnancies and female adult onset of disease. Reproduction 2008; 135: 713-721.

[339] Baillie-Hamilton PF. Chemical toxins: A hypothesis to explain the global obesity epidemic. J Altern Compl Med 2002; 8: 185-92.

[340] Drahl C. Weighing options. Chem Eng News 2009; 87: 11-16.

[341] Newbold RR, Padilla-Banks E, Snyder RJ, Philips TM, Jefferson WN. Developmental exposure to endocrine disruptors and the obesity epidemic. Reprod Toxicol 2007; 23: 290-96.

[342] Newbold RR, Padilla-Banks E, Jefferson WN, Heindel JJ. Effects of endocrine disruptors on obesity. Intern J Androl 2008; 31: 201-208.

[343] Newbold RR, Padilla-Banks E, Jefferson WN. Environmental estrogens and obesity. Mol Cell Endocrinol 2009; 304: 84-9.

[344] Newbold RR. Impact of environmental endocrine disrupting chemicals on the development of obesity. Hormones 2010; 9: 206-17.

[345] Hatch EE, Nelson JW, Stahlhut RW, Webster TF. Association of endocrine disruptors and obesity: perspectives from epidemiological studies. Intern J Androl 2010; 33: 324-32.

[346] Montgomery MP, Kamel F, Saldana TM, Alavanja MCR, Sandler DP. Incident diabetes and pesticide exposure among licensed pesticide applicators: Agricultural health study. Am J Epidemiol 2008; 167: 1235-46.

[347] Elobeid MA, Allison DB. Putative environmental-endocrine disruptors and obesity: a review. Curr Opin Endocrinol Diabetes Obes 2008; 15: 403-408.

[348] Heindel JJ, vom Saal FS. Role of nutrition and environmental endocrine disrupting chemicals during the perinatal period on the aetiology of obesity. Mol Cell Endocrinol 2009; 304: 90-6.

[349] Casals-Casas C, Feige JN, Desvergne B. Interference of pollutants with PPARs: endocrine disruption meets metabolism. Intern J Obesity 2008; 32: S53-S61.

[350] Odermatt A. Corticosteroid-dependent hypertension: environmental influences. Swiss Med Wkly 2004; 134: 4-13.

[351] Odermatt A, Gumy C, Atanasov AG, Dzyakanchuk AA. Disruption of glucocorticoid action by environmental chemicals: Potential mechanisms and relevance. J Steroid Biochem Mol Biol 2006; 102: 222-31.

[352] Grün F, Blumberg B. Endocrine disruptors as obesogens. Mol Cell Endocrinol 2009; 304: 19-29.

[353] Swedenborg E, Rüegg J, Mäkelä S, Pongratz I. Endocrine disruptive chemicals: mechanisms of action and involvement in metabolic disorders. J Mol Endocriol 2009; 43: 1-10.

[354] Lee HK. Persistent organic pollutants and epidemic of diabetes and metabolic syndrome. J Diabetes Invest 2010; 1: 121-2.

[355] Chen J-Q, Brown TR, Russo J. Regulation of energy metabolism pathways by estrogens and estrogenic chemicals and potential implications in obesity associated with increased exposure to endocrine disruptors. Biochim Biophys Acta 2009; 1793: 1128-43.

[356] Latini G, Marcovecchio ML, Del Vecchio A, Gallo F, Bertino E, Chiarelli F. Influence of environment on insulin sensitivity. Environ Int 2009; 35: 987-93.

[357] Grün F, Blumberg B. Perturbed nuclear receptor signaling by environmental obesogens as emerging factors in the obesity crisis. Rev Endocr Metab Disorders 2007; 8: 161-71.

[358] Sugden MC, Holness MJ. Role of nuclear receptors in the modulation of insulin secretion in lipid-induced insulin resistance. Biochem Soc Trans 2008; 36: 891-900.

[359] Alonso-Magdalena P, Vieira E, Soriano S, Menes L, Burks D, Quesada I, Nadal A. Bisphenol A exposure during pregnancy disrupts glucose homeostasis in mothers and adult male offspring. Environ Health Persp 2010; 118: 1243-50.

[360] Lang IA, Galloway TS, Scarlett A, Henley WE, Depledge M, Wallace RB, Melzer D. Association of urinary bisphenol A concentration with medical disorders and laboratory abnormalities in adults. JAMA 2009; 300: 1303-10.

[361] vom Saal SF, Meyers JP. Bisphenol A and risk of metabolic disorders. JAMA 2009; 300: 1353-5.

[362] Fernández M, Bourguignon N, Lux-Lantos V, Libertun C. Neonatal exposure to bisphenol A and reproductive and endocrine alterations resembling the polycystic ovarian syndrome in adult rats. Environ Health Persp 2010; 118: 1217-22.

[363] Mendiola J, Jorgensen N, Andersson A-M, Calafat AM, Ye X, Redmon JB, Drobnis EZ, Wang C, Sparks A, Thurston SW, Liu F, Swan SH. Are environmental levels of bisphenol A associated with reproductive function in fertile men? Environ Health Persp 2010; 118: 1286-1291.

[364] Eveilard A, Mselli-Lakhai L, Mogha A, Lasserre F, Polizzi A, Pascussi J-M, Guillou H, Martin PGP, Pineau T. Di-(2-ethylhexyl)-phthalate (DEHP) activates the constitutive androstane receptor (CAR): A novel signaling pathway sensitive to phthalates. Biochem Pharmacol 2009; 77: 1735-46.

[365] Le Maire A, Grimaldi M, Roecklin D, Dagnino S, Vivat-Hannah V, Balaguer P, Bourguet W. Activation of RXR-PPAR heterodimers by organotin environmental endocrine disruptors. EMBO Rep 2009; 10: 367-73.

[366] Nakanishi T. Potential toxicity of organotin compounds *via* nuclear receptor signaling in mammals. J Health Sci 2007; 53: 1-9.

[367] Nakanishi T. Endocrine disruption induced by organotin compounds; organotins function as a powerful agonist for nuclear receptors rather than an aromatase inhibitor. J Toxicol Sci 2008; 33: 269-76.

[368] Grün F, Blumberg B. Environmental obesogens: Organotins and endocrine disruption *via* nuclear receptor signaling. Endocrinol 2006; 147 (suppl.): S50-S55.

[369] Terrell ML, Manatunga AK, Small CM, *et al.* A decay model for assessing polybrominated biphenyl exposure among women in the Michigan long-term PBB study. J Exp Sci Environ Epidemiol. 2008; 18: 410-20.

[370] Betts KS. Perfluoroalkyl acids: What is the evidence telling us? Environ Health Persp 2007; 115: A250-A256.

[371] Stahlhut RW, van Wijngaarden E, Dye TD, Cook S, Swan SH. Concentrations of urinary phthalate metabolites are associated with increased waist circumference and insulin resistance in adult U.S. males. Environ Health Persp 2007; 115: 876-82.

[372] LaKind JS, Wilkins AA, Berlin Jr. CM. Environmental chemicals in human milk: a review of levels, infant exposure and health, and guidance for future research. Toxicol Appl Pharmacol 2004; 198: 184-208.

[373] Brucker-Davis F, Ducot B, Wagner-Mahler K., *et al.* Environmental pollutants in maternal milk and cryptorchidim. Gynécol Obstét Fert 2008; 36: 840-7.

[374] Horng C-T, Chao H-R, Chang C-M, Agoramoorthy G, Tzeng T-F, Shieh P-C. Polybrominated diphenyl ethers in human milk in Taiwan. Asian J Chem 2010; 22: 2869-78.

[375] Abraham MH, Gil-Lostes J, Fatemi M. Prediction of milk/plasma concentration ratios of drugs and environmental pollutants. Eur J Med Chem 2009; 44: 2452-8.

[376] Cummings JA, Clemens LG, Nunez AA. Mother counts: how effects of environmental contaminants on maternal care could affect the offspring and future generations. Frontiers Neuroendocrinol 2010; 31: 440-51.

[377] Schiavone A, Kannan K, Horii Y, Focardi S, Corsolini S. Polybrominated diphenyl ethers, polychlorinated naphthalenes and polycyclic musks in human fat from Italy: Comparison to polychlorinated biphenyls and organochlorine pesticides. Environ Pollut 2010; 158: 599-606.

[378] Julvez J, Grandjean P. Neurodevelopmental toxicity risks due to occupational exposure to industrial chemicals during pregnancy. Indust Health 2009; 47: 459-68.

[379] Prasse C, Schlüsener MP, Schulz R, Ternes TA. Antiviral drugs in wastewater and surface waters: A new pharmaceutical class of environmental relevance? Environ Sci Technol 2010; 44: 1728-35.

[380] Metcalfe CD, Chu S, Judt C, *et al*. Antidepressants and their metabolites in municipal wastewater, and downstream exposure in an urban watershed. Environ Toxicol Chem 2010; 29: 79-89.

[381] Nillos MG, Chajkowski S, Rimoldi JM, Gan J, Lavado R, Schlenk D. Stereoselective biotransformation of permethrin to estrogenic metabolites in fish. Chem Res Toxicol 2010; 23: 1568-75.

CHAPTER 9

Multi-Analyte Immunoassays for Water Monitoring

G. Proll*

Institute of Physical and Theoretical Chemistry (IPTC) Eberhard Karls University of Tuebingen

Abstract: Clean water, its secure delivery to consumers, and protection of resources are among the most important tasks for humans in future. To protect water resources and control water quality, it is necessary to develop fast, sensitive, cost-effective, and easy-to-use analytical systems capable of measuring a variety of small organic pollutants in aqueous samples.

Immunoassays use antibodies as a versatile analytical tool and are nowadays introduced into many different applications. The predominant testformats in the past have been the RIA (radioimmunoassay) and ELISA (enzyme linked immune sorbent assay). Together with the developments in the area of biosensors, the need for automated immunoassays carried out at the heterogeneous phase has lead to the development of new assay formats. Usually, these systems combine the approaches of various immunoassays with Flow Injection Analysis (FIA) systems and different fluorescence or label-free transduction technologies.

This chapter is dedicated to the application of antibodies in multi-analyte immunoassays for water monitoring with a focus on their application in fluorescence based optical biosensors. This includes practical aspects during assay development like affinity, cross-reactivity, and the validation process. In addition, a strategy to use antibodies with high cross reactivities (*e.g.* to the chemical group of estrogens) for the detection of sum concentrations will be explained as well as a strategy to reduce matrix effects caused by dissolved organic carbon.

Keywords: Antibodies, Immunoassays, Multi-Analyte.

INTRODUCTION

Fully automated immunoassays for trace analytics are an interesting analytical method for water monitoring. The intention is to create optical biosensors capable for the continuous quantification of small organic compounds as a cost effective alternative to lab based classical analytics. These sensors should allow for a quick analysis without the need of labor-intensive sample pre-treatments or enrichment steps. Although fully automated immunoassays are well established *e.g.* in the area of *in vitro* diagnostics, their successful introduction into the area of environmental analysis as commercial products has not yet been realized.

The development of multi-analyte immunoassays for water monitoring has to meet several specific requirements related to practicability and to the behavior of antibodies during these assays. If practicability is not just limited to the question of feasibility but also takes into account commercial aspects the list of requirements is very ambitious. For example a quasi-continuous measurement mode will only be possible with a regeneration step of the sensor after each single measurement. Therefore, it is necessary to create a specific sensor surface which is chemically stable during these procedures. In addition, the detection of small molecules is difficult in testformats where the small molecule has to be recognized by two antibodies *e.g.* sandwich assay. One possible testformat which fulfills these requirements is the binding inhibition test. It is important to select antibodies which meet the essential individual properties that are related to the used testformat. For example the affinity constant and especially the dissociation rate constant of an antibody for

***Address correspondence to G. Proll:** Institute of Physical and Theoretical Chemistry (IPTC) Eberhard Karls University of Tuebingen; http://barolo.ipc.uni-tuebingen.de; E-mail: guenther.proll@ipc.uni-tuebingen.de

Eline P. Meulenberg (Ed)

a competitive testformat should not be too high. On the other hand non-competitive testformats will achieve lowest limits of detection with antibodies offering extremely high affinities. The complex interrelationship between affinity constant, achievable limit of detection, working range, and cross-reactivity has to be taken into account.

This chapter is focused on the theoretical background of the above mentioned important antibody properties supplemented by experimental data to follow the transfer into real life applications.

AFFINITY

Immunoassays make use of the natural phenomenon of the specific interaction between an antibody and its antigen. This biomolecular interaction is characterized by a very high affinity and high specificity. However, the individual affinity constant of an analytical antibody and its affinity to other molecules than its antigen/immunogen, the so called cross-reactivity, are important parameters during immunoassay development.

The sum of the weak interaction forces involved in this biomolecular interaction process leads to specific affinity constant as described by the law of mass action. This interaction is sensitive to temperature, salt concentration, and pH. The law of mass action for this reaction is given by:

$$Ab + Ag \underset{k_{diss}}{\overset{k_{ass}}{\rightleftarrows}} AbAg$$

$$K = \frac{k_{ass}}{k_{diss}} = \frac{[AbAg]}{[Ab][Ag]}$$

The equilibrium constant K is equivalent to the affinity constant and can be calculated as the ratio between the association rate constant k_{ass} and the dissociation rate constant k_{diss}. Typical affinity constants for antibodies are between 10^6 and 10^{10} $\mathrm{Lmol^{-1}}$. This variation range is mainly caused by different dissociation rate constants. For the determination of the affinity constant, a binding inhibition test (see section 5) can be performed providing information about the test mid point of the calibration curve. At this point, corresponding to a specific antigen concentration, 50% of the antibody binding sites (paratopes) are inhibited by the antigen (or analyte). The correlation between the initial concentration of active antibody molecules and the antigen concentration can be used to form the law of mass action as following [1]:

$$K = \frac{[AbAg]}{[Ab][Ag]} = \frac{[AbAg]}{([Ab]_0 - [AbAg])([Ag]_0 - [AbAg])} \qquad \textbf{eq. 1}$$

The antibody molecules usually used within immunoassays belong to the IgG class and provide two paratopes per molecule. Therefore, it is necessary to introduce a distribution function like the binomial distribution. If the two paratopes of an antibody molecule bind to their epitopes independently, it is possible to write

$$[Ab]_c = \frac{[AbAg]^2}{2[Ab]_0} \qquad \textbf{eq. 2}$$

with $[Ab]_0$ as the paratope concentration, $[AbAg]$ antibody-antigen complex, and $[Ab]_v$ as the concentration of antibody molecules with completely occupied paratopes. The test mid point is characterized by 50% occupied paratopes, and therefore the ratio of completely occupied antibody molecules corresponds to one fourth of the paratope concentration.

$$[Ab]_c = \frac{1}{4}[Ab]_0 \qquad \textbf{eq. 3}$$

From equation 2 and 3 the concentration of the complex $[AbAg]_{tmp}$ at the test mid point can be calculated according to:

$$[AkAg]_{TMP} = \frac{1}{\sqrt{2}}[Ak]_0 \qquad \textbf{eq. 4}$$

Together with eq. 1 the affinity constant can be written as:

$$K = \frac{\frac{1}{\sqrt{2}}[Ab]_0}{\left([Ab]_0 - \frac{1}{\sqrt{2}}[Ab]_0\right)\left([Ag]_{0,tmp} - \frac{1}{\sqrt{2}}[Ab]_0\right)} = \frac{\frac{1}{\sqrt{2}}}{\left(1-\frac{1}{\sqrt{2}}\right)\left([Ag]_{0,tmp} - \frac{1}{\sqrt{2}}[Ab]_0\right)} \qquad \textbf{eq. 5}$$

$$= \frac{\frac{1}{\sqrt{2}}}{\left(1-\frac{1}{\sqrt{2}}\right)\frac{1}{\sqrt{2}}\left(\sqrt{2}[Ag]_{0,tmp} - [Ab]_0\right)} = \frac{\left(1-\frac{1}{\sqrt{2}}\right)^{-1}}{\sqrt{2}[Ag]_{0,tmp} - [Ab]_0} \qquad \textbf{eq. 6}$$

$$= \frac{2+\sqrt{2}}{\sqrt{2}[Ag]_{0,tmp} - [Ab]_0} \qquad \textbf{eq. 7}$$

The affinity constant can be determined according to equation 7 from a calibration curve using the analyte concentration at the test mid point $[Ag]_{0,\ tmp}$ and the initial antibody concentration $[Ab]_0$. This calculation is only valid for monoclonal antibodies, because only identical paratopes can be considered. In addition, the measurements during the calibration have to be performed under mass transport limited conditions to exclude effects coming from kinetic effects during the interaction processes at the surface. For polyclonal antibodies a mixture of different paratopes has to be taken into account. However, the following presented data are based on the calculated affinity constants for a polyclonal antibody according to equation 7 in terms of simplification. In this case, the estimated affinity constants for polyclonal antibodies should be denominated as mean affinity constant or avidity, although the underlying affinity distribution is not symmetric.

CROSS REACTIVITY

Although the interaction of a paratope with its epitope is very specific, the same paratope can bind to other epitopes offering structural similarities. This phenomenon is called cross reactivity and has always to be taken into account when using antibodies as the analytical tool in immunoassays. Thereby, this effect is often much stronger for polyclonal antibodies because they represent a mixture of paratopes with different affinities. To quantify this effect, the binding of an antibody to structural similar antigens is usually given as the relative cross reactivity in percent (*%CR*). Therefore, 100% basis is given by the interaction of the antibody to its primary antigen/immunogen. The determination of *%CR* can be done by a titration experiment of the antibody with its primary antigen compared to the same experiment carried out with the potential cross reactive molecule. The *%CR* can now be calculated from the test mid points according to [2, 3]:

$$\%CR = \frac{c_{PAtmp}}{c_{CAtmp}} \cdot 100 \qquad \textbf{eq. 8}$$

with c_{PAtmp}: concentration of the primary antigen at the test mid point

c_{CAtmp}: concentration of the cross reactive antigen at the test mid point

MULTI-ANALYTE IMMUNOASSAYS

In the presence of multiple cross reactive antigens and/or antibodies each individual antibody-antigen interaction takes place in competition to each other resulting in a complex equilibrium. The mathematical description of this situation was introduced by [4-6] based on the following assumptions: 1) each individual reaction is reversible and in equilibrium according to the law of mass action. 2) each paratope (*P*) competes independently for univalent antigens *(A)*. 3) no reactions take place other than:

$$A_i + P_j \rightleftharpoons A_i P_j \qquad \textbf{eq. 9}$$

$i = 1, 2, ., n \; j = 1, 2, ., m$

with n as the number of different cross reactive antigens and m as the number of different paratopes. The resulting complex equilibrium can be described as:

$$K_{A_i,P_j} = \frac{c_{A_iP_j}}{c_{fA_i} \cdot c_{fP_j}} \qquad \textbf{eq. 10}$$

i = 1, 2, ., n j = 1, 2, ., m

$$c_{tA_i} = c_{fA_i} + \sum_{j=1}^{m} c_{A_iP_j} \qquad \textbf{eq. 11}$$

$$c_{tB_j} = c_{fB_j} + \sum_{i=1}^{n} c_{A_iP_j} \qquad \textbf{eq. 12}$$

with $K_{Ai,Pj}$: affinity constant for each partial reaction.

c_{fAi}: free equlibrium concentration of antigen *i*.

c_{fPj}: free equlibrium concentration of paratope *j*.

c_{tAi}: total concentration of antigen *i*.

c_{tPj}: total concentration of paratope *j*.

c_{AiPj}: equilibrium concentration of the complex consisting of analyte *i* and paratope *j*.

Combining equations (10) to (12) results in system of n equations:

$$c_{tA_i} = c_{fA_i} + \sum_{j=1}^{m} \frac{K_{A_i,P_j} c_{tP_j} c_{fA_i}}{1 + \sum_{k=1}^{n} K_{A_k,P_j} c_{fAk}} \qquad \textbf{eq. 13}$$

$i = 1, 2, ., n$

Based on the numerical solution of this system of n nonlinear equations using the concentration of the free paratopes (c_{fBj}) at known values for c_{tAi}, c_{tPj}, and $K_{Ai,Pj}$, it is possible to calculate c_{fPj} according to:

$$c_{fP_j} = \frac{c_{tP_j}}{1+\sum_{i=1}^{n} K_{A_i,P_j} c_{fA_i}} \qquad \text{eq. 14}$$

$j = 1, 2, ., m$

The presented general description of any complex ligand-binding system can be used to characterize cross reactive antibodies as a tool for immunoassays to detect a special group of antigens/analytes as a sum concentration. This idea of group specific antibodies can be very helpful in water analysis. For example, the measurement of the total concentration of estrogenic compounds can be achieved with just one antibody. A prerequisite therefore is an antibody with similar cross reactivities and affinity constants to the structural similar group of antigens. An example to this immunoassay strategy based on a group specific antibody will be given in section 7.

BINDING INHIBITION TEST

In general immunoassays are used to qualitatively or quantitatively detect a molecule in a sample *via* specific biomolecular interaction. The different testformats of immunoassays can be distinguished according to several characteristics. Usually the first criterion is dedicated to the introduction of a solid phase. It is distinguished between homogeneous assays carried out in solution and heterogeneous assays where the reaction takes place at a surface. Furthermore, immunoassays are differentiated in competitive and non-competitive reactions and/or according to the introduced transduction method which can be based on labels (*e.g.* fluorescence) or label-free transduction [7].

In water samples, many analytes of interest are small organic compounds. Therefore, testformats making use of simultaneous binding of two paratopes to two epitopes on the same analyte molecule fail in many cases because of sterical problems due to the small size. In addition, testformats which enable fully automated measurements and a regeneration of the senor surface are preferable. For the latter this means that chemically stable sensor surfaces have to be used. This can be achieved by immobilizing the chemical stable interaction partner of an immunoreaction which in this case is of course the small organic molecule. The testformat which fits to these requirements is the so called binding inhibition test, a heterogeneous and non competitive immunoassay which can be combined with a flow injection analysis system for automation. Together with Total Internal Reflection Fluorescence (TIRF) as the transduction method it is possible to set-up multi-analyte biosensors for the trace analytics of small organic compounds [8].

The scheme of a binding inhibition test performed under continuous flow conditions is shown in Fig. **1**. In a first step prior to the measurement the antibody is mixed with the sample and pre-incubated for several minutes until the equilibrium according to the law of mass action is reached. The next step is the incubation phase where this reaction mixture is pumped over the sensor surface which carries covalently immobilized antigen-derivatives at a very high surface loading. This is necessary to guarantee mass transport limited conditions during the incubation phase. Here, each antibody molecule with at least one free paratope (which comes in contact with the heterogeneous phase because of diffusion) can bind to an epitope on the surface. Therefore, the rate-determining step is the diffusion of the antibody molecules to the surface according to Fick`s Law. This reaction under continuous flow does not change the equilibrium in the bulk mixture and therefore this testformat is non-competitive.

In combination with TIRF as the transduction method the antibodies are labeled with a fluorescent dye. After completion of the incubation phase it is now possible to read out the amount of surface bound antibody molecules *via* the fluorescence intensity. It is important to notice, that the measured signal is inversely related to the antigen/analyte concentration which means that for the blank measurement the highest fluorescence signal is observed.

A typical calibration curve for an immunoassay performed with this testformat is shown in Fig. **2**. The shape of the calibration curve follows the typical sigmoidal curve progression using a semi logarithmic plot. Compared to other assays developed for monoclonal antibodies this calibration curve shows broad working range and a smaller slope at the inflection point. Following the rules of the FDA [9] for immunoassay validation, a four parameter logistic approximation was applied according to:

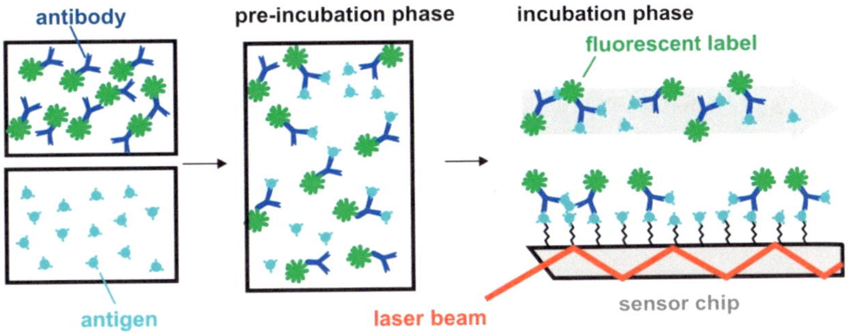

Figure 1: Principle of the binding inhibition assay testformat performed with TIRF as the transduction method.

$$y = \frac{A_1 - A_2}{1 + \left(\frac{x}{x_0}\right)^p} + A_2 \qquad \textbf{eq. 15}$$

With A_1: upper asymptote.

A_2: lower asymptote.

x: analyte concentration.

x_0: test mid point (analyte concentration at inflection point).

p: slope at test mid point after logarithmic transformation.

A_1 is the upper asymptote and A_2 the lower one. The range between A_1 and A_2 is the dynamic signal range. The inflection point is given by the variable x_0 and represents the analyte concentration, which corresponds to a decrease of 50 % of the dynamic signal range – the Inhibitory Concentration 50 % (IC_{50}). The slope of the tangent in this point is given by the parameter p.

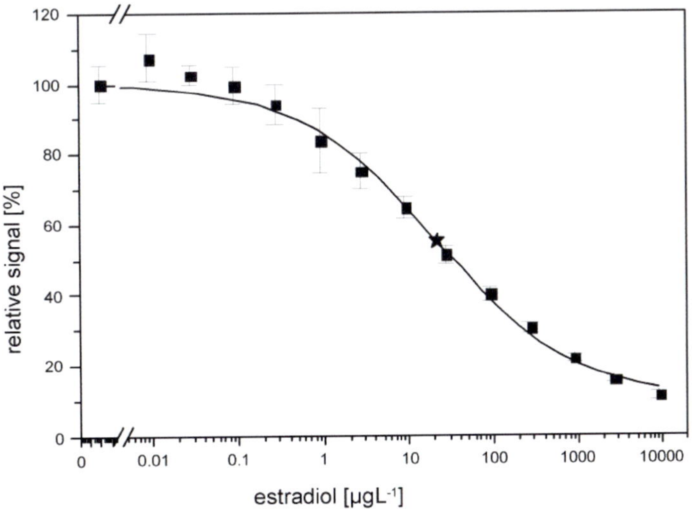

Figure 2: Calibration of the *a-E* antibody (0, 3 µgmL^{-1}) for estradiol. The sensor chip was modified with $E_{1,\,17}$CMO for the TIRF based read out using the binding inhibition assay as the testformat.

The Limit Of Detection (LOD) can be calculated according to the guidelines of analytical chemistry [10] as the corresponding concentration to the signal which is 3 times the standard deviation of the blank signal SD_{blank}. The Limit Of Quantification (LOQ) uses 10 times SD_{blank}. A real alternative is the use of the 95% Confidence Belt and the associated Minimum Detectable Concentration (MDC) and Reliable Detection Limit (RDL), which can easily be calculated for the sigmoidal calibration curves. Furthermore, the approximation of the logistic function is used to calculate the corresponding analyte concentration at the test mid point *[Ag]0, tmp*, which corresponds to the inflection point of the calibration curve. This value can be used to calculate the affinity constant according to equation 7.

These statistical tools are the basis for estimating the validation parameters of a calibration experiment. The complete validation procedure of a new immunoassay for water monitoring carried out with a fully automated biosensor should undergo the same four step validation procedure as usually performed for other techniques:

1. Lab based calibration and replica measurement spiked buffer samples.
2. Measurement of spiked real water samples and comparison to classical analytical methods (ideally carried out by an accredited laboratory).
3. Ring trial together with accredited laboratories.
4. Field test in comparison with accredited laboratories.

GROUP SPECIFIC ANTIBODIES

For monitoring water quality it is important to get a quick overview of several emerging parameters *e.g.* pesticides. Therefore, an analytical method for the quantification of pesticides in water samples must be able to detect and quantify concentrations at the given EU limit for drinking water of 0.1 μgL^{-1} [11, 12]. Because of their high impact on the aquatic fauna and humans even at low concentrations, hormones and their derivatives are of great importance. Up to now there are no limits for hormones or other EDCs. However, because of the no-effect-levels of hormonal active compounds it is necessary to have Limits Of Detection (LOD) in the low nanogram per liter range. The quantification of estrogens at very low concentrations can be performed with the above described biosensor principle. The introduction of a polyclonal antibody with similar affinities to the important members of the estrogen-group follows this idea of screening the water samples by measuring the sum concentration of estrogens rather than quantifying dozens of individual substances in individual immunoassays.

The following data are based on experiments with a polyclonal anti-total-estrogen ($a\text{-}E_t$) antibody from sheep, which offers high cross reactivities to all relevant estrogenic compounds. Using a TIRF biosensor and the binding inhibition test as the testformat, affinity constants for different estrogenic compounds can be calculated according to equation 7 (see Table **1**) on the basis of a set of calibration experiments. The active antibody concentration was determined by label-free reflectometric interference spectroscopy measurements. Corresponding cross reactivities are shown in Fig. **3**.

Table 1: Mean affinity constants of the $a\text{-}E_t$ antibody to different antigens.

Analyte	***K [Lmol⁻¹]***
estradiol	$4, 46\ 10^9$
estrone	$4, 30\ 10^9$
ethinylestradiol	$5, 39\ 10^9$
estriol	$3, 32\ 10^7$
bisphenol A	$4.99\ 10^5$
diethylstilbestrol	$2.01\ 10^6$
genistein	$3, 44\ 10^5$

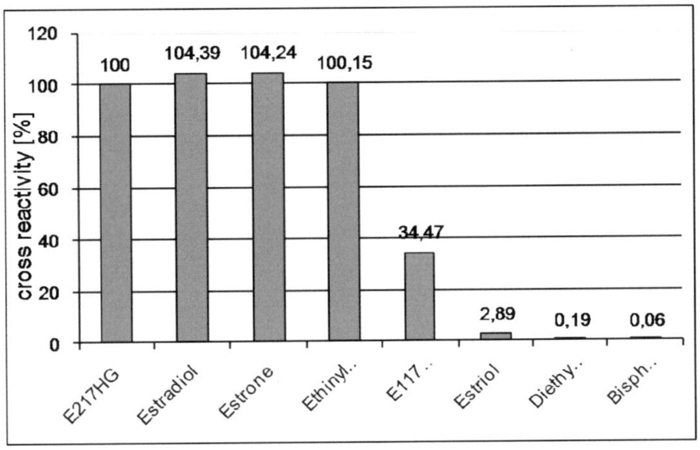

Figure 3: Cross reactivity of the *a-Et* antibody to different estrogens. The immunogen E_217HG (estradiol-17-O-hemiglutarat) was set to 100%.

To verify the performance of this highly cross reactive $a\text{-}E_t$ antibody regarding sum-concentration measurements it is necessary to correlate multi-analyte measurements with the mathematical considerations as described in section 4. Therefore, the expected signals for measurements of complex mixtures of estradiol, ethinylestradiol, estrone, estriol, and diethylstilbestrol at known concentrations are calculated and compared to the measured signals. For the calculation of the measurement signals a reference point is needed. Therefore the concentration of estrone resulting in a 50% inhibition of the paratopes was calculated and measured.

It can be shown that it is possible to calculate the measurements signal for any composition of a complex mixture. For this system the maximum error was below 7%. Therefore, it can be concluded that it is possible to introduce antibodies as a tool for the measurement of sum concentrations at reasonable accuracy. However, the bottleneck of this method is the availability of antibodies offering suitable properties in terms of a homogeneous cross reactivity to the relevant members of a compound class like the estrogens.

MATRIX EFFECTS

In the area of water monitoring, negative effects on the analytical performance of an immunoassay due to the matrix present have always to be taken into account. On the one hand it is possible that analyte molecules adsorb on matrix components and/or particles and therefore are not accessible for the immunoreactions. On the other hand the antibody molecules can be detracted from the active antibody concentration by interaction with these components, or the underlying bio-molecular interaction is disturbed. In the latter case it can be helpful to introduce a standardized matrix into the calibration procedure to simulate real life conditions. This approach follows the recommendations of the FDA to perform the calibration of an immunoassay under matrix conditions which correspond to the respective sample matrix.

One of the most important matrix component in water samples is Dissolved Organic Carbon (DOC). This heterogeneous class of molecules is always present at highly variable concentrations in any surface water sample. The influence of different DOC levels on the analytical performance of immunoassays depends on the testformat, and in particular on the used antibody. To avoid false-negative outcomes during environmental monitoring, a strategy for matrix-referenced correction of results can be applied. Therefore, a synthetic organic carbon standard (DOC standard according to ISO/CEN EN1484) can be introduced during the calibration and validation process. Typical concentrations for DOC are between 10 and 40 mgL^{-1}. In practice the additional presence of DOC results in changed fluorescence signals during biosensor measurements. Interestingly, experiments with real life water samples show much better recovery rates when this reference method is applied as demonstrated together with classical analytical technologies provided by an accredited laboratory [13]. During this study samples from different surface water bodies at different estrone spiking levels have been analyzed by a TIRF based biosensor. The binding inhibition test was performed with a monoclonal anti-estrone antibody. For all samples the Recovery Rates (RR) for different estrone spiking levels have been calculated according to the AOAC International guidelines based on the validation parameters of the buffer-calibration. Especially the RR for the estrone levels between 1.8 and 4.5 ng mL^{-1} were outside of the recommended 70-120% range. After correction of the mean values by measurement of DOC spiked blanks, the RR were reevaluated for estrone spiked samples. Interestingly, all corrections based on different DOC spiking levels resulted in valid RR for the 1.8 ng L^{-1} estrone spiking level (results are summarized in Fig. **4**). With the DOC referencing in this study it was possible to improve especially the RR in the lower nano-gram per liter range for estrone. This is important with respect to the low no-effect levels of hormones. However, it might be advantageous to adjust the DOC correction to the known concentration of DOC in the specific water sample.

In general, this principle of introducing the matrix into the calibration procedure leads to more reliable and robust results compared to approaches only focused on improving other parameters during immunoassay development like surface chemistry or recognition elements.

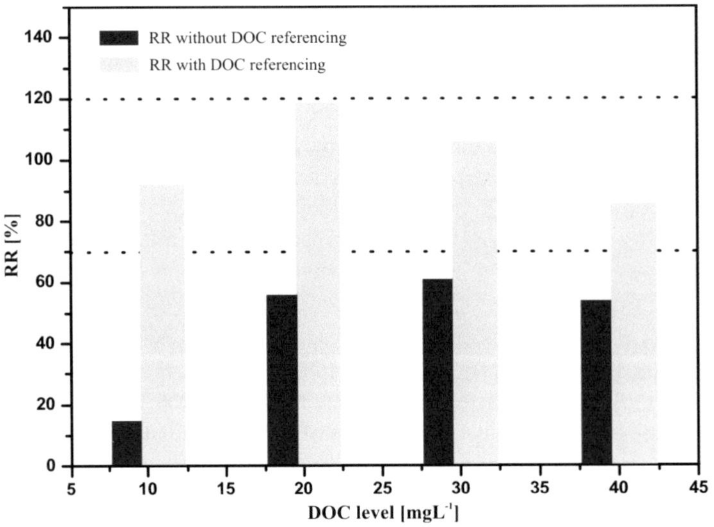

Figure 4: RR for water samples spiked with 1.8 ng mL^{-1} estrone at different DOC levels between 10 and 40 mg L^{-1}. RR without DOC referencing dark grey, RR with DOC referencing light grey.

REFERENCES

[1] Piehler J, Brecht A, Giersch T, Hock B, Gauglitz G. Assessment of affinity constants by rapid solid phase detection of equilibrium binding in a flow system. J. Immunol. Methods 1997; 201: 189-206.

[2] Abraham GE. Solid-phase radioimmunoassay of estradiol-17 beta. J. Clin. Endo 1969; 29: 866-870.

[3] Oubina A, Gascon J, Barcelo D. Multianalyte effect in the determination of cross-reactivities of pesticide immunoassays in water matrices. Analytica Chimica Acta 1997; 341: 121-130.

[4] Feldman HA, Rodbard D, Levine D. Mathematical Theory of Cross-Reactive Radioimmunoassay and Ligand-Binding Systems at Equilibrium. Anal Biochem 1972; 45: 530-556.

[5] Feldman HA. Mathematical Theory of Complex Ligand-Binding Systems at Equilibrium: Some Methods for Parameter Fitting. Anal Biochem 1972; 48: 317-338.

[6] Blomberg KR. Mathematical Theory of Complex Ligand-Binding Systems Applied to Free Triiodothyronine Immunoassays. Anal. Chem 1991; 63: 2581-2586.

[7] Gauglitz G, Vo-Dinh T., editors. Handbook of Spectroscopy Vol. 2, Berlin: Wiley-VCH; 2003.

[8] Tschmelak J, Proll G, Riedt J, *et al.* Automated Water Analyser Computer Supported System (AWACSS) - Part II: Intelligent, remote-controlled, cost-effective, on-line, water-monitoring measurement system. Biosens Bioelectron. 2005; 20(8): 1509-1519.

[9] Food and Drug Administration. Guidance for Industry Bioanalytical Method Validation. U.S. Department of Health and Human Services, Center for Drug Evaluation and Research (CDER), Center for Veterinary Medicine (CVM). 2001.

[10] Inczedy J, Lengyel T, Ure AM., editors. Compendium of Analytical Nomenclature. Definitive Rules 1997, "The Orange Book", 3rd ed., Oxford: Blackwell Science; 1998.

[11] Council Directive 98/83/EC of 3 November 1998 on the quality of water intended for human consumption

[12] World Health Organization. Guidelines for Drinking Water Quality, 3rd Edition. World Health Organization, Geneva, Switzerland, 2003.

[13] Tschmelak J, Proll G, Gauglitz G. Improved strategy for biosensor based monitoring of water bodies with diverse organic carbon levels. Biosens Bioelectron 2005; 21: 979-983.

CHAPTER 10

Principles and Applications of Immunoaffinity Chromatography

Abby J. Jackson, Matthew R. Sobansky and David S. Hage*

Department of Chemistry, University of Nebraska, Lincoln, NE 68588-0304, USA

Abstract: Immunoaffinity Chromatography (IAC) is a type of liquid chromatography that uses the highly specific binding of antibodies for the retention of a target. This approach can be used in a myriad of techniques for the selective purification, concentration and/or analysis of target compounds. This chapter discusses the basic components of an IAC method, including the support, stationary phase, immobilization technique, and proper sample application and elution conditions. Several applications of IAC are also considered. These applications include immunoextraction, immunodepletion, chromatographic immunoassays, and post-column immunodetection. A wide range of targets that have been isolated or measured by these techniques are listed. Related methods based on antibody mimics are also discussed.

Keywords: Antibodies, Immunoaffinity Chromatography.

INTRODUCTION

Immunoaffinity chromatography (IAC) combines the high specificity of antibody-antigen interactions with the use of liquid chromatography. IAC is a subcategory of affinity chromatography that makes use of antibodies or antibody-related molecules as the stationary phase. The strong and selective binding that is typically present between antibodies and their targets, as well as the ability to produce antibodies against a wide range of targets, has made antibodies popular in use as immobilized ligands for affinity chromatography and related methods [1-4].

The earliest known use of IAC in the selective purification of compounds from biological samples dates back to 1935. In this early work, D'Allesandro and Sofia adsorbed specific antigens onto kaolin and charcoal for the isolation of antibodies that were associated with syphilis and tuberculosis [5]. A year later, Landsteiner and coworkers immobilized haptens onto chicken erythrocyte stroma by the diazo coupling for use in isolating antibodies [6]. In 1951, Campbell immobilized albumin to *p*-aminobenzylcellulose for antibody purification [7]. There are now thousands of modern-day reports that have used IAC for the isolation of chemicals and biochemicals [1, 3, 4, 8-12] and in a wide variety of analytical applications [2, 4, 9, 11-21].

This chapter will examine the main components of an IAC method and discuss how the strong and specific nature of antibody-target binding can be used in liquid chromatographic systems. This discussion will include a look at the support materials, immobilization methods, and application or elution techniques that are commonly employed in IAC. Various applications of IAC will then be presented. These applications will include on/off elution methods, immunoextraction, immunodepletion, chromatographic immunoassays, and post-column immunodetection. A wide range of targets that have been isolated or measured by these techniques will also be given. Finally, a brief discussion of related methods based on antibody mimics will be provided.

BASIC COMPONENTS OF IAC

Stationary Phases in IAC

IAC uses an antibody-related ligand as the stationary phase to create a separation method that makes use of the selective binding ability of an antibody with its target. It has been estimated that between 10^7 and 10^9

***Address corresponding David S. Hage:** Department of Chemistry, University of Nebraska, 704 Hamilton Hall, Lincoln, NE 68588-0304, USA; Fax: +1 402 472 9402. E-mail: dhage@unlserve.unl.edu different types of antibodies are produced by the human body, each capable of binding to a different target antigen [3]. This feature makes it possible to generate antibodies for IAC against a wide array of targets. Either polyclonal antibodies or monoclonal antibodies can be used in IAC methods. Polyclonal antibodies tend to be used when tight binding is desired or if some cross-reactivity is needed for more than one compound in the same class of targets. Monoclonal antibodies tend to have more specific binding but also tend to have lower affinities than polyclonal antibodies. The association equilibrium constants for these interactions under physiological conditions are often in the range of 10^6 to 10^{12} M^{-1} [21]. This strong binding is a result of the combined effects of such forces as ionic interactions, hydrogen bonding, hydrophobic interactions and van der Waals forces [3]. Adjusting the extent of these forces is useful in later eluting retained compounds from IAC columns, as is discussed later in this chapter.

Supports for IAC

Early work with IAC was carried out by using low-performance supports such as carbohydrate-related materials (*i.e.*, agarose or cellulose) or synthetic organic supports (*i.e.*, acrylamide polymers, copolymers or derivatives, polymethacrylate derivatives, and polyethersulfone matrixes). While the low cost of these materials has continued to make these supports popular in modern IAC applications involving target purification, these materials also have several limitations. The limitations of these supports include slow mass transfer properties (*i.e.*, poor efficiency) and instability at high pressures, and issues with stability during storage, which tend to limit the usefulness of these supports in HPLC systems. Antibodies can be used with HPLC systems in a method known as High-Performance Immunoaffinity Chromatography (HPIAC) if the support material is sufficiently rigid and efficient, and can withstand the pressures and flow rates used in these systems [22]. Supports commonly used for HPIAC include derivatized silica [23], glass [24], azalactone beads [25], methacrylate polymeric supports [26], and polystyrene-based perfusion media [27].

There are other considerations to also consider when choosing a support for IAC [1-3]. The support should have low non-specific interactions for sample components and be easily modifiable for antibody attachment. When using a porous material, both the size of the pores and the ability of the antibody to access the support's surface for immobilization need to be considered. Supports with small pores tend to have a high surface area for immobilization, but a large fraction of this area may be inaccessible to the antibodies. Supports with large pores do not have problems with accessibility, but they also have less surface area than supports with smaller pores. As a result, maximum antibody immobilization is often observed for supports with pore sizes between 300 and 500Å, which is approximately three to five times the diameter of the antibody [28]. The ability of the target to enter the pores and reach the immobilized antibodies also should be determined on a case-by-case basis.

IAC is usually carried out using particulate supports and packed-bed columns. However, other materials and formats have also been recently used in IAC. These alternative forms of media have included affinity disks, affinity fibers, and affinity monoliths [22, 29]. Some unique features of these materials are their improved mass transfer properties and good flow properties when compared to particulate supports. These properties have made these supports of interest in both target purification and in rapid analytical methods based on IAC [20].

Immobilization Methods for IAC

When creating a support for IAC, the ideal situation is to have the antibodies or binding agents attached to the support in a way that does not alter their binding activity or hinder their accessibility to a target [30]. Antibodies can be immobilized onto supports through a variety of techniques, ranging from covalent attachment to adsorption by binding to a secondary ligand. Covalent attachment methods are the most common approach in IAC and can use various functional groups for immobilization. Antibodies can be immobilized through free amine groups by using supports that are activated with agents such as *N*, *N*'-carbonyldiimidazole, cyanogen bromide, *N*-hydroxysuccinimide, or tresyl chloride/tosyl chloride. Supports that have been treated to produce reactive epoxide or aldehyde groups on their surfaces can also be used for antibody immobilization through amine groups [25, 31, 32]. Although the use of amine groups for immobilization is one of the easiest methods to attaching antibodies to a solid support, the presence of many amine groups on each antibody can lead to random orientation of the immobilized antibodies and blocking of their binding sites. These effects, in turn, can lead to actual or apparent loss of some antibody activity [33].

In order to create more active supports, antibodies or F_{ab} fragments can be covalently immobilized through more site-selective methods. When F_{ab} fragments are generated, free sulfhydryl groups are created on these fragments that can be utilized for immobilization. This type of attachment can be carried out by using techniques such as the divinylsulfone, epoxy, iodoacetyl/bromoacetyl, malemide, or tresyl chloride/tosyl chloride methods [25, 31, 32]. Antibodies can also be selectively immobilized through the carbohydrate residues that are located in their F_c regions. Mild oxidation of the antibody can generate aldehyde groups in these carbohydrate residues that can then be reacted with a hydrazide- [34] or amine-containing support for immobilization [25, 31].

Non-covalent antibody immobilization can be achieved by using a secondary ligand to adsorb the antibody onto a support. A common technique for accomplishing this type of immobilization is to employ the strong binding that occurs between biotin and avidin or streptavidin, which has an association equilibrium constant in the range of 10^{13}-10^{15} M^{-1}. One way of using this system for IAC is to incubate antibodies with *N*-hydroxysuccinimide-*D*-biotin at pH 9, which creates biotinylated antibodies that can be adsorbed to a support containing avidin or streptavidin [35, 36]. The biotin-avidin/streptavidin linkage can withstand many types of elution conditions without dissociation. It should be noted that if the antibodies are biotinylated through an amine-based coupling method, problems with loss of antibody activity can again occur. This problem can be minimized by using hydrazide-biotin to react with aldehyde residues that are created from mild oxidation of an antibodies carbohydrate residues in the F_c region [37].

Another approach for indirectly immobilizing an antibody is based on the strong interactions which take place between protein A or protein G and the F_c regions of many antibodies [3]. This binding is strong until physiological conditions (pH 7.0-7.4), but decreasing the surrounding solution to approximately pH 2-3 will cause these interactions to weaken and allow release of the adsorbed antibodies. This approach to immobilization is useful when high antibody activity is needed, and frequent replacement of antibodies on the IAC support is desired. One limitation of this method is that the frequent release and replacement of adsorbed antibodies will require a much larger amount of antibodies for long-term studies than traditional immobilization methods. This problem can be minimized by cross-linking the antibodies to the protein A or protein G by using carbodiimide [38] or dimethyl pimelimidate [39, 40].

Application and Elution Conditions for IAC

In IAC the application buffer is generally chosen to promote fast and efficient binding of the desired target compound to the immobilized antibodies [3]. Optimum binding for antibodies typically occurs at a physiological pH. The strong binding that occurs for many antibodies under these conditions is not amenable for the use of isocratic elution unless relatively low affinity antibodies (*i.e.*, those with association equilibrium constants less than 10^6 M^{-1}) are present [41-43]. Usually the retained targets are instead released from the antibodies by applying an elution buffer in a stepwise gradient. However, more gradual or non-linear gradients can also be utilized. Fig. **1** shows a typical scheme by which an IAC column can be used to selectively bind and elute analytes from a sample. This particular scheme is based on a step gradient in going from the original application buffer to an elution buffer and is also known as the "on/off" mode of IAC [3].

One of the most popular techniques for eluting retained compounds in IAC is to alter the pH of the mobile phase [2, 3]. This is often done by applying an acidic buffer (*e.g.*, pH 1-3, with pH 2-3 being most common) to the column. Alkaline elution conditions are not favorable for work in IAC that uses supports such as silica or glass beads due to the instability of these materials at a pH greater than 8.0 [2, 44, 45]. While altering the pH of the mobile phase allows for easy elution of most compounds from antibodies, there is also a risk of possibly denaturing the immobilized antibodies or altering pH-sensitive targets when using this approach. However, many IAC systems have been shown to be quite stable when using moderate pH changes (*e.g.*, going from pH 7.0-7.5 to 2.5-3.0) [2, 3].

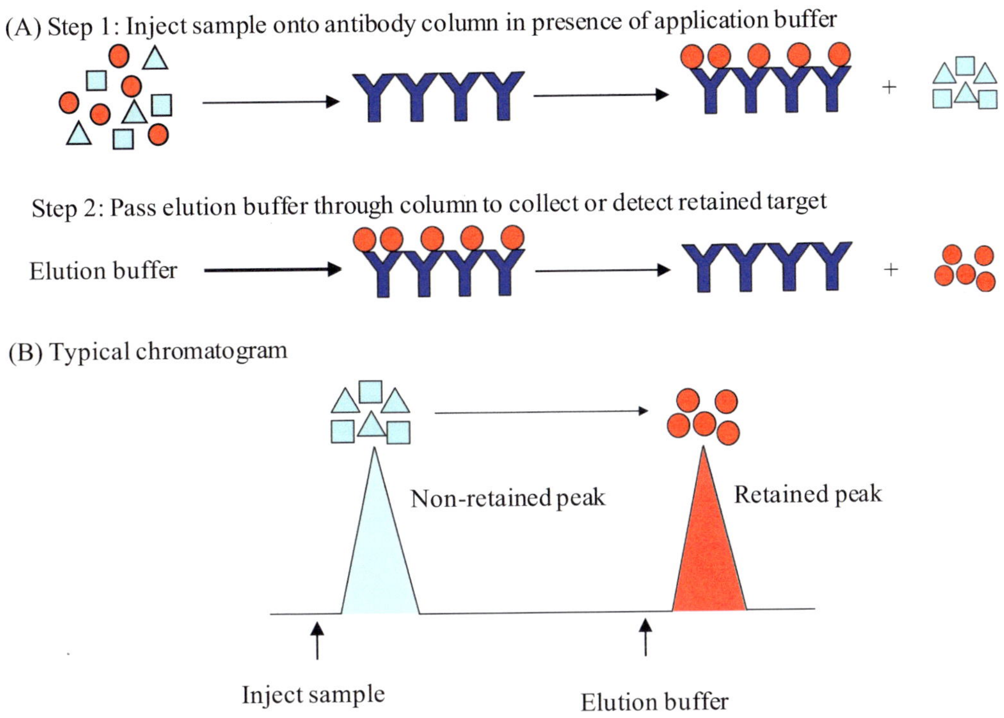

Figure 1: (A) The on/off mode of immunoaffinity chromatography (IAC) and **(B)** an example of general chromatogram that is obtained with this approach. The circles in (A) represent the target analyte, while the squares and triangles represent non-retained sample components.

Elution with chaotropic agents often yields effective results for IAC without the danger of denaturation that is associated with a change in pH [3]. Chaotropic salts such as thiocyanate (SCN^-), trifluoroacetate (CF_3COO^-), perchlorate (ClO_4^-), iodide (I^-) and chloride (Cl^-) can disrupt the structure of water around the target or antibody and reduce hydrophobic interactions. These agents are shown to be effective for target elution when applied at concentrations between 1.5 and 8 M. The relative elution strength for these agents is as follows: $SCN^- > CF_3COO^- > ClO_4^- > I^- > Cl^-$ [46].

Organic modifiers can also be added to the mobile phase for the elution of targets in IAC [3]. In this case, care must be taken to make sure that the concentration of the organic additives is not too high and does not permanently denature the antibodies in the IAC column. For example, the addition of an organic modifier such as methanol has shown to decrease the capacity of some IAC columns. While this denaturation and loss of capacity is not always permanent, regeneration for the IAC can sometimes take several days. Therefore, if harsh elution conditions are required, the capacity of the IAC column should be much larger than the actual amounts of target that are to be measure or isolated to avoid this effect [47].

APPLICATIONS OF IAC

IAC has been utilized in many applications that ranged from preparative work to trace analysis. IAC has also been used analytical methods in techniques that involve both direct and indirect target detection. In addition, IAC has been coupled with techniques such as High-Performance Liquid Chromatography (HPLC), Gas Chromatography (GC), Mass Spectrometry (MS), and Capillary Electrophoresis (CE). These methods will be discussed in more detail in the following sections.

Traditional IAC Methods

The most common and simplest technique that is typically used in IAC is the on/off elution mode [1-3]. In this format (as illustrated earlier in Fig. **1**), the sample of interest is injected onto the IAC column under conditions in which the target has a strong binding to the antibodies immobilized in the column. Only the target and closely-related compounds are usually retained on the IAC column in this format, while other sample components are not retained. After the non-retained sample components have been washed away, an elution buffer is passed through the column. This elution buffer is used to disrupt binding between the target and immobilized antibodies, allowing the target to dissociate and be collected or detected as it elutes from the column. The primary advantage of this format is the speed and simplicity of the technique, especially when it is carried out as part of an HPLC system.

As shown in Fig. **1(b)**, the on/off mode of IAC gives a chromatogram that often contains only two peaks. The first peak in this chromatogram corresponds to all non-retained sample components that elute during the sample application step. The second peak represents the analytes that are originally retained by the IAC column and later eluted when the elution buffer is passed through the column. In this format it is often easy to obtain baseline resolution between the non-retained and retained peaks by changing the time at which the elution buffer is applied. This is another advantage of the on/off mode of IAC that makes this technique appealing for both preparative and analytical applications.

The on/off of IAC has been commonly used in biochemistry and other fields for the examination of specific targets in complex mixtures. Proteins, glycoproteins, carbohydrates, lipids, bacteria, viral particles, drugs, and environmental agents have all been isolated using this format of IAC [1, 3, 4, 8-12]. The use of step elution in the on/off mode is also popular in HPIAC because of its speed and ability to product sharp peaks for the eluting targets. This approach can even be used in the direct detection of targets if they are present at sufficient levels in the sample. The detection method in this approach will depend on the limit of detection that is required and may be based on absorbance measurements, fluorescence, mass spectrometry, pulsed amperometric detection, or radiolabel detection, to name a few possibilities [2]. In general, direct detection works best with targets that dissociate from the IAC column within a few minutes. Targets with longer elution times and broader peaks are best analyzed by an alternative approach, such as immunoextraction coupled with Reversed-Phase Liquid Chromatography (RPLC), as described in the next section.

Immunoextraction and Immunodepletion

Immunoextraction refers to the use of IAC to remove a specific target from a mixture of components in a sample prior to analysis by a second method [2, 15, 48]. This technique has been found to be extremely useful in many areas of science. Immunoextraction is routinely used for the preparative isolation of target compounds in biochemistry and can be utilized for sample treatment prior to the use of analytical methods such as HPLC, GC, MS, or CE [1-3].

Immunoextraction can also be employed in both off-line and on-line formats. Off-line immunoextraction methods are often the easiest approach for combining IAC with other techniques. Off-line immunoextraction has been coupled with other analytical methods for the analysis of urine, food, water and soil extracts. Examples of analytes that have been examined by this approach include α_1-anti-trypsin, atrazine, benzylpenicilloyl-peptides, bovine serum albumin, carbendazim, chloramphenicol, cortisol, clenbuterol and phenytoin, and others [2, 3]. Methods utilizing off-line immunoextraction typically combine this method with Solid-Phase Extraction (SPE). In method, antibodies are immobilized on a low-performance support packed into a small disposable syringe or cartridge. The immunoaffinity cartridge is then conditioned with the application buffer or other necessary solvents prior to application of the sample. Following the removal of non-retained components, an elution buffer is applied to the immunoaffinity cartridge, and the target is collected as it elutes. The collected fraction may then be further treated to make it compatible with a second technique for analysis. Examples of this pretreatment include drying and reconstituting the target in a solvent compatible with HPLC analysis or derivatization of the target to increase its volatility for analysis by GC [2].

In addition to being able to remove the target from a sample matrix, off-line immunoextraction also offers the ability to concentrate a target prior to analysis. This may be accomplished by applying a large sample volume to the immunoaffinity support without exceeding the capacity of this material. The essentially irreversible binding of most targets to immobilized antibodies under typical application conditions results in high retention and focusing of the target based on the IAC support. The later elution of the target with a small volume of elution buffer will lead to an increase in the effective concentration of the target. If additional concentration of the target is still needed, the eluted fraction can be collected, dried, and reconstituted in a small volume of a suitable solvent [2].

A large number of on-line immunoextraction methods have also been reported [2, 3, 15, 17, 18]. In these methods, the IAC column is often used for sample pretreatment prior to the detection, measurement, or characterization of a target. This approach can be performed with a variety of methods (*e.g.*, size-exclusion chromatography, ion-exchange chromatography, CE, MS, or GC), but the direct coupling of immunoextraction with RPLC has been of particular interest. The relative ease with which an immunoextraction column can be incorporated into an HPLC system makes this combination appealing as a means of automating sample pretreatment and reducing the time required for this process. In addition, the high reproducibility seen with modern HPLC systems gives on-line immunoextraction a better precision than off-line immunoextraction methods [2].

A general scheme for utilizing on-line immunoextraction coupled with RPLC is shown in Fig. **2.** In this type of system, a sample is first injected on the immunoextraction column in the presence of an appropriate application buffer. The non-retained compounds are diverted during the injection process to a waste container prior to switching the immunoextraction column on-line with an RPLC column. When the immunoextraction column is switched on-line with a small RPLC precolumn, an elution buffer is applied to dissociate the retained targets. As these targets elute from the immunoextraction column they enter and are concentrated at the head of an RPLC precolumn. Following the removal of all targets from the immunoextraction column, this column is switched back off-line and regenerated with the application buffer before another sample is injected. At the same time, the RPLC precolumn is placed on-line with a longer analytical RPLC column and the targets are eluted through these columns by increasing the organic modifier content of the mobile phase. This step allows the eluting targets to be separated based on their differences in polarity and to be monitored by an on-line detector. On-line immunoextraction coupled with RPLC has been used to measure targets in many types of samples, including food extracts [49], bodily fluids [50-57], cell extracts [58] and environmental samples [59, 60]. This approach has also been used with a wide range of targets that range for herbicides and drugs to proteins [2, 15, 17].

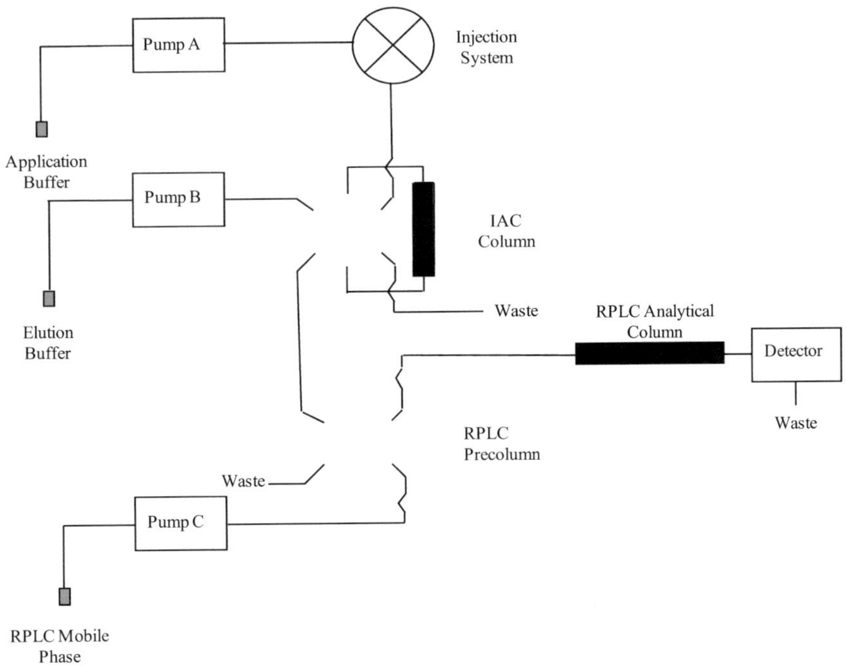

Figure 2: Design of a system for on-line immunoextraction coupled with reversed-phase liquid chromatograph (RPLC).

The method of immunodepletion is closely related to immunoextraction. This technique utilizes an IAC support to remove an abundant target from a sample matrix prior to the use of a second method for the analysis of less abundant components in the sample. This technique is often used in proteomics to remove highly and moderately abundant proteins from samples to aid in the analysis of lower abundance proteins. This approach provides the ability to simultaneously deplete multiple high-abundance proteins in a highly selective manner, a feature which is not possible with other methods such as precipitation, SPE, ultracentrifugation, molecular weight separations, or separations based on differences in isoelectric points [61-66].

Chromatographic-Based Immunoassays

Chromatographic (or flow-injection) immunoassays are another way in which IAC can be utilized as an analytical tool. This technique makes use of immobilized antibody, or antigen, in a column to perform various competitive- or non-competitive immunoassay formats. The competitive-binding immunoassays involve the competition between a target analyte present in the sample matrix and a labeled analyte analog for a limited amount of antibodies that can bind either the native or labeled species. Following a competition for binding sites, the bound analyte and labeled analog are separated from the free portion of each that remains in solution. The amount of labeled analog that is present in either the bound or free faction is then measured. The absence of any unlabeled analyte results in the maximum possible amount of labeled analog in the bound fraction. An increase in the amount of unlabeled analyte results in a decrease in the level of bound labeled analog. The result is a mechanism in which the amount of analyte in the sample can be measured indirectly.

Competitive binding immunoassays can be performed by IAC through the use of several possible formats, such as a simultaneous injection immunoassay [67-98], a sequential injection immunoassay [99-110], or a displacement immunoassay [111, 112] (see Table **1** for a list of reported applications). The simultaneous injection immunoassay is the most common type of competitive binding immunoassay in IAC. This method is performed by mixing the labeled analog with the sample and injecting both this and the analyte simultaneously onto an IAC column. The labeled analog (A*) and the analyte (A) then compete for binding sites on the immobilized antibodies. The competition between A* and A results in an alteration of the amount of labeled analog that is detected in the bound and/or non-retained fractions [21]. Calibration curves for this method are generally prepared by plotting the relative response of the labeled analog (B/B_o) versus the concentration of analyte in the sample, where B is the amount of labeled analog that is bound in the presence of a given amount of analyte and B_o is the amount of labeled analog that is bound in the absence of any analyte. This type of calibration curve will have a maximum value of one when no analyte is present and should approach zero at high analyte concentrations if no non-specific binding is present between the labeled analog and the column [68, 69].

Table 1: Examples of IAC-based Competitive Binding Immunoassays.

Simultaneous Injection Immunoassays			
Target [c]	***Detection Method***	***Assay Characteristics***	***Ref.***
Human transferrin	Fluorescence	Range, <500 μg/mL	[72]
Transferrin	Fluorescence	Limit of detection, 25 μg/mL	[71]
Adrenocorticotropic hormone	Fluorescence	Range, 0.2-10 mg/L	[70]
Testosterone	Fluorescence	Limit of detection, 0.5 μg/mL	[78]
Theophylline	Fluorescence	Limit of detection, 0.3 ng/mL; Range, <500 μg/L	[79]
Atrazine	Fluorescence	Limit of detection, 2.1 μg/mL; Range, 2.1–50 μg/L	[80]
Cephalexin	Electrochemical	Limit of detection, 1 μg/L	[75]
Immunoglobulin G [IgG]	Absorbance	Limit of detection, 333 zmol	[73]
Theophylline	Electrochemical	Limit of detection, 25 ng/mL	[77]
Anti-Bovine serum albumin	Fluorescence	Limit of detection, 0.2 nM; Linear range, 0.4-0.8 nM	[81]

Table 1: cont....

Human serum albumin	Thermometric	Limit of detection, 10^{-10} M	[74]
Theophylline	Fluorescence	Limit of detection, 3 μg/L; Range, 3-75 μg/L	[67]
Pullulanase, IgG, antithrombin	Fluorescence		[76]
IgG	Fluorescence	Limit of detection, 155 ng/mL	[88]
IgG	Fluorescence	Limit of detection, 4 x 10^{-9}M	[89]
Gentamicin	Fluorescence	Limit of detection, 200 ng/mL; Working range, 250-5000 ng/mL	[90]
IgG	Fluorescence	Linear range: 1-5 μg/L	[87]
Insulin	Thermometric	Limit of detection, 0.025 μg/mL; Working range, 0.05-2 μg/mL	[86]
Carbaryl	Fluorescence	Limit of detection, 20 ng/L	[83]
Atrazine	Fluorescence	Limit of detection, 75 ng/L	[82]
Isoproturon	Absorbance	Limit of detection, 0.09 μg/L	[84]
Gentamicin	Thermometric	Range, 10-400 μg/L	[85]
IgG	Electrochemical		[91]
Digoxin	Chemiluminescence	Limit of detection, 0.2 ng/mL	[92]
IgG	Chemiluminescence	Limit of detection, 7 fmol	[93]
Theophylline	Fluorescence		[98]
Theophylline	Fluorescence	Range, 0.025-0.04 mg/L	[96, 144]
Theophylline, caffeine	Fluorescence	Range, 3 x 10^{-5}–3 x 10^{-8} M	[145]
Antitheophylline	Fluorescence	Range, 4 x 10^{-7}–6 x 10^{-9} M	[145]
Methotrexate	Radioactivity	Range, 1-100 μg/L	[95]
Thyroxine	Electrochemical	Limit of detection, 25 μg/L; Linear range, 25-50 μg/L	[94]
Cortisol	Fluorescence	Range, 1-60 μg/dL	[97]
Sequential Injection Immunoassays			
Imazethapyr	Fluorescence	Limit of detection, 500 ppb	[104]
Imazethapyr	Fluorescence	Limit of detection, 0.5 ppb	[104]
IgG	Thermometric	Range, 10-400 μg/mL	[110]
IgG	Thermometric	Limit of detection, 33 pmol	[99]
Digoxin	Electrochemical	Limit of detection, 10 pg/mL; Range, 10-1000 pg/mL	[100]
Atrazine	Fluorescence	Range, 0.02-0.3 μg/L	[101]
Atrazine	Fluorescence	Range, 0.03-0.5 μg/L	[102]
Human serum albumin	Electrochemical		[108]
α-Amylase	Absorbance		[109]
Anti-IgG	Chemiluminescence	Limit of detection, 1 fmol	[106]
Imazethapyr	Fluorescence	Limit of detection, 0.1 ppb	[105]
Imazethapyr	Fluorescence	Range, 0.1-100 ng/mL	[103]
Displacement Immunoassays			
Cocaine, benzoylecgonine	Fluorescence		[145]
TNT, Dinitrotoluene	Fluorescence	Limit of detection, 2.5 ng/mL; Range, 20-1200 ng/mL	[146]

Table 1: cont....

Cocaine, benzoylecgonine	Fluorescence		[147]
2, 4-Dinitrophenol	Radioactivity	Limit of detection, 140 nM; Linear range, 570-4600 nM	[112]
2, 4-Dinitrophenol	Fluorescence	Linear range, 290-2300 nM	[112]
Cortisol	Fluorescence	Dynamic range, 12.5-1250 pmol	[148]
Polychlorinated biphenyls	Fluorescence	Limit of detection, 4 ppm; Linear range, 4-20 µg/mL	[149]
Transferrin, human serum albumin	Absorbance		[150]

Sequential injection immunoassay is another type of competitive binding immunoassay that is utilized in IAC. This method is performed by injecting a sample containing the analyte onto a column containing immobilized antibodies, followed by the subsequent injection of a labeled analog of the analyte. This situation again creates competition between A* and A for binding sites on the immobilized antibodies and results in alteration of the amount of labeled analog that is detected in the bound and/or non-retained fractions. A calibration curve can be generated in this method by using the same procedure as already described for a simultaneous injection immunoassay. The primary advantage of a sequential injection immunoassay versus a simultaneous injection immunoassay is that the labeled analog never comes into contact with the analyte, which eliminates matrix effects during detection of the labeled analog. This effect allows for improved reproducibility, a wider range of suitable detection formats, and lower background signals for the sequential injection format. In addition, the sequential injection format tends to give a lower limit of detection than the simultaneous injection format because the analyte has an increased opportunity to bind to the column. One drawback of a sequential injection immunoassay versus a simultaneous injection immunoassay is its narrower dynamic range [107]. The wider dynamic range in a simultaneous injection immunoassay is a result of the increased ability of the analyte to compete with the labeled analog when they are applied to the immunoaffinity column at the same time.

A third type of competitive binding immunoassay that can be performed by IAC is a displacement immunoassay. In this method, an IAC column is saturated with a labeled analog of the analyte prior to the injection of a sample. As the sample is injected, the analyte can displace any labeled analog that is momentarily free in solution. The eluted labeled analog gives a peak with a response that is proportional to the amount of analyte in the sample. An advantage of this method is that several samples can be injected onto an IAC column that is loaded with the labeled analog before regeneration is necessary [111]. Injection of multiple samples without regeneration requires that enough labeled analog remains bound after each injection to give a consistent and measurable response. As a result, IAC columns with large capacities are preferred in this format. The stability of the signal in a displacement immunoassays will also depend on the rate of dissociation of the labeled analog from the immobilized antibodies [111, 112]. Slow flow rates tend to increase the displacement effect in these assays as the longer contact times between the sample and column allow for more labeled analog to dissociate.

Non-competitive immunoassays, or immunometric assays can also be performed by using IAC. Two types of non-competitive immunoassays in IAC are one-site immunometric methods [113-129] and sandwich immunoassays [73, 130-138] (see examples in Table **2**). One-site immunometric assays are performed by incubating a sample with a known excess of labeled antibodies that are specific for the target. This mixture is then applied to a column containing an immobilized analog of the target analyte. The column binds and removes the unbound portion of labeled antibodies while allowing antibodies bound to target to pass through non-retained. Detection can be performed by measuring the response of the non-retained labeled antibodies or by monitoring the amount of retained antibodies that dissociate from the column during the elution step. The signal for the bound labeled fraction is directly proportional to the amount of target in the original sample. A calibration curve is created by plotting the relative response of the bound, labeled antibody fraction versus the amount of target in the sample. A one-site immunometric assay can be used to detect both large and small targets and a multitude of elution conditions can be used with the immobilized analog columns. The primary difficulty in operation of these assays is obtaining affinity ligands with the required activity and purity to create an assay in which all the excess agent binds to the affinity column and gives a low background signal [129].

Table 2. Examples of IAC-Based Non-Competitive Binding Immunoassays.

One-Site Immunometric Assays			
Target	***Detection Method***	***Assay Characteristics***	***Ref.***
Granulocyte colony-stimulating factor	Fluorescence	Limit of detection, 1.5 ng/120 μL	[113]
Digoxin and metabolites	Fluorescence	Limit of detection, 2 x 10^{-10} M	[114]
Digoxin and metabolites	Fluorescence	Limit of detection, 160 pg/mL; Linear range, 0.2–2 nmol/L	[115]
Digoxin	Fluorescence	Limit of detection, 200 fmol	[116]
Digoxigenin	Fluorescence	Limit of detection, 50 fmol; Linear range, 50–1000 fmol	[117]
Digoxin	Fluorescence	Limit of detection, 0.025 nM	[117]
Digoxigenin	Fluorescence	Limit of detection, 0.01 nM	[117]
Interleukin-10	Fluorescence	Limit of detection, 40 fmol	[118]
Digoxin	Absorbance	Limit of detection, 0.2 μg/L	[119]
2, 4-D	Electrochemical	Limit of detection, 0.25 μg/L	[120]
Digoxigenin	Electrochemical	Limit of detection, 0.5 amol; Linear range, 0.38–7.7 fmol	[121]
α-[Difluoromethyl]-ornithine	Fluorescence	Limit of detection, 200 amol; Linear range, 5 x 10^{-11}–2.5 x 10^{-9} M	[122]
Fatty acid-binding protein	Absorbance	Range, 1–12 μg/L and 12–2000 μg/L	[123]
Thyroxine	Chemiluminescence	Limit of detection, 10^{-11} M	[124]
4-Amino-L- and D-phenylalanine	Chemiluminescence	Limit of detection, 1.76 pmol/mL	[125]
17-Estradiol	Fluorescence		[126]
α-Fetoprotein	Fluorescence	Limit of detection, 0.1 ng/mL; Linear range, 0.5–60 ng/mL	[127]
Terbutryn	Grating coupler	Limit of detection, 15 μg/L; Linear range, 20–200 μg/L	[128]
Sandwich Immunoassays			
Thyroid-stimulating hormone	Absorbance	Range, 0–0.29 nM	[130]
Human chorionic gonadotropin	Fluorescence	Range, 0–66.6 ng/mL	[130]
Human serum albumin	Fluorescence	Limit of detection, 0.001 mg/mL	[151]

Table 2: cont….

Parathroid hormone, interleukin-5	Fluorescence	Limit of detection, 10 nM; Linear range, <250 μM	[131]
Immunoglobulin G [IgG]	Absorbance	Limit of detection, 3 fmol; Range, 3.33 – 130 fmol	[73]
IgG	Fluorescence	Linear range, 0.5–50 pmol/L	[132]
Human serum albumin	Electrochemical	Range, 1-10 mg/mL	[133]
Anti-IgG	Electrochemical	Range, 3-225 fmol	[91]
IgG	Electrochemical	Range, 5-400 ng/mL	[135]
IgG	Chemiluminescence	Range, 0.2–20 fmol	[136]
Parathyroid hormone	Chemiluminescence	Limit of detection, 0.24 pM; Linear range, 0.24–67 pM	[137]

Sandwich immunoassays (also known as two-site immunometric assays) use two different antibodies that can each bind the target of interest (see Fig. **3**). One of the antibodies is immobilized to the support material in an IAC column and is used to extract target from an injected sample. The second antibody is labeled for detection and is either mixed with the sample prior to application or applied to the column directly after the target is bound to the IAC column. The binding of target by the two antibodies creates a "sandwich" complex in the column. After this complex has been created, an elution buffer is applied and the target and labeled antibodies are eluted. Measurement of the labeled antibodies that elute gives a response that is directly proportional to the amount of target. Calibration curves for sandwich immunoassays are prepared by plotting the relative response of the retained, labeled antibodies against the amount of target in the sample. Sandwich immunoassays are capable of giving a linear response over a broad range of analyte concentrations [2, 21]. The main disadvantage of the sandwich immunoassay is that only large targets (*e.g.*, high mass peptides, proteins and biomacromolecules) can be measured by this approach because the target must be able to bind two antibodies simultaneously. Another disadvantage of this format is the added cost of utilizing two different antibodies per analyte [2, 21].

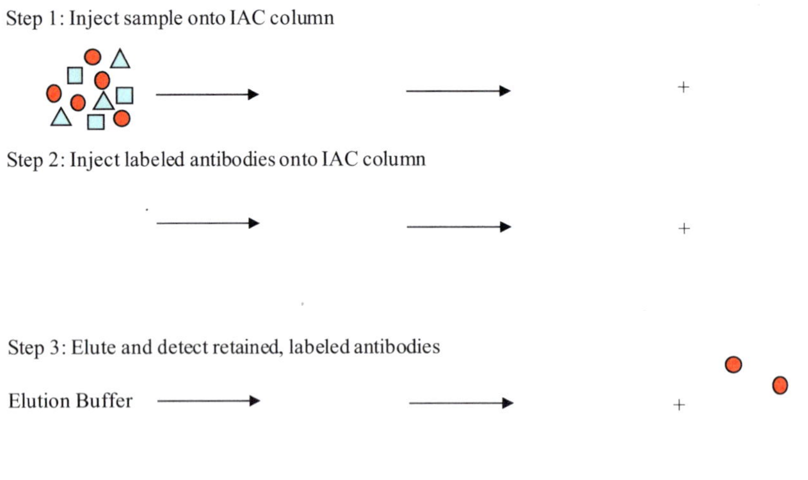

Figure 3: General format for a sandwich immunoassay.

Post-Column Immunodetection

IAC columns can also be utilized to monitor the presence of a specific target that is eluting from other chromatographic columns. This approach is often referred to as immunodetection or post-column immunodetection [2, 21]. This technique typically involves the use of a post-column reactor and an immobilized antibody or antigen column that is attached to the exit of an analytical HPLC column. Immunodetection can be performed using either direct or indirect detection by using a chromatographic-based immunoassay, such as discussed in the previous section.

Fig. **4** illustrates a typical post-column immunodetection system. As the target elutes from the analytical column, it is mixed with an excess labeled antibodies which can bind to the target. The excess, unbound labeled antibodies are removed by then using a column that contains an immobilized analog of the target. Bound, labeled antibodies pass through the analog column and give a signal that is proportional to the eluting target's concentration. When performing post-column immunodetection it is important to ensure that the eluent from the analytical column is adjusted to allow for maximum antibody binding in the post-column reactor. This requires that the pH and ionic strength be adequate for antibody binding to the analog column and that the amount of any organic modifiers be minimized to appropriate levels to allow this binding to occur [2, 21]. This type of detection has been used for various applications, including the quantitation of growth-hormone-releasing factor, digoxin, digoxigenin and human granulocyte colony-stimulating factor [3].

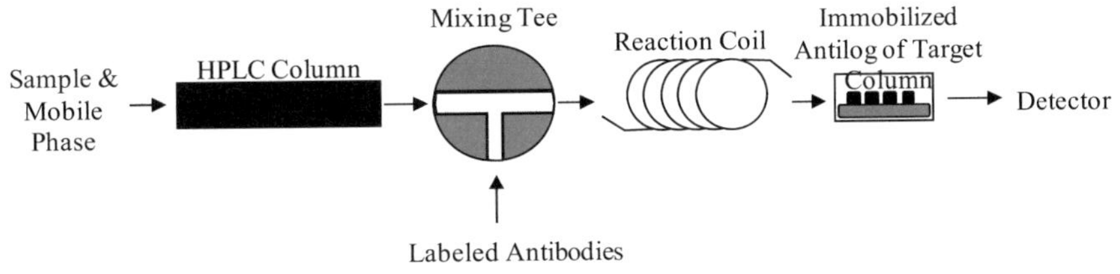

Figure 4: General design of a system for post-column immunodetection.

Related Methods and Antibody Mimics

In recent years, antibody mimics have been successfully utilized as alternative ligands in affinity chromatography. Two types of antibody mimics are aptamers and molecular imprints. Aptamers are polymers of nucleotides with well-defined sequences and three-dimensional structures. Studies have shown that a large number of aptamers can be generated randomly in an oligonucleotide library and the ligands that bind to a given analyte can be selectively enriched for use in affinity chromatography [139-141]. Aptamers are appealing ligands for this work because they can be designed for a specific analyte, they are relatively stable, and they can provide moderate to high selectivity when binding to targets [139-143].

A molecular imprint is an affinity ligand that is incorporated into the internal structure of the support in an affinity column. These supports are usually made by combining the analyte of interest with a series of monomers that contain side chains capable of interacting with the target. As these interactions take place, the monomers are fixed in position about the target during the polymerization process. Following polymerization, the support is ground into a powder and the target used for the imprinting is released by a wash with solvent. The imprinted support is then packed into a column. The result is an affinity support with a known specificity and binding/elution properties [142, 143]. Like aptamers, molecular imprints can be custom designed for a given target, can be stable over long periods of time, and can provide moderate-to-high selectivity for targets [139-143].

CONCLUSIONS

This chapter has discussed the general principles of IAC and has shown how antibodies and antibody mimics can be utilized in affinity columns. The supports and immobilization methods that are utilized in preparing columns for IAC were discussed. The design of IAC methods and the choice of application and elution conditions were also considered. Many formats and applications of IAC were described and examples of these formats were presented. It was shown in this discussion how the highly specific nature of IAC makes this a valuable tool in many areas for both sample analysis and target purification.

ACKNOWLEDGMENTS

This work was supported, in part, by the National Institutes of Health (NIH) under grants R01 GM044931 and R01 DK069629.

DISCLOSURE

Portions of this review have been previously published in A.C. Moser and D.S. Hage, "Immunoaffinity chromatography: an introduction to applications and recent developments", Bioanalysis, 2 (2010) 769-790.

REFERENCES

[1] Moser AC, Hage DS. Immunoaffinity chromatography: an introduction to applications and recent developments. Bioanalysis 2010; 2: 769-90.

[2] Hage DS. Survey of recent advances in analytical applications of immunoaffinity chromatography. J Chromatogr B 1998; 715: 3-28.

[3] Hage DS, Phillips TM. Immunoaffinity Chromatography. In: Hage DS, Ed. Handbook of Affinity Chromatography. New York, Taylor & Francis, 2006; Chap. 6.

[4] Phillips TM. High performance immunoaffinity chromatography. LC Mag 1985; 3: 962-72.

[5] D'allesandro G, Sofia F. The adsorption of antibodies from the sera of syphilitics and tuburculosis patients. Z Immunitats 1935; 84: 237-50.

[6] Landsteiner K, Scheer JVD. Cross reactions of immune sera to azoproteins. J Exp Med 1936; 63: 325-39.

[7] Campbell DH, Luescher E, Lerman LS. Isolation of antibody by means of a cellulose-protein antigen. Proc Natl Acad Sci USA 1951; 37: 575-8.

[8] Subramanian A. Immunoaffinity chromatography. Mol Biotechnol 2002; 20: 41-7.

[9] Weller MG. Immunochromatographic techniques - a critical review. Fres J Anal Chem 2000; 366: 635-45.

[10] Carlton GJ. Immunosorbent separations. Methods Enzymol 1985; 104: 381-7.

[11] Gallant SR. Immunoaffinity chromatography of proteins. Methods Mol Biol 2004; 251: 103-9.

[12] Zolotarjova N, Boyes B, Martosella J. Immunoaffinity Depletion of High-Abundant Proteins for Proteomic Sample Preparation. In: Smejkal GB, Lazarev A, Eds. Separation Methods in Proteomics. Boca Raton, CRC Press, 2006; pp. 63-79.

[13] De Frutos M, Regnier FE. Tandem chromatographic-immunological analyses. Anal Chem 1993; 65: 17A-25A.

[14] Peoples MC, Karnes HT. Microfluidic immunoaffinity separations for bioanalysis. J Chromatogr B 2008; 866: 14-25.

[15] Hage DS, Nelson MA. Chromatographic immunoassays. Anal Chem 2001; 73: 198A-205A.

[16] Hage DS, Clarke W. Immunoaffinity Chromatography in Clinical Analysis. In: Aboul-Enein HY, Ed. Separation Techniques in Clinical Chemistry. New York, Marcel Dekker, 2003; pp. 361-387.

[17] Nelson MA, Hage DS. Environmental Analysis by Affinity Chromatography. In: Hage DS, Ed. Handbook of Affinity Chromatography. New York, Taylor & Francis, 2006; Chap. 19.

[18] Goryacheva IY, Rusanova TY, Burmistrova NA, De Saegar S. Immunochemical methods for the determination of mycotoxins. J Anal Chem 2009; 64: 768-85.

[19] Jiang T, Mallik R, Hage DS. Affinity monoliths for ultrafast immunoextraction. Anal Chem 2005; 77: 2362-72.

[20] Hage DS, Rollag JG, Thomas DH. Analysis of atrazine and its degradation products in water by tandem high-performance affinity chromatograph and reversed-phase liquid chromatography. ACS Symp Ser 1997; 657: 118-32.

[21] Moser AC, Hage DS. Chromatographic Immunoassays. In: Hage DS, Ed. Handbook of Affinity Chromatography. New York, Taylor & Francis, 2006; Chap. 29.

[22] Gustavsson P, Larsson PO. Support Materials for Affinity Chromatography. In: Hage DS, Ed. Handbook of Affinity Chromatography. New York, Taylor & Francis, 2006; Chap. 2.

[23] Schiel JE, Mallik R, Soman S, Joseph KS, Hage DS. Applications of silica supports in affinity chromatography. J Sep Sci 2006; 29: 719-37.

[24] Phillips TM. Measurement of recombinant interferon levels by high performance immunoaffinity chromatography in body fluids of cancer patients on interferon therapy. Biomed Chromatogr 1992; 6: 287-90.

[25] Hage DS. Affinity Chromatography. In: Katz E, Eksteen R, Shoenmakers P, Miller N, Eds. Handbook of HPLC. New York, Marcel Dekker, 1998; Chap. 13.

[26] McConnell JP, Anderson DJ. Determination of fibrinogen in plasma by high-performance immunoaffinity chromatography. J Chromatogr 1993; 615: 67-75.

[27] Zou H, Zhang Y, Lu P, Krull IS. Perfusion immunoaffinity chromatography and its application in analysis and purication of biomolecules. Biomed Chromatogr 1996; 10: 122-6.

[28] Clarke W, Beckwith JS, Jackson A, Reynolds B, Karle EM, Hage, DS. Antibody immobilization to high-performance liquid chromatography supports. Characterization of maximum loads capacity for intact immunoglobulin G and F_{ab} fragments. J Chromatogr A 2000; 888: 13-22.

[29] Mallik R, Hage DS. Affinity monolith chromatography. J Sep Sci 2006; 29: 1686-704.

[30] Kim H, Hage DS. Immobilization Methods for Affinity Chromatography. In: Hage DS, Ed. Handbook of Affinity Chromatography. New York, Taylor & Francis, 2006; Chap. 3.

[31] Hermanson GT, Mallia AK, Smith PK. Immobilized Affinity Ligand Techniques. New York, Academic Press, 1992.

[32] Larsson PO. High-performance liquid chromatography. Methods Enzymol 1984; 104: 212-23.

[33] Kortt AA, Oddie GW, Iliadies P, Gruen LC, Hudson PJ. Nonspecific amine immobilization of ligand can be a potential source of error in Biacore binding experiments and may reduce binding affinities. Anal Biochem 1997; 253: 103-11.

[34] Ruhn PF, Garver S, Hage DS. Development of dihydrazide-activated silica supports for high-performance affinity chromatography. J Chromatogr A 1994; 669: 9-16.

[35] Bayer EA, Wilcheck M. The use of avidin-biotin complex as a tool in molecular biology. Methods Biochem Anal 1980; 26: 1-45.

[36] Hage DS, Bian M, Burks R, Karle E, Ohnmacht C, Wa C. Bioaffinity Chromatography. In: Hage DS, Ed. Handbook of Affinity Chromatography. New York, Taylor & Francis, 2006; Chap. 5.

[37] O'Shannessy DJ, Quarles RH. Labeling of the oligiosaccharide moieties of immunoglobulins. J Immunol Methods 1987; 99: 153-61.

[38] Phillips TM, Queen WD, More NS, Thomspon AM. Protein A-coated glass beads: universal support medium for high-performance affinity chromatography. J Chromatogr 1985; 327: 213-9.

[39] Schneider C, Newman RA, Sutherland DR, Asser U, Greaves MF. A one-step purification of membrane proteins using a high efficiency immunomatrix. J Biol Chem 1982; 257: 10766-9.

[40] Sisson TH, Castor CW. An improved method for immobilizing IgG antibodies of protein A-agarose. Immunol Methods 1990; 157: 215-20.

[41] Zopf D, Ohlson S, Dakour J, Wang W, Lundblad A. Analysis and purification of oligosaccharides by high-performance liquid affinity-chromatography. Methods Enzymol 1989; 179: 55-64.

[42] Dakour J, Lundblad A, Zopf D. Separation of blood group A-active oligosaccharides by high-pressure liquid affinity chromatography using a monoclonal antibody bound to concanavalin A silica. Anal Biochem 1987; 161: 140-3.

[43] Purchades R, Maquieira A. Recent developments in flow injection immunoanalysis. Crit Rev Anal Chem 1996; 26: 195-218.

[44] Ibarra N, Caballero A, Gonzales E, Valdes R. Comparison of different elution conditions for the immunopurification of recombinant hepatitis B surface antigen. J Chromatogr B 1999; 735: 271-7.

[45] Cong J, Thompson VF, Goll DE. Immunoaffinity purification of the calpains. Protein Exp Purif 2002; 25: 283-90.

[46] Sica V, Puca GA, Molinari M, Buonaguro FM, Bresciani F. Effect of chemical perturbation with sodium thiocyanate on receptor-estradiol interaction: a new exchange assay at low temperature. Biochem 1980; 19: 83-88.

[47] Delaunay N, Pichon V, Hennion MC. Immunoaffinity solid-phase extraction for the trace-analysis of low-molecular-mass analytes in complex sample matrices. J Chromatogr B 2000; 745: 15-37.

[48] De Frutos M, Regnier FE. Tandem chromatographic-immunological analyses. Anal Chem 1998; 65: 17A-25A.

[49] Newkirk DK, Benson RW, Howard PC, *et al.* Online immunoaffinity capture, coupled with HPLC and electrospray ionization mass spectrometry, for automated determination of fumonisins. J Agric Food Chem 1998; 46: 1677-88.

[50] Itoh M, Kominami G. On-line immunoaffinity extraction followed by high-performance liquid chromatography and radioimmunoassay for a novel retinobenzoic acid. J Immunoassay Immunochem 2001; 22: 213-23.

[51] Holtzapple CK, Buckley SA, Stanker LH. Determination of fluoroquinolones in serum using an on-line clean-up column coupled to high-performance immunoaffinity-reversed-phase liquid chromatography. J Chromatogr B 2001; 754: 1-9.

[52] Creaser CS, Feel SJ, Houghton E, Seymour M. Immunoaffinity chromatography combined online with high-performance liquid chromatography-mass spectrometry for the determination of corticosteroids. J Chromatogr A 1998; 794: 37-43.

[53] Flurer CL, Novotny M. Dual microcolumn immunoaffinity liquid chromatography: an analytical application to human plasma proteins. Anal Chem 1993; 65: 817-21.

[54] Farjam A, Brugman AE, Lingeman H, Brinkman UAT. On-line immunoaffinity sample pretreatment for column liquid chromatography: evaluation of desorption techniques and operating condtions using an anti-estrogen immuno-precolumn as a model system. Analyst 1991; 116: 891-6.

[55] Radabaugh MR, Nemirovsky OV, Misko TP, Aggarwal P, Mathews WR. Immunoaffinty liquid chromatography-tandem mass spectrometry detection of nitrotyrosine in biological fluids: development of a clinically translatable biomarker. Anal Biochem 2008; 308: 68-76.

[56] Berna M, Schmalz C, Duffin K, *et al.* Online immunoaffinity liquid chromatography/tandem mass spectrometry determination of a type II collagen peptide biomarker in rat urine: investigation of the impact of collision-induced dissociation fluctuation on peptide quantitation. Anal Biochem 2006; 356: 235-43.

[57] Hoos JS, Sudergat H, Hoelck JP. Selective quatitative bioanalysis of proteins in biological fluids by on-line immunoaffinity chromatography-protein digestion-liquid chromatography-mass spectrometry. J Chromatogr B 2006; 830: 262-9.

[58] Roberts DW, Churchwell MI, Beland FA, *et al.* Quantitative analysis of etheno-2'-deoxycytidine DNA adducts using on-line immunoaffinity chromatography coupled with LC/ES-MS/MS detection. Anal Chem 2001; 73: 303-9.

[59] Nelson MA, Papastavros E, Dodlinger M, Hage DS. Environmental analysis by on-line immunoextraction and reversed-phase liquid chromatography: optimization of the immunoextraction/RPLC interface. J Agric Food Chem 2007; 55: 3788-97.

[60] Rollag JG, Beck-Westermeyer M, Hage DS. Analysis of pesticide degradation products by tandem high-performance immunoaffinity chromatography and reversed-phase liquid chromatography. Anal Chem 1996; 68: 3631-7.

[61] Hao P, Ren Y, Xie Y. Label-free relative quantification method for low-abundance glycoprotein in human serum by microTOF-q. J Chromatogr B 2009; 877: 1657-66.

[62] Cellar NA, Karnoup AS, Albers DR, *et al.* Immunodepletion of high abundance proteins coupled on-line with reversed-phase liquid chromatography: a two-dimensional LC sample enrichment and fractionation technique for mammalian proteomics. J Chromatogr B 2009; 877: 79-85.

[63] Dowling P, O'Driscoll L, Meleady P. 2-D Difference gel electrophoresis of the lung squamour cell carcinoma versus normal sera demonstrates consistent alterations in the levels of ten specific proteins. Electrophoresis 2007; 28: 4302-10.

[64] Lai X, Bacallao RL, Blazer-Yost BLL, *et al.* Characterization of the renal cyst fluid proteome in autosomal dominant polycystic kidney disease (ADPKD) patients. Proteomics Clin Appl 2008; 2: 1140-52.

[65] Chromy BA, Gonzales AD, Perkins J. Proteomic analysis of human serum by two dimensional differential gel electrophoresis after depletion of high-abundant proteins. J Proteome Res 2004; 3: 1120-7.

[66] Yu KH, Rustgi AK, Blair IA. Characterization of proteins in human pancreatic cancer serum using differential gel electrophoresis and tandem mass spectrometry. J Proteome Res 2005; 4: 1742-51.

[67] Garcinuno RM, Fernandez P, Perez-Conde C, *et al.* Development of a fluoroimmunosensor for theophylline using immobilized antibody. Talanta 2000; 52: 825-832.

[68] Hage DS, Thomas DH, Beck MS. Theory of a sequential addition competitive binding immunoassay based on high-performance immunoaffinity chromatography. Anal Chem 1993; 65: 1622-30.

[69] Hage DS, Thomas DH, Chowdhuri AR, Clarke W. Development of a theoretical model for chromatographic-based competitive binding immunoassays with simultaneous injection of sample and label. Anal Chem 1999; 71: 2965-75.

[70] Martin-Esteban A, Fernandez P, Perez-Conde C, *et al.* New fluorescence immunoassay for adrenocortitropic hormone determination using flow injection analysis. Anal Quim Int Ed 1996; 92: 37-40.

[71] Palmer DA, Fernandez-Hernando P, Miller JN. A model online flow injection fluorescence immunoassay using a protein A immunoreactor and Lucifer yellow. Anal Lett 1993; 26: 2543-53.

[72] Ren X. Flow injection fluoroimmunoassay for human transferrin using a protein A immunoreactor. Anal Lett 1994; 27: 1067-74.

[73] De Frutos M, Paliwal SK, Regnier FE. Liquid chromatography based enzyme-amplified immunological assays in fused-silica capillaries at the zeptomole level. Anal Chem 1993; 65: 2159-63.

[74] Mattiasson B, Borrebaeck C, Sanfridson B, Mosbach K. Thermometric enzyme linked immunosorbent assay: TELISA. Biochim Biophys Acta 1977; 483: 221-7.

[75] Meyer U, Zhi ZL, Meusel M, *et al.* Automated stand-alone flow injection immunoanalysis system for the determination of cephalexin in milk. Analyst 1999; 124: 1605-10.

[76] Middendorf C, Schultze B, Freitag R, *et al.* Online immunoanalysis for bioprocess control. J Biotech 1993; 31: 395-403.

[77] Palmer DA, Edmonds TE, Seare NJ. Flow-injection immunosensor for theophylline. Anal Lett 1993; 26: 1425-39.

[78] Palmer DA, Evans M, Miller JN, French MT. Rapid fluorescence flow injection immunoassay using a novel perfusion chromatographic material. Analyst 1994; 119: 943-7.

[79] Rico CM, Fernandez MDP, Gutierrez AM, *et al.* Development of a flow fluoroimmunosensor for determination of theophylline. Analyst 1995; 120: 2589-91.

[80] Turiel E, Fernandez P, Perez-Conde C, *et al.* Flow-through fluorescence immunosensor for atrazine determination. Talanta 1998; 47: 1255-61.

[81] Wang Q, Luo G, Wang Y, Yeung WSB. Sandwich immunoassay for monoclonal antibody using protein G immunoaffinity capillary chromatography and diode laser induced fluorescence detection. J Liq Chromatogr Rel Tech 2000; 23: 1489-98.

[82] Gascon J, Oubina A, Ballesteros B. Development of a highly sensitive enzyme-linked immunosorbent assay for atrazine. Performance evaluation by flow injection immunoassay. Anal Chim Acta 1997; 347: 149-62.

[83] Gonzalez-Martinez MA, Morais S, Puchades R, Maquineria A, Abad A, Montoya A. Development of an automated controlled-pore glass flow-through immunosensor for carbaryl. Anal Chim Acta 1997; 347: 199-205.

[84] Katmeh MF, Godfrey AJM, Stevenson D, Aherne GW. Enzyme immunoaffinity chromatography - a rapid semi-quatitative immunoassay technique for screening the presence of isoproturon in water sampels. Analyst 1997; 122: 481-6.

[85] Mattiasson B, Svensson K, Borrebaeck C, Jonsson S, Kronvall G. Non-equilibrium immunoassay of gentamicin. Clin Chem 1978; 24: 1770-3.

[86] Mecklenburg M, Lindbladh C, Li H, Mosbach K, Danielsson B. Enzymic amplification of a flow-injected thermometric enzyme-linked immunoassay for human insulin. Anal Biochem 1993; 212: 388-93.

[87] Pollema CH, Ruzicka J. Flow injection renewable surface immunoassay: a new approach to immunoanalysis with fluorescence detection. Anal Chem 1994; 66: 1825-31.

[88] Pollema CH, Ruzicka J, Christian GD, Lernmark A. Sequential injection immunoassay utilizing immunomagnetic beads. Anal Chem 1992; 64: 1356-61.

[89] Valencia-Gonzalez MJ, Diaz-Garcia ME. Flow-through fluorescent immunosensing of IgG. Ciencia 1996; 4: 29-40.

[90] Yang HH, Zhu QZ, Qu HY, Chen XL, Chen MT, Xu JG. Flow injection fluorescence immunoassay for gentamicin using sol-gel-derived mesoporous biomaterial. Anal Biochem 2002; 308: 71-6.

[91] De Alwis U, Wilson GS. Rapid heterogeneous competitive electrochemical immunoassay for IgG in the picomole range. Anal Chem 1987; 59: 2786-9.

[92] Dreveny D, Seidl R, Gubitz G, Michalowski J. Development of solid-phase chemiluminescence immunoassays for digoxin comparing flow injection and sequential injection techniques. Analyst 1998; 123: 2271-6.

[93] Hacker A, Hinterleitner M, Shellum C, Guebitz G. Development of an automated flow injection chemiluminescence immunoassay for human immunoglobulin G. Fres J Anal Chem 1995; 352: 793-6.

[94] He Z, Jin W. Capillary electrophoresis enzyme immunoassay with electrochemical detection for thyroxine. Anal Biochem 2003; 313: 34-40.

[95] Kamel R, Landon J, Forrest GC. A fully automated, continuous-flow radioimmunoassay for methotrexate. Clin Chem 1980; 26: 97-100.

[96] Locascio-Brown L, Plant AL, Chelser R, Kroll M, Ruddel M, Durst RA. Liposome-based flow-injection immunoassay for determining theophylline in serum. Clin Chem 1993; 39: 386-91.

[97] Schmalzing D, Nashabeh W, Fuchs M. Solution-phase immunoassay for determination of cortisol in serum by capillary electrophoresis. Clin Chem 1995; 41: 1403-6.

[98] Yap WT, Locascio-Brown L, Plant AL, Choquette SJ, Horvath V, Durst RA. Lipsome flow injection immunoassay: model calculations of competitive immunoreactions involving univalent and multivalent ligands. Anal Chem 1991; 63: 2007-11.

[99] Brandes W, Maschke HE, Scheper T. Specific flow injection sandwich binding assay for IgG using protein A and a fusion protein. Anal Chem 1993; 65: 3368-71.

[100] Kaneki P, Xu Y, Kumari A, Halsall HB, Heineman WR, Kissinger PT. Electrochemical enzyme immunoassay using sequential saturation technique in a 20-ml capillary: digoxin as a model analyte. Anal Chim Acta 1994; 287: 253-8.

[101] Kramer P, Schmid R. Flow injection immunoanalysis (FIIA) - a new immunoassay format for the determination of pesticides in water. Biosens Bioelectron 1991; 6: 239-43.

[102] Kramer PM, Schmid RD. Automated quasi-continuous immunoanalysis of pesticides with a flow injection system. Pesticide Sci 1991; 32: 451-62.

[103] Lee M, Durst RA. Determination of imazethapyr using capillary column flow injection liposome immunoanalysis. J Agric Food Chem 1996; 44: 4032-6.

[104] Lee M, Durst RA, Wong RB. Comparison of liposome amplification and fluorophor detection in flow-injection immunoanalysis. Anal Chim Acta 1997; 354: 23-8.

[105] Lee M, Durst RA, Wong RB. Development of flow-injection liposome immunoanalysis (FILIA) for imazethapyr. Talanta 1998; 46: 841-59.

[106] Liu H, Yu JC, Bindra DS, Givens RS, Wilson GS. Flow injeciton solid-phase chemiluminescent immunoassay using a membrane-based reactor. Anal Chem 1991; 63: 666-9.

[107] Nelson MA, Reiter WS, Hage DS. Chromatographic competitive binding immunoassays: a comparison of the sequential and simultaneous injection methods. Biomed Chromatogr 2003; 17: 188-200.

[108] Nilsson M, Haakanson H, Mattiasson B. Process monitoring by flow-injection immunoassay: evaluation of a sequential competitive binding assay. J Chromatogr 1992; 597: 383-9.

[109] Nilsson M, Mattiasson G, Mattiasson B. Automated immunochemical binding assay (flow-ELISA) based on repeated use of an antibody column placed in a flow-injection system. J Biotech 1993; 31: 381-94.

[110] Scheper T, Brandes W, Maschke H, Ploetz F, Mueller C. Two FIA-based biosensor systems studied for bioprocess monitoring. J Biotech 1993; 31: 345-56.

[111] Kusterbeck AW, Wemhoff GA, Charles PT. A continuous flow immunoassay for rapid and sensitive detection of small molecules. J Immunol Methods 1990; 135: 191-7.

[112] Whelan JP, Kusterbeck AW, Wemhorr GA, Brendhorst R, Ligler FS. Continuous-flow immunosensor for detection of explosives. Anal Chem 1993; 65: 3561-5.

[113] Miller KJ, Herman AC. Affinity chromatography with immunochemical detection applied to the analysis of human methionyl granulocyte colony stimulating factor in serum. Anal Chem 1996; 68: 3077-82.

[114] Irth H, Oosterkamp AJ, Tjaden UR, VanderGreef J. Strategies for online coupling of immunoassays to HPLC. Trends Anal Chem 1995; 14: 355-61.

[115] Oosterkamp AJ, Irth H, Beth M, Unger KK, Tjaden UR, VanderGreef J. Bioanalysis of digoxin and its metabolites using direct serum injection combine with liquid chromatography and online immunochemical detection. J Chromatogr B 1994; 653: 55-61.

[116] Irth H, Oosterkamp AJ, VanderWelle W, Tjaden UR, VanderGreed J. Online immunochemical detection in liquid chromatography using fluorescein-labeled antibodies. J Chromatogr 1993; 633: 65-72.

[117] Lindgren A, Emneus J, Marko-Varga G, Irth H, Oosterkamp A, Eremin S. Optimization of a hetergeneous non-competitive flow immunoassay comparing fluorescein, peroxidase and alkaline phosphatase as labels. J Immunol Methods 1998; 211: 33-42.

[118] Kjellstrom S, Emneus J, Marko-Varga G. Flow immunochemical bio-recognition detection for the determination of interleukin-10 in cell samples. J Immunol Methods 2000; 246: 119-130.

[119] Freytag JW, Lau HP, Wadsley JJ. Affinity-column-mediated immunoenzymometric assays: influence of affinity-column ligand and valency of antibody-enzyme conjugates. Clin Chem 1984; 30: 1494-8.

[120] Wilmer M, Trau D, Renneberg R, Spener F. Amperometric immunosensor for the detection of 2,4-dichlorophenoxyacetic acid (2,4-D) in water. Anal Lett 1997; 30: 515-25.

[121] Lovgren U, Kronkvist K, Backstrom B, Edholm LE, Johansson G. Design of non-competitive flow injection enzyme immunoassays for determination of haptens. Application of digoxigenin. J Immunol Methods 1997; 208: 159-68.

[122] Gunaratna PC, Wilson GS. Noncompetitive flow injection immunoassay for a hapten alpha-(difluoromethyl)ornithine. Anal Chem 1993; 65: 1153-7.

[123] Kaptein WA, Korf J, Cheng S, Yang M, Glatz JFC, Renneberg R. Online flow displacement immunoassay for fatty acid-binding protein. J Immunol Methods 1998; 217: 103-11.

[124] Aref'ev AA, Vlasenko SB, Eremin SA, Osipov AP, Egorov AM. Flow-injection enzyme immunoassay of haptens with enhanced chemiluminescence detection. Anal Chim Acta 1990; 237: 285-9.

[125] Silvaieh H, Schmid MG, Hofstetter O, Schurig V, Gubitz G. Development of enantioselective chemiluminescence flow- and sequential-injection immunoassays with alpha-amino acids. J Biochem Biophys Methods 2002; 53: 1-14.

[126] Locascio-Brown L, Choquette SJ. Measuring estrogens using flow injection immunoanalysis with liposome amplification. Talanta 1993; 40: 1899-904.

[127] Wang R, Lu X, Ma W. Non-competitive immunoassay for alpha-fetoprotein using micellar electrokinetic capillary chromatography and laser-induced fluorescence detection. J Chromatogr B 2002; 779: 157-62.

[128] Bier FF, Jockers R, Schmid RD. Integrated optical immunosensor for s-triazine determination: regeneration, calibration and limitations. J Chromatogr A 1994; 680: 93-8.

[129] Oates MR, Clarke W, Zimlich A, Hage DS. Optimization and development of a high-performance liquid-chromatography-based one-site immunometric assay with chemiluminescence detection. Anal Chim Acta 2002; 470: 37-50.

[130] Johns MA, Rosengarten LK, Jackson M, Regnier FE. Enzyme-linked immunosorbent assays in a chromatographic format. J Chromatogr A 1996; 743: 195-206.

[131] Hayes MA, Polson NA, Phyre AN, Garcia AA. Flow-based microimmunoassay. Anal Chem 2001; 73: 5896-902.

[132] Wang Q, Wang Y, Luo G, Yeung WSB. Feasibility study of enzyme-amplified sandwich immunoassay using protein G capillary affinity chromatography and laser induced fluorescence detection. J Liq Chromatogr Rel Tech 2001; 24: 1953-63.

[133] Karube I, Matsunaga T, Satoh T, Suzuki S. A catalytic immunoreactor for the amperometric determination of human serum albumin. Anal Chim Acta 1984; 156: 283-7.

[134] De Alwis WU, Wilson GS. Rapid subpicomole electrochemical enzyme immunoassay for immunoglobulin G. Anal Chem 1985; 57: 2754-6.

[135] Lee IH, Meyerhoff ME. Rapid flow-injection sandwich-type immunoassays of proteins using an immobilized antibody reactor and adenosine deaminase-antibody conjugates. Anal Chim Acta 1990; 229: 47-55.

[136] Shellum C, Guebitz G. Flow-injection immunoassays with acridinium ester-based chemiluminescence detection. Anal Chim Acta 1989; 227: 97-107.

[137] Hage DS, Kao PC. High-performance immunoaffinity chromatography and chemiluminescent detection in the automation of a parathyroid hormone sandwich immunoassay. Anal Chem 1991; 63: 586-95.

[138] Yoshikawa T, Terishima M, Katoh S. Immunoassay using HPLAC and fluorescence-labeled antibodies. J Ferm Bioeng 1995; 80: 200-3.

[139] McGown LB, Joseph MJ, Pitner JB, Vonk JB, Linn CP. The nucleic acid ligand: a new tool for moelcular recognition. Anal Chem 1995; 67: 663A-8A.

[140] Turek C, Gold L. Systematic evolution of ligans bay exponential enrichment: RNA ligands to bacteriphage T4 DNA polymerase. Science 1990; 249: 505-10.

[141] Ellington AD, Szostk JW. *In vitro* selection of RNA molecules that bind specific ligands. Nature 1990; 346: 818-22.

[142] Kriz D, Ramstrom O, Mosbach K. Molecular imprinting: new possibilities for sensor technology. Anal Chem 1997; 69: 345A-9A.

[143] Sellergren B. Nonconvalent molecular imprinting: antibody-like molecular recognition in polymeric network materials. Trends Anal Chem 1997; 16: 310-9.

[144] Durst RA, Locascio-Brown L, Plant AL. Automated liposome-based flow-injection immunoassay system. GBP Monographs 1991; 14: 181-90.

[145] Wemhoff GA, Rabbany SY, Kusterbeck AW, Ogert RA, Bredehorst R, Ligler FS. Kinetics of antibody-binding at solid-liquid interfaces in flow. J Immunol Methods 1992; 156: 223-30.

[146] Rabbany SY, Kusterbeck AW, Bredehorts R, Ligler FS. Effect of antibody density on the displacement kinetics of a flow immunoassay. J Immunol Methods 1994; 168: 227-34.

[147] Kronkvist K, Lovegren U, Svenson J, Edholm LE, Johansson G. Competitive flow injection enzyme immunoassay for steriods using a post-column reaction technique. J Immunol Methods 1997; 200: 145-53.

[148] Charles PT, Conrad DW, Jacobs MS, Bart JC, Kusterbeck AW. Synthesis of a fluorescent analog of polychlorinated biphenyls for use in a continuous flow immunosensor assay. Bioconj Chem 1995; 6: 691-4.

[149] Cassidy SA, Janis LJ, Regnier FE. Kinetic chromatographic sequential addition immunoassays using protein A affinity chromatography. Anal Chem 1992; 64: 1973-7.

[150] Hage DS, Taylor B, Kao PC. Intact parathyroid hormone: performance and clinical utility of an automated assay based on high-performance immunoaffinity chromatography and chemiluminescence detection. Clin Chem 1992; 38: 1494-500.

[151] Hage DS, Walters RR. Dual-column determination of albumin and immunoglobulin G in serum by high-performance affinity chromatography. J Chromatogr 1987; 386: 37-49.

CHAPTER 11

Lateral Flow Assays

Geertruida A. Posthuma-Trumpie and Aart van Amerongen*

Wageningen UR Food & Biobased Research, Biomolecular Sensing & Diagnostics, P.O. Box 17, 6700 AA Wageningen, The Netherlands

Abstract: A simple version of immunochemical-based methods is the Lateral Flow Assay (LFA). It is a dry chemistry technique (reagents are included); the fluid from the sample runs through a porous membrane (often nitrocellulose) by capillary force. Typically the membrane is cut as a strip of 0.5*5 cm. In most cases, coloured colloidal nanoparticles serve as a label. The method is very user-friendly, as only the liquid sample has to be added. Results are available within 5-15 minutes and after evaluation of the signal by visual inspection, a desktop scanner with image analysis software, or a dedicated reader, the used strips can be discarded. With respect to the specificity, sensitivity and efficiency the technology is heavily dependent on the recognition of the analyte by the corresponding antibody. Lateral flow assays are mainly used for qualitative or semi-quantitative detection of (un)wanted substances in the biomatrix or the environment. The technology requires a minimum of resources and skills of the operator. Many applications already reached the market. We will address here a bit of history and the general principle of the technique, and critical parameters influencing the performance of the assay. Amongst those are the material of the membrane, the sample pad, the conjugate pad and the absorbent pad, properties of currently used labels, formats of the tests and properties of good recognition elements. Processing of the results will be discussed as well.

Keywords: Antibodies, Lateral Flow Immunoassays, Strip Tests.

1. INTRODUCTION

This chapter reports on Lateral Flow Assays (LFA). LFAs have become very popular during the last decade, as is shown in a recent survey [1]. LFAs are based on the principle of immunochromatography where the specific interaction of antigen and antibody is responsible for the response. LFAs are especially designed for single use at point of care/need, *i.e.*, outside the laboratory, and are important for user-friendly diagnostic purposes. LFAs, are prefabricated strips of a carrier material containing dry reagents that are activated by applying the fluid sample. They are used (i) in phytopathology, medical and veterinary practice aimed to indicate the cause of an infection, ascertain pregnancy, or failure of internal organs (*e.g.*, heart attack, renal failure or diabetes) (Table **S1**); (ii) to ascertain the safety of food and feed or the environment for presence of toxic compounds or allergens (Table **S2**); (iii) in forensic studies, including abuse of (illicit) drugs (Table **S3**). These assays are often incorrectly referred to as "dipsticks". Real dipstick assays are based on the immunoblotting principle and do not rely on lateral fluid flow through a membrane. In this chapter lateral flow (immuno)assays are evaluated and, therefore, reference to dipsticks that are lateral flow assays will be named LFAs. Applications for which an on/off signal is sufficient, are excellently suited for this technology. The best-known application is the pregnancy test [2, 3]. Results usually come within 10-20 minutes. The current generation of LFAs combines high sensitivity and selectivity with ease of use. In most cases sensitivity and selectivity are achieved by using miniaturized thin-layer chromatography and analyte-specific antibodies or DNA/RNA specific sequences, and by labelling the analyte or the recognition element.

2. HISTORY OF THE ASSAY FORMAT

Originally the technique was called Sol Particle Immunoassay (SPIA) [2]. The assay format in Lateral Flow Immunoassay (LFIA) is comparable to Enzyme Immunoassay (EIA), although it does not replace that assay format. In fact, first reports on LFIAs showed the use of the same components as in EIAs, although in this

***Address correspondence to Aart van Amerongen:** Wageningen UR Food & Biobased Research, Biomolecular Sensing & Diagnostics, P.O. Box 17, 6700 AA Wageningen, The Netherlands; Tel. +31 317 480 164; E-mail: aart.vanamerongen@wur.nl

Eline P. Meulenberg (Ed)

particular case the antibody/antigen was coated on a chromatographic paper strip [5]. In doing so, the technology took advantage of the chromatographic principle and, in addition, of the immunological recognition system. The first labels were the enzymes used for EIAs [5, 6], but were replaced soon by particulate labels [2, 3]. Nowadays when presenting a new methodology on LFIAs, the performance of the new system is often compared to the performance of EIAs [4, 7-10].

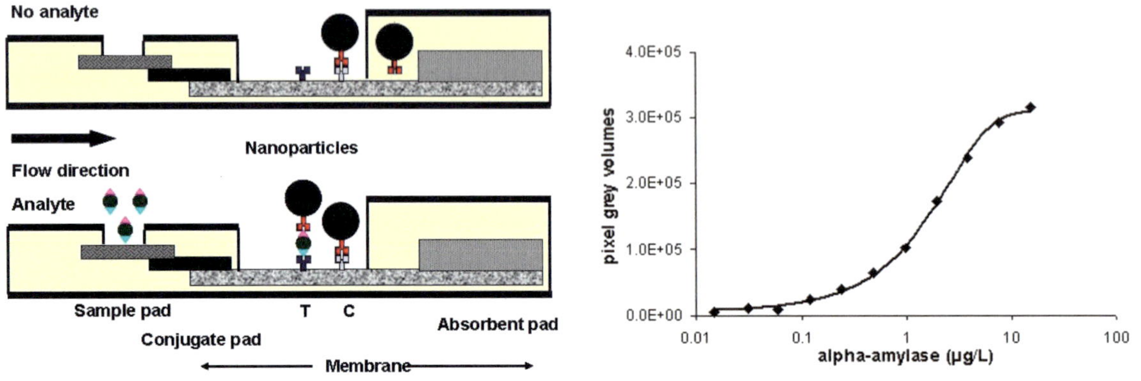

Figure 1: Lateral flow immunoassay in sandwich format. a) scheme of the recognition and response process (not to scale) test-line T (primary antibody) and control line C (tertiary antibody) are indicated, secondary antibody is conjugated to reporting nanoparticles and is dried in the conjugate pad; b) typical calibration curve of α-amylase, details are given in [4], reproduced with permission.

3. GENERAL PRINCIPLE OF LATERAL FLOW ASSAY

The lateral flow assay is based on a chromatographic principle, where sample analyte can compete with labelled analyte for immobilised recognition element binding sites, or sample analyte can compete with immobilized analyte for labelled recognition element binding sites (Fig. **1**).

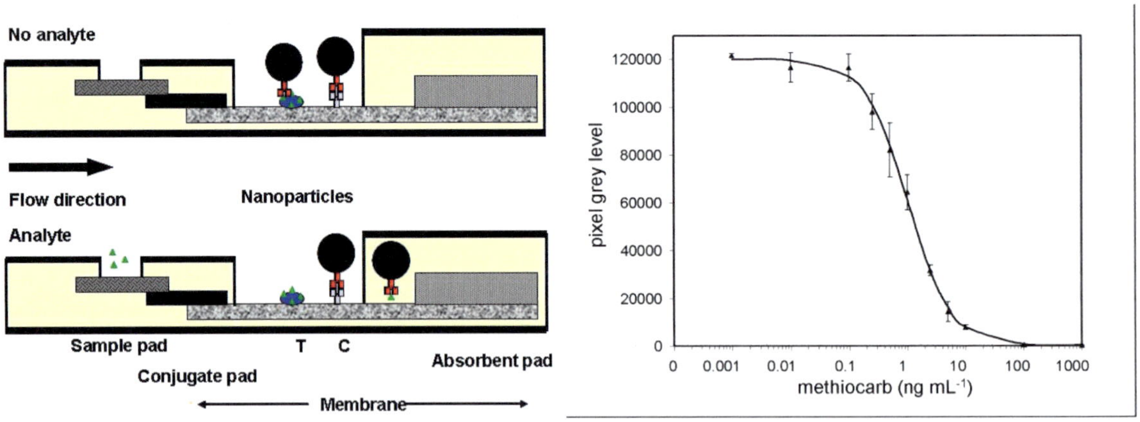

Figure 2: Lateral flow immunoassay in inhibition format. a) scheme of the recognition and response process, T: test-line analyte conjugated to a protein, C: control-line (secondary antibody) (not to scale) primary antibody is conjugated to reporting nanoparticles and dried in the conjugate release pad; b) typical calibration curve of methiocarb; details are given in .[11], reproduced with permission.

In most cases anti-analyte antibodies are used as recognition elements. For high molecular mass analytes the format may be of the sandwich type, but for low molecular mass analytes (haptens) the format is restricted to the inhibition format (Fig. **2**), although direct hapten LFAs can be developed by using anti-idiotypic antibodies [12, 13], or by applying the apposition system [14].

It is also possible to use nucleic acid hybridisation as recognition element, called Nucleic Acid Lateral Flow Assay (NALF) [15]. A combination of nucleic acid and antigen-antibody interaction is also possible, and is called Nucleic Acid Lateral Flow Immunoassay (NALFIA). In this last format the application of tag-labelled primers enables the sandwiching of amplicon between binding proteins on the membrane and on the coloured nanoparticles [16, 17] (Fig. **3**).

4. COMPONENTS OF THE ASSAY FORMAT

Antibody. The antibody is the workhorse of every immunochemical application. This is especially true for LFAs as the interaction time between antigen and antibody is usually very short. The antibody needs to have optimal binding characteristics to enable the test to be sensitive, specific, and efficient.

Membrane materials. The test is made of a porous polymeric membrane cut to an appropriate size, *e.g.* 5*0.5 cm, equipped with a plastic backing. The membrane used as strip material is a very important part of the test system. Most often this strip material is made of nitrocellulose [18-29], available from, *e.g.*, GE Healthcare (Whatman), Sartorius, Pierce, or MilliPore. Several other polymeric materials are also available, *e.g.*, nylon [30] (MilliPore), polyethersulfone [31, 32] (Pall Biosciences), polyethylene [33] (Porex) or fused silica (Fusion5, Whatman), but these are used less often. A slight tendency to use polyethersulfone material was observed in the NALF format. This material comes in different pore sizes, usually indicated by the time it takes for a fluid front to travel a distance of 4 cm, called the capillary rise time or wicking rate (min/4 cm). Not only the capillary forces of the carrier material are important, but also the binding capacity for proteins, which is necessary for sequential selection, reaction and detection.

Material of the sample pad, conjugate release pad and adsorbent pad. The sample pad can be used to perform multiple tasks, of which the promotion and even distribution of the sample to the conjugate pad is most important. The sample pad can also be impregnated with, *e.g.*, proteins, detergents, viscosity enhancers and buffer salts to influence the ionic conditions and flow rate of the sample. Such additions serve, for example, to increase the sample viscosity, to increase the reaction time at the conjugate pad, or even to chemically modify the target compound in the sample for binding at the test-line. The pores in the sample pad can be distributed symmetrically (homogeneously or inhomogeneously), or asymmetrically, providing an initial filter to remove coarse material, *e.g.*, whole cells. Asymmetrical pore size distribution can be used to trap cells in the pad. (see, *e.g.*, Pall Ahlstrom (Cytosep) [4, 34, 35], or Advanced Microdevices Pvt, India [21]). The material of the sample pad is often chosen in advance in accordance with the aim of the test and the properties of the sample. Optimisation is usually not reported.

The conjugate release pad, made of cross-linked silica is in close contact with the strip material and the sample application pad. Labelled analyte(s) or recognition element(s) (depending on the application) are dried on this pad and after addition of the (buffer-diluted) sample, this material will dissolve in the fluid; the formation of specific interactions will be initiated here and will continue during the chromatographic process.

The primary function of the absorbent pad is to drain off the fluid from the membrane. When an absorbent pad is used, the amount of sample can be increased, resulting in an increased sensitivity. Most often cellulose filters are used.

Labels. Nowadays many labels are used, often these are made of coloured (nano)particles, but enzyme labels are being applied as well. In that case there is no strict single-step assay, as the substrate of the enzyme has to be added in a second step [36-38]. Nanoparticles are used in the majority of cases, particularly based on gold [1]. Other materials are less frequently applied such as colloidal carbon [39], coloured latex particles [40-42], Europium-labelled silica nanoparticles [43, 44], quantum dots [45], electro-active [46-48] or fluorescent labelled liposomes [31, 49, 50], selenium [51], up-converting phosphor reporters [52, 53], magnetic particles [54-59], Raman-active tags [60], or even a fluorophore [34]. Original applications published in the scientific press between 2005-2009 are summarised in supplementary material Tables **S1-S3**.

Optimisation. To optimise the assay, several parameters need to be investigated. Choosing the right strip material, sample pad, conjugate release pad and adjustment of the position of the test-line is usually done, as illustrated in [11, 26, 61, 62]. When the inhibition format is used, labelling of the reporter nanoparticle with secondary antibodies, *i.e.* antibodies against the species of the primary antibodies will not only increase the sensitivity, but will also diminish the amount of the primary antibody and cut the price substantially. Furthermore, especially when polyclonal antibodies are used, one special batch will last much longer. This is done by titrating the, often expensive, primary antibody and labelling the, often less expensive, secondary antibody [26, 63]. In this case, a tertiary antibody has to be used at the control line, often also of low cost.

Another item of concern is the blocking procedure. Wetting agents are added in the casting procedure during manufacturing of the strips to ensure a proper flow during the test. Several reports mention a blocking procedure, as is commonly done during EIA tests, after spraying the test and the control line on the strip [37, 62, 64]. In that case these wetting and flow properties can be lost. It is advisable to add the blocking agent in the dilution buffer of the sample instead. Careful choice of the blocking agent is advisable as shown in [11, 26, 62].

However, all optimisation of these materials is to no avail when one of the materials chosen from the market, *e.g.* membrane, antibody, antigen preparation, or blocking procedure does not perform as requested.

5. PREPARATION AND ASSEMBLY OF THE STRIP

To develop LFAs the minimal requirements in a research laboratory are a sprayer and a cutter to cut the strips that come as a sheet or on a roll. The preparation starts with the immobilisation of the capture agent on the strip. Strips can be ordered with a backing of a polymer film; otherwise one has to stick the strip material to a backing first. The material is cut to an appropriate size, *e.g.* 20*5 cm and the capture reagent for the test-line and the control line (if applicable) is dissolved in a low salt buffer of high pH, *e.g.* 5 mM borate buffer pH 8.5 to an appropriate concentration, *e.g.* between 100 and 1000 μg mL^{-1}. The solutions are sprayed on the strip at appropriate distances from the bottom by using, *e.g.*, piezoelectric dispensing using a Biodot or Kinematic sprayer, or a gas-driven TLC sprayer such as the Linomat IV or V (Camag). Another option is to pipet 1 μL of the solution for initial research. After spraying, the strip is dried at 37 °C for at least 2 hrs, or overnight. Separately, the sample and conjugate pads are being prepared. Together with the absorbent pad these pads are placed in particular positions on the polymeric membrane. Subsequently, a backing card is applied to the strip and the resulting assemblage is cut into sticks, for example 5*0.5 cm using a guillotine cutter (Scheme. **S1**, supplementary material). Certain levels of automation can be applied [65], although this is usually not the case in a research environment. *Protocol.* Application of a drop of the fluid sample, often diluted in running buffer, or dipping the strip into the sample, initiates a flow through the porous membrane, whereby the fluid dissolves the conjugate. At the test-line, specific reactions give the required response.

It is also possible to evaluate the presence or absence of more than one analyte as shown in Refs. [16, 17, 24, 55, 66-73]. However, the number of lines on one strip is usually limited to 2-5 mainly due to physical limitations of the LFA strip format.

6. LATERAL FLOW IMMUNOASSAY

The LFIA technique is used in the form of an immunostrip, simply dipped into the fluid sample, or mounted in a device for easier handling. On this membrane at least one test-line and a control line have been sprayed. The test-line can be made up of anti-analyte antibody (primary antibody) or antigen, which in case of a hapten is conjugated to a protein. The control line is made up of immunoglobulin (IgG) raised against the animal species of the labelled antibody. The sample pad, conjugate pad, and/or the control line can be present, or may be omitted. Another option is to dehydrate the labelled conjugate in a test tube and add the sample and the strip to the test tube [4, 16].

For analytes with more than one epitope the sandwich format is applicable (Fig. **1**). In this format the test-line can be prepared using one analyte-specific, preferably polyclonal, antibody. The sample is mixed with a solution of a second anti-analyte antibody, labelled with coloured or fluorescent nanoparticles. This antibody can be different from the first and monoclonal, or both antibodies can be the same. Analyte in the sample will bind during the initial chromatographic process and a free epitope can bind to the immobilized antibody at the test-line. The response is directly proportional to the amount of analyte in the sample (Fig. **1**).

In the inhibition LFIA format the response is negatively correlated to the analyte concentration (*e.g.*, more analyte present results in less signal; no analyte present gives the highest signal) (Fig. **2**). Two layouts are possible: (i) antibody is sprayed at the test-line, a mixture of sample analyte and labelled analyte is applied and both compete for binding sites on the antibody; (ii) a conjugate of the analyte to a protein is sprayed at the test-line, a mixture of labelled antibody and sample analyte is applied, giving the sample analyte a head start for binding to the antibody. The preferred layout is dependent on the particular application.

7. NUCLEIC ACID LATERAL FLOW (IMMUNO) ASSAY

In this format, recognition of the analyte (DNA or RNA specific for the micro-organism or other species) is performed by a combination of DNA/RNA hybridisation or binding during or after the amplification process and in case of NALFIA label-specific antibodies. Several layouts are possible.

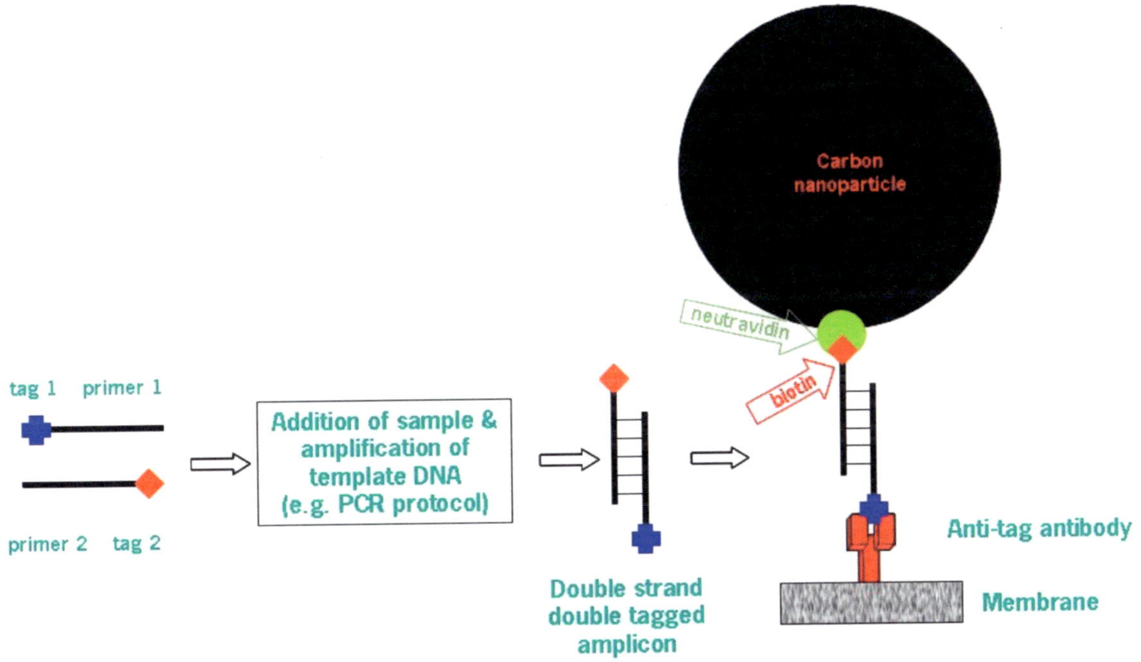

Figure 3: Principle of nucleic acid lateral flow assay (not to scale). Two tagged primers are used to amplify the template sequence by, *e.g.*, PCR or NASBA resulting in 2-side tagged amplicons. Amplicons are sandwiched between the distinghuising anti-tag antibody and the avindin-labelled reporting nanoparticle.

In a typical layout using the NALFIA format and developed for the detection of pathogenic bacteria, template DNA or RNA was amplified by using the Polymerase Chain Reaction (PCR) [17, 74], the Nucleic Acid Sequence-Based Amplification (NASBA) [75], or the Loop-Mediated Isothermal Amplification (LAMP) [76] with sets of tag-labelled primers or probes. As an example the following set up is possible: Discriminative antibodies raised against particular tags (DNP, FITC, Texas Red, *etc.*) are sprayed as the test-lines and bind their respective tags that are part of the final, specific amplicons through incorporation of the primer or binding of the probe. The other tag is biotin and is also part of the final amplicon through incorporation of the other primer or binding of the other probe. Streptavidin-labelled nanoparticles will recognize the second tag. Hence, the amplicons are sandwiched between the discriminating anti-tag antibody immobilised on the strip and the avidin-coated reporter resulting in a coloured response (Fig. **3**) [16, 17].

A layout without antibodies is possible as well. One capture probe with complementary sequence is labelled with a T_{20} tail and covalently immobilized on the strip material using UV irradiation. The reporting nanoparticle, in this case gold, is covalently coupled to the other capturing complementary sequence [15]. After amplification of the required sequence, the strip is inserted into a amplicon solution (diluted with running buffer).

Another strategy is employed when a reporter probe is made of labelled liposomes (with a fluorescent compound *via* an amide bond). If the specific DNA or RNA sequence is present this will hybridise with both the capture sequence immobilised on the membrane and the reporter sequence, giving a linear response with the concentration of the amplified sequence [75].

8. EVALUATION OF THE RESULTS

As stated in the introduction, results are often evaluated by visual inspection. However, this can only be done when coloured labels are used (gold, carbon or latex particles). Even then there may be reasons to store the results in a digital way for comparison or quantification. Digitising can be done in several ways, *e.g.*, by using a CCD camera [3], a desktop scanner [22] or a dedicated strip reader [77, 78]. Strip readers are obligatory when results of fluorescent [43], or magneto-resistive labels [56] need to be evaluated. Commercial readers can be obtained from, *e.g.*, ESE, Forsite Diagnostics, Romer Labs Singapore, Charm or Biodot. In a literature survey made by Drs J. Gordon and G. Michel on behalf of FIND Diagnostics [1] it became clear that semi-quantitative evaluation is often not reported. From that evaluation report the performance of carbon nanoparticles using a flatbed scanner and image analysis software was outstanding in sensitivity (low picomolar), ease of use and price.

As a trend in recent publications it can be observed that more quantification is reported nowadays [11, 16, 58, 73, 77, 79-81].

REFERENCES

[1] Gordon J, Michel G. Analytical sensitivity limits for lateral flow immunoassays. Clin Chem 2008; 54: 1250-1.

[2] Leuvering JHW, Thal PJHM, van der Waart M, Schuurs AHWM. Sol particle immunoassay (SPIA). J Immunoass Immunochem 1980; 1: 77-91.

[3] van Amerongen A, van Loon D, Berendsen LBJM, Wichers JH. Quantitative computer image analysis of a human chorionic gonadotropin colloidal carbon dipstick assay. Clin Chim Acta 1994; 229: 67-75.

[4] Koets M, Sander I, Bogdanovic J, Doekes G, van Amerongen A. A rapid lateral flow immunoassay for the detection of fungal alpha-amylase at the workplace. J Environ Monit 2006; 8: 942-6.

[5] Litman DJ, Hanlon TM, Ullman EF. Enzyme channeling immunoassay: A new homogeneous enzyme immunoassay technique. Anal Biochem 1980; 106: 223-9.

[6] Pappas MG, Hajkowski R, Hockmeyer WT. Dot enzyme-linked immunosorbent assay (Dot-ELISA): a micro technique for the rapid diagnosis of visceral leishmaniasis. J Immunol Methods 1983; 64: 205-14.

[7] Cazacu AC, Greer J, Taherivand M, Demmler GJ. Comparison of lateral-flow immunoassay and enzyme immunoassay with viral culture for rapid detection of influenza virus in nasal wash specimens from children. J Clin Microbiol 2003; 41: 2132-4.

[8] Nielsen K, Yu WL, Kelly L, Bermudez R, Renteria T, Dajer A, *et al.* Development of a lateral flow assay for rapid detection of bovine antibody to *Anaplasma marginale*. J Immunoass Immunochem 2008; 29: 10-8.

[9] Salomone A, Mongelli M, Roggero P, Boscia D. Reliability of detection of *Citrus tristeza virus* by an immunochromatographic lateral flow assay in comparison with ELISA. J Plant Pathol 2004; 86: 43-8.

[10] Wang S, Quan Y, Lee N, Kennedy IR. Rapid determination of Fumonisin B_1 in food samples by enzyme-linked immunosorbent assay and colloidal gold immunoassay. J Agr Food Chem 2006; 54: 2491-5.

[11] Blažková M, Micková-Holubová B, Rauch P, Fukal L. Immunochromatographic colloidal carbon-based assay for detection of methiocarb in surface water. Biosens Bioelectron 2009; 25: 753-8.

[12] Barnard G, Osher J, Lichter S, Gayer B, De Boever J, Limor R, *et al.* The measurement of progesterone in serum by a non-competitive idiometric assay. Steroids 1995; 60: 824-9.

[13] Winger LA, Dessi JL, Self CH. Enhanced specificity for small molecules in a convenient format which removes a limitation of competitive immunoassay. J Immunol Methods 1996; 199: 185-91.

[14] Self CH, Thompson S, Winger LA. Non-competitive immunoassay for small molecules - the anti-complex, selective and apposition systems. In: Wild D, editor. The Immunoassay Handbook. 3rd ed. Amsterdam: Elsevier Ltd; 2005. pp. 41-7.

[15] Aveyard J, Mehrabi M, Cossins A, Braven H, Wilson R. One step visual detection of PCR products with gold nanoparticles and a nucleic acid lateral flow (NALF) device. Chem Commun 2007; 4251-3.

[16] Blažková M, Koets M, Rauch P, van Amerongen A. Development of a nucleic acid lateral flow immunoassay for simultaneous detection of *Listeria* spp. and *Listeria monocytogenes* in food. Eur Food Res Technol 2009; 229: 867-74.

[17] Mens PF, van Amerongen A, Sawa P, Kager PA, Schallig HDFH. Molecular diagnosis of malaria in the field: development of a novel 1-step nucleic acid lateral flow immunoassay for the detection of all 4 human *Plasmodium* spp. and its evaluation in Mbita, Kenya. Diagn Micr Infec Dis 2008; 61: 421-7.

[18] Fong WK, Modrusan Z, McNevin JP, Marostenmaki J, Zin B, Bekkaoui F. Rapid solid-phase immunoassay for detection of methicillin-resistant *Staphylococcus aureus* using cycling probe technology. J Clin Microbiol 2000; 38: 2525-9.

[19] Jin S, Chang ZY, Ming X, Min CL, Wei H, Sheng LY, *et al.* Fast dipstick dye immunoassay for detection of immunoglobulin G (IgG) and IgM antibodies of human toxoplasmosis. Clin Diagn Lab Immun 2005; 12: 198-201.

[20] Kim YM, Oh SW, Jeong SY, Pyo DJ, Choi EY. Development of an ultrarapid one-step fluorescence immunochromatographic assay system for the quantification of microcystins. Environ Sci Technol 2003; 37: 1899-904.

[21] Leung W, Chan CPY, Bosgoed F, Lehmann K, Renneberg I, Lehmann M, *et al.* One-step quantitative cortisol dipstick with proportional reading. J Immunol Methods 2003; 281: 109-18.

[22] Lönnberg M, Carlsson J. Quantitative detection in the attomole range for immunochromatographic tests by means of a flatbed scanner. Anal Biochem 2001; 293: 224-31.

[23] Mansfield MA. The use of nitrocellulose membranes in lateral-flow assays. In: Wong RC, Tse HY, Eds. Drugs of Abuse: Humana Press; 2005. pp. 71-85.

[24] Oku Y, Kamiya K, Kamiya H, Shibahara Y, Ii T, Uesaka Y. Development of oligonucleotide lateral-flow immunoassay for multi-parameter detection. J Immunol Methods 2001; 258: 73-84.

[25] Paek S-H, Lee S-H, Cho J-H, Kim Y-S. Development of rapid one-step immunochromatographic assay. Methods 2000; 22: 53-60.

[26] Posthuma-Trumpie GA, Korf J, van Amerongen A. On the development of a competitive lateral flow immunoassay for progesterone: Influence of coating conjugates and buffer components. Anal Bioanal Chem 2008; 392: 1215-23.

[27] van Dam GJ, Wichers JH, Ferreira TMF, Ghati D, van Amerongen A, Deelder AM. Diagnosis of schistosomiasis by reagent strip test for detection of circulating cathodic antigen. J Clin Microbiol 2004; 42: 5458-61.

[28] Zhang G-P, Guo J-Q, Wang X-N, Yang J-X, Yang Y-Y, Li Q-M, *et al.* Development and evaluation of an immunochromatographic strip for trichinellosis detection. Vet Parasitol 2006; 137: 286-93.

[29] Zhu Y, He W, Liang Y, Xu M, Yu C, Hua W, *et al.* Development of a rapid, simple dipstick dye immunoassay for schistosomiasis diagnosis. J Immunol Methods 2002; 266: 1-5.

[30] Buechler KF, Moi S, Noar B, McGrath D, Villela J, Clancy M, *et al.* Simultaneous detection of seven drugs of abuse by the Triage panel for drugs of abuse. Clin Chem 1992; 38: 1678-84.

[31] Edwards KA, Baeumner AJ. Optimization of DNA-tagged dye-encapsulating liposomes for lateral-flow assays based on sandwich hybridization. Anal Bioanal Chem 2006; 386: 1335-43.

[32] Kalogianni DP, Goura S, Aletras AJ, Christopoulos TK, Chanos MG, Christofidou M, *et al.* Dry reagent dipstick test combined with 23S rRNA PCR for molecular diagnosis of bacterial infection in arthroplasty. Anal Biochem 2007; 361: 169-75.

[33] Fernandez-Sanchez C, McNeil CJ, Rawson K, *et al.* One-step immunostrip test for the simultaneous detection of free and total prostate specific antigen in serum. J Immunol Methods 2005; 307: 1-12.

[34] Choi S, Choi EY, Kim DJ, Kim JH, Kim TS, Oh SW. A rapid, simple measurement of human albumin in whole blood using a fluorescence immunoassay (I). Clin Chim Acta 2004; 339: 147-56.

[35] Verheijen R, Osswald IK, Dietrich R, Haasnoot W. Development of a one step strip test for the detection of (Dihydro)streptomycin residues in raw milk. Food Agr Immunol 2000; 12: 31-40.

[36] Kim MS, Doyle MP. Dipstick immunoassay to detect enterohemorrhagic *Escherichia coli* O157:H7 in retail ground beef. Appl Environ Microbiol 1992; 58: 1764-7.

[37] Sananikone K, Delwiche MJ, BonDurant RH, Munro CJ. Quantitative lateral flow immunoassay for measuring progesterone in bovine milk. T ASAE 2004; 47: 1357-65.

[38] Watanabe H, Satake A, Kido Y, Tsuji A. Monoclonal-based enzyme-linked immunosorbent assay and immunochromatographic assay for enrofloxacin in biological matrices. Analyst 2002; 127: 98-103.

[39] van Amerongen A, Wichers JH, Berendsen LBJM, Timmermans AJM, Keizer GD, van Doorn AWJ, *et al.* Colloidal carbon particles as a new label for rapid immunochemical test methods: Quantitative computer image analysis of results. J Biotechnol 1993; 30: 185-95.

[40] Danks C, Barker I. On-site detection of plant pathogens using lateral-flow devices. EPPO Bulletin 2000; 30: 421-6.

[41] Hasegawa T, Asaeda A, Hamaguchi Y, Numazaki K. Development of rapid diagnostic reagents for measles. Hybridoma 2009; 28: 241-9.

[42] Nielsen K, Yu WL, Lin M, Davis SAN, Elmgren C, MacKenzie R, *et al.* Prototype single step lateral flow technology for detection of avian influenza virus and chicken antibody to avian influenza virus. J Immunoass Immunochem 2007; 28: 307-18.

[43] Song X, Knotts M. Time-resolved luminescent lateral flow assay technology. Anal Chim Acta 2008; 626: 186-92.

[44] Xia X, Xu Y, Zhao X, Li Q. Lateral flow immunoassay using Europium chelate-loaded silica nanoparticles as labels. Clin Chem 2009; 55: 179-82.

[45] Lingerfelt BM, Mattoussi H, Goldman ER, Mauro JM, Anderson GP. Preparation of quantum dot-biotin conjugates and their use in immunochromatography assays. Anal Chem 2003; 75: 4043-9.

[46] Lee KS, Kim T-H, Shin M-C, Lee W-Y, Park J-K. Disposable liposome immunosensor for theophylline combining an immunochromatographic membrane and a thick-film electrode. Anal Chim Acta 1999; 380: 17-26.

[47] Sippy N, Luxton R, Lewis RJ, Cowell DC. Rapid electrochemical detection and identification of catalase positive micro-organisms. Biosens Bioelectron 2003; 18: 741-9.

[48] Yoon C-H, Cho J-H, Oh H-I, Kim M-J, Lee C-W, Choi J-W, *et al.* Development of a membrane strip immunosensor utilizing ruthenium as an electro-chemiluminescent signal generator. Biosens Bioelectron 2003; 19: 289-96.

[49] Roberts MA, Durst RA. Investigation of liposome-based immunomigration sensors for the detection of polychlorinated biphenyls. Anal Chem 1995; 67: 482-91.

[50] Wen H-W, Borejsza-Wysocki W, DeCory TR, Durst RA. Development of a competitive liposome-based lateral flow assay for the rapid detection of the allergenic peanut protein Ara h1. Anal Bioanal Chem 2005; 382: 1217-26.

[51] Lou S, Patel C, Ching S, Gordon J. One-step competitive immunochromatographic assay for semiquantitative determination of lipoprotein(a) in plasma. Clin Chem 1993; 39: 619-24.

[52] Zijlmans HJMAA, Bonnet J, Burton J, Kardos K, Vail T, Niedbala RS, *et al.* Detection of cell and tissue surface antigens using up-converting phosphors: a new reporter technology. Anal Biochem 1999; 267: 30-6.

[53] Kuningas K, Rantanen T, Ukonaho T, Lovgren T, Soukka T. Homogeneous Assay Technology Based on Upconverting Phosphors. Anal Chem 2005; 77: 7348-55.

[54] Gao W, Li X, Zeng L, Peng T. Rapid isothermal detection assay: a probe amplification method for the detection of nucleic acids. Diagn Micr Infec Dis 2008; 60: 133-41.

[55] Koets M, van der Wijk T, van Eemeren JTWM, van Amerongen A, Prins MWJ. Rapid DNA multi-analyte immunoassay on a magneto-resistance biosensor. Biosens Bioelectron 2008; 24: 1893-8.

[56] Taton K, Johnson D, Guire P, Lange E, Tondra M. Lateral flow immunoassay using magnetoresistive sensors. J Magn Magn Mater 2009; 321: 1679-82.

[57] Wang Y, Xu H, Wei M, Gu H, Xu Q, Zhu W. Study of superparamagnetic nanoparticles as labels in the quantitative lateral flow immunoassay. Mat Sci Eng C 2009; 29: 714-8.

[58] Xu Q, Xu H, Gu H, Li J, Wang Y, Wei M. Development of lateral flow immunoassay system based on superparamagnetic nanobeads as labels for rapid quantitative detection of cardiac troponin I. Mat Sci Eng C 2009; 29: 702-7.

[59] Tang D, Sauceda JC, Lin Z, Ott S, Basova E, Goryacheva I, *et al.* Magnetic nanogold microspheres-based lateral-flow immunodipstick for rapid detection of aflatoxin B2 in food. Biosens Bioelectron 2009; 25: 514-8.

[60] Doering WE, Piotti ME, Natan MJ, Freeman RG. SERS as a foundation for nanoscale, optically detected biological labels. Adv Mater 2007; 19: 3100-8.

[61] Girotti S, Eremin S, Montoya A, Moreno M, Caputo P, D'Elia M, *et al.* Development of a chemiluminescent ELISA and a colloidal gold-based LFIA for TNT detection. Anal Bioanal Chem 2010; 396: 687-95.

[62] Kolosova AY, Sibanda L, Dumoulin F, Lewis J, Duveiller E, Van Peteghem C, *et al.* Lateral-flow colloidal gold-based immunoassay for the rapid detection of deoxynivalenol with two indicator ranges. Anal Chim Acta 2008; 616: 235-44.

[63] O'Keeffe M, Crabbe P, Salden M, Wichers J, van Peteghem C, Kohen F, *et al.* Preliminary evaluation of a lateral flow immunoassay device for screening urine samples for the presence of sulphamethazine. J Immunol Methods 2003; 278: 117-26.

[64] Edwards KA, Baeumner AJ. Liposome-enhanced lateral-flow assays for the sandwich-hybridization detection of RNA. In: Rasooly A, Herold KE, Eds. Biosensors and Biodetection. Totowa, New Jersey, USA: Humana Press; 2009. pp. 185-215.

[65] Carlberg D. Lateral-Flow Assays - assembly and automation. In: Wong RC, Tse HY, Eds. Drugs of Abuse. Totowa, New Jersey, USA: Humana Press; 2005. pp. 99-114.

[66] Abrams WR, Barber CA, McCann K, Tong G, Chen Z, Mauk MG, *et al.* Development of a microfluidic device for detection of pathogens in oral samples using upconverting phosphor technology (UPT). Ann NY Acad Sci 2007; 1098: 375-88.

[67] Corstjens PLAM, Chen Z, Zuiderwijk M, Bau HH, Abrams WR, Malamud D, *et al.* Rapid assay format for multiplex detection of humoral immune responses to infectious disease pathogens (HIV, HCV, and TB). Ann NY Acad Sci 2007; 1098: 437-45.

[68] Goryacheva IY, De Saeger S, Eremin SA, Van Peteghem C. Immunochemical methods for rapid mycotoxin detection: Evolution from single to multiple analyte screening: A review. Food addit contam A 2007; 24: 1169 - 83.

[69] Greenwald R, Esfandiari J, Lesellier S, Houghton R, Pollock J, Aagaard C, *et al.* Improved serodetection of *Mycobacterium bovis* infection in badgers (*Meles meles*) using multiantigen test formats. Diagn Micr Infec Dis 2003; 46: 197-203.

[70] Kolosova A, De Saeger S, Sibanda L, Verheijen R, Van Peteghem C. Development of a colloidal gold-based lateral-flow immunoassay for the rapid simultaneous detection of zearalenone and deoxynivalenol. Anal Bioanal Chem 2007; 389: 2103-7.

[71] Kranthi KR, Davis M, Mayee CD, Russell DA, Shukla RM, Satija U, *et al.* Development of a colloidal-gold based lateral-flow immunoassay kit for "quality-control' assessment of pyrethroid and endosulfan formulations in a novel single strip format. Crop Prot 2009; 28: 428-34.

[72] Zhang C, Zhang Y, Wang S. Development of multianalyte flow-through and lateral-flow assays using gold particles and horseradish peroxidase as tracers for the rapid determination of carbaryl and endosulfan in agricultural products. J Agr Food Chem 2006; 54: 2502-7.

[73] Zhang M-Z, Wang M-Z, Chen Z-L, Fang J-H, Fang M-M, Liu J, *et al.* Development of a colloidal gold-based lateral-flow immunoassay for the rapid simultaneous detection of clenbuterol and ractopamine in swine urine. Anal Bioanal Chem 2009; 395: 2591-9.

[74] van Amerongen A, Koets M. Simple and rapid bacterial protein and DNA diagnostic methods based on signal generation with colloidal carbon particles. Rapid methods for biological and chemical contaminants in food and feed. 1 ed. Wageningen, The Netherlands: Wageningen Academic Publishers; 2005. pp. 105-26.

[75] Zaytseva NV, Montagna RA, Lee EM, Baeumner AJ. Multi-analyte single-membrane biosensor for the serotype-specific detection of Dengue virus. Anal Bioanal Chem 2004; 380: 46-53.

[76] Tomlinson JA, Dickinson MJ, Boonham N. Rapid detection of *Phytophthora ramorum* and *P. kernoviae* by two-minute DNA extraction followed by isothermal amplification and amplicon detection by generic lateral flow device. Phytopathology 2010; 100: 143-9.

[77] Molinelli A, Grossalber K, Krska R. A rapid lateral flow test for the determination of total type B fumonisins in maize. Anal Bioanal Chem 2009; 395: 1309-16.

[78] Niedbala RS, Feindt H, Kardos K, Vail T, Burton J, Bielska B, *et al.* Detection of analytes by immunoassay using up-converting phosphor technology. Anal Biochem 2001; 293: 22-30.

[79] Drygin Y, Blintsov A, Osipov A, Grigorenko V, Andreeva I, Uskov A, *et al.* High-sensitivity express immunochromatographic method for detection of plant infection by tobacco mosaic virus. Biochemistry (Moscow) 2009; 74: 986-93.

[80] Li L, Zhou L, Yu Y, Zhu Z, Lin C, Lu C, *et al.* Development of up-converting phosphor technology-based lateral-flow assay for rapidly quantitative detection of hepatitis B surface antibody. Diagn Micr Infec Dis 2009; 63: 165-72.

[81] Tippkötter N, Stückmann H, Kroll S, Winkelmann G, Noack U, Scheper T, *et al.* A semi-quantitative dipstick assay for microcystin. Anal Bioanal Chem 2009; 394: 863-9.

CHAPTER 12

Trends and Perspectives in Immunosensors

Caroline Viguier[1,2,‡], Carol Crean[1,‡] and Richard O'Kennedy[1]

[1]School of Biotechnology and Biomedical Diagnostics Institute, National Centre for Sensor Research, Dublin City University, Dublin 9, Ireland and [2]Enfer Scientific Unit T, M7 Business Park, Newhall, Naas, Co. Kildare, Republic of Ireland

Abstract: Immunosensors are devices that comprise both a biomolecular recognition system, such as an antibody and its corresponding antigen, and a transducer to translate the high affinity and specific binding event into a physical signal.

Antibodies are produced by an immunological response to the presence of a foreign substance called an antigen. Antibodies may be immobilised onto a variety of platforms including bulk planar surfaces and nanoparticles by either covalent or adsorption strategies. Different interfaces between the bio-components and the detector are available to monitor in 'real-time' the signal generated by biological interactions. The transducers detect, for example, the change in electron transfer, absorbance, fluorescence, refractive index, mass change or heat transfer as the antibody binds to the antigen of interest. Such analytical devices have allowed a wide range of analytes to be identified and quantified such as pathogens, toxins, environmental food contaminants and disease biomarkers.

The demand for sensitive, rapid, and 'on-site' techniques has taken advantage of the latest advances in microfluidics and nanotechnology. This chapter will highlight current trends in immobilisation, micro/nano-fluidics/and transducers utilised. A number of examples outlining the exploitation of these elements in immunosensors and their successful applications will be described.

Keywords: Antibodies, Immunosensors.

1. INTRODUCTION

Conventional immunoassays such as Enzyme-Linked Immunosorbent Assay (ELISA) can be complex and laborious to perform. They are often time-consuming, need to be carried out by highly-trained staff with expensive and specialised equipment, and thus are difficult to automate. Long incubation steps are required for the analytes to diffuse from the solutions to the solid platform and for the antibody (Ab)-antigen interaction to reach equilibrium. In addition, they involve numerous washing steps to ensure the absence of any non-specific binding. The small ratio between the low platform surface and the large volume of the different solutions can also affect the sensitivity and efficiency of the assay.

Immunosensors are a good alternative to traditional immunoassays. They use a recognition element such as an Ab or antigen in combination with a transducer. They allow the observation and analysis of the Ab-antigen interaction in 'real-time', with or without the need for a label. The binding is detected on the platform, either directly or indirectly, by a transducer providing a signal when the reaction occurs. The two main formats used for immunosensors are sandwich and competitive assays. When immobilising the Ab, it is of crucial importance that the method of immobilisation maintains the stability and activity of the Ab. Immunosensors can be used to monitor the presence of the Ab or antigen and either the Ab or the antigen can be immobilised or labelled depending on the assay requirements.

The basic structure of an Ab is a Y-shaped molecule made of two heavy (H) and two light (L) polypeptide

[*]**Address correspondence to Carol Crean:** School of Biotechnology and Biomedical Diagnostics Institute, National Centre for Sensor Research, Dublin City University, Dublin 9, Ireland; E-mail: c.crean@surrey.ac.uk
[‡]CV and CC contributed equally.

chains held together by disulfide linkages (-S-S-). Each chain consists of constant (C) and variable (V) regions (Fig. **1**). The H chain is composed of a variable region (VH), responsible for binding to the antigen, and three constant regions (CH1, CH2 and CH3). The light chain is made of one variable region (VL) and one constant region (CL). The antibody binds to the antigen through the variable light (VL) and heavy (VH) domains forming the hyper-variable regions of the antibody, known as the Complementarity Determining Regions (CDRs).The selection of the Ab to be used on the immunosensor is a crucial step to develop a sensitive and reliable assay. The chosen Ab must be specific, have a stable interaction with its target and be able to detect the antigen at the required concentration range. The development of specific Abs involves immunising living hosts by injecting a foreign substance, the antigen, leading to an immunological response. Polyclonal, monoclonal and recombinant Abs can all be used for the development of immunosensors. Polyclonal Abs, generated by multiple plasma cells, are cheap and easy to produce and can recognise a large number of epitopes. On the other hand, they can lack specificity. Monoclonal Abs are specific to an individual epitope as they are generated using hybridoma technology. Cheaper but less stable, recombinant Abs are the product of phage display technology. Genetic engineering and biopanning of Ab libraries allow for the selection of highly specific and sensitive recombinant Abs [1].

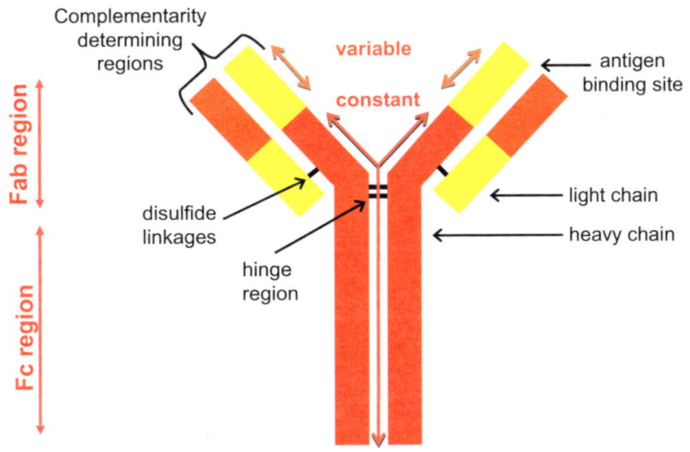

Figure 1: Schematicrepresentation of an immunoglobulin G (IgG). The antibody structure is made of two heavy and two light chains held together by disulfide linkages.

Immunosensors use optical, electrochemical and mass transducers. For each situation and each compound to be analysed, adaptation of the different types of immunosensor may be required. Several factors can affect the practicality of an immunosensor design. It will need to be optimised in order to reach a high level of sensitivity, efficiency, accuracy and reproducibility. Ease-of-use and low production cost targets need to be reached in addition to meeting the market demands and complying with regulatory authorities.

2. IMMOBILISATION OF RECOGNITION ELEMENTS

The attachment of a capture Ab or antigen to an assay surface requires careful consideration. Both the nature of the assay system and the substrate used will determine the strategies required for Ab immobilisation. Immobilisation of active recognition molecules at high-density to the sensor surface is one of the most critical steps in biosensor development. This aspect of immunosensor design will determine whether the immobilised Ab is correctly oriented to favourably interact with the target antigen with minimal steric hindrance.

Entire Ab's have estimated molecular dimensions of 15 x 7 x 3.5 nm, while the smallest Ab fragments, *i.e.* single-domain Ab fragments, are only 4 x 2.5 x 3.5 nm (Fig. **2**) [2]. Whole Ab's when immobilised may tilt due to the presence of the Fc region, or lie on their side, leaving the antigen binding sites close to the assay surface [3]. Pronounced steric hindrance may result, in particular if the antibody reacts with a large-molecular-weight antigen. Ideally, specific recognition of the target antigen should occur at the lowest possible concentration. Therefore, the smaller the Ab fragment, the more can be immobilised onto the surface. This increased Ab fragment density should theoretically result in enhanced detection sensitivity of the target antigen. Cho *et al.* [3] experimentally confirmed this when an enhanced binding capacity was reported from an assay using Fab fragments compared to full Abs (Fig. **2**). The authors carried out a sandwich-type immunoassay for the cardiac biomarker, Troponin I (cTnI), where the detection limits were 1.01 and 0.13 ng mL^{-1}, for the full Ab and Fab fragment respectively. The authors attribute the different analytical performances to variable Ab densities on the assay surface, caused by the differing packing ability of full versus fragmented Abs.

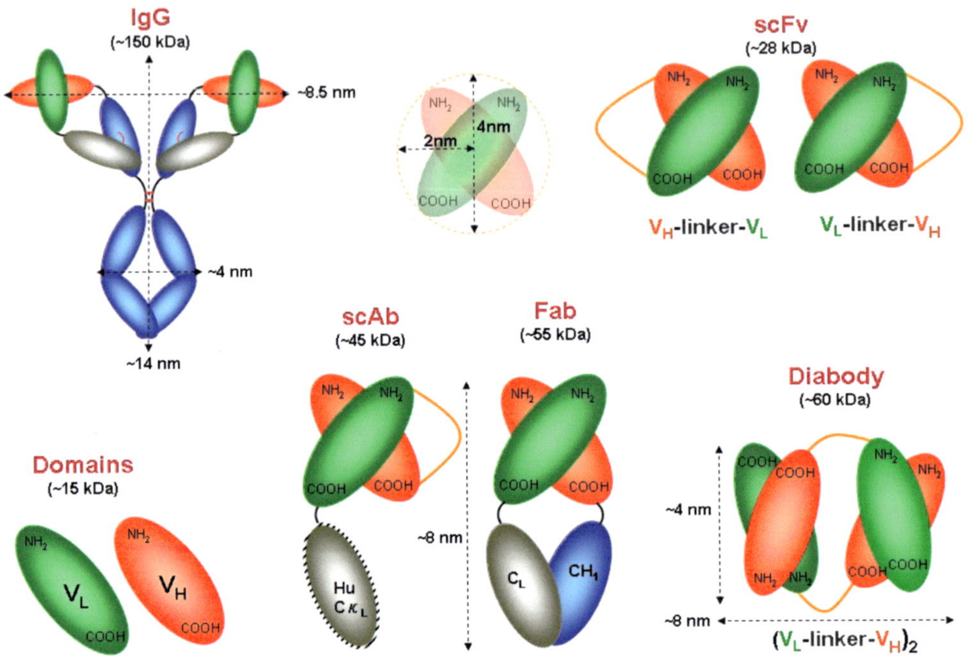

Figure 2: Formats of recombinant Abs: The scFv fragment consists of the VH (red) and VL (green) chains connected by a flexible linker at their terminal ends. A scAb fragment incorporates an additional constant light chain added to the terminal of VL. The Fab fragment contains the VH (red) and VL (green) chains with both constant heavy (blue) and light (grey) chains. Figure adapted from [1].

Unfortunately, proteins and Abs in particular, may lose their biological activity when immobilised on a surface. This can be due to a change in conformation when binding with the assay surface and/or unfavourable orientation of the active site. Non-specific adsorption of Abs on surfaces also frequently causes inactivation. Furthermore, Ab modification, such as engineering or labelling, can diminish the antigen binding ability. Binding may be particularly diminished if the modification occurs on antigen binding sites, which is often the case for random chemical tagging of Abs. The ideal choice of immobilisation method should not significantly change the ability of the Ab to bind its target antigen.

The spacer between the Ab and the immobilisation surface also plays a role in the final Ab–antigen interaction [4]. Direct conjugation of Abs to surfaces often hinders antigen binding (steric hindrances) and limits the mobility of the bound Abs. Immobilising Abs *via* flexible spacer chains can lead to target antigens being captured twice as efficiently as directly-linked Abs [4]. This technology is adapted by Biacore (GE Healthcare) where they use carboxymethylated dextran as a linker, which is attached to a gold sensor surface. Ab or antigen binding to the dextran layer results in a high binding capacity giving a high sensor response, which Biacore recommends as "advantageous for capture assays".

Several strategies are used to immobilise capture Abs on solid surfaces including physical adsorption, covalent attachment, entrapment within a polymer matrix, directed immobilisation and Ab engineering for improved surface affinities (Table **1** and Fig. **3**).

Table 1: Advantages and disadvantages of Ab immobilisation methods.

Immobilisation Method	Advantages	Disadvantages
Adsorption	Simple method of immobilisation No Ab modification High level of immobilisation achieved	Random orientation Ab denaturation Non-specific protein binding Leakage of Ab from surface
Covalent coupling	Stable immobilisation Commercially available surfaces	Random orientation Ab modification, possible denaturation
Ab fragment tag	Oriented immobilisation	Surface stability
Ab-binding proteins	Oriented immobilisation No Ab modification	Surface stability
Ab fragment fusions	Oriented immobilisation Surface stability	Compatibility between Ab fragment and fusion partner

2.1. Physical Adsorption

Although rather uncontrollable, physical adsorption is the simplest method of protein binding on a surface. It can occur through hydrophilic, hydrophobic or both types of interactions between Abs and the sensor surface. Surfaces used include glass and other silica particles, polystyrene and silicone plastics, nitrocellulose and nylon membranes, and also metallic surfaces such as gold and silver [5]. In addition, these surfaces may be further modified to improve adhesion including poly-L-lysine/nitrocellulose coating or organosilane modification of glass and plastic surfaces (*e.g.* cyanosilane or 3-aminopropyltriethoxysilane (APTES)). Such immobilisation processes can lead to random orientation of the absorbed Abs. In addition, Abs may interact with the adsorptive surface in such a way that the antigen-binding site is not available which impedes antigen detection.The hydrophobic interactions which drive passive adsorption of antibodies can reportedly reduce the number of functional sites or activities by more than 90% [6-8]. Using adsorption as the method of immobilisation also has the disadvantage that the biomolecule can easily desorb from the surface during use.

Another form of non-covalent immobilisation of Abs involves conducting polymer films such as polyaniline, polypyrrole and polythiophene. Immobilisation generally involves entrapment within the polymer matrix, where the Ab is co-immobilised with the polymer onto a sensor surface from a monomer solution. However, this can lead to denaturation of the Ab and also result in a large population of Abs that are inaccessible because they are buried deep within the polymer film. To solve this, many authors have used an electrochemical adsorption technique. This is achieved by applying a potential to the polymer electrode surface, which enhances electrostatic interactions with the polymer backbone and the Ab, thereby, facilitating immobilisation [9].

Adsorption methods, despite their drawbacks, have been used in many applications due to their simplicity with no modifications of Abs required. Novel surfaces for Ab adsorption with improved orientation have recently been reported. Surfaces covered with calixarene derivatives have been demonstrated to capture Abs with a proper orientation [10, 11]. In addition, Zn^{II} metal complexes have been used for Ab adsorption [12, 13]. Mercaptohexadecanoic acid (MHA) was patterned on a thin-film gold substrate followed by coordination of the carboxylic acid groups of MHA to Zn^{II} ions. The authors report how these Zn^{II} ions can immobilise Abs (*e.g.* chicken IgY and mouse IgM) that generally have a low affinity for Ab-binding proteins A, G, A/G, or L. However, they are unclear how the Abs are immobilised by the metal ions or even how these methods achieve partial orientation.

2.2. Covalent Attachment

Covalent attachment of biomolecules to surfaces ensures sufficient immobilisation without leaching of the biomolecule from the substrate surface during use. Such covalent binding of proteins to a biosensor surface represents a rational and robust approach. One of the most commonly used methods for covalent immobilisation couples the Abs randomly *via* their free amino-groups to an activated sensor surface (Fig. **3**). Chemical coupling agents, such as carbodi-imides and succinimidyl esters, may be used to activate carboxylic acids on sensor surfaces. Amines or alcohols can be activated by isothiocyanates, epoxides, glutaraldehyde or other aldehydes. Oxidation of alcohols is achieved with periodate to yield aldehydes, which react readily with amines (Fig. **3**). In addition, conversion of alcohols to a highly reactive ester by cyanogen bromide allows for further reaction with amines present in the Ab. Another approach is to use what are termed hetero-bifunctional linkers. Hetero-bifunctional cross-linking reagents contain two different reactive groups, thereby, providing a means of covalently linking two dissimilar target groups (*e.g.* groups on the sensor surface with groups on the protein). A wide variety of these linkers are commercially available to cover the broad range of functional groups necessary.

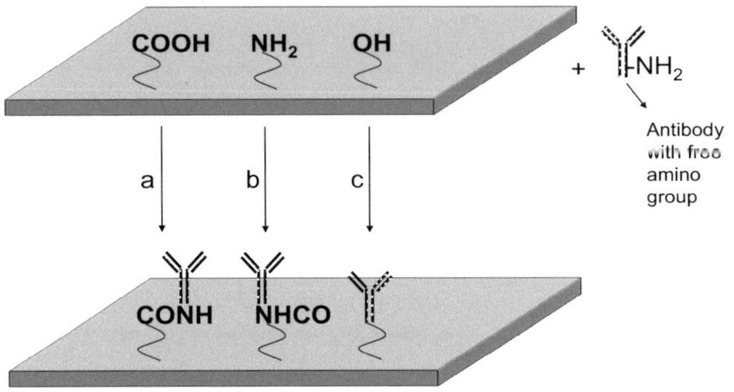

Figure 3: Scheme showing covalent immobilisation of antibodies to sensor surfaces *via* their free amino-groups. Reaction (a) involves activation of carboxylic acids (COOH), achieved with carbodi-imides and succinimyl esters. Reaction (b) shows amine surfaces (NH_2), which can be activated using isothiocyanates, epoxides or aldehydes. Reaction (c) shows alcohol surfaces which can be activated using periodate oxidation, isothiocyanates, epoxides, aldehydes and cyanogen bromide.

The chemistry for surface activation on glass and gold is also well established. In the case of glass surfaces, organosilanes are often employed. The silane part of the organosilane will react with the glass leaving the organo functional group available for conjugation to the protein. One of the most commonly used is the amino-silane 3-aminopropyltriethoxysilane (APTES), while other derivatives include aldehyde silane and epoxy silane [14]. Other authors have used amino-silanes combined with a bi-functional N-hydroxysuccinimide (NHS) or a mercapto-silane combined with maleimido-NHS [14]. In relation to gold surfaces, these are generally functionalised using a thiol or amino bi-functional cross-linker, which will attach to the gold, leaving another reactive group free to bind the protein of interest [15].

Although highly stable, Abs covalently-linked through amino groups are randomly oriented with their antigen binding capacities reported as 2–3-fold lower compared to those of well-oriented Abs [3, 16]. Strategies available for the covalent site-specific oriented immobilisation of Abs exist using the carbohydrate chains of Abs for immobilisation [17]. One simple oriented immobilisation strategy involves chemically coupling the Ab directly onto the transducer surface, *e.g.* a non-coated gold surface and available thiol (–SH) groups on the probe [18, 19]. However, these methods require chemical treatments of an Ab prior to immobilisation, such as carbohydrate oxidation and disulfide bond reduction, which may detrimentally alter it. Enzymatic digestion of an Ab followed by chemical reduction has yielded Fab fragments with exposed active sulfhydryl groups. Direct bonding between the sulfhydryl group and a gold surface, as well as thiol-specific cross-linking on non-metallic surfaces has been reported [20, 21].

There are several advantages to using the directional immobilisation processes. Ideally, the surface-coupling site is at a distant position from the antigen-capturing site, thereby, allowing the antigen-binding domains accessibility to the analyte. Bonroy *et al.* [22] showed for a particular Ab-antigen pair that the optimized fragment type combined with an oriented immobilisation of Fab fragments led to a greater than two-fold increase of the antigen-binding signals compared to randomly covalent immobilised full-size Abs.

A commonly used affinity-based method for orienting Abs specifically onto surfaces involves attachment of biotinylated Abs onto a (strept)avidin-modified surface. While technically this does not involve covalent binding, the dissociation constants of biotin-avidin and biotin-streptavidin interactions are some of the largest association energies observed for non-covalent interactions (of the order of 10^{-15} mol L^{-1}). The use of this type of immobilisation crucially retains the biological function of the immobilised Ab [23]. Abs can be biotinylated randomly or by oriented labelling procedures. Much higher loading densities were achieved with randomly biotinylated scFvs than full size Abs, leading to improved biosensor sensitivity and specificity [24]. Site-directed biotinylation of Abs at their hinge region was developed to orient the immobilisation of Abs which showed consistently enhanced detection capabilities compared to randomly biotinylated Abs [25].

Several reports have demonstrated DNA-directed Ab immobilisation whereby single-stranded DNA-Ab conjugates were immobilised onto complementary DNA surfaces [26-28]. This allows directed immobilisation without the use of harsh chemicals and incubation procedures. Human chorionic gonadotropin (hCG) was measured to levels as low as 0.1 ng mL^{-1} using DNA-directed Ab immobilisation on gold surfaces compared to an LOD of 5 ng mL^{-1} using directly coupled Abs on gold surfaces. This is an example of where linker chemistry in assays is key; the long, stable, flexible linker of DNA between the Ab and the gold sensing surface was, according to the authors, a likely contributor to the observed high sensitivity.

2.3. Antibody-Binding Proteins

Oriented immobilisation can also be achieved *via* an intermediate layer as an alternative to direct chemical coupling (Fig. **4**). An elegant example of this is to employ Ab-binding proteins such as protein A or G. These proteins bind specifically to Abs through their non-antigenic (Fc) regions, which leaves the antigen binding sites of the immobilised Ab available for binding. Such Ab-binding proteins have been extensively used to capture Abs on biosensor surfaces with their antigen-binding site maximally exposed to the solution and thus remaining fully functional. While the binding capacity of protein A is predominantly limited to three human IgG subclasses (IgG 1, 2 and 4), protein G has specificity for subclasses of Abs from many species. In addition, genetic engineering has enabled the production of a fusion protein, protein A/G that combines IgG binding domains of both protein A and protein G.Higher sensing abilities are regularly exhibited for immunoassays employing Ab-binding proteins for Ab immobilisation compared to those using conventional methods such as random covalent immobilisation [29, 30]. Although there is the additional step of immobilising the Ab-binding protein on the surface prior to Ab immobilisation, Ab-binding proteins can be genetically engineered and easily prepared in large quantities, providing many options for immobilisation. For example, a protein G layer was engineered to contain cysteines, which formed a more ordered film on bare gold compared to a control protein G layer [31]. This genetically engineered protein G layer allowed the immobilisation of approximately 4-fold more Abs compared to the control.

Ab fragments can also be genetically fused to a range of proteins and subsequently immobilised onto an assay surface. Fusion of Ab fragments to a common immobilisation domain will allow for identical orientation of all Abs. Pleschberger *et al.* [32] fused a bacterial S-layer protein to a nanobody (single chain Ab). This fusion protein self-assembled onto solid surface with the nanobody pointing outwards from the protein lattice surface into the solution. A similar approach was used to fuse scFvs with pIII surface protein, allowing a more sensitive detection to be achieved [33]. Fusion of Ab fragments with proteins such as beta-galactosidase, maltose-binding protein, calmodulin-binding protein, chitin-binding domain, cellulose-binding domain or glutathione-S-transferase is also possible. These fusion proteins (*e.g.* maltose-binding protein) on the Ab fragments allow for oriented immobilisation on surfaces containing the fusion partner (*e.g.* maltose).

In order to facilitate purification, most recombinant Ab fragments are expressed with an affinity tag. This tag may also be used for immobilisation onto a sensor surface (Fig. **4**). Histidine (his-tag) fused Ab fragments may be non-covalently immobilised onto Ni^{2+} or gold surfaces. ScFv fragments may also be engineered to contain two histidines where the scFvs are bound in a proper orientation, can retain antigen-binding affinity, and in addition, may be coupled at a high surface concentration [34]. Replacing the standard single his-tag with a double his-tag on scFvs has led to significantly enhanced binding onto Ni^{2+}-nitrilotriacetic acid-coated substrates [35].

In biomaterial science, Abs with a high affinity for certain material types would be advantageous as they could be used to immobilise probes on biosensor surfaces. Ab fragments that bind to the biodegradable polymer polyhydroxybutyrate, have been generated by phage display, thereby, allowing site-directed oriented immobilisation of Ab fragments on this biomaterial [36]. By grafting material-binding peptides into loops of the complementarity determining regions of Abs, fragments with binding affinity and specificity for non-biological inorganic material surfaces (*e.g.* gold) have been generated [37].

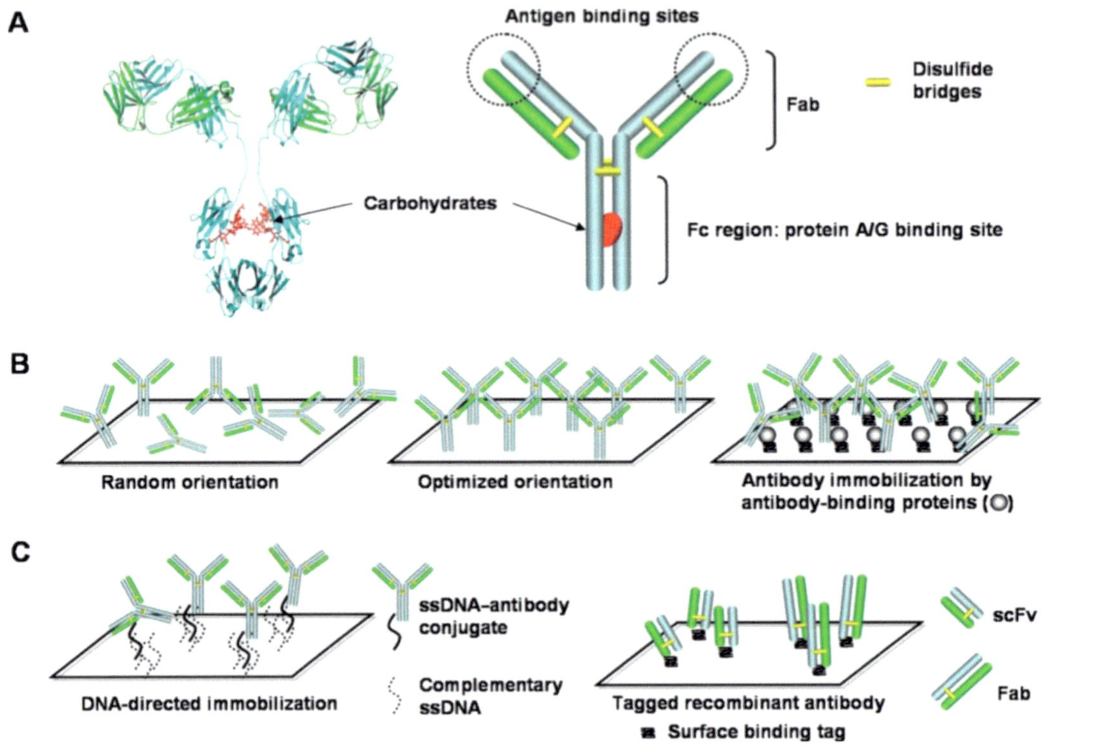

Figure 4: Schematic of different immobilisation strategies employed in immunosensors [2]. Reproduced with permission from Wiley-VCH Verlag GmbH.

3. IMMUNOSENSORS

3.1. Electrochemical

The oldest and most commonly used transducers are electrochemical. Electrical detection methods are appealing because of their low cost, low power consumption, ease of miniaturization, and potential multiplexing capability [38, 39]. The basis of these detection systems stems from a binding-induced change in some electrical property of the circuit of which the sensor is a vital component. A number of attributes of electrochemistry make it popular as a detection technique in immunosensing. The high sensitivity of electrochemical transducers and sample independence of turbidity and colour make them the transducer of choice for many researchers. Since most Abs and antigens in immunosensors are unable to act as redox partners, a label is often conjugated to one of the components of the immunocomplex to promote an electrochemical reaction. The electrochemical signal produced is then quantitatively related to the amount of analyte present in a sample. Potentiometry, amperometry, and electrochemical impedance spectroscopy are among the electrochemical detection techniques most often used with immunoassay systems and immunosensors. The fundamental principles of these techniques are presented, followed by discussions based on some recent work and trends in these areas.

3.2. Potentiometric Sensors

Based on the Nernst equation, potentiometric sensors measure a change in potential of a system. Potentiometric immunosensors depend on a change in potential between two electrodes due to a specific interaction between an Ab and its antigen [40]. One of the main disadvantages of this type of detection is the relatively small change in potential that arises from the interaction between an Ab and its antigen. Furthermore, interferences in the sample may prevent this small signal from being successfully detected. Such sensors, therefore, often have compromised sensitivity. A recent example of a potentiometric immunosensor involves using a polypyrrole coated screen-printed electrode [41]. Ab immobilisation on the polypyrrole layer was achieved by either direct adsorption or by binding a biotinylated Ab to streptavidin-coated polypyrrole. Incubation of this immuno-electrode was carried out in solutions containing either hepatitis B surface antigen or the cardiac marker, Troponin I. A sandwich immunoassay was completed by introducing a signal Ab labelled with Horse Radish Peroxidase (HRP). Potentiometric measurements were performed in 0.01 M Phosphate Buffer Saline (PBS) (pH 7.4) with o-phenylenediamine dihydrochloride added to initiate the enzymatic reaction. A deliberate separation of the immunoreaction from the detection step was employed to minimise matrix interferences. The change in potential was found to be proportional to the concentration of analyte in the sample. The sensitivities for hepatitis B surface antigen and troponin I were reported to be 50 fmol L^{-1} and 0.4 pmol L^{-1}, respectively.

3.3. Amperometric Sensors

Amperometric sensors measure the current produced by the oxidation or reduction of an electroactive species (which is monitored at a specific potential). The magnitude of the current can be related to the analyte concentration. To promote an electrochemical reaction at the sensor surface, a label must be introduced to the immuno-complex since both Ab and antigen are not intrinsically electroactive. Enzyme labels including the oxidoreductase, HRP, and the hydrolytic enzyme Alkaline Phosphatase (AP) are frequently used. The magnitude of the current from the redox reaction involving the enzyme can then be quantitatively related to the analyte concentration. A major advantage of enzyme labels is the amplification of the signal that can be detected as a result of the catalytic effect even when a minute quantity of enzyme is used. However, a drawback of the enzymatic signal-generating scheme described above is that it is an indirect detection technique.

In some amperometric immunosensors, the enzyme may be located some distance away from the electrode surface. In addition to this, the redox active site of an enzyme is usually covered by an insulating protein layer and therefore may not undergo direct electron transfer reactions at an electrode surface. In otheramperometric immunosensors, the presence of interfering substances in biological samples may require using an alternative electron transfer pathway. These two issues may be overcome with a redox-active species called an electron transfer mediator. Often used in analytical chemistry, electron transfer mediation is a well-known technique for overcoming limitations of electron transfer at metal electrodes.Mediatorsact as ashuttle to transfer electrons between the redox centre of theelectrode active materials(such as the peroxidase enzyme, HRP or glucose oxidase) and the surface of the electrode.A typical example of a mediator includes ferrocene and its derivatives. An electrochemical immunosensor using a mediator and single walled carbon nanotube forests as the electrode surface was demonstrated in a competitive immunoassay for detecting biotin-HRP and unlabelled biotin. In this competitive assay, labelled and unlabelled antigens competed for binding sites on the anti-biotin capture Ab [42]. The mediator chosen for this system was hydroquinone, used to facilitate a catalytic reduction of hydrogen peroxide by transferring electrons between HRP and the peroxide. LODs of 2.5 nM and 16 μM were achieved for biotin-HRP and unlabelled biotin, respectively.

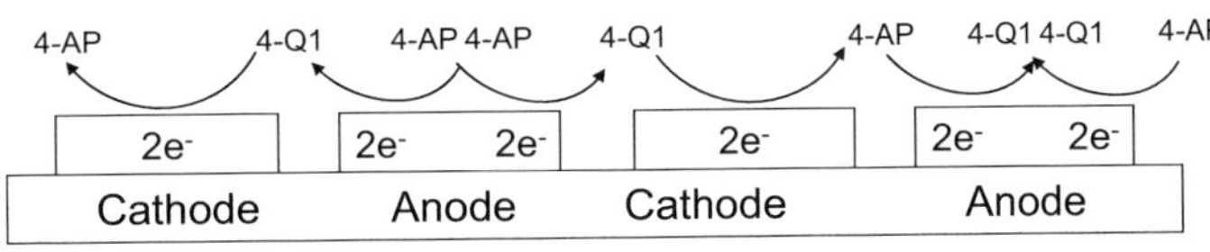

Figure 5: Scheme showing how interdigitated electrodes work. Redox cycling between 4-AP and 4-QI occurs at adjacent electrodes (denoted Anode and Cathode).

Generally, the development of electrochemical immunosensors involves the immobilisation of an immunocomplex on an electrode, followed by detection *via* the immunocomplex label at the same electrode. Interdigitated array (IDA) microelectrodes have gained popularity as transducers in electrochemical immunoassays. A simple IDA consists of a pair of interdigitated microelectrode "fingers". When an IDA is used as a sensing electrode in a voltammetric experiment, the two interdigitated electrodes are usually held at different potentials to achieve redox cycling of the electroactive species to be detected.

Redox cycling at interdigitated electrodes is illustrated in (Fig. **5**) where an oxidizing potential is applied to one of the two IDA electrodes (denoted Anode) to promote the oxidation of 4-aminophenol (4-AP) to 4-quinone imine (4-QI). Then, 4-QI diffuses to the adjacent electrode held at a more negative potential (denoted Cathode), where it is reduced to 4-AP, which can then undergo another oxidation at the next adjacent electrode. Major advantages of this redox cycling are lower LODs and improved sensitivity achieved by enhancing the Faradaic current relative to the background current, resulting in an improved signal-to-noise ratio. Thomas *et al.* used an IDA consisting of 25 pairs of platinum microelectrodes as a detector in immunoassays for mouse IgG [43]. Four-fold signal amplification was obtained compared to single-electrode detection, with an LOD of 3.5 fmol mouse IgG.

3.4. Electrochemical Impedance Spectroscopy

Changes occur in the interfacial charge, capacitance, resistance, mass, and thickness at an immunosensor surface upon binding of an antigen by an immobilised Ab. Electrochemical Impedance Spectroscopy (EIS) is a method for probing the features of an electrode surface modified by such immunocomplexes. In EIS, sensing is accomplished by measuring changes in the resistance and/or capacitance of the electrode–solution interface upon binding of a target molecule to a receptor functionalized surface [38, 39]. EIS does not require the use of enzyme labels to report binding events which contrasts with other electrical measurements, such as amperometry, potentiometry and voltammetry.

Recent developments in EIS report using alternative electrode materials such as electrically conducting polymers [44, 45] and nanoparticles [46, 47]. Additionally, electrode geometry has proven important with interdigitated electrode arrays providing improved sensitivity [39, 48]. Impedance-based sensors have been used to monitor protein–carbohydrate [49] and protein–protein [50, 51] interactions. For example, Yu *et al.* [52] reported multiplexed protein monitoring with an array of gold electrodes.Immobilised on the gold electrodes were human IgG (hIgG), rat IgG (rIgG), human globin and bovine serum albumin. This array was incubated with goat anti-hIgG Ab, goat anti-rIgG Ab, anti-human globin Ab and a mixture of the three Abs. Formation of an antigen-Ab complex significantly changed the electron transfer resistance of the electrodes allowing detection of the four Abs.

3.5. Trends in Electrochemical Immunosensors

Nanomaterial-enhanced electrochemical immunosensors are currently a hot topic with the rapid growth in this area being driven by a need for analytical devices requiring smaller sample volumes, decreased power consumption and improved performances. Due to their dimensions, nanostructured materials display unique properties not traditionally observed in bulk materials. Characteristics such as increased surface area along with enhanced electrical properties make them suitable for sensing applications. In addition, nanomaterials are comparable in size to many biomacromolecules. Therefore, their nanodimensions exploit the possibility of bringing these materials into close proximity with proteins, enabling them to act as one dimensional channels for electron transfer in proteins.

Based on their unique electrical and catalytic properties, nanoparticles can perform various roles in electrochemical sensing systems. They can be used for the immobilisation or labelling of biomolecules, the catalysis of electrochemical reactions, the enhancement of electron transfer, or even act as a reactant. Due to their excellent conductivity and catalytic properties metal nanoparticles are ideal "electronic wires" for enhancing the electron transfer between redox centres in proteins and electrode surfaces. For example, gold nanoparticles (Au NPs) can exhibit excellent catalytic activity due to their relative high surface area to volume ratio, and their interface-dominated properties, which significantly differ from their bulk counterparts [53] (Table **2**).

Table 2: LODs of amplified electrochemical bioassays.

Assay	Target	LOD[a]	Ref.
Au(III) ion	IgG	3 pM	[54]
Oligonucleotide (purine base)	IgG	13 fM	[55]
CNT-ALP[b]	IgG	3 fM	[56]
CNT-HRP[c]	PSA	100 fM	[57]
AuNP-Ab	IgG	7 aM	[58]
AuNP-Ab-hydrazine	IgG	670 aM	[59]
AuNP–polymer complex	IgG	1 fM	[60]

[a] Limit of detection, [b] CNT-ALP (carbon nanotube-alkaline phosphatase), [c]CNT-HRP (carbon nanotube-horseradish peroxidase).

By means of direct electrochemical detection of Au NPs, Ko *et al.* [61] have reported a multiplex immuno-biosensor to detect cancer biomarkers including prostate specific antigen (PSA). Au NPs act as catalysts in the reduction of silver ions to metallic silver, which is deposited onto the gold nanoparticles, thereby enlarging the particles. The growing size of the particles connects them to each other, forming an electrical bridge; thus, decreasing the resistance between electrodes. This biosensor could detect PSA at an LOD of 10 pg mL^{-1}. Another immuno-biosensor for the rapid detection of PSA uses a different technique of integrating an immuno-chromatographic strip with Screen-Printed Electrodes (SPE). This acts as an electrochemical transducer for stripping analysis of metal ions released from captured Quantum Dot (QD) labels. It was found that this biosensor showed high sensitivity with a LOD of 20 pg mL^{-1} [62].

Carbon Nanotubes (CNTs) can also be used to develop highly sensitive and specific nanoscale immunosensors [63]. Examples of where CNTs were used to amplify detection of PSA in serum include CNTs carrying Numerous Horseradish Peroxidase (HRP) enzyme labels and secondary Abs [64, 65]. The secondary Ab and HRP label were covalently linked to CNTs at high ratios of 1:200 in place of singly labelledsecondary Abs in a sandwich immunoassay [66]. This amplification strategy improved the LOD 100-fold to 4 pg mL-1 and the sensitivity by 800-fold, compared to conventional ELISA. These results highlight the excellent promise CNTs show in ultrasensitive immunoassay research in proteomics and systems biology.

In addition to electrochemical sensors using CNTs as an electrode substrate, sensors based on transistor arrangements using CNTs have been developed [67]. Single Wall Carbon Nanotubes (SWNTs) are the most likely candidate for miniaturising electronics beyond the micro-electromechanical scale currently used in electronics. They exhibit electrical properties not shared by their multi-walled counterparts and certain sizes of SWNT act as semiconductors. The intrinsic bandgap in semiconducting SWNTs (typically 0.5 eV, but this is diameter-dependent) allows them to be used as nanosized semiconducting channels in Field-Effect Transistors (FETs) (Table **3**) [68]. Since FET-based biomolecular detection does not employ fluorescence, electrochemical, or magnetic tags, it has been termed as “label-free” methodology [69-71]. FETs generally consist of a substrate (gate), two microelectrodes (source and drain), and a SWNT (or SWNT network) that bridges the electrodes. Usually SWNTs are grown directly *via* Chemical Vapour Deposition (CVD) or cast from a dispersion onto a substrate either before or after the electrodes are patterned [72]. Single-nanotube FETs require arduous screening of devices to eliminate metallic SWNTs. This need is obviated for nanotube networks cast from dispersions, where the 2 to 1 ratio of semiconducting to metallic SWNTs renders the likelihood of forming a continuous metallic pathway between source and drain unlikely. Sensing is based on the fact that the current flow in SWNT FETs is extremely sensitive to the binding of biomolecules and produces a detectable signal. A wide variety of applications for CNT FETs have been investigated including the detection of proteins, Ab-antigen interactions, glucose, DNA and DNA hybridization. The LOD for the sensing of proteins or protein-protein interactions has generally been in the range of 100 pM to 100 nM [73].

An SWNT-FET immunoassay typically involves first immobilising an Ab, thus providing a recognition site for the target antigen. The current–voltage characteristics or conductance of the Ab-modified SWNT-FET are measured prior to antigen binding. Following exposure to the antigen, the conductance of the SWNT-

FET device is again measured [74].To detect IgE 50-amino-modified aptamers immobilised on a CNT-FET were used [75]. The net current change increased with the IgE concentration and an LOD for IgE of 250 pM was reported. Li *et al.* [76] studied the detection of PSA with an FET comprised of a network of SWNTs. The authors measured the electronic interaction of an anti-PSA Ab capturing PSA antigen. The interaction is thought to be a charge-transfer mechanism with a reported limit of detection of 14 pM, at a signal-to-noise ratio of 2. Table **3** summarises SWNT-FET biosensors showing how pM LOD for Ab–antigen binding [73, 77] have been achieved.

Table 3: SWNT-FET biosensor configuration tabulated against receptor Ab, target antigen, LOD and signal amplification [68].

Receptor	Target	SWNT Configuration	CNT Fabrication	SD Fabrication	Gate	LOD	Signal Amplification
Ab (SpA, hCG)	Antigen (IgG, β-hCG)	Mat	CVD (Fe)	Cr-Au Shad-Mask/Evap	Liquid	1pM	SB area increase
Ab (SpA, BT, U1A)	Antigen (IgG, SP, mAbs)	Mat	CVD (Fe)	Ti-Au Shad-Mask/Evap	Liquid	100nM-100pM	N/R
Ab (BT)	Antigen (SP)	Single/few	CVD (Fe)	Ti-Au PhotoL/Evap	Bottom	N/R	N/R
Ab (anti-CEA)	Antigen (CEA)	Single/few	CVD (Fe, alumina)	Ti-Au PhotoL/Evap	Liquid	300fM	N/R

CVD: chemical vapour deposition; PhotoL: photolithography; Evap: evaporation; Shad-mask: Shadow mask; SB: Schottky barrier; N/R: not reported; SpA; specific protein A, derived from *Staphylococcus aureus*; hCG: human chorionic gonadotropin; IgG: rabbit immunoglobulin G; β-hCG: mouse Ab; BT: biotin; SP: streptavidin; U1A: human autoantigen, a prototype target of the autoimmune response in patients with systemic lupus erythematosus and mixed connective tissue diseases; mAb: monoclonal Ab; CEA: carcinoembryonic antigen; anti-CEA: CEA Ab.

3.6. Optical Immunosensors

Due to ever improving technologies, the field of optical immunosensors is progressing rapidly. The methods involved are based on detecting the interactions between antigens and their specific Abs through changes in optical characteristics such as absorption, fluorescence, chemiluminescence and refractive index among others.Optical immunosensors can be classified into two categories according to direct or indirect detection of the binding event. Direct/label-free sensors monitor Ab-antigen interactions which generate a measurable signal. These methods do not require any additional reagents and can work in complex matrices. However, they may be limited by low molecular weight analyte detection and by being prone to non-specific interactions. On the other hand, indirect optical methods necessitate the incorporation of suitable labels such as fluorophores onto the Ab or antigen to monitor the binding event. This leads to assays with higher specificity and sensitivity but the labelling steps can be labour-intensive, the reagents involved expensive and the reaction may subsequently affect Ab binding reactions.Optical immunosensors often use an evanescent wave generated at the interface between two media with different optical properties, the sensor platform and the sample, to sense the binding events. The signal measured is correlated with the concentration of the analyte in the sample. A variety of transducers are available such as Surface Plasma Resonance (SPR) and Total Internal Reflection Fluorescence (TIRF).

3.7. Direct Optical Detection

The main types of direct optical immunosensor detectors are based on grating-couplers, Mach-Zehnder interferometers and SPR [78-81].Some of the most sensitive optical immunosensors involve SPR, an optoelectronic phenomenon, first observed by Wood in 1902 [82]. SPR immunosensors use electromagnetic waves, also called surface plasmons, to probe interactions between the analyte in solution and its recognition element immobilised on a thin metal film usually made from gold.The wave's oscillation occurs and propagates at the interface between two transparent media of different refractive index such as glass and a metal. When plane polarised light, of appropriate wavelength and angle, illuminates thc metal film, *via* a hemispherical optical prism, the light is reflected back into the metal layer and partly refracted to the sample solution. The energy from the incident photons is absorbed and generates the surface plasmons (Fig. **6**).Above a critical angle of incidence, no light passes into the sample solution and Total Internal Reflection (TIR) occurs. When the light is totally internally reflected, an evanescent wave is created at the interface close to the metal layer. The evanescent wave penetrates the thin film and excites the electromagnetic surface plasmon wave, with the intensity of the wave depending on the angle of incidence [83, 84]. SPR occurs as the surface plasmons absorb some of the light energy from the evanescent field, which corresponds to a match between the energy and momentum of the incident light and the energy and momentum of the surface plasmons. The energy of the incident light is transferred to the plasmons, which can be observed as a marked drop in the total internal reflection light intensity reflected from the sensor surface at a specific angle (SPR angle θ). The resonance angle is sensitive to the refractive index of the solution adjacent to the sensor surface. Interactions between the recognition elements and their analytes change the mass at the surface of the chip but also the refractive index. Those variations affect the velocity, and, therefore, the momentum of the surface plasmons, causing a shift of the resonance to a longer wavelength and a change in the incident angle at which resonance occurs.

Different formats of SPR immunosensors exist. Direct, sandwich and competitive inhibition assays have all been developed using the technology (Fig. **6**). In direct immunoassays, the recognition element is the Ab immobilised onto the metal layer and the change in mass and in resonance angle due to its interaction with an antigen is correlated to the concentration of the analyte. Guidi *et al.* [85] demonstrated the detection of insulin-like growth factor-1 in milk using a SPR direct assay. Since milk spoils quickly, real-time monitoring of the milk samples is preferable to time-consuming methods such as ELISA. SPR sandwich assays involve an additional Ab to the one immobilised on the sensor surface, improving its sensitivity compared to direct assays as the antigen is then recognised and captured by two Abs. Teramura *et al.* [86] developed an SPR sandwich assay to detect alpha-fetoprotein, a major tumour marker for hepatocellular tumour, in human plasma at the ng level necessary for clinical diagnosis. However, competitive inhibition assays are the method of choice forsmall-moleculedetection. Such assays can sometimes involve the conjugation of the antigen to a carrier protein for immobilisation on the sensor surface. The Ab is pre-incubated with the antigen and the mixture injected over the sensor surface. The free Ab is then separated from the bound Ab. The concentration of the free Ab is inversely proportional to the concentration of the antigen. Competitive inhibition assays have been used to detect a wide range of small-molecule antigens as small as 250-500 Da [87].

The advantages of SPR immunosensors are that the same chip can be used several times; these SPR assays do not necessitate any labelling and can monitor in 'real-time' the binding events of small molecules with a very high sensitivity. They can give information on kinetics, affinity and concentration of the target analytes. However, the equipment required can be bulky and expensive, but emerging technologies will lead to significant reductions in size. SPR assays have found many applications in different fields such as biomedical diagnostics [88, 89], and drug discovery [90, 91].

3.8. Indirect Optical Detection

Immunosensors with indirect optical detection involve the labelling of recognition elements, used to sense the Ab/antigen interaction. Those labels will fluoresce, luminesce or absorb the light. Different strategies have been developed to use such labelled biomolecules with the most popular being the addition of a fluorophore.

Total Internal Reflection Fluorescence (TIRF) is based on total internal reflection happening between optically dense media joined to the recognition elements and optically less dense sample solutions containing the target molecule. At large angles of incidence, the excitation beam reflects into the glass and generates an evanescent wave at the interface with the sample. The wave can only excite the elements present on the TIRF surface. It has a maximum intensity at the surface,which is reduced with increasing distance from the surface [92]. These sensors demonstrate high sensitivity and can avoid separation and extraction steps from complex matrices such as body fluids [93, 94]. As an example, studies were carried out using TIRF immunosensors to evaluate the concentration of bovine progesterone, a reproductive hormone present in raw milk [95, 96]. The assay was designed as a competitive-inhibition test with progesterone attached on the sensor surface and a monoclonal anti-progesterone Ab used as the biological recognition element. The LOD was 0.04 ng mL^{-1} and this immunosensor for progesterone could be utilised as a reproductive management instrument. Albrecht *et al.* [97] developed an assay for the detection of C-Reactive Protein (CRP), an inflammation marker using TIRF. A binding-inhibition and a sandwich assay were developed. The concentration of CRP in normal blood is usually between 1 to 10 mg L^{-1} but can reach 40 mg L^{-1} with a viral infection and 500 mg L^{-1} with a bacterial infection. The immunosensor had an LOD of 0.44 mg mL^{-1} and 0.13 mg mL^{-1} for the sandwich and inhibition assay respectively. Thus, they have the potential to contribute to the realisation of a diagnostic test for CRP.

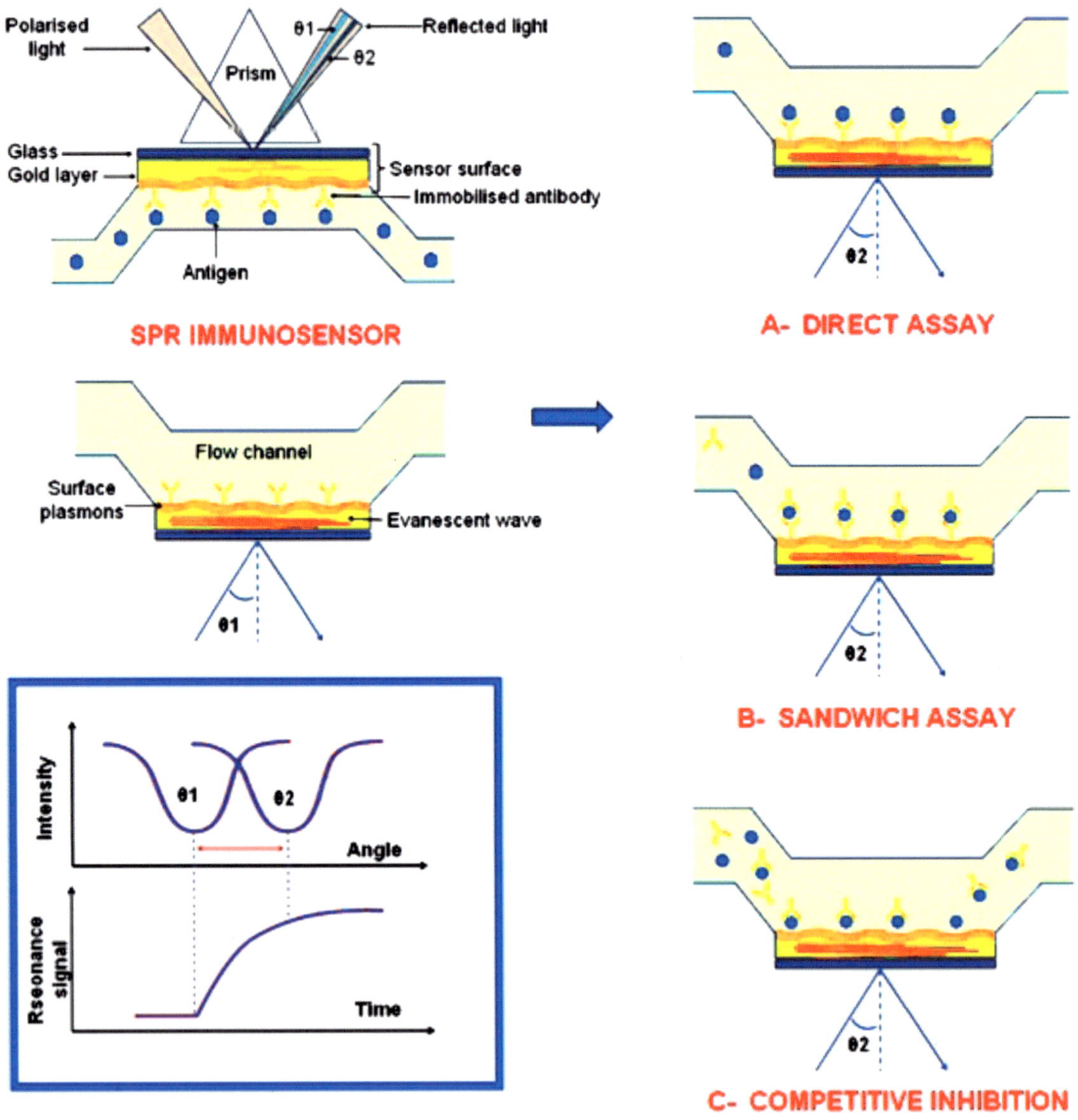

Figure 6: SPR phenomenon representation. The binding interaction between the Ab and the antigen results in a mass change at the surface of the sensor leading in a change in refractive index (θ1 to θ2). The three main assay formats are: (A) direct assay, (B) sandwich assay and (C) competitive inhibition assay.

There are also examples of optical immunosensors using evanescent wave effects coupled to optic fibres. The optic fibre is a perfect transducer to combine with fluorescent signals increasing the efficiency of light collection. When light illuminates an optic fibre, a small proportion escapes from the surface of the fibre generating an evanescent wave interface between the optic fibre and the sample of interest. The evanescent zone extends along the length of the fibre sensor and decreases in intensity exponentially from the sensor surface. At an appropriate wavelength, fluorescent entities, such as labelled Abs present in the evanescent wave, can absorb energy and fluoresce. Part of the fluorescence is refracted into the fibre and detected. Both direct and sandwich assay formats have been used. For the sandwich assay, the antigen is recognised by both a capture Ab immobilised onto the fibre surface and a second labelled detection Ab added to the solution. If there is no antigen present, no fluorescence is observed. However, if there is antigen present, the detection Ab fluoresces due to its excitation by the evanescent wave. Long *et al.* [98] developed a fluorescent fibre-optic immunosensor for the detection of microcystin-LR in water samples. The inhibition assay was carried out with the level of Abs binding to microcystin-LR-ovalbumin conjugate covalently immobilised to the fibre optic surface depending on the concentration of microcystin-LR in the water samples. The LOD was 0.03 mu g L^{-1} and the quantitative detection range 0.1-10.1 mu g L^{-1}. These immunosensors have advantages in that they are sensitive, specific and inexpensive. In addition, they are not prone to electromagnetic interference, offer 'real-time' monitoring of the binding events and can be easily miniaturised [99, 100].

Fluorescent capillary fill immunosensors have also been developed. They consist of two sheets of glass held apart at a distance of 100 μm and between which the reagents are immobilised and the binding reactions take place (Fig. 7). The sample enters the device by capillary action. Once inside, the analyte present in the sample matrix has to compete with the fluorescently-labelled antigens for the binding sites of the Abs that are immobilised on the glass. When the fluorescently-labelled analyte is trapped on the glass plate in the sample matrix, the fluorophores within the evanescent field are excited. The fluorescence formed in the capillary is quantified by scanning the capillary with light to excite the fluorophore labels. The photons, emitted at angles smaller than the critical angle, are trapped in the capillary walls and the light leaving the capillary is detected and the level of photons correlated to the concentration of the analyte. Sensitivities of 3 ng mL^{-1} and 0.5 ng mL^{-1} have been obtained for hCG in serum and estrone-3-glucuronide in urine, respectively [101-103]. More recently, Petrou *et al.* [104] developed a similar system to simultaneously determine the level of three hormones, follitropin, hCG and prolactin, in human serum, which levels are important for the diagnosis of fertility and development disorders. In that case, the immunosensor was made from a plastic capillary. The LOD was 1.3 μgL^{-1}, 2.3 IUL^{-1} and 3.6 IUL^{-1} for prolactin, follitropin and hCG, respectively, which are appropriate levels for the determination of these analytes in human serum.

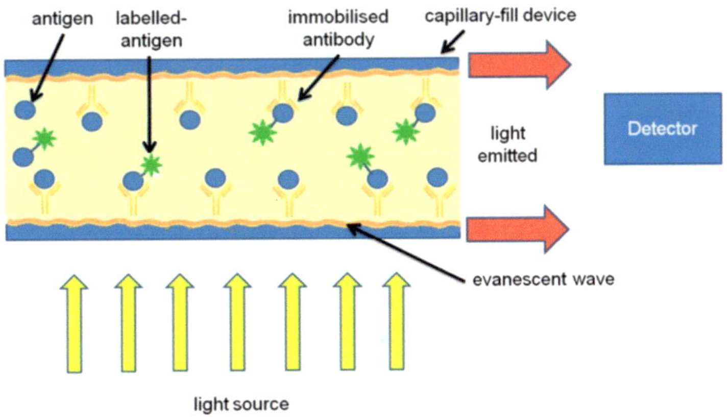

Figure 7: Schematic representation of the fluorescence-based detection capillary fill immunosensor.

Planar waveguide immunosensors employ evanescent illumination to excite fluorophores at the surface of a waveguide. They differ from fibre optic sensors by collecting the emitted light perpendicular to the waveguide while fibre optic immunosensors collect the emitted light at the end of the fibre. Planar waveguide immunosensors have been used to perform analysis on sample assays in parallel. Rowe-Taitt *et al.* [105] demonstrated using a cocktail of fluorescent Abs on a single sensor substrate the simultaneous detection of six biohazardous analytes: cholera toxin (from *Vibrio cholerae*), *Staphylococcus aureus* enterotoxin B, ricin, *Bacillus anthracis*, *Francisella tularensis*, and *Brucella abortus*.

Another type of fluorescence-based immunosensor employs fluorescence polarization; it is based on the increase in fluorescence polarisation of small labelled antigens (tracer) added to the sample (Fig. **8**). When the tracer is free, its volume is small, its rotation fast and its fluorescence polarisation low. The fluorescence increases when it interacts with its specific Ab leading to a larger volume of the tracer-Ab complex and to a slower rotation. However, in the presence of the target antigen, the antigen competes with the tracer for binding with the Ab and the polarization signal decreases. The higher the concentration of unlabelled antigen present in the sample, the less bound tracer is present and, consequently, the lower the polarization of the fluorescent emitted light. These sensors use fluorophores and are very precise with a coefficient of correlation below 5 %. However, they can be prone to light scattering interferences [106]. Gachoz *et al.* [107] developed a fluorescence polarization immunoassay for the detection of mycotoxins such as ochratoxin A, aflatoxin B1 and zearalenone. The LOD of the mycotoxins was 1 ng mL^{-1}, thus, below the acceptable maximum residue limit in food. Wang *et al.* [108] developed an immunoassay for the detection of the antibiotic, sulfamethazine (LOD of 41 ng mL^{-1}), with a value available in just 5 minutes.

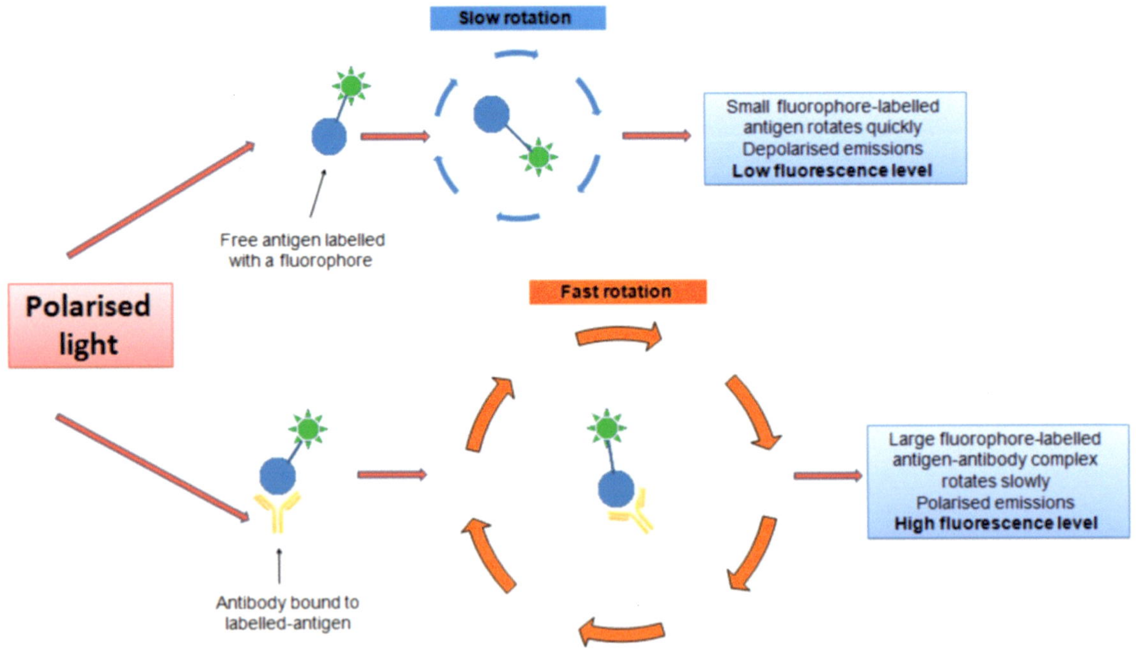

Figure 8: Basic representation of the concept of a fluorescence polarisation immunoassay.

Chemiluminescence and Quantum Dots (QDs) have also received increasing interest for labelling Abs in the development of immunosensors. Chemiluminescent immunosensors use enzyme labels. The light emitted from the bound enzyme-labelled to the Ab/antigen is transmitted to a photomultiplier. Chemiluminescent detection possesses several advantages such as the relatively simple instrumentation required, very low LODs and a wide dynamic range [109]. Chemiluminescent optical fibre-immunosensors have been developed for the detection of *Brucella* with a LOD of*Brucella* smooth-A-O-chain antigen of 1.098 ng mL^{-1} corresponding to about 305 cfu mL^{-1}*Brucella* cells [110]. Salama *et al.* [111] reported an assay for the detection of Abs specific to GIPC-1, a protein involved in ovarian and breast cancer. The antigen was immobilised onto the optic fibre and a standard curve was built using a human monoclonal anti-GIPC-1 Ab purified from breast cancer patients, with a LOD of 30 pg mL^{-1}. This chemiluminescent fibre-optic immunosensor had an LOD 50 times lower than a chemiluminescent ELISA, and approximately 500 times lower than a colorimetric ELISA for the detection of GIPC-1.

QDs are ultrasensitive colloidal nanocrystals with unique photophysical properties [112]. They offer advantages over molecular dyes by being brighter, resistant to photo bleaching and amenable to multiplexed detection [113]. They can be conjugated to Abs by replacing thiol acids present on the QD surface with the Ab or using linker molecules such as biotin and streptavidin. They have been used, for example, to label Abs specific for total Prostate Specific Antigen (PSA) [114]. QD sensors have great potential as a diagnostic tool for prostate cancer detection with an LOD of 0.25 ng mL^{-1} in human serum samples.

3.9. Mechanical Immunosensors

3.9.1. Mass-Detecting Immunosensors

Piezoelectric immunosensors are based on the analysis of binding events between antigens and Abs though mass increase at the surface of piezoelectric materials such as quartz crystal (Fig. **9**). The quartz crystal resonates at a particular oscillation frequency when subjected to an electric field. Changes in resonance frequency are measured, which correspond to the mass increase on the chip surface during the interaction. The relationship between the mass and frequency was established by the Saurbrey equation; the higher the mass, the lower is the frequency [115].

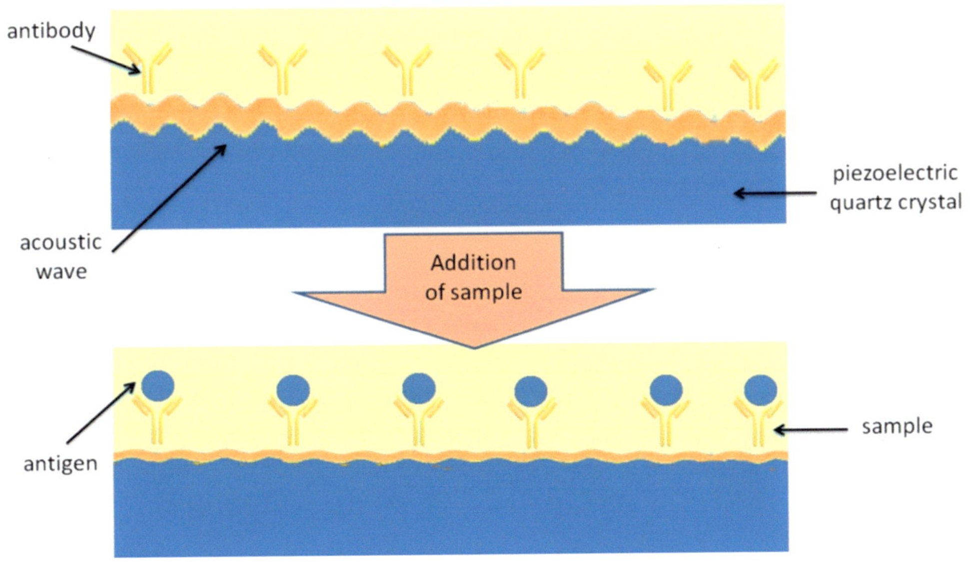

Figure 9: Basic principle of piezoelectric transduction in an immunoassay.

Two major types of piezoelectric transducer exist: the Quartz Crystal Microbalance (QCM), also called bulk acoustic wave and the Surface Acoustic Wave (SAW) transducers. With the first type, resonance happens in the whole crystal mass while for the latter resonance only occurs on its surface. The QCM can resonate at a frequency up to 30 MHz due to the stability of the crystal mechanical structure while the SAW frequency can go up to 200 MHz and they are thus expected to be more sensitive to the Ab-antigen interaction than QCM [116, 117]. The first piezoelectric transducer was developed in 1972 by Shons and Dorman for the detection of IgG in bovine serum [118]. Such transducers show real potential for 'point-of-care' diagnostics. Recent studies reported the development of a QCM immunosensor to detect CRP based on an indirect competition assay. It aimed to detect CRP, a biomarker for heart disease, hypertension and inflammation. The sensor detected a wide concentration range of 0.130–25,016 ng mL^{-1} of CRP with an LOD of 0.130 ng mL^{-1}. Also, the intensity of the signal could be increased by introducing a streptavidin coated gold nanoparticle increasing the sensitivity of the assay [119, 120]. Lee *et al.* [121] developed an immunosensor using a SAW transducer to demonstrate the detection of hepatitis B surface Abs that are present during the late phase of the virus infection. The immunosensor showed binding-specificity to the Ab and a LOD below 10 pg μL^{-1}. It could also detect the Ab in blood samples.

Piezoelectric immunosensors are popular as they are affordable and easy to use. They do not require the need to label Abs or antigens and can detect antigens down to the pg range. However, with piezoelectric systems, non-specific binding on the surface of the crystal can lead to erroneous results.

3.9.2. Micro-Cantilever Immunosensors

Benefitting from Atomic Force Microscope (AFM) technology, microcantilever biosensors are an emerging sensor technique. This technique utilisesbending of the microcantilever (which changes its resonant frequency)due to specific biomolecular interactions and recording of either optical or electronic signals.Vibrational frequency changes that are caused by molecules adsorbed on a microcantilever are referred to as "curling" due to the adsorption stress on one side of the cantilever. Molecular binding events on cantilevers may be transduced *via* deflection of the cantilever [122] or a change in the resonance frequency of the cantilevers (Fig. **10**) [123]. The simplest method is a change in deflection, which is measured by reflecting a laser beam off the back of the cantilever and measuring its position with a photodiode. Cantilever deflection has been applied for detection of the pesticide DDT with an LOD of 10 nM [124]. A competitiveimmunoassay was carried out using a synthetic hapten conjugated with BSA and its specific Ab. Clinically relevant concentrations of myoglobin with an LOD of 85 $ngmL^{-1}$was detected by Raiteri *et al.* using a monoclonal anti-myoglobin Ab [125]. Using micro-cantilevers Wu *et al.* [126] detected PSA with an LOD of 0.2 ng mL^{-1} in serum containing 1 mg mL^{-1} albumin and plasminogen. The same research group, using very large arrays of up to 960 individually readable microcantilevers, demonstrated sensitive protein detection [127]. Monitoring the change in the resonance frequency on binding of an analyte is the principle behind resonance-based transduction of microcantilevers [123]. This is by far the most sensitive method, even if significantly more complex than that for deflection-based detection [122]. Using this more sensitive resonance-based measurement strategy, PSA with an LOD of 10 $pgmL^{-1}$was detected [128].

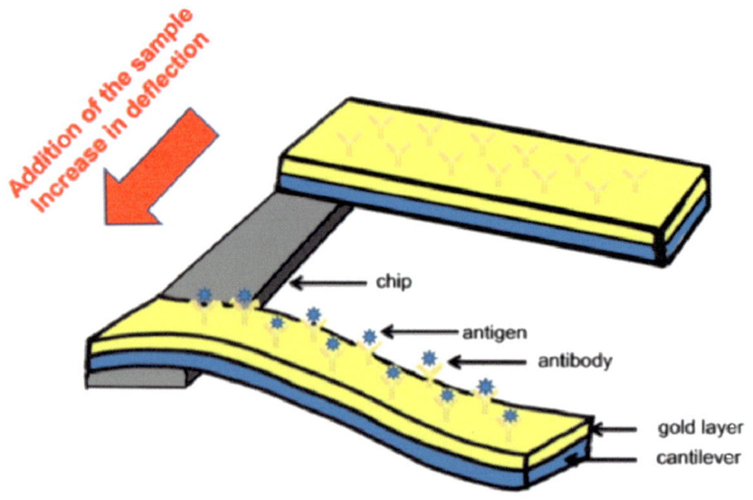

Figure 10: Schematic representation of a micro-cantilever immunoassay.

The incorporation of piezoelectric materials into microcantilevers can also be used to monitor the presence of biomolecules. Binding events on the cantilever surface are transduced by bending of the cantilever, which then generates an electric current in an attached piezoelectric element [129]. Piezoelectric-modified microcantilevers may be operated in both deflection-based and resonance-based modes. Analyte binding to the cantilever surface causes the cantilever to deflect, consequently depolarising the material and generating a current. A piezoelectric nanomechanical cantilever was fabricated by Lee *et al.* for the labelfree detection ofPSA with anLOD of 10 pg mL^{-1} [130].

Currently microcantilever-based sensors are an appealing method for sensitive, label-free detection of biomolecules. The major advantages of microcantilever sensors overtraditional transducers such as the QCM exist in their superior sensitivity toanalytes. LODs are at least comparable to those for SPR. The ease of cantilever functionalisation allows for systems as varied as single molecules to whole cells to be studied. In addition, the ability to micro-fabricate compact arrays of cantileversfacilitates simultaneous and high throughput measurements [128, 131].

4. MINIATURISATION OF IMMUNOSENSORS

Intensive work has been directed toward the miniaturisation of immunosensors. The miniaturisation of assays will lead to the development of cheaper and more portable instruments, which can be used as point-of-care devices for diseases diagnosis. It will also facilitate research applications in areas such as environmental monitoring with the opportunity to carry out analysis in the field. Microfluidic platforms offer great potential for the integration of immunoassays. Microfluidics will aid the reduction of sample volumes, some of which are not always available in large quantities (*e.g.* bodily fluids), and of expensive reagents such as Abs and enzymes [132]. Both samples and reagents can be added to the structures down to the nanolitre scale and transferred from one chamber to the next as they are going through a series of reactions. These steps can involve separation, mixing, incubation, washing steps and enzyme reactions with substrates necessary for the immunoassay [133]. It may also ease the automation of reactions alleviating the human error involved in the loss of accuracy and lowering the energy requirements of the assay [134].

The use of microfluidic devices will also lead to improved analytical efficiency by shortening the time required to carry out the reaction. This is due to larger surface-to-volume ratios and improved mass transport efficiency. However, this advantage can also increase the level of non-specific binding of the antigen and of its Ab outside the detection area. This problem can be alleviated by carrying out appropriate surface modifications depending on the choice of chip fabrication material. Microfluidic platforms can be made from various substrates such as silicon, glass and polymers. Early devices were mainly fabricated with silicon. Polymers are now more commonly used due to their cheaper material and fabrication cost as well as their superior optical properties. Polymers, such as polydimethylsiloxane (PDMS), polycarbonate (PC), polymethylethacrylate (PMMA), and cyclo-olefins such as Zeonor, show considerable advantages such as their low cost and ease-of-use. PDMS allows for the rapid fabrication of prototypes and can be sealed and bound to other structures made from different materials [135, 136]. With the aid of injection moulding technology, PMMA, a thermoplastic polymer, is even faster to use for chip fabrication, while cyclo-olefin polymers show excellent optical properties [137].

To remove any non-specific binding, surface modifications such as blocking steps with BSA can be necessary depending on the material selected [138]. Abs can be immobilised on hydrophobic substrates by adsorption. Due to the instability of Abs immobilised by adsorption, other surface chemistries have been developed to covalently bind the Abs to the platform [139-145]. The Abs and antigens can also be immobilised onto micro-beads added to the device. The beads offer a large surface area where added functional groups allow for the conjugation of Abs or antigens. They also allow for the easy transportation of Abs/antigens over the platform using pressure or electric fields [146, 147].

Microfluidic platforms can vary in size and shape but are typically made of channels and reaction chambers of small dimensions. Fluids have to be mixed efficiently and transferred between the different channels and reaction chambers of the structure in a controlled way. Flow behaviour of fluids inside a microchannel is laminar but pumps and valves can be used to control the circulation of the samples and reagents [148,149]. In centrifugal microfluidic immunosensors (*e.g.* Centrifugal Devices (CD)), the circulation of the fluid relies on the hydrophilicity of the surface substrate. The sequential release of the fluids depends on the centrifugal and capillary forces; when spinning the device, the centrifugal force overcomes the capillary force in the valves [150, 151]. An advantage of the CD is that centrifugal pumping eliminates the need for pumps requiring large power supplies to drive the fluids. Structures such as siphons and capillary burst valves can also be added to the design to regulate the microfluidic flow of the different solutions [152]. For example, capillary burst valves prevent the circulation of the fluid forming a barrier when the channel section expands abruptly. Sandwich, direct and competitive immunoassays have been developed on CDs [153-155]. This makes these devices perfect candidates to be used in the field.

The successful development of an immunoassay involves a signal with a strong enough intensity to be detected. Microfluidic sensors mainly use optical and electrochemical transducers. Fluorescence optical systems are preferred over light absorbance ones due to their higher sensitivity on small platforms [156]. There are also reports of small immunosensors using SPR [157, 158], chemiluminescence [159], light scattering [160] and electrochemical systems [161].

5. CONCLUSION

In conclusion, over the last 30 years, emerging technologies have led to the development of rapid immunosensors available for food quality, heath and environmental monitoring. These assays demonstrate high sensitivities and specificities due to the progress in Ab development and allow the real-time monitoring of Ab-antigen interactions. This in conjunction with the diversity of transducers available has led to a rapid growth of research in immunoassay techniques. However, the assays available to date are largely more suited to research laboratories than to commercialisation. Novel microfluidic techniques permit the future miniaturisation of existing immunosensors which should lead to faster, cheaper and more sensitive assays. This will help to feed the need for automation of the tests developed and to a larger utilisation of immunosensors in modern applications such as point-of-care diagnostics.

REFERENCES

[1] Conroy PJ, Hearty S, Leonard P, O'Kennedy RJ. Antibody production, design and use for biosensor-based applications. Semin Cell Dev Biol 2009; 20: 10-26.

[2] Jung Y, Jeong JY, Chung BH. Recent advances in immobilization methods of antibodies on solid supports. Analyst 2008; 133: 697-701.

[3] Cho IH, Paek EH, Lee H, *et al.* Site-directed biotinylation of antibodies for controlled immobilization on solid surfaces. Anal Biochem 2007; 365, 14-23.

[4] Cao T, Wang A, Liang X, *et al.* Investigation of spacer length effect on immobilized *Escherichia coli* pili-antibody molecular recognition by AFM. Biotechnol Bioeng 2007; 98: 1109-22.

[5] Pavlickova P, Schneider EM Hug H. Advances in recombinant antibody microarrays. Clin Chim Acta 2004; 343: 17-35.

[6] Butler JE, Ni L, Nessler R, *et al.* The physical and functional behaviour of capture antibodies adsorbed on polystyrene. J Immunol Methods 1992; 150: 77-90.

[7] Butler JE. Solid supports in enzyme-linked immunosorbent assay and other solid-phase immunoassays. J Immunol Methods 2000; 22: 4-23.

[8] Davies J, Dawkes AC, Haymes AG, *et al.* A scanning tunnelling microscopy comparison of passive antibody adsorption and biotinylated antibody linkage to streptavidin on microtiter wells. J Immunol Methods 1994; 167: 263-9.

[9] Morrin A, Ngamna O, Killard AJ, *et al.* An amperometric enzyme biosensor fabricated from polyaniline nanoparticles. Electroanalysis 2005; 17: 423-30.

[10] Lee Y, Lee EK, Cho YW, *et al.* ProteoChip: A highly sensitive protein microarray prepared by a novel method of protein immobilization for application of protein-protein interaction studies. Proteomics 2003; 3: 2289-304.

[11] Ahn EH, Kang DK, Chang SI, *et al.* Profiling of differential protein expression in angiogenin-induced HUVECs using antibody-arrayed ProteoChip. Proteomics 2006; 6: 1104-9.

[12] Vega RA, Maspoch D, Shen CK, *et al.* Functional antibody arrays through metal ion-affinity templates. Chem Bio Chem 2006; 7: 1653-7.

[13] Muir BW, Barden MC, Collett SP, *et al.* High-throughput optimization of surfaces for antibody immobilization using metal complexes. Anal Biochem 2007; 363: 97-107.

[14] Kusnezow W, Hoheisel JD. Antibody microarrays: promises and problems. BioTechniques 2002; 33: S14-23.

[15] Hahn HW, Bakry R, Huck CW, *et al.* Current advances in antibody immobilization on different surfaces and beads. Current Proteomics 2008; 5: 115-28.

[16] Kang JH, Choi HJ, Hwang SY, *et al.* Improving immunobinding using oriented immobilization of an oxidized antibody. J Chromatogr A 2007; 1161: 9-14.

[17] Franco EJ, Hofstetter H, Hofstetter O. A comparative evaluation of random and site-specific immobilization techniques for the preparation of antibody-based chiral stationary phases. J Sep Sci 2006; 29: 1458-69.

[18] Ionescu RE, Jaffrezic-Renault N, Bouffier L, *et al.* Impedimetric immunosensor for the specific 'label-free' detection of ciprofloxacin antibiotic. Biosens Bioelectron 2007; 23: 549-5.

[19] Neves-Petersen MT, Snabe T, Klitgaard S, *et al.* Photonic activation of disulfide bridges achieves oriented protein immobilization on biosensor surfaces. Protein Sci 2006; 15: 343-51.

[20] Kim BY, Swearingen CB, Ho JA, *et al.* Direct immobilization of Fab' in nanocapillaries for manipulating mass-limited samples. J Am Chem Soc 2007; 129: 7620-6.

[21] Vikholm-Lundin I, Albers WM. Site-directed immobilisation of antibody fragments for detection of C-reactive protein. Biosens Bioelectron 2006; 21: 1141-8.

[22] Bonroy K, Frederix F, Reekmans G, *et al.* Comparison of random and oriented immobilisation of antibody fragments on mixed self-assembled monolayers. J Immunol Methods 2006; 312: 167-81.

[23] Zaco E, Pividori MI, Alegret S. Electrochemical biosensing based on universal affinity biocomposite platforms. Biosens Bioelectron 2006; 21: 1291-1301.

[24] Shen Z, Yan H, Parl FF, Mernaugh RL, Zeng X. Recombinant antibody piezoimmunosensors for the detection of cytochrome P450 1B1. Anal Chem 2007; 79: 1283-9.

[25] Cho IH, Paek EH, Lee H, *et al.* Site-directed biotinylation of antibodies for controlled immobilization on solid surfaces. Anal Biochem 2007; 365: 14-23.

[26] Boozer C, Ladd J, Chen S, Jiang S. DNA-directed protein immobilization for simultaneous detection of multiple analytes by surface plasmon resonance biosensor. Anal Chem 2006; 78: 1515-9.

[27] Bailey RC, Kwong GA, Radu CG, Witte ON, Heath JR. DNA-encoded antibody libraries: a unified platform for multiplexed cell sorting and detection of genes and proteins. J Am Chem Soc 2007; 129: 1959-67.

[28] Boozer C, Ladd J, Chen S, *et al.* DNA directed protein immobilization on mixed ssDNA/Oligo(ethylene glycol) self-assembled monolayers for sensitive biosensors. Anal Chem 2004; 76: 6967-72.

[29] Danczyk R, Krieder B, North A, *et al.* Comparison of antibody functionality using different immobilization methods. Biotechnol Bioeng 2003; 84: 215-23.

[30] Bilitewski U. Protein-sensing assay formats and devices. Anal Chim Acta 2006; 568: 232-47.

[31] Lee JM, Park HK, Jung Y, *et al.* Direct immobilization of protein G variants with various numbers of cysteine residues on a gold surface. Anal Chem 2007; 79: 2680-7.

[32] Pleschberger M, Saerens D, Weigert S, *et al.* An S-layer heavy chain camel antibody fusion protein for generation of a nanopatterned sensing layer to detect the prostate-specific antigen by surface plasmon resonance technology. Bioconjug Chem 2004; 15: 664-71.

[33] Nanduri V, Bhunia AK, Tu SI, Paoli GC, Brewster JD. SPR biosensor for the detection of *L. monocytogenes* using phage-displayed antibody. Biosens Bioelectron 2007; 23: 248-52.

[34] Shen Z, Mernaugh RL, Yan H, *et al.* Engineered recombinant singlechain fragment variable antibody for immunosensors. Anal Chem 2005; 77: 6834-42.

[35] Steinhauer C, Wingren C, Khan F, *et al.* Improved affinity coupling for antibody microarrays: engineering of double-(His)6-tagged single framework recombinant antibody fragments. Proteomics 2006; 6: 4227-34.

[36] Watanabe H, Tsumoto K, Taguchi S, *et al.* A human antibody fragment with high affinity for biodegradable polymer film. Bioconjug Chem 2007; 18: 645-51.

[37] Hattori T, Umetsu M, Nakanishi T, *et al.*Grafting of material-binding function into antibodies. Functionalization by peptide grafting. Biochem Biophys Res Commun 2008; 365: 751-7.

[38] Lisdat F, Schafer D. The use of electrochemical impedance spectroscopy for biosensing. Anal Bioanal Chem 2008; 391: 1555-67.

[39] Daniels JS, Pourmand N. Label-free impedance biosensors: opportunities and challenges. Electroanalysis 2007; 19: 1239-57.

[40] Marco MP, Barcelo D. Environmental applications of analytical biosensors. Meas Sci Technol 1996; 7: 1547-62.

[41] Purvis D, Leonardova O, Farmakovsky D, Cherkasov V. An ultrasensitive and stable potentiometric immunosensor. Biosens Bioelectron 2003; 18: 1385-90.

[42] O'Connor M, Kim SN, Killard AJ, *et al.* Mediated amperometric immunosensing using single walled carbon nanotube forests. Analyst 2004; 129: 1176-80.

[43] Thomas JH, Kim SK, Hesketh PJ, Halsall HB, Heineman WR. Microbead-based electrochemical immunoassay with interdigitated array electrodes. Anal Biochem 2004; 328: 113-22.

[44] Darain F, Park D-S, Park J-S, Shim Y-B. Development of an immunosensor for the detection of vitellogenin using impedance spectroscopy. Biosens Bioelectron 2004; 19: 1245-52.

[45] Tully E, Higson SP, O'Kennedy R. The development of a 'label-less' immunosensor for the detection of *Listeria monocytogenes* cell surface protein, Internalin B. Biosens Bioelectron 2008; 23: 906-12.

[46] Chen X, Wang Y, Zhou J, *et al.* Electrochemical impedance immunosensor based on three-dimensionally ordered macroporous gold film. Anal Chem 2008; 80: 2133-40.

[47] Li C-Z, Liu Y, Luong JHT. Impedance sensing of DNA-binding drugs using gold substrates modified with gold nanoparticles. Anal Chem 2005; 77: 478-85.

[48] Dharuman V, Grunwald I, Nebling E, *et al.* Label-free impedance detection of oligonucleotide hybridisation on interdigitated ultramicroelectrodes using electrochemical redox probes. Biosens Bioelectron 2005; 21: 645-54.

[49] La Belle JT, Gerlach JQ, Svarovsky S, Joshi L. Label-free impedimetric detection of glycan-lectin interactions. Anal Chem 2007; 79: 6959-64.

[50] Du Y, Li BL, Wei H, Wang YL, Wang EK. Multifunctional label-free electrochemical biosensor based on an integrated aptamer. Anal Chem 2008; 80: 5110-7.

[51] Evans D, Johnson S, Laurenson S, *et al.* Electrical protein detection in cell lysates using high-density peptide-aptamer microarrays. J Biol 2008; 7: 3.1-11.

[52] Yu X, Xu D, Lv R, Liu Z. An impedance biosensor array for label-free detection of multiple antigen-antibody reactions. Front Biosci 2006; 11: 983-90.

[53] Shipway AN, Lahav M, Willner I. Nanostructured gold colloid electrodes. Adv Mater 2000; 12: 993-8.

[54] Dequaire M, Degrand C, Limoges B. An electrochemical metalloimmunoassay based on a colloidal gold label. Anal Chem 2000; 72: 5521-8.

[55] Wang J, Liu G, Munge B, Lin L, Zhu Q. DNA-based amplified bioelectronic detection and coding of proteins. Angew Chem Int Ed 2004; 43: 2158-61.

[56] Wang J, Liu G, Jan MR. Ultrasensitive electrical biosensing of proteins and DNA: carbon-nanotube-derived amplification of the recognition and transduction events. J Am Chem Soc 2004; 126: 3010-11.

[57] Yu X, Munge B, Patel V, *et al.* Carbon nanotube amplification strategies for highly sensitive immunodetection of cancer biomarkers. J Am Chem Soc 2006; 128: 11199-11205.

[58] Das J, Abdul Aziz M, Yang H. A nanocatalyst-based assay for proteins: DNA-free ultrasensitive electrochemical detection using catalytic reduction of *p*-nitrophenol by gold-nanoparticle labels. J Am Chem Soc 2006; 128: 16022-3.

[59] Das J, Jo K, Lee JW, Yang H. Electrochemical immunosensor using *p*-aminophenol redox cycling by hydrazine combined with a low background current. Anal Chem 2007; 79: 2790-6.

[60] Shiddiky MJA, Aminur Rahman M, ShimY-B. Hydrazine-catalyzed ultrasensitive detection of DNA and proteins. Anal Chem 2007; 79: 6886-90.

[61] Ko YJ, Maeng JH, Ahn Y, *et al.* Microchip-based multiplex electro-immunosensing system for the detection of cancer biomarkers. Electrophoresis 2008; 29: 3466-76.

[62] Lin YY, Wang J, Liu G, Wu H, Wai CM, Lin Y. A nanoparticle label/immunochromatographic electrochemical biosensor for rapid and sensitive detection of prostate-specific antigen. Biosens Bioelectron 2008; 23: 1659-65.

[63] Rusling JF, Sotzing G, Papadimitrakopoulos F. Designing nanomaterial-enhanced electrochemical immunosensors for cancer biomarker proteins. Bioelectrochemistry 2009; 76: 189-94.

[64] Yu X, Munge B, Patel V, *et al.* Carbon nanotube amplification strategies for highly sensitive immunodetection of cancer biomarkers. J Am Chem Soc 2006; 128: 11199-205.

[65] Wang J, Liu G, Jan MR. Ultrasensitive electrical biosensing of proteins and DNA: carbon-nanotube derived amplification of the recognition and transduction events. J Am Chem Soc 2004; 126: 3010-11.

[66] Wang JX, Li MX, Shi ZJ, Li NQ, Gu ZN. Direct electrochemistry of cytochrome c at a glassy carbon electrode modified with single-wall carbon nanotubes. Anal Chem 2002; 74: 1993-7.

[67] Lin YY, Wang J, Liu G, *et al.* A nanoparticle label/immunochromatographic electrochemical biosensor for rapid and sensitive detection of prostate-specific antigen. Biosens Bioelectron 2008; 23: 1659-65.

[68] Kim SN, Rusling JF, Papadimitrakopoulos F. Carbon nanotubes for electronic and electrochemical detection of biomolecules. Adv Mater 2007; 19: 3214-28.

[69] Chen RJ, Bangsaruntip S, Drouvalakis KA, *et al.* Noncovalent functionalization of carbon nanotubes for highly specific electronic biosensors. Proc Natl Acad Sci (USA) 2003; 100: 4984-9.

[70] Star A, Tu E, Niemann J, *et al.* Label-free detection of DNA hybridization using carbon nanotube network field-effect transistors. Proc Natl Acad Sci (USA) 2006; 103: 921-6.

[71] Zheng G, Patolsky F, Cui Y, Wang WU, Lieber CM. Multiplexed electrical detection of cancer markers with nanowire sensor arrays. Nature Biotechnol 2005; 23: 1294-301.

[72] Stokes P, Khondaker SI. Local-gated single-walled carbon nanotube field effect transistors assembled by AC dielectrophoresis. Nanotech 2008; 19: 175202/1-4.

[73] Rusling JF, Zhang Z. Designing Functional Biomolecular Films on Electrodes, Vol 111, New York: Marcel Dekker 2003.

[74] Lu F, Gu L, Meziani MJ, *et al.* Advances in bioapplications of carbon nanotubes. Adv Mater 2009; 21: 139-52

[75] Maehashi K, Katsura T, Kerman K, *et al.* Label-free protein biosensor based on aptamer-modified carbon nanotube field-effect transistors. Anal Chem 2007; 79: 782-7.

[76] Li C, Currelli M, Lin H, *et al.* Complementary detection of prostate-specific antigen using In_2O_3 nanowires and carbon nanotubes. J Am Chem Soc 2005; 127: 484-5.

[77] Byon HR, Choi HC. Network single-walled carbon nanotube-field effect transistors (SWNT-FETs) with increased schottky contact area for highly sensitive biosensor applications. J Am Chem Soc 2006; 128: 2188-9.

[78] Luff BJ, Wilkinson JS, Piehler J, *et al.* Integrated optical Mach-Zehnder biosensor. J Lightwave Technol 1998; 16: 583-92.

[79] Kim N, Park IS, Kim WY. Salmonella detection with a direct-binding optical grating coupler immunosensor. Sens Actuators B 2007; 121: 606-15.

[80] Shankaran DR, Gobi KV, Miura N. Recent advancements in surface plasmon resonance immunosensors for detection of small molecules of biomedical, food and environmental interest. Sens Actuators B 2007; 121: 1-30.

[81] Gutiérrez-Gallego R, Bosch J, Such-Sanmartín G, Segura J. Surface plasmon resonance immunoassays - a perspective. Growth Horm IGF Res 2009; 19: 388-98.

[82] Wood RW. Philos. Mag. 1902; 4: 396-402.

[83] Maier, S.A. Maier, Plasmonics: Fundamentals and Applications (1st ed.). New York: Springer 2007.

[84] Zhang LM, Uttamchandani D. Optical chemical sensing employing surface plasmon resonance. Electron Lett 1988; 24: 1469-70.

[85] Guidi A, Laricchia-Robbio L, Gianfaldoni D, Revoltella R, Del Bono G. Comparison of a conventional immunoassay (ELISA) with a surface plasmon resonance-based biosensor for IGF-1 detection in cows' milk. Biosens Bioelectron 2001; 16: 971-7.

[86] Teramura Y, Iwata H. Label-free immunosensing for α-fetoprotein in human plasma using surface plasmon resonance. Anal Biochem 2007; 365: 201-7.

[87] Wear MA, Patterson A, Malone K, *et al.* A surface plasmon resonance-based assay for small molecule inhibitors of human cyclophilin A. Anal Biochem 2005; 345:214-26.

[88] Jung SH, Jung JW, Suh IB, *et al.* Analysis of C-reactive protein on amide-linked N-hydroxysuccinimide - Dextran arrays with a spectral surface plasmon resonance biosensor for serodiagnosis. Anal Chem 2007; 79: 5703-10.

[89] Byrne B, Stack E, Gilmartin, O'Kennedy RJ. Antibody-based sensors: principles, problems and potential for detection of pathogens and associated toxins. Sensors 2009; 9: 4407-45.

[90] Kuroda Y, Saito M, Sakai H, Yamaoka T. Rapid characterization of drug-drug interaction in plasma protein binding using a surface plasmon resonance biosensor. Drug Metab Pharmacokinet 2008; 23: 120-7.

[91] Myszka DG, Rich RL. Implementing surface plasmon resonance biosensors in drug discovery. Pharm Science Technol Today 2000; 3: 310-07.

[92] Piervincenzi RT, Reichert WM, Hellinga HW. Genetic engineering of a single-chain antibody fragment for surface immobilisation in an optical biosensor. Biosens Bioelectron 1998; 13: 305-12.

[93] Schuderer J, Akkoyun A, Brandenburg A, Bilitewski U, Wagner E. Development of a multichannel fluorescence affinity sensor system. Anal Chem 2000; 72: 3942-8.

[94] Schult K, Katerkamp A, Trau D, *et al.* Disposable optical sensor chip for medical diagnostics: new ways in bioanalysis. Anal Chem 1999; 71: 5430-5.

[95] Tschmelak J, Kappel N, Gauglitz G. TIRF-based biosensor for sensitive detection of progesterone in milk based on ultra-sensitive progesterone detection in water. Anal Bioanal Chem 2005; 382: 1895-1903.

[96] Kappel ND, Proll F, Gauglitz G. Development of a TIRF-based biosensor for sensitive detection of progesterone in bovine milk. Biosensens and Bioelectron 2007; 22: 2295-300.

[97] Albrecht C, Kaeppel N, Gauglitz G. Two immunoassay formats for fully automated CRP detection in human serum. Anal Bioanal Chem 2008; 391: 1845-52.

[98] Long F, He M, Zhu AN, Shi HC. Portable optical immunosensor for highly sensitive detection of microcystin-LR in water samples. Biosens Bioelectron 2009; 24: 2346-51.

[99] Thompson VS, Maragos CM. Fiber-optic immunosensor for the detection of fumonisin B1. J Agric Food Chem 1996; 44: 1041-6.

[100] Maragos CM., Thompson VS. Fiber-optic immunosensor for mycotoxins. Nat. Toxins 1999; 7: 371-6.

[101] Deacon JK, Thomson AM, Page AL, *et al.* An assay for human chorionic gonadotropin using the capillary fill immunosensor. Biosens Bioelectron 1991; 6: 193-9.

[102] Robin GA, Attridge JW, Deacon JK, Whiteley SC. The fluorescent capillary fill device. Sens Actuators B Chem 1993; 11: 235-8.

[103] Robinson GA. Optical immunosensing systems meeting the market needs. Biosens Bioelectron 1991; 6: 183-91.

[104] Petrou PS, Kakabakos SE, Christofidis I, Argitis P, Misiakos K. Multi-analyte capillary immunosensor for the determination of hormones in human serum samples. Biosens Bioelectron 2002; 17: 261-8.

[105] Rowe-Taitt CA, Hazzard JW, Hoffman KE, *et al.* Simultaneous detection of six biohazardous agents using a planar waveguide array biosensor. Biosens Bioelectron 2000; 15: 579-89.

[106] Smith DS, Eremin SA. Fluorescence polarization immunoassays and related methods for simple, high-throughput screening of small molecules. Anal Bioanal Chem 2008; 391: 1499-507.

[107] Gachok IV, Bondarenko AP, De Saeger S, *et al.* Multi-detection of mycotoxins by fluorescence polarization immunoassay. Toxicol Lett 2008; 180: S28.

[108] Wang Z, Zhang S, Ding S, Eremin SA, Shen J. Simultaneous determination of sulphamerazine, sulphamethazine and sulphadiazine in honey and chicken muscle by a new monoclonal antibody-based fluorescence polarisation immunoassay. Food Addit Contam Part A Chem Anal Control Expo Risk Assess 2008; 25: 574-82.

[109] Baeyens WRG, Schulman SG, Calokerinos AC, *et al.* Chemiluminescence-based detection: principles and analyticalapplications in flowing streams and in immunoassays. J Pharm Biomed Anal 1998; 17, 941.

[110] Liebes Y, Amir L, Marks RS, Banai M. Chemiluminescent optical fiber immunosensor detection of *Brucella* cells presenting smooth-A antigen. Sens Actuators B 2009; 140: 568-76.

[111] Salama O, Herrmann S, Tziknovsky A, *et al.* Chemiluminescent optical fiber immunosensor for detection of autoantibodies to ovarian and breast cancer-associated antigens. Biosens Bioelectron 2007; 22: 1508-16.

[112] Jorge PAS, Martins MA, Trindade T, Santos JL, Fahari F. Optical fiber sensing using quantum dots. Sensors 2007; 7: 3489-3534.

[113] Bruchez M, Moronne M, Gin P, Weiss S, Alivisatos AP. Semiconductor nanocrystals as fluorescent biological labels. Science 1998; 281: 2013-6.

[114] Kerman K, Endo T, Tsukamoto M, *et al.* Quantum dot-based immunosensor for the detection of prostate-specific antigen using fluorescence microscopy. Talanta 2007; 71: 1494-9.

[115] Sauerbrey G. Verwendung von Schwingquarzen zur Wägung dünner Schichten und zur Mikrowägung. Zeitschrift für Physik A Hadrons and Nuclei, Springer Berlin/Heidelberg. 1959; 155: 206-222.

[116] Lin Z, Yip CM, Joseph IS, Ward MD. Operation of an ultrasensitive 30-MHz quartz crystal microbalance in liquids. Anal Chem 1993; 65: 1546-51.

[117] Lee BS, Lee JN, Park JM, *et al.* A fully automated immunoassay from whole blood on a disc. Lab Chip 2009; 9: 1548-55.

[118] Shons A, Dorman F, Najarian J. An immunospecific microbalance. J Biomed Mater Res 1972; 6: 565-70.

[119] Kim N, Kim DK, Cho YJ. Gold nanoparticle-based signal augmentation of quartz crystal microbalance immunosensor measuring C-reactive protein. Current Applied Physics, In Press, Accepted Manuscript, Available online 21 February 2010.

[120] Kim N, Kim DK, Cho YJ. Development of indirect-competitive quartz crystal microbalance immunosensor for C-reactive protein. Sens Actuators B 2009; 143: 444-8.

[121] Lee HJ, Namkoong K, Cho EC, *et al.* Surface acoustic wave immunosensor for real-time detection of hepatitis B surface antibodies in whole blood samples. Biosensens Bioelectron 2009; 24: 3120-5.

[122] Lavrik NV, Sepaniak MJ, Datskos PG. Cantilever transducers as a platform for chemical and biological sensors. Rev Sci Instrum 2004; 75: 2229-53.

[123] Ilic B, Czaplewski D, Zalalutdinov M, *et al.* Single cell detection with micromechanical oscillators. J Vac Sci Technol B 2001; 19: 2825-8.

[124] Alvarez M, Calle A, Tamayo J, *et al.* Development of nanomechanical biosensors for detection of the pesticide DDT. Biosens Bioelectron 2003; 18: 649-53.

[125] Raiteri R, Grattarola M, Butt HJ, Skladal P. Micromechanical cantilever-based biosensors. Sens Actuators B 2001; 79: 115-126.

[126] Wu GH, Datar RH, Hansen KM, Thundat T, Cote RJ, Majumdar A. Bioassay of prostate-specific antigen (PSA) using microcantilevers. Nature Biotechnol 2001; 19: 856-60.

[127] Yue M, Stachowiak JC, Lim H, Datar R, Cote R, Majumdar A. Label-free protein recognition two-dimensional array using nanomechanical sensors. Nano Lett 2008; 8: 520-4.

[128] Lee JH, Hwang KS, Park J, Yoon KH, Yoon DS, Kim TS. Immunoassay of prostate-specific antigen (PSA) using resonant frequency shift of piezoelectric nanomechanical microcantilever. Biosens Bioelectron 2005; 20: 2157-62.

[129] Ivanov T, Gotszalk T, Grabiec P, Tomerov E, Rangelow IW. Thermally driven micromechanical beam with piezoresistive deflection readout. Microelectron Eng 2003; 67-68: 550-6.

[130] Lee JH, Hwang KS, Park J, Yoon KH, Yoon DS, Kim TS. Immunoassay of prostatespecific antigen (PSA) using resonant frequency shift of piezoelectric nanomechanical microcantilever. Biosens Bioelectron 2005; 20: 2157-62.

[131] Dutta P, Tipple CA, Lavrik NV, *et al.* Enantioselective sensors based on antibody-mediated nanomechanics. Anal Chem2003; 75: 2342-2348.

[132] Knight HJ. I shrunk the lab. Nature 2002; 418: 474-5.

[133] Diercks AH, Ozinsky A, Hansen CL, Spotts JM, Rodriguez DJ, Aderem A. A microfluidic device for multiplexed protein detection in nano-liter volumes. Anal Biochem 2009; 386: 30-5.

[134] Bange A, Halsall HB, Heineman WR. Microfluidic immunosensor systems. Biosens Bioelectron 2005; 20: 2488-2503.

[135] Fu AY, Chou HP, Spence C, Arnold FH, Quake SR. An integrated microfabricated cell sorter. Anal Chem 2002; 74: 2451-7.

[136] Thorsen T, Maerkl SJ, Quake SR. Microfluidic Large Scale Integration. Science 2002; 298: 580-4.

[137] Schift H, David C, Gabriel M, *et al.* Nanoreplication in polymers using hot embossing and injection molding. Microelec Eng 2000; 53: 171-4.

[138] Tang D, Yuan R, Chai Y. Magnetic control of an electrochemical microfluidic device with an arrayed immunosensor for simultaneous multiple immunoassays. Clin Chem 2007; 53: 1323-9.

[139] Butler JE, Ni L, Nessler R, *et al.* The physical and functional behavior of capture antibodies adsorbed on polystyrene. J Immunol Methods 1992; 150: 77-90.

[140] Davies J, Dawkes AC, Haymes AGR, *et al.* A scanning tunnelling microscopy comparison of passive antibody adsorption and biotinylated antibody linkage to streptavidin on microtiter wells. J Immunol Methods 1994; 167: 263-9.

[141] Butler JE. Solid supports in enzyme-linked immunosorbent assay and other solid-phase immunoassays. Methods Mol Med 2004; 94: 333-72.

[142] Makamba H, Kim JH, Lim K, Park N, Hahn JH. Surface modification of poly(dimethylsiloxane) microchannels. Electrophoresis 2003; 24: 3607-19.

[143] Talapatra A, Rouse R, Hardiman G. Protein microarrays: challenges and promises. Pharmacogenomics 2002; 3: 527-36.

[144] Seurynck-Servoss SL, Baird CL, Rodland, KD, Zangar RC. Surface chemistries for antibody microarrays. Front Biosci 2007; 12: 3956-64.

[145] Wen X, He H, Lee LJ. Specific antibody immobilization with biotin-poly(L-lysine)-g-poly(ethylene glycol) and protein A on microfluidic chips. J Immunol Methods 2009; 350: 97-105.

[146] Martinez NA, Schneider RJ, Messina GA, Raba J. Modified paramagnetic beads in a microfluidic system for the determination of ethinylestradiol (EE2) in river water samples. Biosens Bioelectron 2010; 25: 1376-81.

[147] Lee YF, Lien KY, Lei HY, Lee GB. An integrated microfluidic system for rapid diagnosis of dengue virus infection. Biosens and Bioelectron 2009; 25: 745-52.

[148] Gao X, Jiang L, Su X, Qin J, Lin B. Microfluidics and miniaturization microvalves actuated sandwich immunoassay on an integrated microfluidic system. Microfluidics and miniaturisation 2009; 30: 2481-87.

[149] Luo Y, Qin JH, Lin BC. Methods for pumping fluids on biomedical lab-on-a-chip. Front Biosci 2009; 14: 3913-24.

[150] Honda N. Simultaneous multiple immunoassays in a compact disc-shaped microfluidic device based on centrifugal force. Clinical Chemistry 2005; 51: 1955-61.

[151] Lee BS, Lee JN, Park JM, *et al.* A fully automated immunoassay from whole blood on a disc. Lab Chip 2009; 9: 1548-55.

[152] Nashida N, Satoh W, Fukuda J, Suzuki H. Electrochemical immunoassay on a microfluidic device with sequential injection and flushing functions. Biosens Bioelectron. 2007; 22: 3167-73.

[153] Gao X, Jiang L, Su X, Qin J, Lin B. Microvalves actuated sandwich immunoassay on an integrated microfluidic system. Electrophoresis. 2009; 30: 2481-7.

[154] Lai S, Wang S, Luo J, Lee LJ, Yang ST, Madou MJ. Design of a compact disk-like microfluidic platform for enzyme-linked immunosorbent assay. Anal Chem 2004; 76: 1832-7.

[155] Arévalo FJ, Messina GA, Molina PG, Zón MA, Raba J, Fernández H. Determination of progesterone (P4) from bovine serum samples using a microfluidic immunosensor system. Talanta 2010; 80: 1986-92.

[156] Bunyakul N, Edwards KA, Promptmas C, Baeumner AJ. Cholera toxin subunit B detection in microfluidic devices. Anal Bioanal Chem 2009; 393: 177-86,

[157] Kurita R, Yokota Y, Sato Y, Mizutani F, Niwa O. On-chip enzyme immunoassay of a cardiac marker using a microfluidic device combined with a portable surface plasmon resonance system. Anal Chem 2006; 78: 5525-31.

[158] Luo YQ, Yu F, Zare RN. Microfluidic device for immunoassays based on surface plasmon resonance imaging. Lab Chip 2008; 8: 694-700.

[159] Bhattacharyya A, Klapperich CM. Design and testing of a disposable microfluidic chemiluminescent immunoassay for disease biomarkers in human serum samples. Biomed Microdevices 2007;9: 245-51.

[160] Heinze BC, Song JY, Lee CH, Najam A, Yoon JY. Microfluidic immunosensor for rapid and sensitive detection of bovine viral diarrhea virus. Sens Actuators B Chem 2009; 138: 491-496.

[161] Messina GA, Panini NV, Martinez NA, Raba J. Microfluidic immunosensor design for the quantification of interleukin-6 in human serum samples. Anal Biochem 2008; 380: 262-7.

[162] Dequaire M, Degrand C, Limoges B. An electrochemical metalloimmunoassay based on a colloidal gold label. Anal Chem 2000; 72: 5521-8.

[163] Wang J, Liu G, Munge B, Lin L, Zhu Q. DNA-based amplified bioelectronic detection and coding of proteins. Angew Chem Int Ed 2004; 43: 2158-61.

[164] Wang J, Liu G, Jan MR. Ultrasensitive electrical biosensing of proteins and DNA: carbon-nanotube-derived amplification of the recognition and transduction events. J Am Chem Soc 2004; 126: 3010-11.

[165] Yu X, Munge B, Patel V, *et al.* carbon nanotube amplification strategies for highly sensitive immunodetection of cancer biomarkers. J Am Chem Soc 2006; 128: 11199-11205.

[166] Das J, Abdul Aziz M, Yang H. A nanocatalyst-based assay for proteins: DNA-free ultrasensitive electrochemical detection using catalytic reduction of *p*-nitrophenol by gold-nanoparticle labels. J Am Chem Soc 2006; 128: 16022-3.

[167] Das J, Jo K, Lee JW, Yang H. Electrochemical immunosensor using *p*-aminophenol redox cycling by hydrazine combined with a low background current. Anal Chem 2007; 79: 2790-6.

[168] Shiddiky MJA, Aminur Rahman M, ShimY-B. Hydrazine-catalyzed ultrasensitive detection of DNA and proteins. Anal Chem 2007; 79: 6886-90.

CHAPTER 13

Immunoelectrochemistry for the Detection of Clinical Biomarkers

Sonia Centi[a,*] and Marco Mascini[b]

[a]Università degli Studi di Firenze, Dipartimento di Fisiopatologia Clinica, Viale G. Pieraccini, 6 - 50139 Firenze and [b]Università degli Studi di Firenze, Dipartimento di Chimica, Polo Scientifico, via della Lastruccia 3, 50019 Sesto Fiorentino, Firenze, Italy

Abstract: Immunoassays are based on the molecular recognition occurring between an antigen and its antibody. They can be set up in a variety of formats (sandwich or competitive assays). The main differences between them are the immobilised species (antibody or target analyte), the number of experimental steps involved, and in which order the different reagents are exposed to the surface. The choice of the format depends on the molecular size of the analyte, the availability of reagents and the cost. Radioimmunoassays (RIA), fluorescence immunoassays (FIA) and enzyme immunoassays (EIA) are well established in clinical diagnostics. For the development of hand held devices which can be used for point of care measurements, electrochemical immunoassays are optimal alternative to existing immunochemical tests.

In this chapter, the current status of research in electrochemical immunoassays is considered. Primary attention was focused on label-free and enzyme-labelled immunosensors, and the analytical performance of these devices are discussed. Moreover, the use of magnetic beads as new materials for immunoassays coupled with electrochemical transduction is also described. Examples of such devices used for the detection of some biomarkers in clinical analysis are reported.

Keywords: Antibodies, Immunoelectrochemical Sensors, Biomarkers.

1. INTRODUCTION

Immunoassay based on the detection of antibody-antigen interaction is one of the most important analytical techniques, with many applications in clinical diagnosis and in experimental laboratories, since it enables the specific detection of small amounts of target molecules in biological samples [1, 2].

Immunoassays are based on the reaction of an analyte or antigen (Ag) with a selective antibody (Ab) to give a product (Ag-Ab) to detect. The reagents are in a state of equilibrium which is characterised by the law of mass action [3].

In recent years, together with or in place of antibodies, other ligands such as aptamers or peptides are more and more used [4-7]. They are ligands able to bind selectively to low-molecular weight molecules or to macromolecules. The interest in such molecules as ligands is related to their ease of preparation and to the fact that they don't need to use animals for their production. Both aptamers and peptides are produced by chemical synthesis and purified to a very high degree by eliminating the batch-to-batch variation found when using antibodies and, by chemical synthesis, modifications can be introduced enhancing the stability, affinity and specificity of the molecules.

Many types of technical labels have been used in immunoassays, including radioactivity, enzymes, fluorescence, luminescence and phosphorescence [8-13]. Each of these labels has advantages, but the most common label for clinical, food and environmental analysis is the use of enzymes and colorimetric substrates [14-16].

Nevertheless, electrochemical methods are increasingly applied to immunoassays [17-20]. Electrochemical

*Address correspondence to Sonia Centi: Università degli Studi di Firenze, Dipartimento di Fisiopatologia Clinica, Viale G. Pieraccini, 6 - 50139 Firenze; E-mail: Sonia.Centi@unifi.it

Eline P. Meulenberg (Ed)

detection in immunoassay overcomes problems associated with other modes of detection [21]. For example, the short half-life of radioactive reagents, concerns of health hazards, while limited sensitivity in the analysis of coloured or turbid samples is achieved in immunoassays coupled with optical detection. In this case, electrochemical immunoassays offer a fast, simple, and cheap detection method that is free of these problems.

In this context immunosensors, which are a particular family of biosensors, give the possibility of direct monitoring of immunoreactions, providing opportunity to gain new insight into antigen-antibody reaction kinetics and to develop rapid assay devices having wide applications [22]. Similar to conventional immunoassays, these devices are based on the principles of solid-phase immunoassay, with either antibody or antigen immobilised at the sensor surface. An extensive range of analytes can be detected and measured by immunosensors [23, 24].

2. CONVENTIONAL IMMUNOASSAYS

Immunoassays are based on the specific antibody-antigen interaction measured by the affinity constant which is a quantitative measurement of the affinity between the two reagents and range from 10^6-10^{12} M^{-1}. Generally, antibodies with affinity constants of 10^8 M^{-1} are used in immunoassays [25].

Immunoassays can be used to determinate either antibody or antigen concentration. To monitor the interaction, one of the species is conjugated with one the many available labels. In general, in an immunoassay, one of the reaction partners, antibody or antigen, is bound to a surface and the binding of the second immunoreagent is detected by measuring the concentration of the attached label. Various assay formats are used for different applications and are briefly discussed in the following section..

Immunoassays can be catalogued in these categories:

1. Enzyme immunoassay (EIA). Enzyme-Linked Immunosorbent Assays (ELISAs) are the most commonly used format for analysis. The factors, that have contributed to the success of this format, are the speed, sensitivity, selectivity and the no use of radioactive materials.

2. Radioimmunoassay (RIA).

3. Fluorescent immunoassay (FIA).

Immunoassays are well established in many fields of analytical interest for screening purposes or accurate results: in fact they are cheap, sensitive and allow many simultaneous analyses.

3. IMMUNOASSAY FORMATS

Immunoassays can be set up in a variety of formats and the most important are competition and sandwich formats. The main difference between the two formats is the immobilised species, such as antibody, antigen or hapten conjugate, the number of layers used. The decision which of the formats is used for a particular analytical problem is influenced by the nature of the analyte, the cost and availability of antigen and antibody and required sensitivity.

The sandwich assay is used when the molecular target has multiple epitopes, that is able to bind more than one antibody simultaneously; this is possible when the epitopes are sufficiently well spatially separated. This means that a large antigen is required and small haptens, such as polychlorinated biphenyls (PCBs) or Polycyclic Aromatic Hydrocarbons (PAHs), cannot be detected by sandwich assays.

In a direct sandwich assay, a first antibody (called capture antibody) is immobilised on the solid phase, then the antigen (analyte) is added. The solid phase is washed to remove the unreacted reagents and then incubated with a labelled detection antibody, able to react with another epitope. After the washing step, the amount of detection antibody bound to solid phase is detected. Fig. **1** shows a schematic representation of a sandwich assay.

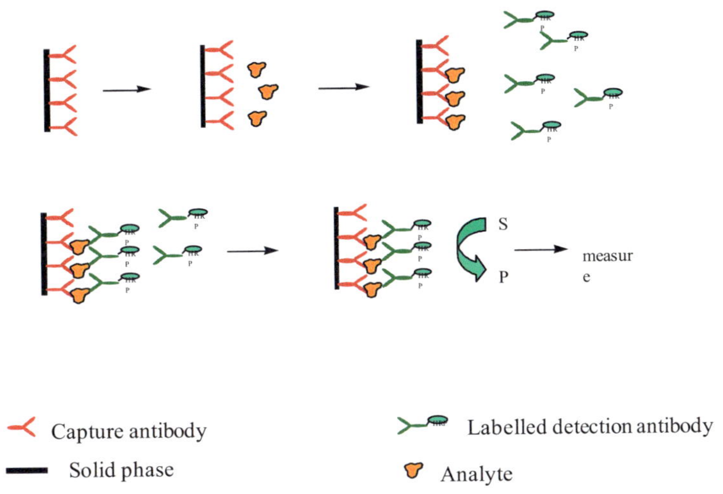

Figure 1: Sandwich assay scheme.

A competitive assay is generally used when the target analyte has only one epitope and involves a competition reaction between two reagents for a third one.

In a indirect competitive assay, the solid phase is modified by the immobilisation of a spacer-linked antigen and the labelled antibody and the free antigen (analyte) are added. The free antigen and that bound to the solid phase compete for the antibody binding sites. The extent of the affinity reaction is detected by adding a secondary-labelled antibody able to bind the first one, as showed in (Fig. **2**). When the concentration of the labelled antibody is kept constant, an increasing analyte concentration occupies more and more binding sites. This means that less labelled antibody can bind to the surface bound antigen. Increasing analyte concentrations cause decreasing signals.

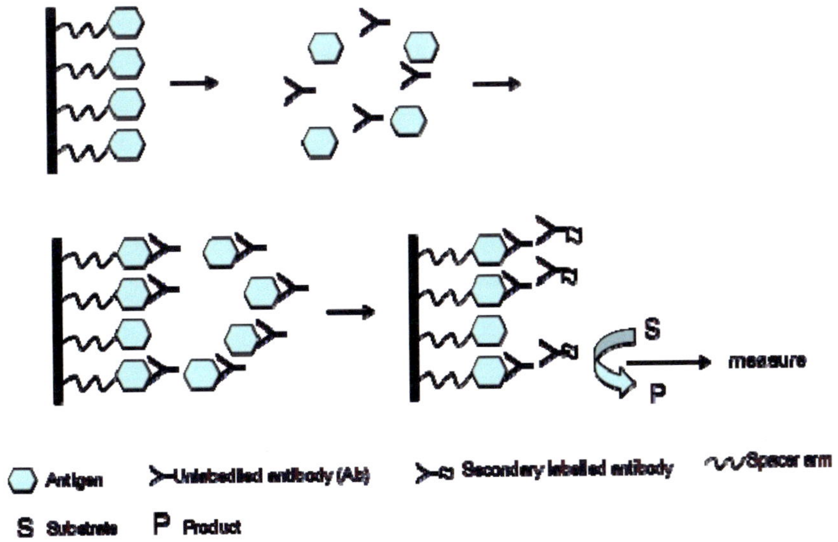

Figure 2: Scheme of an indirect competitive immunoassay.

In a direct competitive assay (Fig. **3**) the solid phase is modified by immobilisation of the specific antibody and free and labelled antigen are added. The concentration of the labelled antigen is kept costant. Free antigen is added in a dilution series or as an unknown sample. Free and labelled antigen molecules compete for the binding site of the immobilised antibody. High analyte concentrations occupy most of the binding sites and result in a low signal.

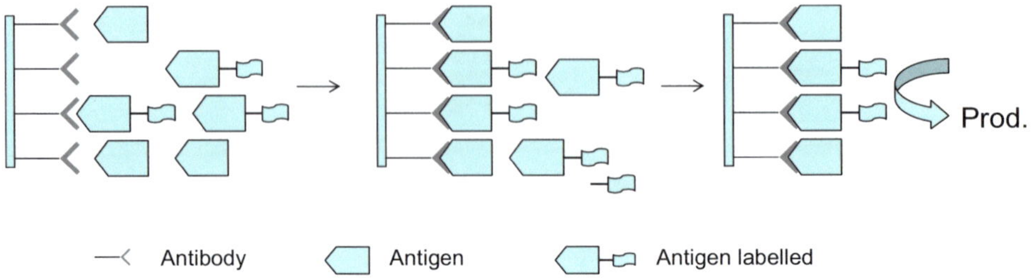

Figure 3: Scheme of direct competitive immunoassay.

4. IMMUNOSENSORS

Immunosensors are affinity biosensors and are defined as analytical devices that detect the binding of an antigen to its specific antibody by coupling the immunochemial reaction to the surface of a device known as a transducer. They have been the subject of increasing interest mainly because of their potential application as an alternative immunoassay technique in areas such as clinical diagnostics [26, 27] environmental and food control [28, 29]. They are miniaturised analytical devices which selectively detect analytes and provide a concentration-dependent signal.

Electrochemical immunosensors, based on the electrochemical detection of immunoreaction, have been widely reported. They employ either antibodies or their complementary binding partners (antigens and haptens) as biorecognition elements coupled with electrochemical transducers (electrodes, field effect transistors), which represent the most developed area in biosensing. Thus, antibodies provide specificity while electrochemical measuring procedures offer high detection sensitivity and low cost of the resulting sensors and instrumentation [30, 31].

Electrochemical transducers can be divided into potentiometric (field-effect transistors and ion-selective electrodes) and amperometric (metal and graphite electrodes) detectors. In the latter mode, current is measured at a constant potential. The widespread use of the above-mentioned immunosensors is due not only to the high sensitivity and selectivity required for immunoassay, but also to the fact that instruments based on these detectors are comparatively inexpensive and small in size.

Electrochemical detection of immunoreactions can be performed both with and without labelling. A frequently used format in electrochemical immunosensing is based on an amperometric detection, in which proteins are labelled with an enzyme producing an electroactive product from an added substrate. Detection without labelling can be also performed, usually by cyclic voltammetry or by impedimetric measurements. These methods are able to detect a change in capacitance and/or resistance of the electrode induced by binding of protein. In the next sections, a more detailed description of new strategies in label-free and labelled immunosensors development is presented.

4.1. Screen-Printed Immunosensors

In recent years, the interest for development of rapid, inexpensive and disposable immunosensors in fields such as clinical, environmental and food analysis is increasing. For this reason screen-printing technology is gaining consideration and importance in analytical chemistry, especially in the field of immunosensing. The most common disposable immunosensors are those produced by thick-film technology. A thick-film biosensor configuration is based on the layers deposition of inks or pastes sequentially onto an insulating support or substrate; the ink is forced through a screen onto a substrate and the open mesh pattern in the screen defines the pattern of the deposited ink. Screen-printing allows the fast mass production of highly reproducible electrodes at low cost for disposable use.

A variety of screen-printed thick-film devices can be fabricated as a base for disposable electrochemical immunosensors, DNA sensors and enzyme electrodes (Fig. **4**).

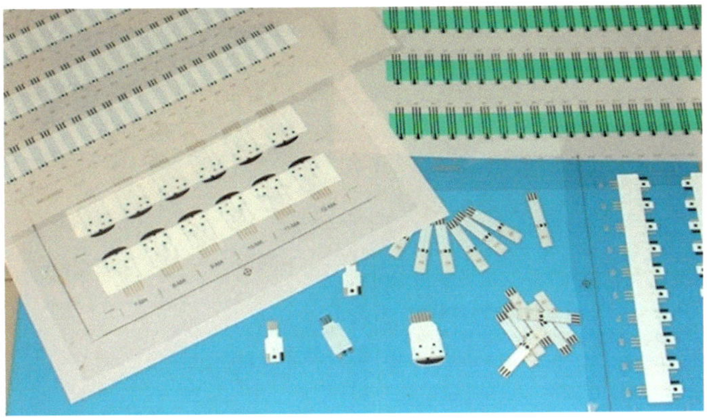

Figure 4: Some screen-printed electrodes.

The most well-known application of screen-printed electrode technology has been in the clinical analysis of blood glucose levels in people with diabetes. Historically, glucose sensing has dominated the biosensor literature and has delivered huge commercial successes to the field. The combination of a fungal enzyme (glucose oxidase) with an electrochemical detector has effectively met the needs of the person with diabetes [32].

5. ELECTROCHEMICAL IMMUNOMAGNETIC SENSORS

Unlike electrochemical immunosensors characterised to have the sensing element in intimate contact with the transducer, the electrochemical immunomagnetic sensors show the sensing element not directly immobilised on the transducer but on a different support.

As described above, electrochemical immunosensors are usually based on the use of a reagent enzyme-labelled that generates an electroactive product which can be detected at the electrode surface using, for example, a voltammetric method. The main advantage of this method is the formation of a relatively high local concentration of the enzyme product, leading to a significant signal amplification. By the way, the use of the electrode surface as solid phase as well as electrochemical transducer can present some problems: a shielding of the surface by bio-specifically bound antibody molecules can cause hindrance in the electron transfer, resulting in a reduced signal from voltammetric analysis and so a loss of sensitivity. Among the different ways that can be used to improve the sensitivity of the system, an interesting approach could involve the screen-printed electrodes use only for the transduction step, whereas the affinity reaction could be performed using another physical support.

The use of magnetic beads as solid phase is another possibility, widely documented in literature [33-36]. The use of such support to perform the immunoassay allows to obtain a high yield of solid phase-antibody binding and of the affinity reaction: in fact the probability that antibodies meet the magnetic beads or the antibody-coated magnetic beads meet the analyte is very high keeping the solution under stirring. After molecular recognition on the magnetic beads, it is possible to build up the immunosensing surface by localizing the immunomagnetic beads on the working electrode area of a screen-printed electrode with the aid of a magnet and perform the electrochemical measurement.

This approach allows to separate the steps relative to the immunoreaction from the step of electrochemical detection and for this reason the working electrode surface is easily accessible by enzymatic product, which diffuse onto bare electrode surface. Using this strategy, finding the optimum conditions for the immunoassay on the magnetic beads and for electrochemical detection on the transducer (carbon screen-printed electrodes) is much easier than in the usual one (electrode) surface systems, because optimum conditions for immunoassay do not conform with those for electrochemical detection and viceversa [36] (Fig. **5**).

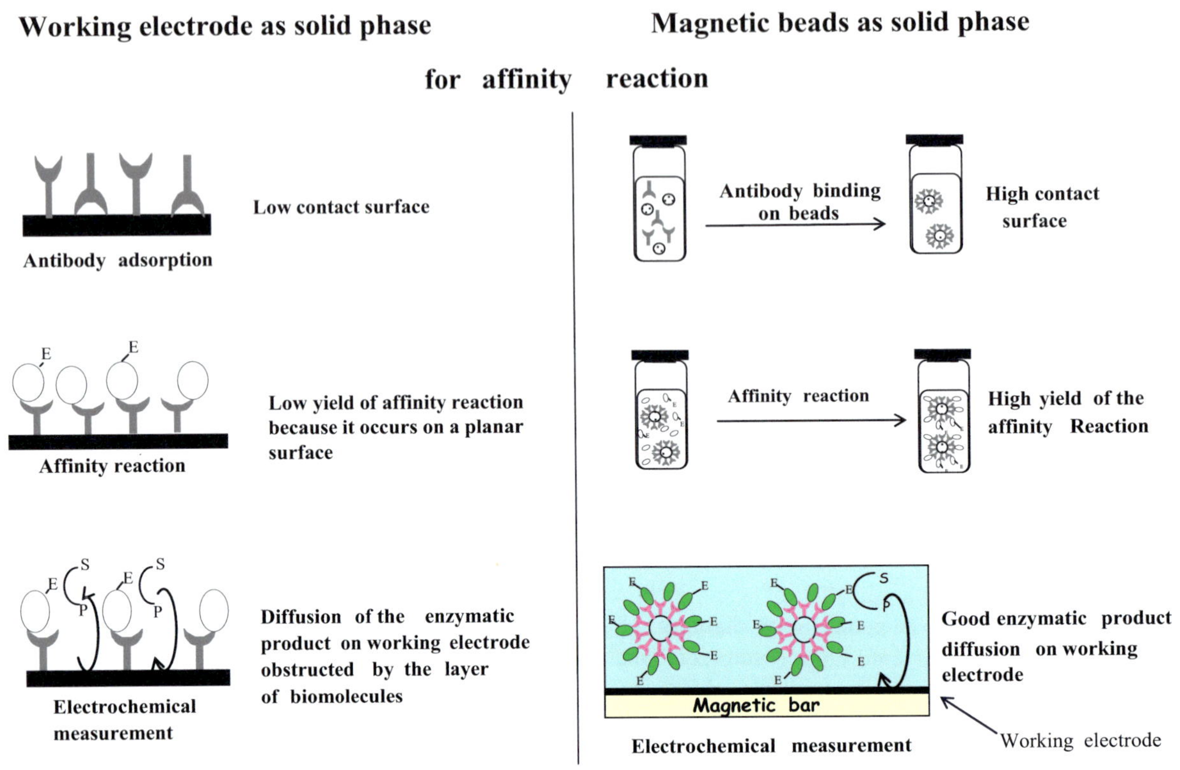

Figure 5: Main advantages related to the use of magnetic beads.

6. LABEL-FREE IMMUNOSENSORS

Label-free immunosensors are very attractive because they allow real-time measurement without any additional hazardous reagents, and in addition the direct detection approach simplifies the sensing protocol. Direct detection without labelling can be performed by potentiometry, amperometry, impedimetry, and also by pulsed amperometric detection [37]. All these methods have been used from long time for electrochemical immunoassays development.

6.1. Potentiometric Immunosensors

After the publication of Janata's work [38] there was a wide interest in potentiometric immunoassays. This work was based on the prerequisite that, since proteins are polyelectrolytes in aqueous solutions and an antibody is a protein, the binding of antibodies to antigens affects the electric charge of the system. Thus, the potential difference between a working electrode with immobilised antibodies and a reference electrode depends on the concentration of free antigens [39]. This approach, based on the use of immunoelectrodes, was rapidly used in the subsequent decades. The design of immunoelectrodes is similar to that of ion-selective electrodes. The detected response may be proportional to the logarithm of the analyte concentration or to the logarithm of the concentration of an immuno-complex. As example, Tang and coworkers [40] developed a novel fabrication method for a potentiometric immunosensor by using a combination of gold nanoparticles, gelatin, and Nafion as immobilisation matrices.

In the first step of this approach, a Nafion membrane was immobilised on a platinum disk electrode surface. This was then removed to parch with infrared light for 20 min. After washing with water, a mix of gold nanoparticles and hepatitis B antibody ($HBsAb_1$) was subsequently deposited onto the functionalised electrode surface, so that $-NH_3^+$ groups on antibody molecules can interact by electrostatic attraction with $-SO_3^-$ groups present on the Nafion membrane. Finally, the modified electrode was dipped into a gelatin solution and quickly removed to be stored at 4 °C for at least 24 h before use. Nanometer-sized gold colloids play an important role, similar to that of a conducting wire or an electron-conducting tunnel, making it easier for electron transfer to take place [40]. The detection of the antigen hepatitis B (HBsAg) was finally performed by potentiometric measurements, based on the change in the potentiometric response before and after the antigen-antibody reaction. Although considered advantageous from the operative point of view, potentiometric methods are still suffering from major problems of sensitivity (which is inferior to that of amperometric transducers) and nonspecific effects of binding or signalling (influences from other ions present in the sample). Especially, the low signal-to-noise ratio, due to interferences coming e. i. from ionic strength variations, causes analytical problems which are difficult to overcome. Thus, a trend away from potentiometric immunosensors has been observed in the last few years [41].

6.2. Amperometric Immunosensors

In amperometric-based immunosensors the detection is based on the change in charge on the electrode surface during the affinity binding reaction [37]. An example of a label-free amperometric immunosensor was reported by He and coworkers [42], who applied it to the detection of carcinoembryonic antigen (CEA). This immunosensor was constructed by immobilising the anti-CEA antibody on a Glassy Carbon Electrode (GCE) modified with a film of gold nanoparticles and with nano-Au/chitosan composite. To prepare it, a porous film of gold nanoparticles (NG) was firstly formed by immersing the GCE into the 100 mg l^{-1} $HAuCl_4$ solution and by applying a constant potential of −0.2 V for 60 s. The modified electrode (NG/GCE) was washed with water. Then, 25 µl of gold nanoparticles/chitosan composite solution was pipetted onto the surface of the NG/GCE. The casting solution was allowed to dry at 4 °C overnight. At this point, the modified electrode (nano-Au/Chit/NG/GCE) was washed with water and then immersed in the anti-CEA solution at 4 °C for 12 h. The resulting electrode was incubated in BSA solution (w/w, 0.25%) about 1 h at 35 °C in order to block possible remaining active sites and avoid the non-specific adsorption. The main steps for construction of the immunosensor are shown in (Fig. **6**).

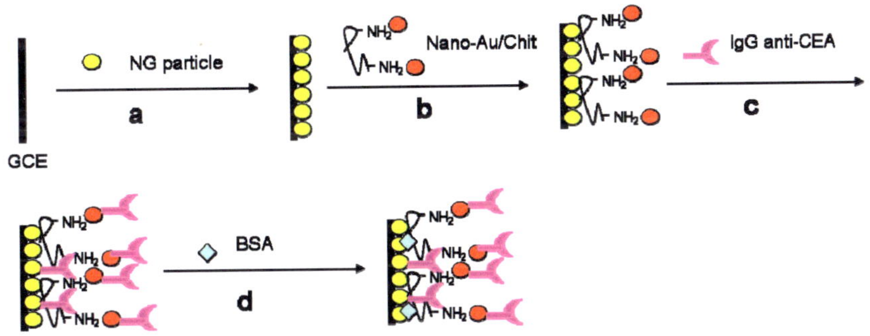

Figure 6: Main steps related to the immunosensor fabrication process: a) formation of porous NG film, b) casting of nano-Au/Chitosan composite, c) adsorption of anti-CEA, d) blocking of non-specific active sites with BSA. From He *et al.*, 2008 [42].

The interaction of the antibody with various concentrations of antigen was detected; measurements were carried out by cyclic voltammetry. The immunosensor showed a high sensitivity (1310 nA/ng/mL) and a good correlation for detection of CEA in the range 0.2-120 ng mL^{-1} with a detection limit of 0.06 ng mL^{-1} estimated at a signal to noise ratio of 3. An additional advantage was the immunosensor regeneration. After completing each assay, the sensor can be immersed in a 4 M urea solution for about 10 min to dissociate the antigen-antibody complex.

6.3. Impedimetric Immunosensors

Impedance Spectroscopy (IS) is a powerful method of analysing the electrical resistance of a system and is sensitive to surface phenomena and changes of bulk properties, for this reason it is a valuable method in electrochemical research [43]. Considering the detection of biorecognition reactions, IS is a valuable tool for characterising surface modifications, such as those that occur during the immobilisation of biomolecules on the transducer surface. The application of Electrochemical Impedance Spectroscopy (EIS) in biorecognition processes has been reported by many authors [44, 45]. In EIS measurements, the electrode impedance is monitored as a function of the frequency of an applied alternative voltage [46]. EIS specifically monitors the current response of an electrochemical system to the application of small amplitude AC signals of varying frequencies. For this reason, the name impedance "spectroscopy" is derived from the fact that the impedance is generally determined at different frequencies rather than just one. A large part of impedance-based immunosensors is based on the antibody modification of a conducting-polymer layer, which coats the surface of an electrode. The interactions between antigens and antibodies result in considerable changes in the capacitive reactance [39].

The construction of impedimetric immunosensors using conducting polymers was investigated in many papers [47-49]. One of the first approaches on that was reported in 1999 by Sargent and Sadik. They investigated the mechanisms of Antibody-Antigen (Ab-Ag) interactions at conducting polypyrrole electrodes using EIS [50]. Anti-Human Serum Albumin (AHSA) antibodies incorporated into a polypyrrole film and its corresponding antigen Human Serum Albumin (HSA) were used to develop a model assay. The binding event between the immobilised antibody and its antigen was characterised by a change in the double layer capacitance and the charge transfer resistance as a function of the frequency. Thus, impedance technique was used for the study of the resistivity variation of the modified electrodes.

An impedimetric immunosensor based on a polypyrrole-modified electrode surface was recently developed [51] and applied to the detection of the antibiotic ciprofloxacin. The antibody anti-ciprofloxacin was covalently bound to an electrogenerated poly(pyrrole-NHS) film. To monitor the interactions between the analyte and its specific immobilised antibody, impedance measurements were recorded between 100 kHz and 50 mHz with an AC amplitude of 10 mV peak to peak with 5 points per decade of frequencies. A bias potential of -1.4 V was applied for biosensor impedance measurements; this value was identified as the optimum bias potential in order to emphasize the influence of the antigen-antibody complex formation on the resistivity of the formed biofilm [47]. The affinity reaction between immobilised antibodies and ciprofloxacin results in an extremely sensitive and specific impedance response (reported as R vs. ciprofloxacin concentration) even with analyte concentrations as low as 10 pg mL^{-1}, coupled with a CV (calculated as average on three tested immunosensors) of 5%. The effect of interfering compounds as tobramycin, ceftriaxone, ofloxacin and norfloxacin on the immunosensor response was also investigated, and no significant changes in the impedimetric responses were observed.

7. ELECTROCHEMICAL IMMUNOSENSORS BASED ON ENZYME LABELLING

Electrochemical immunosensors with an enzymatic label are widely used because they combine the specificity of the antigen-antibody recognition to the advantages of the enzyme-amplified signal. They rely on the use of an enzyme label that generates an electroactive product close to the electrode surface; the formation of a relatively high local concentration of the enzyme product generated by the high enzyme turnover leads to a significant signal amplification. This approach has found various applications both in clinical field [52-58]. Some examples of enzyme-labelled electrochemical immunosensors applied to the detection of clinical biomarkers are described.

The rapid quantification of Prostate Specific Antigen (PSA) in human serum samples was reported by Panini and coworkers [56], who described the development of an immunosensor using a Glassy Carbon Electrode (GCE) modified with multi-walled carbon nanotubes (CNT-GCE) integrated with microfluidic systems. Mouse monoclonal antibodies against PSA were immobilised on the working electrode; prior to the modification, the glassy carbon electrode surface was polished with alumina, rinsed, sonicated into water and then into acetone, and dried in air. Then, one milligram of CNTs was dispersed with the aid of ultrasonic stirring for 45 min in methanol/water (50:50 v/v) in an aqueous 0.1% Nafion solution. Finally, a 20 μL aliquot of this dispersion was dropped on the GC electrode surface and then the solvent was evaporated under an infrared heat lamp.

To carry out the test, PSA in the serum sample was allowed to react with the immobilised anti-PSA antibody. Finally a second Horseradish Peroxidase (HRP) enzyme-labelled antibody specific to PSA was added. HRP, in the presence of hydrogen peroxide catalysed the oxidation of the additional substrate 4-tert-butylcatechol (4-TBC) and its back electrochemical reduction was detected on CNT-GCE at −0.15 V [56].

The electrochemical detection was completed within 1 min and the total assay time was 30 min. The estimated detection limit for the immunosensor was 0.08 μg L^{-1}, where a CV below 5% was obtained.

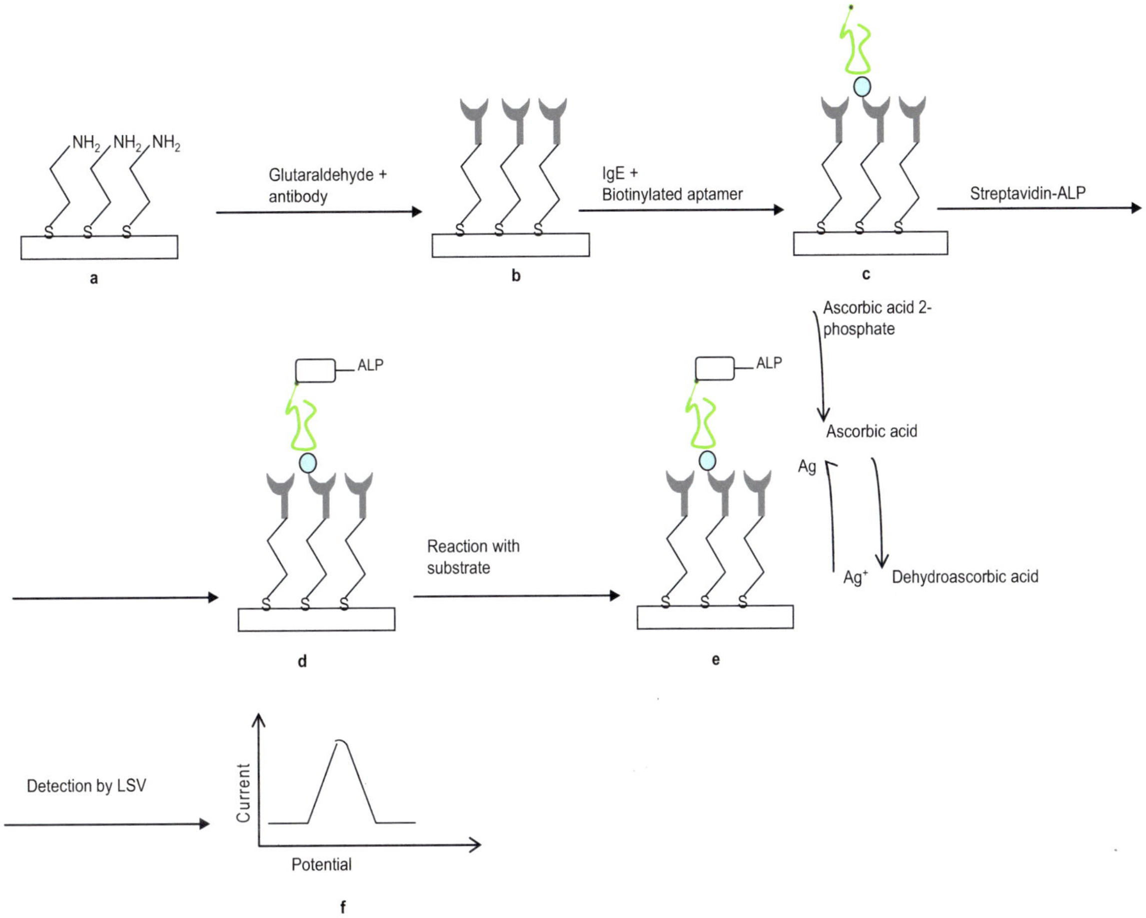

Figure 7: Schematic representation of the elettrochemical sandwich assay developed for the detection of IgE. **a)** binding of cysteamine on a gold electrode and formation of a self-assembled monolayer on it; **b)** immobilisation of IgE polyclonal antibody on the gold electrode; **c)** capture of IgE and binding of the biotynilated aptamer anti-IgE; d) binding with streptavidin-alkaline phosphatise; **e)** enzymatic reaction; **f)** silver detection by Linear Sweep Voltammetry. From Feng *et al.* (2008) [58].

Enzyme signal amplification coupled with semiconductors as transducers were applied to immunosensor development. A simple example based on a sandwich format using human serum IgG as target model has been developed by Zhong *et al.* [53]. An anti-IgG layer was formed on an Indium Tin Oxide (ITO) electrode. After the incubation of the immunoelectrode with a sample containing human serum IgG, a sandwich assay was carried out using anti-IgG antibodies labelled with HRP-doped double codified nanosilica particles (anti-IgG–SiO_2–HRP). The electrochemical detection was finally based on the catalytic reduction of the carried HRP in the nanosilica particles relative to the H_2O_2 system. HRP-doped nanosilica particles possess several merits, such as high catalytic efficiency, good stability due to the exclusion of oxygen by silica encapsulation, and good potential as transducers for several biorecognition binding applications. The extreme catalytic efficiency makes them especially suitable for ultrasensitive bioanalysis without the need for additional reagents or signal amplification steps [53]. With this format the linear range of the developed immunosensor by using anti-IgG–SiO_2–HRP as tracer and tetramethylbenzidine (TMB)/hydrogen peroxide (H_2O_2) as enzyme substrate was 0.01–15 nmol L^{-1} IgG with a detection limit of 5.0 pmol L^{-1}, at a signal to noise ratio of three times the Standard Deviation of the blank (SD) (n = 15), while the assay sensitivity by directly using HRP-labelled anti-IgG as secondary antibodies was 1.0–10 nmol L^{-1} with a detection limit of 0.1 nmol L^{-1} IgG. Authors explain these differences as due to: 1) the amplification of the amperometric signal output, that was mainly ascribed to the excess HRP present in the nanosilica particles; 2) the high surface-to-volume ratio of SiO_2-HRP nanoparticles that could have a higher probability of binding more anti-IgG target; 3) the synthesized nanosilica particles that could accommodate more HRP molecules than that of the standard method, such as standard ELISA. The reproducibility and specificity of the proposed immunoassay method were finally evaluated (average CVs of 5.9, 5.2% respectively) whereas in terms of stability, if stored at + 4°C, the developed system retained 89.1% of its initial response after a storage period of 32 days.

An example of electrochemical sandwich assay for detection of immunoglobulin E (IgE) was reported [58]. The assay was performed coupling an antibody against IgE with an aptamer anti-IgE. Antibody molecules were covalently immobilised as capture probe on gold electrodes *via* a self-assembled monolayer of cysteamine through the glutaraldehyde-based bifunctional linking. After that the target was captured, the biotinylated anti-IgE aptamer was added because it could interact specifically with the analyte, followed by the addition of a streptavidin-alkaline phosphatase (streptavidin-AP) solution. Once biotin-streptavidin recognition occurred, the signal amplification was achieved based on enzymatic silver deposition. Ascorbic acid 2-phosphate was converted by AP into ascorbic acid, a strong reducing agent. It could reduce the silver ions in the solution to silver metal that preferentially deposited on the gold surface of electrodes. The amount of deposited silver, which is proportional to the amount of IgE target bound on the electrode surface, was quantified by linear sweep voltammetry (Fig. **7**). The detection limit calculated using this approach was 0.02 nM of IgE.

7.1. Enzyme-Labelled Electrochemical Immunosensors Based on the Use of Screen-Printed Sensors

One of the main problems associated with immunosensors is their cost, and consequently, the regeneration of the sensing surface by exploiting the reversibility of the antibody/antigen reaction is desirable. However, this regeneration step is time-consuming and gives irreproducible results, particularly when the immunocomplex possess a high affinity constant. Moreover, the drastic regeneration conditions can damage and release the immunoreagent bound to the surface of the transducer. This problem was partially overcome by using disposable transducers such as screen-printed electrodes. This approach finds various applications in clinical field, as demonstrated by the large bibliography production [59-64].

Carbon-based screen-printed electrodes were largely used for immunosensor development owing to easy adsorption of biomolecules on graphite. One interesting example was reported by Pemberton and coworkers, who developed a disposable electrochemical immunosensor based on a competitive assay scheme for the determination of estradiol in human serum extracts [63]. At this purpose, anti-mouse IgG were adsorbed on the carbon surface of a disposable screen-printed electrode and then mouse monoclonal antibody anti-estradiol was added. Competition between estradiol and a fixed concentration of an enzyme-labelled estradiol was then promoted. Alkaline Phosphatase (AP) was used as the enzyme label, coupled with 1-naphthyl phosphate as substrate and Differential Pulse Voltammetry as detection technique.

The calibration curve of estradiol showed a measurable range between 25 and 500 pg/ml with a detection limit of 50 pg/ml. The immunosensor was applied to the determination of estradiol in spiked serum, following an extraction step with diethyl ether. A mean recovery for the method of 102.5% was obtained with a CV of 19%.

Escamilla-Gómez *et al.* developed a voltammetric enzyme dual sensors for simultaneous determination of free and total prostate specific antigen (f-PSA and t-PSA) [62]. In this application, antibodies specific for f-PSA and t-PSA respectively were immobilised on a dual screen-printed electrode based on different materials such as carbon, gold and carbon modified with nanogold. Dual screen-printed carbon electrodes modified with nanogold resulted finally the SPEs with the best analytical characteristics and lead to the most repeatable bioelectrodes. Once the surface was chosen, antibodies were immobilised onto the two working electrodes; then, biotinylated anti-PSA antibody and streptavidin-AP conjugate were used as detection reagents, giving rise to the first simultaneous electrochemical biosensor for free and total PSA. The PSA dual sensor was used to monitor PSA production from three different cultures of human androgen-sensitive prostate tumour cells.

A disposable electrochemical competitive assay for detection of IgE was proposed by Papamichael *et al.* [64]. In this work the IgE antigen was immobilized on the surface of screen-printed electrodes, then a competition step between IgE bound to the electrode surface and IgE in solution for the biotinylated aptamer was left to occur. At this point the streptavidin-alkaline phosphatase conjugate was added to the electrode. p-Aminophenyl phosphate (p-APP) was used as enzymatic substrate and differential pulse voltammetry as electrochemical technique. The results obtained with the electrochemical aptasensor were compared with those based on an ELISA-type assay (ELONA). The aptasensor showed high specificity and selectivity toward IgE with a detection limit of 23 ng/mL, which is a concentration sufficient for detection of IgE in blood considering that the IgE concentration in blood samples of healthy subjects is in the range 240 – 290 ng/mL. Moreover, in this work the stability of the assay performed using the aptamer against IgE was compared with that of the assay carried out with a monoclonal antibody specific for IgE. Authors reported that the assay performed using the aptamer was more stable than that with antibody, considering that aptamers can be easily regenerated also using harsh conditions and are thermo-stable, because the aptamer folding is not affected by the temperature.

8. ELECTROCHEMICAL SENSORS BASED ON THE USE OF MAGNETIC BEADS FOR THE DETECTION OF CLINICAL BIOMARKERS

The use of magnetic beads as an alternative support for biological immobilisation was reported for the first time by Varlan and coworkers [65]. The proposed technique consisted in linking the enzyme immunoconjugate onto the modified magnetic beads and then patterning the particles on a sensor by a thick-film permanent magnet localised in the back side of the sensor (Fig. **8**). This new enzyme entrapment technique takes advantage of the protein covalent bonding features, of the high specific surface area exhibited by the particles and of the possibility to fix the magnetic particles of the latex by the means of a magnetic field. The result is a stable "patterned" enzymatic membrane [65].

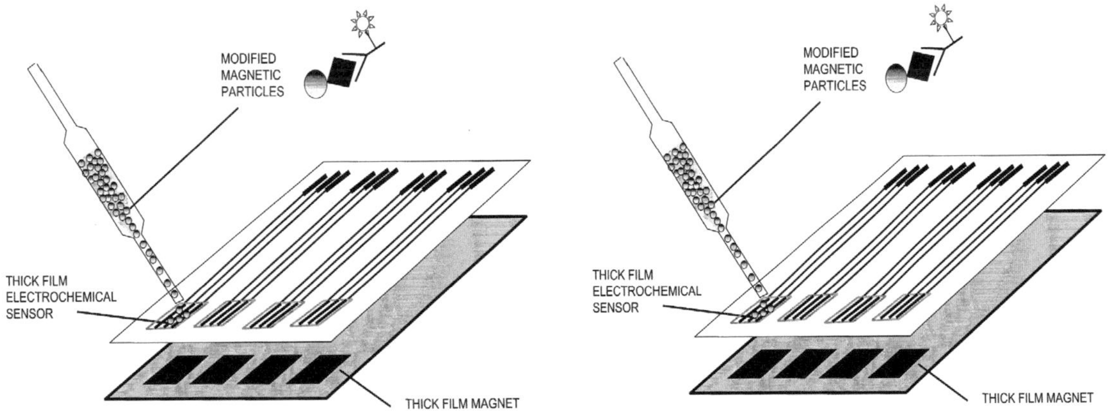

Figure 8: Principle of the electrochemical immunosensor based on the use of magnetic beads. From Varlan *et al.*, 1995 [65].

There are several applications of electrochemical immunosensors based on magnetic beads in the environmental, food and clinical fields, and the number of paper is still growing, demonstrating the current interest of researchers in this area [66-71].

Centi *et al.* [71] developed an electrochemical aptamer-based assay for analysis of C Reactive Protein (CRP) in serum, using a simple target capturing step by aptamer functionalised magnetic beads. CRP is a plasma protein and is among the most expressed proteins in acute phase inflammation cases, being a known biomarker for inflammatory states. The assay was based on a sandwich format in which a RNA aptamer was coupled to a monoclonal antibody and Alkaline Phosphatase (AP) was used as enzymatic label. After the sandwich assay, the modified magnetic beads were captured by a magnet on the surface of a graphite working electrode and the electrochemical detection was thus achieved through the addition of the AP substrate (a-naphthyl-phosphate) and a-naphthol produced during the enzymatic reaction was detected using Differential Pulse Voltammetry (DPV) (Fig. **9**).

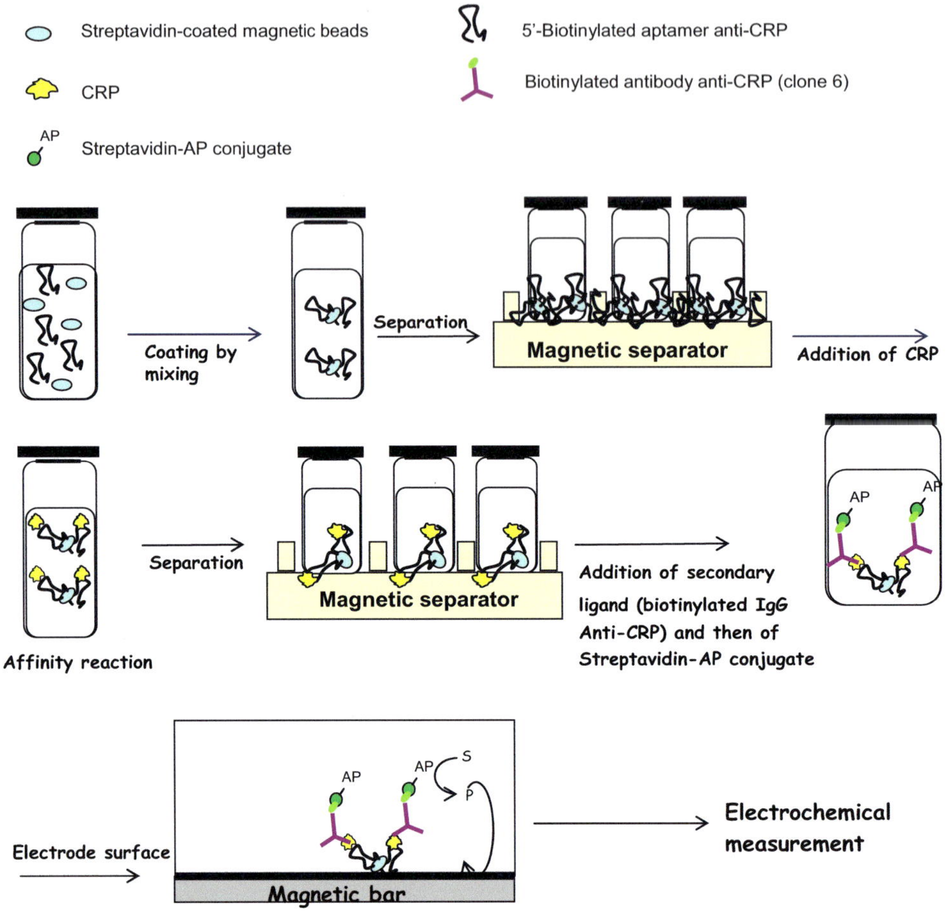

Figure 9: Schematic representation of the electrochemical sandwich assay developed for CRP detection.

The parameters influencing the different steps of the assay were optimized in order to reach the best sensitivity (LOD= 5.4×10^{-2} mg/L) and specificity. The ability of the electrochemical aptamer-based assay to detect CRP in CRP free serum, diluted 1 : 10, was evaluated. CRP free serum was tested alone or spiked with CRP (in the concentration range 0 – 1000 mg/ L), and the corresponding dose response curve covered the whole dynamic range from the region of signal noise to a saturation value. The signal increased with the increased concentration of the analyte and a matrix effect was observed considering the lower currents measured in serum with respect to buffer. Probably this decrease was due to a reduced concentration of CRP available for the binding caused by the interaction with some matrix components. The calculated LOD was 0.2 mg/L. The matrix effect increased the value of the detection limit even if such value is comparable with that reported by the reference method used for CRP detection.

Finally, the assay was applied to the analysis of some serum samples.

9. SUMMARY

Immunoassays are analytical techniques commonly used for screening purposes or quantitative detection of molecules of clinical interest: they are cheap, sensitive and allow many simultaneous analyses. Immunoassay procedures have been optimised for many analytes and commercial kits are available for a wide variety of clinical biomarkers (prostate specific antigen (PSA), C Reactive Protein (CRP), carcinoembryonic antigen (CEA), estradiol, progesterone, *etc.* Despite the high sensitivity and reproducibility of conventional immunoassays such as radioimmunoassays (RIAs) and Enzyme-Linked Immunosorbent Assays (ELISAs), immunological methods have some limitations: in addition to the problems related to short shelf life of ^{125}I-labeled antibody in RIAs, all immunological methods require long analysis times, skilled personnel because of the complicated procedures and do not allow easily to perform the measurement directly "in situ". An alternative strategy are electrochemical immunosensors which are analytical devices able to detect the binding of an antigen to its specific antibody by coupling the immunochemial reaction to an electrochemical transducer. The main characteristics of these devices are low detection limits correlated to the electrochemical measurement, fast analysis times and an excellent specificity and a good reproducibility, which are comparable to those of immunoassays. Moreover, immunosensors are small devices that allows to decentralise the analysis in field and to perform continuous measurements. As examples, the analytical characteristics of the electrochemical immunosensors for the detection of progesterone and CRP are compared with those obtained by the ELISA kits commercially available: for the detection of progesterone, most electrochemical immunosensors present in literature show detection limits (around 0.2 ng/mL) comparable to those of the commercial ELISA kits but shorter analysis time (around 1 h vs. some hours) and a miniaturized apparatus which is more suitable for in field measurements, whereas, for the detection of CRP, most electrochemical immunosensors reported in literature, based on the use of antibodies, show a higher sensitivity than 10 ng/mL which is the detection limit of the ELISA kits called high sensitivity C reactive protein (hs-CRP). Also in the case of CRP, the analysis time of electrochemical immunosensors are faster than those necessary to the ELISA kits. Electrochemical immunosensors have thus opened new scenarios in the field of analytical chemistry because of their ease, sensitivity, selectivity and fast detection.

At the moment, although there are many and many papers concerning the development of electrochemical immunosensors and procedures have been optimised for many analytes especially in clinical field, only few electrochemical immunosensors are commercially available. However, in the last years many companies are funding in this new challenge also thanks to many projects involving this topic.

In this chapter several applications of electrochemical immunosensors for the detection of clinical biomarkers have been reported. Different electrochemical methods (potentiometric, amperometric, impedimetric, voltammetric) have been considered for the detection of molecules of clinical interest such as CEA, PSA, immunoglobulin E (IgE), estradiol, CRP. Moreover, the use of magnetic beads as new materials for immunosensors coupled with electrochemical detection has been also described, together with the use of new molecules as well aptamers as specific biorecognition elements. Examples of the applicability of these devices to solving various analytical problems in clinical field have been reported.

10. CONCLUSIONS

In this chapter several applications of immunoassays for the detection of some clinical biomarkers have been reported. In particular, the current status of research in electrochemical immunoassays is considered. The attractive aspect in electrochemical immunosensor development is related to the combination of the advantages taken from antibody/aptamer-based assays, magnetic beads as solid-phase and electrochemical transduction for the development of simple and fast procedures able to detect analytes of clinical interest in complex biological matrices.

DISCLOSURE

Part of contents reported in this chapter has been published before [72].

REFERENCES

[1] Li X-M, Yang X-Y, Zhang S-S. Electrochemical enzyme immunoassay using model labels. Trends Anal Chem 2008; 27: 543-553.

[2] Franek M, Hruska K. Antibody based methods for environmental and food analysis a review. Vet Med.-Czech 2005; 50: 1-10.

[3] Shan G, Lipton C, Gee SJ, Hammock BD. Immunoassay, biosensors and other nonchromatographic methods. In: Philip WL, Eds. Handbook of Residue Analytical Methods for Agrochemicals. John Wiley & Sons Ltd Publisher 2002, pp. 623-79.

[4] Tombelli S, Minunni M, Mascini M. Aptamers-based assays for diagnostics, environmental and food analysis. Biomol Eng 2007; 24 (2): 191-200.

[5] Keefe A D, Schaub R G. Aptamers as candidate therapeutics for cardiovascular indications. Curr Opin Pharmacol 2008; 8 (2):147-152.

[6] Albrecht C, Fechner P, Honcharenko D, Baltzer L, Gauglitz G. A new assay design for clinical diagnostics based on alternative recognition element. Biosens Bioelectron 2010; 25 (10): 2302-2308.

[7] Choulier L, Enander K. Environmentally sensitive fluorescent sensors based on synthetic peptides. Sensors 2010; 10: 3126-3144.

[8] Takahashi H, Takahashi M, Nagaya H, *et al.* Establishment of a specific radioimmunoassay for bovine interferon τ. Theriogenology 2005; 63 (4):1050-1060.

[9] Gosling JP. Enzyme immunoassay. Immunoassay 1996; 287-308.

[10] Kreuzer MP, O'Sullivan CK, Guilbault GG. Alkaline phosphatase as a label for immunoassay using amperometric detection with a variety of substrates and an optimal buffer system. Anal Chim Acta 1999; 393: 95-102.

[11] Beckman EM, Kawaguchi T, Chandler GT, Decho AW. Development of a microplate-based fluorescence immunoassay using quantum dot streptavidin conjugates for enumeration of putative marine bacteria, Alteromonas sp., associated with a benthic harpacticoid copepod. J Microbiol Methods 2008; 75:441-444.

[12] Yang X, Janatova J, Andrade JD. Homogeneous enzyme immunoassay modified for application to luminescence-based biosensors. Anal Biochem 2005; 336 (1): 102-107.

[13] Liu JM, Zhu GH, Rao ZM, *et al.* Determination of human IgG by solid substrate room temperature phosphorescence immunoassay based on an antibody labeled with nanoparticles containing dibromofluorescein luminescent molecules. Anal Chim Acta 2005; 528:29-35.

[14] Hilborn ED, Carmichael WW, Yuan M, Azevedo SMFO. A simple colorimetric method to detect biological evidence of human exposure to microcystins. Toxicon 2005; 46: 218-221.

[15] Lehmann U, De Courten D, Vandevyver C, *et al.* On-chip antibody handling and colorimetric detection in a magnetic droplet manipulation system. Microelectronic 2007; 84:1669-1672.

[16] Kim J, Jeon M, Paeng K-J, Paeng IR. Competitive enzyme-linked immunosorbent assay for the determination of catecholamine, dopamine in serum. Anal Chim Acta 2008; 619:87-93.

[17] Wilson MS, Rauh RD. Novel amperometric immunosensors based on iridium oxide matrices. Biosens Bioelectron 2004; 19: 693-699.

[18] Ammida NHS, Micheli L, Palleschi G. Electrochemical immunosensor for determination of aflatoxin B1 in barley. Anal Chim Acta 2004; 520: 159-164.

[19] Centi S, Silva E, Laschi S, Palchetti I, Mascini M. Polychlorinated biphenyls (PCBs) detection in milk samples by an electrochemical magneto-immunosensor (EMI) coupled to solid-phase extraction (SPE) and disposable low-density arrays. Anal Chim Acta 2007; 594: 9-16.

[20] Zacco E, Galve R, Marco MP, *et al.* Electrochemical biosensing of pesticide residues based on affinity biocomposite platforms. Biosens Bioelectron 2007; 22: 1707-1715.

[21] Fowler JM, Wong DKY, Halsall HB, Heineman WR. Recent developments in electrochemical immunoassays and immunosensors. Electrochemical Sensors, Biosensors and their Biomedical Applications 2008; 115-143.

[22] Morgan CL, Newman DJ, Price CP. Immunosensors: technology and opportunities in laboratory medicine. Clin Chem 1996; 42: 193-209.

[23] Lin J, Ju H. Electrochemical and chemiluminescent immunosensors for tumor markers. Biosens Bioelectron 2005; 20: 1461-1470.

[24] Jiang X, Li D, Xu X, *et al.* Immunosensors for detection of pesticide residues. Biosens Bioelectron 2008; 23: 1577-1587.

[25] Davies C. Introduction to immunoassay principles. In: Wild D, EDs. The Immunoassay Handbook. The Mac Millian Press Ltd 1994, p. 10.

[26] Wu J, Fu Z, Yan F, Ju H. Biomedical and clinical applications of immunoassays and immunosensors for tumor markers. Trends Anal Chem 2007; 26 (7): 679-688.

[27] Lin J, Ju H. Electrochemical and chemiluminescent immunosensors for tumor markers. Biosens Bioelectron 2005; 20:1461-1470.

[28] Sharma S K, Sehgal N and Kumar A. Biomolecules for development of biosensors and their applications. Curr Appl Phys 2003; 3: 307-316.

[29] Adányi N, Váradi M, Kim N, Szendrö I. Development of new immunosensors for determination of contaminants in food. Curr Appl Phys 2006; 6: 279-286.

[30] Warsinke A, Stöcklein W, Leupold E, *et al.* Electrochemical Immunosensors on the route to proteomic chips. Perspect Bioanal 2005; 1: 451-483.

[31] Medyantseva EP, Khaldeeva EV, Budnikov GK. Immunosensors in biology and medicine: analytical capabilities, problems and prospects. J Anal Chem 2001; 56: 886-900.

[32] Cardosi MF, Turner APF. Recent advances in enzyme-based electrochemical glucose sensors. In: Alberti K and Krall LP, Eds. The Diabetes Annual 5. Elsevier 1990; pp. 254-72.

[33] Solé S, Merkoçi A, Alegret S. New materials for electrochemical sensing III. Beads. Trends Anal Chem 2001; 20 (2):102-110.

[34] Paleček E, Kizek R, Havran L, *et al.* Electrochemical enzyme-linked immunoassay in a DNA hydridization sensor. Anal Chim Acta 2002; 469:73-83.

[35] Alefantis, Grewal P, Ashton J, *et al.* A rapid and sensitive magnetic bead-based immunoassay for the detection of staphylococcal enterotoxin B for high-through put screening. Mol Cell Probes 2004; 1-4.

[36] Centi S, Laschi S, Fránek M, Mascini M. A disposable immunomagnetic electrochemical sensor based on functionalised magnetic beads and carbon-based screen-printed electrodes (SPCEs) for the detection of polychlorinated biphenyls (PCBs). Anal Chim Acta 2005; 538: 205-212.

[37] Warsinke A, Benkert A, Scheller FW. Electrochemical immunoassays. Fresenius J Anal Chem 2000; 366: 622-634.

[38] Janata J. An Immunoelectrode. J Am Chem Soc 1975; 97 (10): 2914-2916.

[39] Medyantseva EP, Khaldeeva EV, Budnikov GK. Immunosensors in biology and medicine: analytical capabilities, problems and prospects. J Anal Chem 2001; 56: 886-900.

[40] Tang DP, Yuan R, Chai YQ, *et al.* Novel potentiometric immunosensor for hepatitis B surface antigen using a gold nanoparticle-based biomolecular immobilization method. Anal Biochem 2004; 333: 345-350.

[41] Luppa PB, Sokoll LJ, Chan DW. Immunosensors—principles and applications to clinical chemistry. Clin Chim Acta 2001; 314: 1-26.

[42] He X, Yuan R, Chai Y, Shi Y. A sensitive amperometric immunosensor for carcinoembryonic antigen detection with porous nanogold film and nano-Au/chitosan composite as immobilization matrix. J Biochem Biophys Methods 2008; 70: 823-829.

[43] Lisdat F, Schäfer D. The use of electrochemical impedance spectroscopy for biosensing. Anal Bioanal Chem 2008; 391: 1555-1567.

[44] Katz E, Willner I. Probing biomolecular interactions at conductive and semiconductive surfaces by impedance spectroscopy: routes to impedimetric immunosensors, DNA-sensors, and enzyme biosensors. Electroanalysis 2003; 15: 913-947.

[45] Rahman MdA, Shiddiky MJA, Park J-S, Shim Y-B. An impedimetric immunosensor for the label-free detection of bisphenol A. Biosens Bioelectron 2007; 22: 2464-2470.

[46] Lucarelli F, Marrazza G, Mascini M. Enzyme-based impedimetric detection of PCR products using oligonucleotide-modified screen-printed gold electrodes. Biosens Bioelectron 2005; 20: 2001-2009.

[47] Ouerghi O, Senillou A, Jaffrezic-Renault N, *et al.* Gold electrode functionalized by electropolymerization of a cyano N-substituted pyrrole: application to an impedimetric immunosensor. J Electroanal Chem 2001; 501: 62-69.

[48] Ouerghi O, Touhami A, Jaffrezic-Renault N, *et al.* Impedimetric immunosensor using avidin-biotin for antibody immobilization. Bioelectrochemistry 2002; 56: 131- 133.

[49] Cooreman P, Thoelen R, Manca J, *et al.* Impedimetric immunosensors based on the conjugated polymer PPV. Biosens Bioelectron 2005; 20: 2151-2156.

[50] Sargent A, Sadik OA. Monitoring antibody-antigen reactions at conducting polymer-based immunosensors using impedance spectroscopy. Electrochimica Acta 1999; 44: 4667-4675.

[51] Ionescu RE, Jaffrezic-Renault N, Bouffier L, *et al.* Impedimetric immunosensor for the specific label free detection of ciprofloxacin antibiotic. Biosens Bioelectron 2007; 23: 549-555.

[52] Wilson MS. Electrochemical Immunosensors for the simultaneous detection of two tumor markers. Anal Chem 2005; 77: 1496-1502.

[53] Zhong Z, Li M, Xiang D, *et al.* Signal amplification of electrochemical immunosensor for the detection of human serum IgG using double-codified nanosilica particles as labels. Biosens Bioelectron 2009; 24: 2246-2249.

[54] Wang Z, Tu Y, Liu S. Electrochemical immunoassay for α-fetoprotein through a phenylboronic acid monolayer on gold. Talanta 2008; 77: 815-821.

[55] Gao Z, Zhang J, Ting B P. A doubly amplified electrochemical immunoassay for carcinoembryonic antigen. Biosens Bioelectron 2009; 24: 1825-1830.

[56] Panini NV, Messina GA, Salinas E, Fernández H, Raba J. Integrated microfluidic systems with an immunosensor modified with carbon nanotubes for detection of prostate specific antigen (PSA) in human serum samples. Biosens Bioelectron 2008; 23: 1145-1151.

[57] Fernandez-Sanchez C, McNeil CJ, Rawson K, Nilsson O. Disposable noncompetitive immunosensor for free and total prostate-specific antigen based on capacitance measurement. Anal Chem 2004; 76: 5649-5656.

[58] Feng K, Kang Y, Zhao J-J, *et al.* Electrochemical immunosensor with aptamer-based enzymatic amplification. Anal Biochem 2008; 378: 38-42.

[59] Wu J, Zhang Z, Fu Z, Ju H. A disposable two-throughput electrochemical immunosensor chip for simultaneous multianalyte determination of tumor markers. Biosens Bioelectron 2007; 23: 114-120.

[60] Escamilla-Gómez V, Campuzano S, Pedrero M, Pingarrón JM. Electrochemical immunosensor designs for the determination of Staphylococcus aureus using 3,3-dithiodipropionic acid di(N-succinimidyl ester)- modified gold electrodes. Talanta 2008; doi: 10.1016/j.talanta.2008.07.045.

[61] Conneely G, Aherne M, Lu H, Guilbault GG. Development of an immunosensor for the detection of testosterone in bovine urine. Anal Chim Acta 2007; 583: 153-160.

[62] Escamilla-Gómez V, Hernández-Santos D, González-García M B, *et al.* Simultaneous detection of free and total prostate specific antigen on a screen-printed electrochemical dual sensor. Biosens Bioelectron 2009; 24: 2678-2683.

[63] Pemberton R M, Mottram T T, Hart J P. Development of a screen-printed carbon electrochemical immunosensor for picomolar concentrations of estradiol in human serum extracts. J Biochem Biophys Methods 2005; 63: 201-212.

[64] Papamichael K I, Kreuzer M P, Guilbault G G. Viability of allergy (IgE) detection using an alternative aptamer receptor and electrochemical means. Sensors and Actuators B 2007; 121: 178-186.

[65] Varlan R, Suls J, Jacobs P, Sansen W. A new technique of enzyme entrapment for planar biosensors. Biosens Bioelectron 1995; 10: XV-XIX.

[66] Lin Y-Y, Liu G, Wai CM, Lin Y. Magnetic beads-based bioelectrochemical immunoassay of polycyclic aromatic hydrocarbons. Electrochem commun 2007; 9: 1547-1552.

[67] Lermo A, Fabiano S, Hernández S, *et al.* Immunoassay for folic acid detection in vitamin-fortified milk based on electrochemical magneto sensors. Biosens Bioelectron 2009; 24: 2057-2063.

[68] Zacco E, Pividori MI, Alegret S, *et al.* Electrochemical magnetoimmunosensing strategy for the detection of pesticides residues. Anal Chem 2006; 78:1780-1788.

[69] Zhuo Y, Yuan P-X, Yuan R, *et al.* Bienzyme functionalized three-layer composite magnetic nanoparticles for electrochemical immunosensors. Biomaterials 2009; 30: 2284-2290.

[70] Centi S, Tombelli S, Minunni M, Mascini M. Aptamer-based detection of plasma proteins by an electrochemical assay coupled to magnetic beads. Anal Chem 2007; 79: 1466-1473.

[71] Centi S, Bonel Sanmartin L, Tombelli S, *et al.* Detection of C Reactive Protein (CRP) in serum by an electrochemical aptamer-based sandwich assay. Electroanalysis 2009; 21(11):1309-1315.

[72] Laschi S, Centi S, Mascini M. Electrochemical arrays coupled with magnetic separators for immunochemistry. Bioanalytical Reviwes 2011, 3:11–25.

CHAPTER 14

Antibody Fragment Engineering and Applications in Diagnosis and Therapeutics

Xuemei Xie, Gabrielle Richard, and John Christopher Hall*

School of Environmental Sciences, University of Guelph, 50 Stone Road East, Guelph, Ontario, Canada, N1G 2W1

Abstract: The advent of innovative recombinant DNA technology has made antibodies a new generation of pharmaceuticals for diagnosis and therapeutics. For the past few decades, minimal antigen-binding fragments, such as Fab (fragment antigen binding), Fv (fragment variable), and single variable domains (sVD), have emerged as credible alternatives to monoclonal antibodies (mAb) in many applications. These recombinant antibody fragments (rAbFs) retain the target specificity and affinity of whole mAbs and have the advantages of economical production, superior biodistribution, easy genetic manipulation and chemical modification to create reagents with required properties for a range of diagnostic and therapeutic applications. To enhance their application efficiency, these fragments have been engineered into multivalent, multispecific, or fusion molecules, or linked to therapeutic payloads (*e.g.* radionuclides, liposomes, toxins, cytokines, enzymes, and anti-sense RNA) that perform a specific function. The advances of selection technologies (*e.g.* phage-, ribosome-, and yeast-display) and the emergence of various production systems (*e.g.* bacteria, yeast, plants, and mammalian cells) have significantly facilitated rAbF development and diversified their applications. This chapter primarily focuses on the current advances in antibody engineering for improving the diagnostic or therapeutic applications of rAbFs.

Keywords: Antibodies, Engineering, Applications, Diagnosis, Therapeutics.

1. INTRODUCTION

The high specificity and affinity of antibodies to target molecules and their distinct structural and functional characteristics make them attractive reagents in scientific research and clinical diagnostics as well as promising drug candidates in therapeutics. Although naturally produced by plasma cells, the need for antibodies in large quantities has encouraged the production of antibodies using heterogeneous expression systems. Hybridoma technology developed by Kohler and Milstein in 1975 [1] opened a new era in antibody engineering and production. Throughout the 1990s, recombinant DNA technologies, especially chimerization and humanization, have improved the clinical application of murine mAbs for the treatments of cancer, autoimmune disease, and infectious disease. Today, mAbs and related molecules are becoming one of the fastest growing classes of pharmaceuticals.

The therapeutic efficacy of intact mAbs in certain applications is limited by their pharmacological characteristics: slow blood clearance that leads to significant exposure to normal tissues and relatively poor tissue penetration that results in inadequate quantities being delivery to the target tissue [2, 3]. Therefore, in the past two decades, efforts to circumvent such limitations have led to the generation of minimal antigen-binding fragments, such as Fab, Fv, and sVD. The small size (15-50 kDa) of these rAbFs makes them potentially more suitable than intact mAbs for certain therapeutic applications where the Fc region-dependent effector functions are not required [*e.g.* in the cases of viral or toxin neutralization [4, 5] and where delivery into tissue is required [6, 7]. The advances of selection technologies (*e.g.* phage-, ribosome-, and microbial surface-display) and the development of new expression systems (*e.g.* bacteria, yeast, plants,

***Address correspondence to John Christopher Hall:** School of Environmental Sciences, University of Guelph, 50 Stone Road East, Guelph, Ontario, Canada, N1G 2W1; Tel: 519-824-4120 Ext. 52740; E-mail: jchall@uoguelph.ca and mammalian cells) for rAbF production at a large scale have enhanced their clinical applications. In recent years, these rAbFs have been engineered in numerous ways to meet various application requirements as well as to improve their application efficacy by reducing immunogenicity [8], increasing functional binding affinity (avidity), improving pharmacokinetic profiles, and/or introducing new effector functions [9]. For example, rAbFs have been constructed into multivalent and multispecific molecules (*e.g.* diabodies, tribodies, tetrabodies, minibodies, fusion proteins, and bispecific antibodies) or immunoconjugates with new therapeutic properties through genetic or chemical fusion to other effector molecules, such as enzymes for prodrug therapy, toxins or cytokines for cancer treatment, viruses for gene therapy, and liposomes for improved drug delivery [9]. All these redesigned rAbFs have improved *in vivo* pharmacokinetics and are promising reagents for diagnosis or drug candidates for immunotherapy; some of these reagents are already in clinical trials [9].

This chapter primarily provides an update on the current development of engineered rAbFs with desired pharmacokinetic and therapeutic properties that specifically target antigens associated with human diseases. The different selection and expression systems for rAbF production are also discussed.

2. STUCTURAL AND FUNCTIONAL FEATURES OF INTACT ANTIBODIES

Antibodies are glycoproteins, which are naturally produced and secreted by mammalian plasma cells, against a wide range of antigens. Among the five distinct classes of antibodies, *i.e.*, IgA, IgD, IgE, IgG, and IgM, IgG is the most abundant Ig and comprising approximately 80% of the total serum Igs. There are four subclasses of IgGs, known as IgG1, IgG2a, IgG2b and IgG3 in mice and IgG1, IgG2, IgG3 and IgG4 in humans. IgGs are widely used in diagnostics and therapeutics because of their long serum half-lives (>20 days) and superior capacity to interact with other components of the immune system [10].

Each IgG contains two molecularly and functionally separable regions: Fab fragments for target recognition and an Fc region for triggering effector functions and regulating both *in vivo* half-life and biodistribution (Fig. **1**). The Fab fragment is composed of the entire light (L) chain and the VH and CH1 domains of the heavy (H) chain, both of which are linked by a disulfide bond. Within the variable domains of both L and H chains, there are three hypervariable regions, denoted as HV1, HV2, and HV3, which combine to form antigen-binding sites at the N-termini of the Fab fragments [11]. These hypervariable regions determine the antigen-binding specificity and affinity by forming a surface complementary to the structure of the epitope on an antigen and thus, are more commonly called the Complementarity Determining Regions (CDRs). Within the same domain, there are also four regions that are quite conserved in amino acid composition and known as the Framework Regions (FR), designated FR1, FR2, FR3, and FR4. The framework regions act as a scaffold to support the CDRs, and are thereby also involved indirectly in antigen recognition.

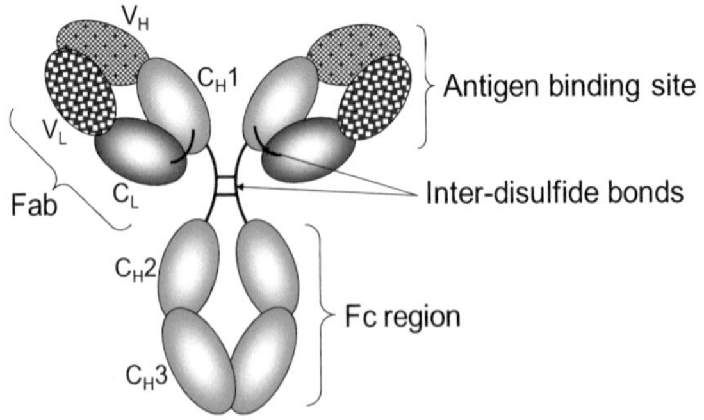

Figure 1: The basic structure of an IgG antibody. Each IgG contains two functionally and molecularly separate modules, the Fab and Fc regions, and is composed of four polypeptide chains: two light (L) chains and two heavy (H) chains. Each L chain is composed of one variable domain (V_L) and one constant domain (C_L), while each H chain consists of one variable domain (V_H) and three constant domains (C_H). Each domain contains about 110 amino acids. Inter-disulfide bonds link the L chain to the H chain and the two H chains together. The variable regions are responsible for the antigen recognition and binding, while the Fc region is essential for the recruitment and activation of immune effectors.

The Fc region contains the paired C_H2 and C_H3 domains of H chains and mediates immune effector functions, including complement activation, opsonic phagocytosis of target cells, and cell-dependent cytotoxicity, *via* interaction with complement and Fc receptors (FcR) expressed on immune effector cells [12]. The Fc region also confers a long serum half-life to IgGs and regulates their biodistribution through interaction with neonatal Fc receptors (FcRn) present on a variety of cells, which rescue IgG from intracellular degradation [13]. The carbohydrate moieties in the C_H2 domain are essential for Fc region-mediated effector functions, which includes prolonging their *in vivo* half-lives [13, 14]. For example, compared to its intact chimeric IgG, ΔC_H2, an aglycosylated IgG lacking carbohydrates in the C_H2 domain, was cleared much faster from circulation and showed enhanced antigen-binding activity but little Antibody-Dependent Cell-Mediated Cytotoxicity (ADCC) and no Complement-Dependent Cytotoxicity (CDC) [15].

Functional differences among antibody isotypes mainly lie on the Fc regions. In mice, IgG2a and IgG2b are the most active in stimulating FcR-mediated effector functions [16, 17], with the phagocytic killing activity generally being IgG2a > IgG3 > IgG2b > IgG1 [17]. In humans, IgG1 and IgG3 are the most efficient at mediating Antibody-Dependent Cell-Mediated Phagocytosis (ADCP), ADCC, as well as CDC, and therefore, are the most suitable for treatments of infectious diseases and cancer. Conversely, IgG4 functions poorly or has no detectable activities and, therefore, is suitable for applications in diagnostics, blocking ligand-receptor interactions, or triggering signal pathway activation [18, 19].

3. rAb VERSUS rAbF

3.1. Production

For the production of functional intact mAbs, the expression systems must possess the mechanisms required for correct protein assembly, post-translational modification (*e.g.* disulfide bond formation and proper glycosylation), and secretion. Therefore, intact mAbs are currently expressed in mammalian cells at a high cost. Less expensive and scalable antibody production systems, such as transgenic animals and plants, which are capable of producing mAbs, have been developed [20-22]. These systems may reduce the costs of mAb production; however, it is time-consuming to build such systems for production of new mAbs. Furthermore, the significant differences in glycosylation patterns generated in plants may affect the effector functions of mAbs [14]. In contrast, since no glycosylation and complicated post-translational modifications are required for the production of antibody fragments, rAbFs with antigen-binding capability and specificity can be economically produced in large quantities using inexpensive prokaryotic (*Escherichia coli*) [23] and lower eukaryotic (yeast) based bioreactors [24].

3.2. Pharmacokinetics and Biodistribution

Several factors affect pharmacokinetics of IgGs, mainly their size, immunogenicity, and binding affinity to FcRn. In general, intact antibodies have better pharmacokinetics than rAbFs in terms of circulating half-lives. The serum half-lives of antibody molecules mainly depend on their size in relation to renal threshold (the approximate 70 kDa) and their charge and conformation [25, 26]. rAbFs have a Molecular Weight (MW) below glomerular cut-off (> 70 kDa) and thus, renal clearance is the major elimination pathway for these molecules. Human IgGs usually have long circulating half-lives, with $t_{1/2}\alpha$ (distribution-phase half-life) values of 18-22 hours and $t_{1/2}\beta$ (terminal-elimination-phase half-life) values of 21-23 days for IgG1, IgG2 and IgG4 [27]. In comparison with intact mAbs, the half-lives of rAbFs are relatively short due to their small size and lack of an Fc region. For example, a humanized IgG administered to rats was relatively long-lived with a $t_{1/2}\alpha$ of 5.8 hours and a $t_{1/2}\beta$ of 104 hours, whereas its Fab was cleared much more rapidly with a $t_{1/2}\alpha$ of 0.3 hours and a $t_{1/2}\beta$ of 23 hours [28]. Similarly, in mice humanized IgGs have half-lives of 22-120 h [5, 29], whereas Fab and scFv have $t_{1/2}\beta$ of only 4-8 [5] and 2-3.5 hours [30], respectively.

Specific sequences in the Fc region of an IgG are also essential for prolonging its circulating time in the serum. The binding of IgG to FcRn prevents it from being degraded by lysosome after being internalized by cells, and then triggers recyclingto the cell surface where the IgG and FcRn dissociate because of the higher pH, after which the IgG is returned to the circulatory system [13]. Due to this FcRn-mediated recycling mechanism, it was shown by Weir *et al.* [31] that an isolated Fc fragment exhibited a half-life similar to that of whole IgG, whereas Fab and $F(ab')_2$ were cleared more quickly. Furthermore, in mutant mice deficient in FcRn, the plasma levels of IgGs were relatively lower compared to those in wild type mice, and administered IgG and Fc fragments had abnormally short half-lives [29, 32]. These studies show the importance of the FcRn-mediated recycling mechanism for extending the circulating time of antibody molecules. Furthermore, Mueller *et al.* [15] showed that carbohydrates attached to C_H2 domain affect the half-lives of IgGs, since an aglycosylated IgG had a similar blood clearance rate as $F(ab')_2$ in tumor-bearing mice and cleared much faster than the corresponding intact IgG. In addition, immunogenicity of antibody molecules can also potentially affect their pharmacokinetics by eliciting anti-antibody immune responses that accelerate the clearance of administered antibodies and thereby reduce their therapeutic efficiency [33].

The size of antibody molecules also has important impact on their biodistribution. Systematic *in vivo* studies revealed that intact IgGs diffused slowly through tumor tissues and were non-uniform in their final distribution due to their large size, which limits quantities found in target tissues. For example, an intact IgG needed 54 h to travel 1 mm in a solid tumor, whereas the corresponding Fab took only 16 h to travel the same distance [34]. Thus, due to the poor tissue penetration of mAbs, immunotherapy is more successful for the treatment of circulating cancer cells than solid tumors. Although rAbFs (*e.g.* Fab, scFv, and sVD) exhibit better pharmacokinetics for tissue penetration, they often exhibit fast dissociation rates and poor retention time on the target because of their monovalent binding, which results in a low tumor versus normal tissue uptake [35-38]. For example, the percentage of the injected dose per gram of solid tumor tissue (ID/g) for an IgG was 3.68% at day 7 with a Localization Index (LI) of 4.38, while only 0.31% of the administered Fab accumulated in target tissue with a LI of 2.58 at day 1 [39]. Similarly, scFvs exhibited a high tumor to normal tissue ratio in xenograft mouse models; however, the absolute quantity of tumor uptake was less than that of intact mAbs [35, 36]. The low tumor retention compromises the efficiency of rAbFs in immunotherapy. For this reason, Fab and scFv are often engineered into dimeric, trimeric, or tetrameric molecules to increase their binding avidity, thereby improving retention time on targets (Fig. **2B** and **2D**) [35, 37, 38, 40].

3.3. Potential Therapeutic Properties

The long serum half-life and the combination of the two functional modules (*i.e.*, Fab and Fc region) of mAbs make them an attractive reagent for immunotherapy. Intact mAbs have practical value for therapeutic applications where a prolonged serum half-life is desirable and Fc region-mediated effector functions (*i.e.*, ADCC, ADCP, and CDC) are required. As stated above, the long serum half-life reduces dosage required for each treatment and frequency of administration, while the Fc region triggers immune effector functions against tumor cells or invading pathogens as well as confers a long serum half-life to IgG. Several mAbs have been approved for cancer treatment, such as Rituxan for non-Hodgkin lymphoma, Campath and Mylotarg for leukemia, Herceptin for breast carcinoma, and Panorex for colon cancer [41].

Not all therapeutic applications require the presence of both the target recognition and the effector function triggering modules. There are certain applications, in which the Fc region-mediated functions are dispensable and even undesirable, and thus rAbFs with antigen binding sites are adequate and even preferred. Examples of such applications are viral and toxin neutralization, receptor blockade, cytokine inactivation, drug delivery, and tumor imaging. For these applications, rAbFs have several advantages over intact mAbs. RAbFs have the advantage of lower immunogenicity when derived from heterologous antibodies because of their small size [42]. For example, most rAbFs do not suffer from the disadvantage of mAbs, which are often of murine origin that may result in Human Anti-Mouse Antibody (HAMA) responses [33, 43, 44], which can reduce the therapeutic efficacy by rapidly removing the administrated antibodies from body. Moreover, because rAbFs do not have an Fc region, and thus do not result in production FcR-expressing immune cells, massive cytokine release and associated toxic effects will not occur [45, 46]. Furthermore, rAbFs can be easily engineered to have functional properties not normally associated with mAbs through chemical coupling or genetic fusion to a variety of molecules with unique effector functions, such as toxins, radionuclides, cytotoxic prodrugs, cytokines, enzymes for prodrug activation and liposomes for improved drug delivery [9]. In this type of settings, rAbFs function as a carrier to deliver the attached therapeutic agents to the target sites.

The small size of rAbFs displaying effective tumor penetration is an advantage not only because they may have high tumor to normal tissue uptake ratios, but they are also rapidly cleared from the circulation through the kidneys, making them desirable as the ideal tumor imaging reagents with low background signal [47] and target-specific drug delivery with reduced toxicity to normal tissues [48]. Indeed, in several studies on tumor imaging, rAbFs have been shown to perform well and even better than intact mAbs [49]. By increasing the size and hence altering the properties of rAbFs as is the case with multivalent molecules (*i.e.*, 80 kDa minibodies), the ideal tumor-targeting agents can be created because they have excellent tissue penetration, high target retention, and yet are no longer cleared rapidly as lower molecular weight rAbFs from the circulation, hence their half-life is significantly improved [35, 37, 38, 40, 50, 51].

4. IMPROVEMENT OF THERAPEUTIC POTENTIAL OF RAbFs

As previously stated, RAbFs are attractive agents in immunotherapy, especially for patients with cancer. However, their therapeutic efficiency is often compromised by low antigen-binding affinity due to monovalent binding, rapid blood clearance due to low MW and inability to recruit host immune effectors due to the lack of Fc region. Several strategies are discussed below to overcome these shortcomings by generating antibody fragment constructs with significantly improved pharmacological profiles and therapeutic properties.

4.1. Engineering with Improved Antigen Binding Avidity

4.1.1. Affinity Maturation

There are two basic approaches used for enhancing the antigen binding affinity of antibody molecules. One approach is to artificially extend the contact regions of the binding site of antibodies [52]. For example, it has been shown that the addition of a random sequence of two, three, or four amino acids to the heavy CDR2 loop of an antibody enhances its binding affinity from a dissociation constant (Kd) of 2.6×10^{-9} to 2.2×10^{-10} [52]. A different approach is to directly improve antigen binding affinity of the binding site of antibodies through mutagenesis of the variable regions, including site-directed mutagenesis, random mutagenesis, and shuffling [53].

In site-directed mutagenesis, specific residues within CDRs or framework regions of heavy and light chains are mutated and then, a library is constructed and screened for high-affinity binders [53]. For example, when this approach was used the affinities of Fabs were increased 1.7 to 4.8 fold, when compared to the original Fabs [54]. In general, mutations in CDRs are more effective than those in framework regions at increasing antigen binding affinity [55].

In addition to using focused mutagenesis of specific regions, libraries containing affinity-improved mutants can be constructed by random mutagenesis, in which mutations are randomly introduced throughout a gene sequence *via* error-prone PCR [56, 57] or by bacterial mutator strains [58]. Error-prone PCR introduces point mutations at low frequency randomly across a gene under low-fidelity polymerization conditions and is an efficient strategy to enhance both specificity and affinity of antibody molecules. The random mutation of the entire V_H and V_L of an anti-estradiol-17β (E_2) scFv by error-prone PCR was shown by Kobayashi *et al.* [59] to improved its detection sensitivity by 10-fold. The point mutation of Fabs, directed against progesterone-BSA and selected from a naïve phage-displayed library *via* error-prone PCR, increased their affinity by 30-fold as compared to unmodified Fabs [60]. Since the Fabs isolated from the mutated library had several point mutations at different locations, it is apparent that different residues can each account for improved affinity. Antibodies with high-affinity can also be selected from a library followed by mutagenesis through amplification in an *E. coli* mutator strain (*i.e.*, MutD5). Such mutator strains introduce single base substitutions either through transversions or transitions at high frequency as compared to normal *E. coli* strains, thus generating a large number of mutant antibodies [58, 61]. By using this technique, the binding affinity of an anti-glycophorin scFv, generated over several rounds of mutagenesis, increased by 100-fold, from 320 nM for the parental scFv to 3.2 nM for the highest-affinity mutant [58].

Shuffling techniques include DNA shuffling [62], chain shuffling [63], and Staggered Extension Process (StEP) [64]. In DNA shuffling, the antibody coding DNA sequence is digested with DNase I and the resulting DNA fragments are randomly reassembled and amplified by PCR, producing antibodies with improved diversity and affinity [59]. A scFv with an off-rate 10,000-fold lower than that of a parental scFv was obtained by four cycles of random fragmentation, reassembly and screening [62]. In chain shuffling, the heavy and light chains of antibodies isolated from an immune library are randomly recombined, thereby generating a large number of recombinant antibodies [63]. Chain shuffling, however, is only suitable for the antibodies isolated from an immune library. Another commonly used approach is combinatorial mutagenesis, by which subsets of residues within CDRs of heavy and light chains or certain discrete spots of the variable domains are randomly mutated, after which the libraries are screened for improved binding affinity; finally, the best mutants of the heavy and light chains are combined to generate high-affinity binders [65]. By using this technique, the binding affinity of an anti-RAGE antibody was increased up to 110-fold compared to that of the unmodified IgG [65]. StEP is a PCR-based method, in which template switching, caused by several cycles of denaturation and shortened extension time, recombines various portions of several parental antibody coding sequences, creating a pool of recombinant genes [64]. By using the StEP approach, the off-rates of scFvs from a mRNA-display library were decreased by more than one order of magnitude and the Kds were improved up to 30-fold, while the antigen-specificity remained unchanged [64]. Since shuffling strategies mimic somatic hypermutation, it is believed that they are more efficient than site-directed or random mutagenesis at generating antibodies with high-affinity [66]. Among the strategies described above, site-directed mutagenesis and error-prone PCR are the most frequently used methods.

4.1.2. Multivalent Designs

In general, the antigen binding avidity of monomeric rAbFs is lower compared to parent antibodies because of monovalent binding. The low antigen binding avidity compromises therapeutic efficiency of rAbFs [35, 36]; therefore, monomeric rAbFs have been constructed into dimeric, trimeric, or tetrameric molecules to increase their binding avidity and improve performance during imaging and immunotherapy (Fig. **2B** and **2D;** Table **1A.**) [31, 40, 67-69]. Various methods have been used to engineer scFvs to create diabodies; the most successful method is to engineer the appropriate short peptide linkers to facilitate dimerization [40, 70]. For example, non-covalent $(scFv)_2$ diabodies have been generated by reducing the linker length to 3-12 residues (Fig. **2B**) [71] and scFv tribodies and tetrabodies (Fig. **2B**) were constructed by further reducing the linker length below 3 residues [69, 72]. When compared to monomeric scFvs, these non-covalently linked multimers had prolonged tumor retention time and a higher tumor-to-blood ratio, as a result of both reduced renal clearance and improved binding avidity [71, 72]. Alternatively, covalent $(scFv')_2$ diabodies can be generated by *in vitro* chemical coupling of scFvs containing either a cysteine residue in the conserved framework regions or an additional C-terminal cysteine [73]. Spontaneous site-specific dimerization in the periplasm of *E. coli* [74] can also be used to produce a disulfide-stabilized Fv (dsFv). These $(scFv')_2$ homodimers had an antigen binding avidity comparable to that of parental mAbs and higher than that of monomeric scFvs and were also more stable than the monomers [74, 75]. The high binding avidity led to improved tumor retention volumes and high tumor-to-blood ratios [69, 74, 75]. Bivalent or multivalent scFvs can also be constructed by genetic fusion to protein dimerizing motifs (*e.g.* amphipathic helices, leucine zipper proteins, transcriptional factor p53 and streptavidin), forming miniantibodies (Fig. **2D**) [40, 70, 76]. Furthermore, scFv monomers have been fused to; i) a Ig C_H3 domain *via* a two amino acid linker, usually leucine and aspartate (LD), to produce a minibody, ii) to the Fc region to produce a bivalent $(scFv)_2$-Fc fusion protein, or iii) to the hinge region of IgG which in turn is fused to a C_H3 domain *via* an additional 10 residues to produce a Flex minibody (Fig. **2D**) [77, 78]. Similarly, divalent and trivalent Fab multimers were also constructed from monomeric Fabs by either chemical conjugation or genetic fusion [31, 67, 79]. As stated earlier, these multimeric antibody molecules usually have binding avidities comparable to those of the parental IgGs and exhibit dramatically prolonged tumor retention time and better target-specific accumulation than monomeric fragments [38, 40, 69, 70, 72, 78].

For example, the tumor localization of ^{99m}Tc-sc$(Fv)_2$ was 7.2% ID/g at 6 h post-administration, whereas the tumor uptake was 19.1% ID/g for ^{99m}Tc-[sc$(Fv)_2$]$_2$ [38]. A tetravalent minibody TNF-TeAb, constructed by fusing human p53 to the C-terminus of an anti-TNF-scFv, showed an enhanced ability to inhibit both receptor binding and cytolytic activity of TNF-α. This tetravalent minibody resulted in a much more significant therapeutic effect than did TNF-scFv in suppressing arthritis progression by attenuating inflammation and destruction in joints and down-regulating pro-inflammatory cytokines and anti-collagen antibody in rats with collagen-induced arthritis [76]. Divalent and trivalent Fab multimers also display enhanced tumor accumulation and internalization properties when compared with parental Fab [31, 67, 79]. Furthermore, shortening the scFv peptide linker to improve non-covalent interaction also improves multimeric scFv stability. An anti-CD22 $(scFv)_2$ diabody with linkers of zero residues in length was substantially more stable than the five-residue form [80]. The high binding avidity, stability, and favorable pharmacokinetics make multivalent antibody fragments promising agents for applications in diagnostics and immunotherapy [69]. Indeed, some have been shown to function well in preclinical studies of tumor imaging and immunotherapy [38, 51, 81].

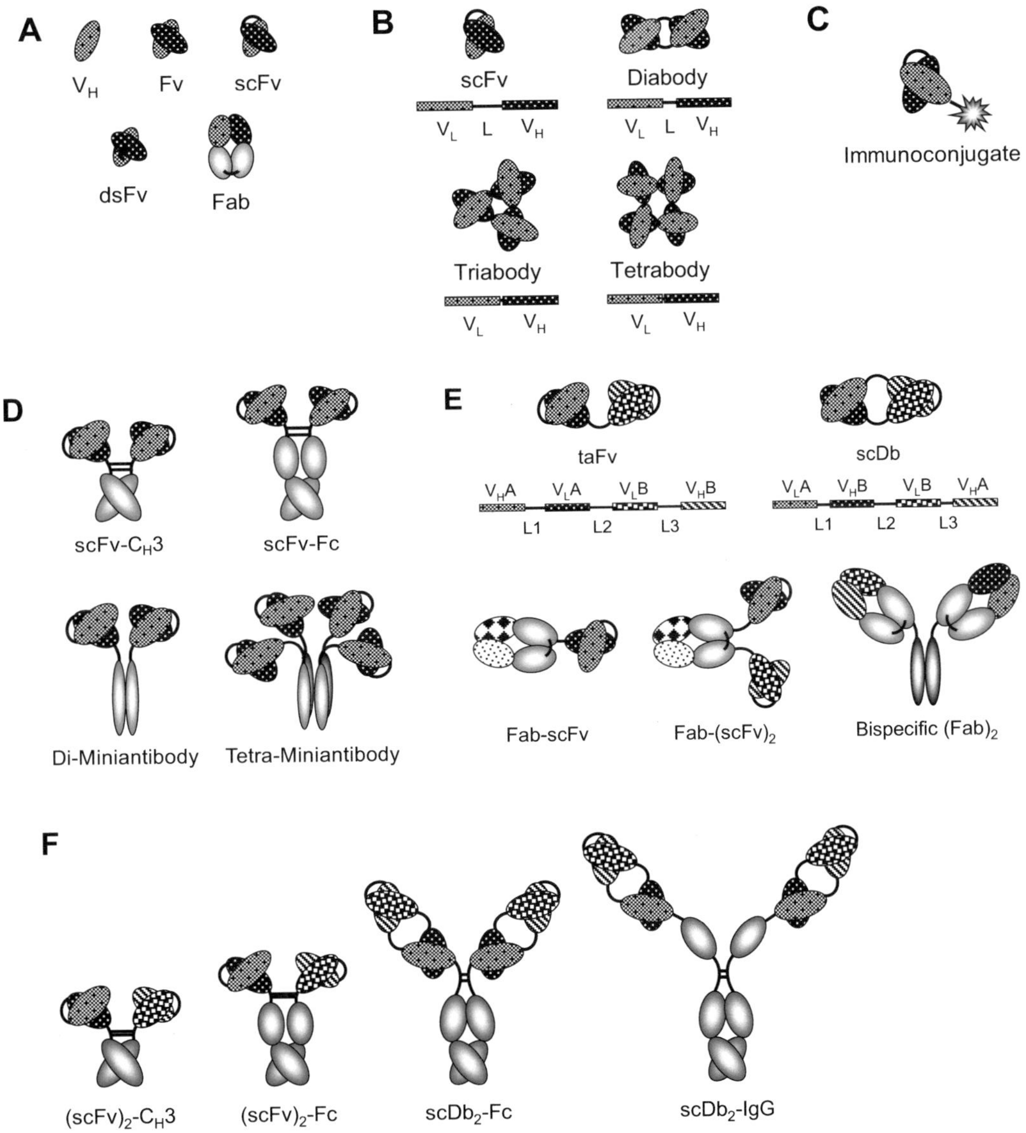

Figure 2: Schematic representation of rAbF constructs. A, monovalent rAbFs. B, scFv-based multivalent rAbFs, engineered by shortening the flexible peptide linkers of scFvs. C, immunoconjuates, constructed by chemically or genetically linking rAbFs to diverse classes of molecules (*i.e.*, toxins, cytokines, radionuclides, or enzymes). D, scFv-based miniantibodies, generated by incorporating several scFvs by either chemical coupling or genetic fusion to an adhesive domain (*i.e.*, C_H3 domain or Fc region of an IgG or leucine zippers). E, scFv- and Fab-based bispecific rAbFs, engineered by genetic fusion of scFv or Fab with different specificities *via* flexible peptide linkers or an adhesive domain. F, IgG-like bispecific molecules, constructed by fusion of rAbFs with different specificities with the C_H3 domain, Fc region, or C_H1-C_H2-C_H3 fragment of an IgG, which are capable of recruiting all effector functions of the Fc isotype.

4.2. Engineering with Improved Pharmacokinetics

4.2.1. PEGylation

Conjugation with hydrophilic polymers is a widely used approach for improving pharmacokinetic profiles of therapeutic proteins, including antibody molecules. The resulting conjugates have been shown to be more stable, less immunogenic and have a longer serum half-life when compared to unmodified molecules [82, 83]. To date, the most successful approach used to improve the pharmacokinetics of antibody molecules is PEGylation, by which polyethylene glycol (PEG) molecules with different MWs are randomly or site-specifically coupled to amino groups of antibody molecules (Fig. **3A**) [83, 84]. PEGylation provides antibody molecules with several advantages, including reduction in immunogenicity, improvement of stability, prolongation of serum half-life, and retention of *in vivo* biological activity[83].

PEGylation increases apparent MW of rAbFs to above the glomerular filtration cutoff, thereby prolonging their half-lives [84]. Preclinical studies showed that PEGylation of Fab and scFv increased their circulation time and promoted efficacy of immunotherapy for a variety of applications [83, 85, 86]. For example, the pharmacokinetic profiles of anti-TNF-α and anti-VEGFR2 di-Fab′ fragments for treatments of rheumatoid arthritis [85] and solid tumor [86], respectively, were significantly improved after PEGylation, with a minimal loss of antigen binding activity. The site-specific PEGylation extended circulation time of scFvs by 30- to 100-fold [30, 87] and sVDs from 20 min to 39 h in mice (I.M. Tomlinson, Domantis, Cambridge, personal communication). PEGylation is also efficient in reducing immunogenicity [84] and enhancing toxin-neutralization [88] or anti-tumor activities [89]. After PEGylated with a PEG (40 kDa), a scFv specific for *Bacillus anthracis* exotoxin had a serum half-life of 108 h, which was longer than that of murine IgG (96 h), and it conferred significant protection in guinea pigs challenged with a relatively high dose of anthrax spores [88]. Site-specific PEGylation also extended the serum half-life an anti-TNF-α Fab from 23 h to 14 days in rheumatoid arthritis patients [90]. An anti-TNF-α Fab-PEG conjugate has completed phase III clinical trials in patients with Crohn's disease [91]. Similarly, after site-specific PEGylation, an anti-platelet GPIIb/IIIa Fab exhibited prolonged circulation time and also effectively inhibited platelet aggregation [89]. By increasing *in vivo* half-lives, PEGylation can also promote tumor localization of the modified molecules. As a result of prolonged serum half-lives, the attachment of a PEG (20 kDa) to an anti-HER2 scFv and to its dimer markedly improved tumor accumulation by 8.5- and 14.5-fold, respectively, when compared to the unmodified molecules 48 h post-administration [69]. PEGylations are suitable not only for monomeric fragments but also for immunoconjugates, thus facilitating delivery of effector molecules to target sites [69, 92-95].

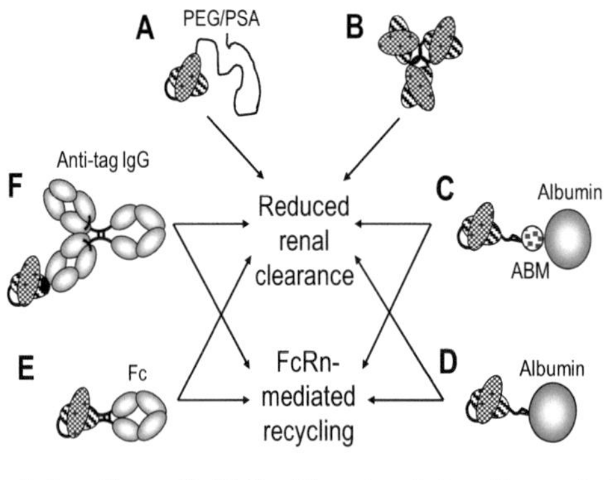

Figure 3: Strategies to prolong circulation time of rAbFs. The circulation time of rAbFs can be increased by attaching them to polyethylene glycol (PEG) or polysialic acids (PSA) (A), multimerization or by (B), fusing them to an albumin-binding moiety (ABM) (C), directly to an albumin (D), the Fc region of an IgG (E), or an eptiope tag recognized by an anti-tag IgG (F). These strategies prolong the circulation time of rAbFs through either reducing the renal clearance by increasing their apparent molecular weights or by FcRn-mediated recycling mechanism by the addition of an Fc region.

Despite significant success in improving pharmacokinetics of therapeutic proteins, studies have shown that PEGylation has several drawbacks. One of the drawbacks is that PEG is not biodegradable; thus, when

PEGylated proteins have an apparent MW above the glomerular filtration cutoff, PEG will accumulate in lysosome of exposed tissues [96]. Furthermore, PEGylated proteins have been found to stimulate the generation of anti-PEG antibodies that may reduce therapeutic efficiency by removing the PEGylated molecules from the body [97]. Fortunately, no adverse effects of PEG immunogenicity have been observed [96]. Moreover, PEGylation have been reported to lead to some loss of antigen-binding activity, even at a low loading. For example, PEGylation with an average of 4 and 10 PEGs per antibody molecule resulted in a 70% and 90% reduction in binding activity, respectively, while attachment with 15 PEGs per antibody led to complete loss of binding activity [84]. Although site-specific PEGylation extended the half-life of an anti-TNF-α scFv by up to 100-fold in mice, its reactivity to target antigen was significantly inhibited as a result of PEGylation [87]. Similarly, PEGylation with a 20 kDa PEG improved tumor-specific uptake of an anti-HER2 scFv, but the scFv-PEG conjugate showed a 5-fold reduction in binding affinity [69]. In the case of intact mAbs, PEGylation also substantially compromised the Fc-mediated effector functions, such as complement fixation and FcR binding. The FcR binding activity was reduced by 16% when 4.4% of amines of an antibody were conjugated with 8 kDa PEG and by greater than 50% when a little over a quarter of amines were modified [84]. These studies demonstrate that PEGylation can influence the antigen-binding and Fc-mediated activities very readily, leading to a marked reduction in therapeutic potency of antibody molecules.

4.2.2. Polysialylation

Another approach commonly used to improve pharmacokinetics of antibody molecules is polysialylation, by which rAbFs are conjugated with the naturally occurring polysialic acids (PSA) of different MWs (Fig. **3A**). PSAs are hydrophilic linear polymers of *N*-acetylneuraminic acid (sialic acid) that abundantly presents on many proteins and cell surfaces [82]. Certain bacteria have evolved to escape host defenses by coating their cell walls with PSAs [98]. The ability of PSA to protect invading bacteria from the host defense has been employed to improve the clinical application efficiency of therapeuticals by preserving both structural integrity and therapeutic activity as well as prolonging serum persistence. Polysialylation is believed to be as effective as PEGylation but without the potential toxicity. Unlike PEG, PSA is biodegradable and exhibits a long half-life of up to 40 h in mice [98]. Conjugation with PSAs can abrogate the immunogenicity of heterogeneous proteins and also increase their stability and persistence in the serum, thus reducing dosages and frequency of administration [82]. In addition, the highly ionic state of PSA also contributes to prolonged serum persistence of conjugated proteins by reducing their loss through the kidneys [99]. These unique properties, especially the low toxicity and natural metabolism, make PSA an attractive alternative to PEG for improving the pharmacokinetic profiles of short-lived therapeutic drugs. For example, conjugation of an anti-tumor Fab with PSA of different MWs increased its half-life by 50- to 80-fold, when compared to the unmodified Fab and also improved its tumor localization [100]. Similarly, polysialylation with a PSA prolonged the circulating half-life of an anti-placental alkaline phosphatase (PLAP) Fab by 5-fold and improved tumor uptake by 3-fold, with only a minor decrease in tumor-to-blood ratios, when compared to the unconjugated Fab [101]. This Fab-PSA conjugate also had a blood bioavailability comparable to that of an intact mAb, and different coupling ratios and length of PSAs to the Fab had a minor effect on its antigen binding activity [101]. A prime consideration when using PSA as a carrier for antibody molecules is the maintenance of their biological functions, such as antigen binding affinity and interactions with FcR or complement in the case of intact mAbs.

4.2.3. Multimerization

As previously stated molecular size has important impact on pharmacokinetics and biodistribution of antibody molecules. Therefore, Fab and scFv monomeric fragments are often engineered into multivalent molecules (*e.g.* diabodies, triabodies, tetrabodies and minibodies) by either chemical or genetic cross-links to improve their pharmakinetic profiles and antigen binding avidity as well (Fig. **2B**, **2D**, **2E**, and **2F**; Fig. **3B;** Table **1A**) [31, 40, 67, 68]. All these multivalent molecules had a higher MW and exhibited a more favorable pharmacokinetics than monomeric parent fragments [69]. For example, a divalent $(scFv)_2$ and tetravalent $[(scFv)_2]_2$ of a mAb CC49 had a $t1/2_\beta$ of 144 min and 307 min, respectively, which was much higher than that of monomeric scFv [38]. Multimerization has been proven to be an effective approach for improving the therapeutic potential of rAbFs through prolongation of their half-lives by increasing the apparent MW and improvement of their antigen binding avidity by increasing the binding valency [69, 102].

4.3. Fusion or Association with Long-Lived Serum Molecules

To prolong the serum persistence of rAbFs, they can be non-covalently associated with naturally occurring long-lived serum proteins, such as albumin (67 kDa) (Fig. **3C** and **3D,** Table **1B**) [103, 104] and IgG (150 kDa) (Fig. **3E** and **3F**) [105]. Albumin was originally used as a carrier for small drugs because it has a long half-life of 19 days in humans as a result of interaction with FcRn at a site different from that of IgG [103]. In recent years, it has also been utilized to extend the half-lives of small rAbFs [103, 104, 106]. By fusion to human serum albumin, the serum half-lives of bispecific rAbFs, *i.e.*, tandem scFv (taFv), diabodies (Db), and single chain diabodies (scDb), which were directed against the tumor antigen carcinoembryonic antigen (CEA) and the T cell receptor complex molecule CD3, were substantially prolonged [104]. The $t_{1/2\alpha}$ was dramatically increased from 5 to 37 min for taFv, from 8 to 43 min for scDb, and from 8 to 117 min for $(scFv)_2$, while fully retaining their binding capacities to both antigens. Alternatively, albumin binding peptides were also used to prolong serum persistence of rAbFs from mins to hours (Fig. **3D**) [107, 108]. When fused to an albumin binding domain, *in vivo* half-life was extended 26-fold to 10.4 h in mouse and 37-fold to 32.4 h in rabbit, as compared to the unmodified Fab [107]. Similarly, after fusion to an albumin binding peptide, the circulation time of a bispecific scDb, specific for cytotoxic Tcells and CEA-expressing tumor cells, was prolonged 5- to 6-fold as compared to unfused scDb [109]. Several human sVDs, specific for mouse, rat and/or human serum albumin, showed serum half-lives that were similar to that of serum albumin and much longer than those (less than 45 min) of control sVDs that had no specificity to albumin [110]. More importantly, the serum half-lives of small drugs and their *in vivo* therapeutic efficacy were dramatically increased after fusion with albumin-binding sVDs [110]. Site-specific conjugation of a Fab′, non-covalent coupling of a bispecific $F(ab')_2$ that binds rat serum albumin, and genetic fusion of a scFv to rat serum albumin substantially extended *in vivo* half-lives of these fragments in rats while retaining the full antigen binding capabilities of their parental molecules [111]. The albumin-conjugated Fab′ had an Area Under the Curve (AUC) 17-fold greater than did the control Fab′conjugated to cysteine, while the AUC of the bispecific $F(ab')_2$ was 8-fold greater than a non-albumin-binding control $F(ab')_2$.

The use of IgG is an attractive alternative to other macromolecular drug carriers for the improvement of pharmacokinetics of small drugs and for the systemic drug delivery to target tissues (Fig. **3F**). The large MW (150 kDa), long circulation half-life ($t_{1/2\beta}$ >21 days in humans), high serum concentration (12 mg/ml), and high binding affinity make IgGs an ideal carrier for drug delivery. For example, following binding to serum IgG, the *in vivo* half-life of a bispecific diabody was extended to 10 h, which was approximately 6-fold higher than that of a non-IgG-binding control diabody [105]. Moreover, the diabody-IgG complex was able to mediate Fc-dependent effector functions, *i.e.*, ADCC, ADCP, and CDC [105]. When immunocomplexed with endogenous IgG, CpG-oligodeoxynucleotides (CpG-ODNs) displayed a substantial increase in systemic exposure by 900-1650 fold and in half-life by 100-300 fold, and a remarkable decrease in systemic clearance by 750-1500 fold and in volume of tissue distribution by 13-37 fold [112]. CpG-ODN-IgG immunocomplexes also showed sustained tumor accumulation and enhanced antitumor activity.

The Fc region of IgGs has been fused with rAbFs to prolong the serum persistence of these molecules *via* increasing their apparent MW and FcRn-mediated recycling mechanism (Fig. **3E**) [12, 13]. Bivalent $(scFv)_2$ fused to the Fc region exhibited longer tumor retention time and increased serum half-lives ranging from 93 h to 12 days when compared to the unmodified scFvs that had a typical half-life of 3.5 h [113, 114]. Alternatively, rAbFs were also fused to IgG C_H3 domains either chemically or genetically to produce minibodies with increased half-lives [3, 77, 115].

In addition to the strategies described above, N-linked glycosylation and modification of the surface charge (isoelectric point, pI) were also used as alternative approaches for half-life extension of small rAbFs [116]. Introduction of N-linked glycosylation into a flanking linker and a C-terminal peptide of a bispecific scDb specific for both CEA and CD3 extended its half-life by 2 to 3-fold [116]. Modification of the pI of rAbFs altered their pharmacokinetics by interfering with their interactions with the kidneys [117, 118]. This strategy was also effective at increasing the tumor uptake of a Fab from 8.3% to 14.8% ID/g [117] and at reducing toxicity of both the scFv and Fv-PE38 immunotoxin without affecting their biological activities [119, 120]. However, other studies showed that the renal uptake and whole body retention of a dsFv [118] and a Fab [117] were reduced by lowering pI.

4.4. Engineering Novel Effector Functions

4.4.1. Immunoconjugates

For some applications, particularly in tumor therapy, rAbFs have been linked chemically or genetically to diverse classes of molecules that provide them with important effector functions, resulting in the formation of immunoconjugates (Fig. **2C**, Table **1B**). These effector molecules include toxins, radionuclides, cytokines, Major Histocompatibility Complexes (MHC), cytotoxic prodrugs, enzymes and liposomes. By conjugation with antibody molecules, these effector molecules can be specifically delivered to target sites, their half-lives can be prolonged, and the possible systemic toxicity to normal tissues can be reduced, which frequently is observed during systemic application of toxins or cytokines alone in cancer treatments [121]. The effector molecule is directed by the antibody to the disease site where it induces target cell-specific destruction. The easy generation and high yield of rAbF-based conjugates together with their potent anti-tumor activity make rAbFs promising vehicles for new generation of cancer therapeutics.

4.5. Immunotoxin

Among immunoconjugates, the most studied are immunotoxins, which consist of a tumor-specific antibody molecule fused to a protein toxin capable of killing target cells once internalized (Fig. **4B**) [122, 123]. Immunotoxins are wildly studied for cancer therapy because of the catalytic nature of protein toxins and their cytotoxic effectiveness with only a limited number of toxin molecules being required to cause cell death. Many protein toxins are composed of two subunits; one has the enzymatic activity , while the other subunit is essential for binding of the toxin to its receptor on the surface of the host cells for subsequent translocation of the enzymatic subunit across the membrane [124]. Once internalized and released from the native toxin, the enzymatic component becomes active and performs the cytotoxic function. For therapeutic applications, these toxins are usually modified to remove their binding subunits to avoid non-specific binding to normal tissues [125] and deglycosylated to escape uptake by liver cells expressing mannose receptors [126]. Furthermore, to achieve the specific targeting and to reduce the systemic cytotoxicity, toxins are usually conjugated with targeting molecules, *i.e.* antibody molecules, growth factors, cytokines, and peptide hormones [127]. Various toxins, mainly ribosome-inactivating or translation-inhibiting polypeptides, have been used in immunotoxin engineering. These include plant toxins (*e.g.* ricin, abrin, gelonin, and saporin) that inactivate ribosomes and fungal (*e.g.* α-sarcin) and bacterial toxins [(*e.g.* *Pseudomonas* exotoxin A (PE) and Diphtheria Toxin (DT)] that inhibit protein synthesis by adenosine diphosphate (ADP) ribosylating elongation factor 2 (EF-2) (Fig. **4B**) [123, 128]. PE and DT are the most commonly used in clinical trials because they can be easily produced in *E. coli* and have greater cytotoxic activities with fewer side effects when compared to plant or fungal toxins [128].

There are several types of antibody-based immunotoxins, with scFvs being most commonly used rAbF platform. A number of immunotoxins, constructed by coupling of plant or bacterial toxins with scFvs directed against various antigens, *i.e.*, CD3, CD22, CD25, CD30, Lewis Y antigen, EGFR, ErbB2/HER2, and mesothelin, have been evaluated for the treatments of hematological malignancies and solid tumors [122, 123, 129, 130]. These immunotoxins were selectively cytotoxic to antigen-positive malignant cell lines and leukemic cells isolated from cancer patients; treatment with these immunotoxins led to significant tumor regression in animals bearing tumor xenografts and high responses in patients with cancers, with several being evaluated in clinical trials [130-134]. For example, anti-CD25 scFv coupled with PE40 or PE38 immunotoxin displayed cytotoxicity only against $CD25^+$ malignant cell lines and leukemic cells isolated from patients [135, 136]; treatment with these immunotoxins resulted in complete tumor regression in mice bearing human $CD25^+$ xenografts [137, 138]. The anti-CD25 scFv-PE38 treatment also caused 100% response in patients with Hairy-Cell Leukemia (HCL) [139] and partial responses in patients with

Chronic Lymphocytic Leukemia (CLL), adult T-cell leukemia (ATL), or Hodgkin Disease (HD) [135]. Similarly, an anti-CD22 dsFv-PE38 immunocojugate not only showed specific cytotoxicity to $CD22^+$ tumor cell lines and leukemic cells from patients with CLL and Non-Hodgkin's Lymphoma (NHL), but also induced complete tumor regression in mice bearing human tumor $CD22^+$ xenografts [139-141]. Furthermore, HCL patients treated with this immunotoxin showed 61% complete remission and 19% partial responses [133, 134, 142]. This immunotoxin is currently in phase I trail for both CLL and pediatric Acute Lymphoblastic Leukemia (ALL) and in phase II trial for HCL.

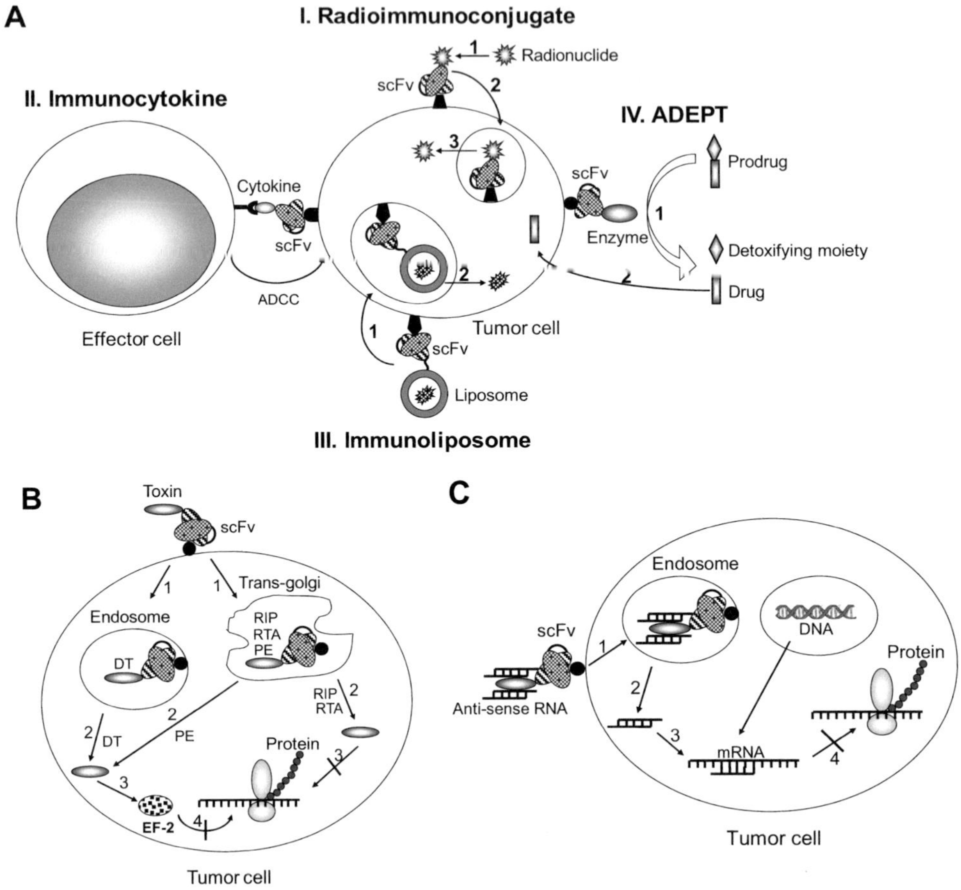

Figure 4: Therapeutic applications of rAbF-based immunoconjugates. Radionuclides (A-I) and toxic drugs embedded in a liposome (A-III) can be directed to tumor cells by rAbFs. Once internalized *via* endocytosis, these molecules are released into the cytosol from endosomes and exert their cytotoxic activities on their targets, resulting in the destruction of tumor cells. Cytokines (*i.e.*, IL-2, 12, 18, TNFα) (A-II) attached to rAbFs can be used to modulate the immune response (*i.e.*, recruitment and activation of immune effector cells) against tumor cells. Alternatively, the antibody-directed enzyme prodrug therapy (ADEPT) (A-IV) approach is used to convert a prodrug to a chemotherapeutic agent in the target site by an enzyme that is delivered to tumor cells *via* an anti-tumor rAbF. B. A bacterial, fungal or plant toxin can be directed to tumor cells by a tumor-specific rAbF and subsequently localized by endocytosis to an endosome in the case of DT (diphtheria toxin) or the ER and trans-Golgi apparatus in the case of PE and plant-derived ribosome-inactivating proteins (RIP). Inside these organelles, the toxin is unattached from rAbF by proteolytic cleavage and then released into the cytosol where it inactivates the protein synthesis machinery of the target cell, leading to cell death. DT and PE inactivate elongation factor-2 (EF-2) and activate caspase 3, whereas RIP cleaves a single adenine base from ribosomal RNA and thereby prevent its binding to EF-2. C. RAbFs can also be used in gene therapy to specifically delivery anti-sense RNAs to tumor cells. After internalization *via* endocytosis and release into the cytoplasm, dsRNA is unwound and the unwound single-stranded antisense RNA represses translation by pairing to partial complementary sites of target mRNAs, inhibiting protein thesis.

scFv-based immunotoxins have high tissue penetration due to their small MW; however, the refolding yields and stability of scFv-toxins were relatively low [143, 144]. Due to these limitations attempts have been made to produce dsFv- and Fab-based immunotoxins. As compared with scFv-toxins, dsFv-toxins were more stable and had higher yields [145, 146]. Similarly, divalent immunotoxins $(Fab\text{-}SWn\text{-}PE38)_2$ and $(Fab\text{-}PE38fl)_2$, generated by a disulfide bond formation between two corresponding monomers, were very stable and had a cytotoxicity on tumor cells 18.8-fold and 2.5-fold higher than that of the monomeric molecules, respectively [147, 148]. In comparison with scFv-toxins, Fab-toxins have two major advantages: higher expression yield (*e.g.* 10-fold higher than that of scFv-toxin and dsFv-toxin) [149, 150] and improved stability (*e.g.* comparable to that of the whole antibody-toxin) [151-154].

The cytotoxic effect of immunotoxins to tumor cells depends on several biochemical properties, including target-binding affinity, internalization ability, intracellular processing and intrinsic toxicity [155]. For example, the difference in the internalization rate resulted in an 11-fold difference in the cytotoxic effect of an anti-ganglioside GD2 immunotoxin in two different tumor cell lines [156]. Despite these promising results in preclinical studies, the potent application of immunotoxins in cancer therapy is frequently hampered by their systemic cytotoxicity (*i.e.*, vascular leak syndrome and hepatocyte injury) and the immunogenicity of the toxins [131]. Several strategies have been utilized to overcome the problems associated with the immunogenicity of toxins; such examples include co-administration of immunosuppressive agents and modifications of toxins [157]. PEGylation of toxins and genetic engineering of humanized toxins have been shown to be promising approaches to reduce the toxin immunogenicity [127, 157, 158].

4.6. Immunocytokine

Immunocytokines are fusion proteins of tumor-specific antibody molecules conjugated to immunostimulatory cytokines, *i.e.*, interleukin (IL)-2, IL-12, IL-15, TNFα, cytotoxic T-lymphocyte antigen (CTLA)-4, interferon (IFN)α, IFNγ, and granulocyte-macrophage colony stimulating factor (GM-CSF) (Fig. **4AII**) [159-165]. Cytokines, secreted by specific cells of the immune system, have pleiotropic activities, including stimulation of growth, differentiation, and activation of normal cells as well as participation in pro- and anti-inflammatory responses, all which depend on the microenvironment [166-168]. Cytokines also have potent anti-tumor activities [169-171]. However, cytokine-based cancer therapy is often compromised by systemic toxicities due to non-specific exposure to normal tissues, which significantly hampers their therapeutic efficiency [172, 173]. To reduce the side effects associated to the systemic action of cytokines and to improve their specific redelivery to target sites, they have been fused to anti-tumor antibody molecules, thus generating immunocytokines. The antibody molecules are used to target coupled cytokines to tumor sites where cytokines recruit and subsequently activate cytotoxic cells such as cytotoxic T lymphocytes (CTL) and natural killer (NK) cells, leading to target cell destruction [162, 165].

Among the cytokines, IL-2 fused with antibody molecules is the most studied [174-177]; several antibody-IL-2 fusion proteins have proven to be effective in preclinical studies for treatments of lung metastases [178, 179] and breast cancer [179, 180], and in phase I clinical trials for the treatments of melanoma and neuroblastoma [181-183]. Some have shown promising results. One such example is an anti-fibronectin scFvL19-IL-12 fusion protein that was found to be more effective than IL-12 alone in several mouse models with different aggressive murine tumors [178, 180]. Immunocytokines of an anti-fibronectin scFv-IL-12 fused with either a p40-p35 heterodimer, p40, or p35 showed excellent tumor targeting and potent anti-tumor activities [184]. Other immunocytokines, *i.e.*, anti-tumor scFv-IL-2, scFv-IL-15, scFv-TNFα, scFv-GM-CSF, and scFv-IFNγ, were demonstrated to exhibit excellent tumor uptake and potent anti-tumor activities, both in subcutaneous and metastatic tumor-based mouse models, *via* the recruitment and activation of $CD8^+$ T cells at target sites [185-189]. An immunocytokine scFvMEL/TNF, specific for the melanoma gp240 antigen, showed impressive cytotoxic effects against human melanoma cell lines *in vitro*, and systemic administration led to potent tumor suppression and complete tumor regression of all lesions in athymic mice bearing established human melanoma xenograft tumors [190]. In another example, an anti-HER2/neu scFv-TNFα immunocytokine was able to elicit HER2/neu signaling, prevent apoptosis, and promote wound healing of injured epithelia *in vitro* [191]. Furthermore, the anti-tumor activity of immunocytokines was enhanced by combination with other effector molecules, *i.e.*, doxorubicin and other immunocytokines [188]. For example, the combination of anti-fibronectin scFv-IL-12 with scFv-TNFα fusion proteins resulted in synergistic anti-tumor activity and led to the eradication of teratocarcinomas grafts in immunocompetent mice and a delayed onset of tumor growth due to the induction of a partial antitumor vaccination effect [192]. In spite of these promising outcomes, poor protein production and adverse immune reactions, *e.g.* tumor lysis syndrome, acute phase response, tissue injury, and vascular leak syndrome, are all potential side effects of cytokine-based therapies, and thus have severely comprised their preclinical evaluation [162].

In addition to using immunocytokines and bispecific antibodies, CTLs can also be redirected to tumor sites by MHC containing antigenic peptides that are linked to tumor-specific rAbFs. For instance, monomeric MHC complex coupled to an anti-TAA Fab selectively induced tumor cell killing by $CD8^+$ T cells through the oligomerization of the MHC on tumor cells [193]. An anti-tumor scFv-MHC fusion inhibited the growth of human tumor xenografts *via* recruitment and activation of CTLs in nude mice injected with large amounts of cloned human T cells [194]. Immunoconjugates, *e.g.* anti-CEA Fab conjugated to MHC-viral peptide (anti-CEA X H-2D(b)/GP33 LCMV peptide) [195, 196] and anti-HER2 Fab conjugated to MHC-viral peptide (anti-HER2 X H-2D(b)/NP366 influenza peptide) [197], were created to deliver the MHC-viral peptides to the surface of cancer cells, subsequently inducing specific tumor cell lysis by the recruitment of T cells. Furthermore, systemic treatment with the Fab-MHC-viral peptides conjugates completely abolished tumor growth in four of five immunocompetent mice infected with the virus [198]. Similarly, systemic administration of an anti-HER2 scFv-αGalCer/sCD1d (non-polymorphic MHC related molecules) immunoconjugate resulted in inhibition of experimental lung metastasis and established subcutaneous tumors, as a result of accumulation and activation of iNKT, NK, and T cells at the tumor site [199]. These systemic studies demonstrate the potential of immunocytokines in cancer therapy.

4.7. Immunoliposomes

Immunoliposomes, constructed by conjugating target-specific antibody molecules with lipids, are used as drug carriers to deliver cytotoxic drug-loaded liposomes to diseased tissues (Fig. **4AIII**) [200, 201]. Liposomes were traditionally used as a drug delivery system in which a drug in aqueous phase is enclosed by a phospholipid membrane bilayer, which assists in formulation of poorly soluble therapeutic drugs for oral or parenteral administration [200, 202]. Due to their short half-lives *via* rapid clearance by phagocytotic cells in the liver, spleen and bone marrow [203, 204], the phospholipid bilayer of liposomes have been conjugated with PEG or gangliosides to prolong their persistence in the serum [205-208]. It is believed that the PEG coating prevents binding of opsonins from physiological fluids, thus avoiding the recognition by phagocytotic cells [203]. PEGylation of liposomes decreased systemic plasma clearance by 200-fold and increased area uner the time-concentration curve by 100-fold [208] and $t1/2\beta$ up to 90 h in human [209]. Further, to improve the target specificity and drug delivery efficiency, liposomes are conjugated with an appropriate targeting vehicle, *i.e.* proteins, peptides, or antibody molecules, *via* amino-reactive homobifunctional cross-linkers or disulfide bonds [205, 210-213].

Some impressive results have been obtained with antibody-directed immunoliposomes. PEGylated-liposomes conjugated with an anti-HER2 Fab' or scFv showed up to 6-fold greater intracellular uptake by cancer cells when compared to liposomes with no associated rAbFs (aka untargeted liposomes), which were found predominantly in extracellular stroma or within macrophages [95]. The anti-HER2 Fab′-targeted PE38 liposomes were more cytotoxic than non-targeted PE38-liposomes in HER2-overexpressing breast cancer cells [212]. Immunoliposomes, composed of an anti-fibroblast activation protein (FAP) scFv coupled to TLP-scTNF-PEG or Mal-PEG-DSPE, successfully delivered conjugated liposomes to FAP-positive cells and further led to internalization of intact liposomes into the endosomal compartment [206]. Similarly, an anti-epithelial cell adhesion molecule (EpCAM) scFv-based immunoliposome was able to specifically target antisense oligonucleotide to the EpCAM-expressing tumor cells, with 10- to 20-fold increased binding when compared to untargeted liposomes [214]. It also enhanced internalization of targeted liposomes and induced apoptosis of EpCAM-positive tumor cells. Furthermore, an anti-endoglin scFv immunoliposome (ILA5) was demonstrated to selectively bind to and subsequently be internalized by human endoglin-expressing endothelial cells *in vitro*. Furthermore, the doxorubicin-loaded ILA5 displayed enhanced cytotoxicity towards endothelial cells than non-targeted liposomes and free doxorubicin [215], demonstrating the potential for vascular targeting in cancer therapy. These studies show that the development of immunoliposomes represents another category for target cell-specific delivery and uptake of encapsulated drugs that holds promise.

4.7.1. Radioimmunotherapeutics

Radioimmunotherapeutics, consisting of target-specific antibody molecules conjugated with radionuclides, are an attractive agent particularly for tumor imaging and therapy (Fig. **4AI**). In general, short-lived radioisotope-labeled rAbFs are used for solid tumor targeting, while long-lived radioimmunotherapeutics are more desirable for tumor therapy. Once again, the small to intermediate size of rAbFs are considered to be suitable molecules for tumor imaging and therapy because of their superior properties of easy tissue penetration, high tumor retention, and rapid blood clearance [216]. These properties facilitate specific targeting of radiation to malignant cells, while minimizing background signals in tumor imaging and destruction of normal cells in tumor therapy. For example, several intermediate-sized rAbFs [*e.g.* diabodies (60 kDa)], labeled with short-lived positron-emitting radioisotopes (*e.g.* ^{123}I, ^{125}I, and ^{111}In), were demonstrated to be effective in targeting solid tumors due to fast blood clearance and rapid tumor uptake [106, 115, 217-220]. They also functioned well in imaging angiogenesis [221] and atherosclerotic plaques [222]. Conversely, larger sized rAbFs [*e.g.* minibodies (90 kDa), Fab′$_2$ dimers (110 kDa), and scFv tetramers (120 kDa)] have been proven to be suitable for tumor therapy in preclinical trials when labeled with long-lived radioisotopes (*e.g.* ^{64}Cu, ^{124}I, and ^{90}Y) because of higher total tumor uptake and faster blood clearance when compared to intact mAb (150 kDa) [50, 67, 81, 217, 219, 223, 224] . Indeed, a single intravenous administration of a ^{90}Y-labeled diabody inhibited growth of established HER2 tumor xenografts in nude mice [223].

In addition to co-administration of rAbFs with coupled radionuclides, a pretargeting approach, in which an anti-tumor rAbF is administered first, then followed by administration of a radioisotopic compound capable of binding to the localized rAbF (Fig. **4AI**), have been shown to perform well in tumor-targeting with higher tumor-to-normal tissue ratios than that obtained with one-step radioimmunotherapy [217, 225-228]. For example, administration of tetrameric [(scFv)$_2$]$_2$-streptavdin fusion proteins, followed by treatment with ^{111}In-DOTA-biotin 24 hours later, showed superior tumor-to-normal tissue ratios of radioactivity; more than 90% of mice bearing lymphoma were cured with minimal toxicity using either antibody conjugate followed by treatment with ^{90}Y-DOTA-biotin [229]. Administration of an anti-CD20 [(scFv)$_2$]$_2$-streptavidin fusion protein, followed by therapy with $^{90}Y/^{111}In$-DOTA-biotin 24 hours later, resulted in 2 complete remissions and one partial response out of 15 patients with B cell NHL [230]. Furthermore, the pretargeting with bispecific F(ab')$_2$ or tri-Fab, specific for both an antigen on tumor cells and a hapten-peptide linked with a diagnostic or therapeutic radionuclide, followed by treatment with a radiolabeled peptide, were very effective at targeting specific tumor cells and showed improved tumor uptake of radio-labeled peptide and enhanced tumor-to-blood ratios when compared with the corresponding radiolabeled IgG [217, 224, 226]. They also displayed enhanced therapeutic efficacy in animal models as compared with ^{90}Y-IgG [217, 224]. Similar results were obtained when tumor cells were pretargeted with a bispecific scFv-Fab (AP39Xm679) specific for both fibronectin and a small peptidic hapten Histamine-Succinyl-Glycine (HSG), followed by subsequent injection of ^{90}Y-hapten-peptide; the resulting therapeutic efficacy in solid tumors was 3-fold greater than that of a directly radiolabeled control scFv [227]. Finally, radioisotope-labeled anti-CEA Fab$_2$ and scFv have been approved by FDA for the imaging of colon cancer metastasis [231]. All these results demonstrate the improved therapeutic efficacy of pretargeting the tumor with BsAbs before radionucleide administration, when compared with conventional therapy using a antibody labeled with the radionucleide.

5. ADEPT

Antibody-Directed Enzyme Prodrug Therapy (ADEPT) is aimed at restricting the anti-tumor effect of a toxic drug to cells targeted by antibodies. In typical ADEPT, antibody molecules are coupled with enzymes that are able to convert non-toxic prodrugs into active drugs at disease sites (Fig. **4AIV**) [232, 233]. ADEPT is a three-phase system. First, an enzyme of choice is specifically localized to target sites by coupling it with a target-specific antibody. Then, another antibody, or some other reagent, is used to inactivate and clear the administered enzyme from the blood but not the targeted tissue. Finally, a non-toxic prodrug is administered and subsequently converted into an active and highly cytotoxic agent in the previously targeted tissues [232, 234]. Three types of enzymes have been used in ADEPT, and include; type I enzymes that are of non-mammalian origin with no mammalian homologues, type II enzymes that are of non-mammalian origin with a mammalian homologue, and type III enzymes that are of mammalian origin [235]. Type I enzymes have the advantage that prodrugs can be designed not to be cleaved by endogenous enzymes, thereby avoiding non-specific cytotoxicity. The major disadvantage of type I enzymes is that they may stimulate an immune response because of their non-mammalian origin, thereby reducing therapeutic efficacy. By contrast, type III enzymes are less immunogenic, but prodrugs designed for these types of enzymes may be cleaved by endogenous enzymes, thus reducing cytotoxic specificity. Type II enzymes have the disadvanges of immunogenicity and induction of non-specific cytotoxicity.

Despite the disadvantages of ADEPT mentioned above, several antibody-enzyme conjugates have been developed and evaluated in animal models [7, 232]. For example, a fusion protein of an anti-CEA diabody with the bioluminescence enzyme *Renilla* luciferase, which is able to catalyze the odidation of D-Luciferin to yield light, was used as a probe to visualize CEA-positive xenografts in mice [236]. Furthermore, an Epidermal Growth Factor Receptor (EGFR)-specific scFv fused to a pro-apoptotic serine protease granzyme B exhibited selective and effective killing of EGFR-positive tumor cells *via* activation of apoptosis pathway through direct activation of caspases and cleavage of central caspase substrates [237]. An A33scFv-CDy conjugate, formed by fusing anti-gpA33 scFv with cytosine deaminase from yeast (CDy) that converts 5-fluorocytosine (5-FC) into 5-Fluorouracil (5-FU), displayed cytotoxicity *in vitro* comparable to that of 5-FU [238, 239] and also had excellent tumor uptake of 87% ID/g 47 h post injection, and a high tumor-to-blood ratio of 8:1 at 67 h post injection [240]. Treatment with this A33scFv-CDy-5-Fc/5-FU ADEPT system resulted in a significant reduction of tumor size in mice [240]. In another example, a humanized anti-CEA scFv successfully delivered a carboxypeptidase G2 enzyme to the tumor site for local activation of the mustard prodrug ZD2767P, with a tumor-to-plasma ratio of 1400:1 and 339:1 in two different animal models [7, 241]. Furthermore, treatment with this conjugate resulted in inhibition of tumor growth and some regressions of established tumor xenografts in both animal models [7] and currently is in phase I clinical trial [241]. Several nanobody-based fusion proteins with enzymes have also been generated. For example, nanobody-β-lactamase [242] and nanobody-GFP [243] immunoconjugates were recently constructed and evaluated for ADEPT and live-cell imaging, respectively. The nanobody-β-lactamase conjugate, formed by coupling a camelid anti-CEA V_HH to a *Enterobacter cloacae* β-lactamase effectively activated a cephalosporin prodrug on the surface of CEA-expressing tumor cells *in vitro*, showed excellent biodistribution profiles *in vivo*, and induced regressions and cures of established tumor xenografts in mice with minimal toxicity [242]. These encouraging preclinical studies indicate the feasibility of ADEPT for cancer treatment. However, most of the enzymes used in ADEPT are of non-human origin and have potential to evoke immune responses. To circumvent possible immunogenicity and to achieve high therapeutic efficacy, it has been proposed that these enzymes be humanized or other methods be used to reduce their immunogenicity [244, 245].

5.1. Gene Therapy

Antibody molecules can also be used for delivering oligonucleotides, *i.e.*, antisense RNA, small interfering RNAs (siRNA) and micro RNA (miRNA), into target cells in gene therapy (Fig. **4C**) [76, 246]. These oligonucleotides have been shown to have high affinity to their target mRNAs, and thus inhibit their functions *in vitro*. Consequently, these antibody/oligonucleotides have potential to be used for down-regulation of numerous intracellular mRNA targets, thereby inhibiting viral replication and tumor growth [246-248]. However, the delivery of these oligonucleotides into target cells has been a key obstacle to their therapeutic application. They are generally delivered to target cells *in vitro via* lipid-mediated transfection or electroporation. However, both delivery methods are not broadly applicable for *in vivo* administration. Currently used approaches for *in vivo* delivery of these therapeutics include formulation in ligand-targeted nanoparticles [249] and in lipid-encapsulated oligonucleotides [250, 251].

The unique properties of high affinity and specific binding of antibodies to their targets make them a valuable carrier for the target-specific delivery of antisense oligonucleotides. For example, an anti-EpCAM scFv-based immunoliposome has successfully delivered an antisense oligonucleotide to tumor cells expressing EpCAM and further induced its internalization by receptor-mediated endocytosis [214]. The intracellular delivery of the antisense oligonucleotide resulted in down-regulation of both bcl-2 and bcl-xL expression at both mRNA and protein levels, leading to enhanced apoptosis of target tumor cells. Recently, siRNAs have been specifically delivered into hepatitis B surface antigen (HBsAg)-positive cells [252] or HER2-expressing cancer cells [253] by a protamine scFv conjugate. The siRNAs delivered by this protamine-scFv conjugate effectively inhibited HBV gene expression and replication in host cells [252]. Similarly, a protamine-Fab fusion protein specifically delivered FITC-labeled siRNAs to HIV-infected cells [6]. The siRNAs induced silencing only in cells expressing the HIV-1 envelope and inhibited HIV replication in HIV-infected primary T cells *in vitro*. Furthermore, an *in vivo* study demonstrated that the protamine-Fab-siRNAs targeted HIV-1 envelope-expressing cells but not normal cells, and further inhibited envelope-expressing subcutaneous tumor growth in mice [253]. An anti CD7 scFv-oligo-9-arginine peptide fusion protein also has been shown to specifically deliver antiviral siRNAs to HIV-infected T cells, leading to the inhibition of viral replication and prevention of disease-associated CD4 T cell loss in HIV-infected NOD/SCIDIL-$2^{-/-}$ mice that were reconstituted with human lymphocytes cells [247]. All these studies demonstrate the applicability of antibody-based delivery system for gene therapy.

Due to the high therapeutic efficiency of toxins, they have been also used for gene therapy, in which a vector carrying the gene encoding a toxin is used to deliver the toxin into target cells [254, 255]. In addition, genes encoding other therapeutic proteins or peptides were also delivered into target cells using the similar system [256, 257]. To date, most studies use either modified viruses or non-specific vectors as vehicles for the delivery of therapeutic genes to target cells [258, 259]. These vectors are less specific and viral vectors often evoke immune responses and therefore, antibody molecules have been used as a component of DNA delivery vector to increase the specificity and efficiency of gene delivery [76, 247, 252, 253, 260, 261]. In this technique, an antibody molecule is usually fused to a human DNA binding protein (*e.g.* human protamine), which contains a nuclear localization signal that directs the DNA-protein complex into the target cells and further into the nucleus where the gene expression takes place. For example, a genetic immunotoxin was constructed by fusion of a human Fab specific for the envelope glycoprotein gp 120 of HIV-1 to a human DNA-binding moiety protamine and further complexed with plasmid DNA encoding the catalytic subunit of *Pseudomonas* exotoxin. The biofunctional fusion protein was specifically delivered into HIV-1-infected cells by receptor-mediated endocytosis and further resulted in selective killing of the target cells [262]. One of the significant advantages of gene therapy is that the immune response elicited against the protein therapeutics can be avoided since they are expressed inside the cell and in addition, the DNA itself is weak or non-immunogenic [263]. The antibody-based delivery system provides a promising avenue for gene therapy despite the challenges of the potential immunogenicity of protein-RNA/DNA complex and the safety and technical hurdles for this technology.

5.2. Bispecific rAbFs

In the past few years, rAbFs have been rebuilt into multivalent bispecific antibodies (BsAbs) to improve their pharmacokinetics and therapeutic efficacy in preclinical and clinical applications (Table **1C**). In most cases, BsAbs are used to redirect cytotoxic effector cells and therapeutic agents to kill target tumor cells. BsAbs are generated by chemical linkage or genetic fusion of two rAbFs with different specificities into a single molecule. They can be engineered to bind simultaneously two adjacent epitopes on the same antigen, thereby increasing their binding avidity [79, 264]. Alternatively, they can be engineered to have two distinct antigen-binding sites (Fig. **2E** and **2F**), with one site binding to an antigen on a target cell and the other binding to a determinant (*e.g.* CD3, CD16, or CD64) on an effector cell (*e.g.* T cells, NK cells, or other mononuclear cells) [264-267]. In this type of construct, BsAbs not only redirect effector cells to target cells but also trigger their activation and lead to effective target cell destruction.

Since first described in 1983 [268], a number of bispecific scFv diabodies (BsDb) have been generated by non-covalent association of two scFvs with different specificities, introducing a disulfide bound into the V_H/V_L interface, or connecting two hybrid scFvs with a peptide linker, all which result in the formation of a single chain diabody (scDb) (Fig. **2E**) [81, 266, 269, 270]. These BsDbs are capable of recruiting a variety of effector cells to the target sites, for instance, retargeting of NK cells *via* CD16 [269, 271-273] or CTLs *via* CD3 or CD28 [81, 267, 274-276] to tumor sites for tumor ablation. For example, BsDbs, targeted to viral surface protein or tumor antigen CD19 and CD3 on T cells, cross-linked CTLs and target cells and further induced T-cell cytotoxicity to virus-infected tumor cells [275] or CD19-positive tumor cells [277], respectively. Other bispecific scFv-based antibodies, *i.e.*, taFv, Db, dsFv-dsFv, and scDb, were able to retarget CTLs to tumor cells, leading to tumor cell destruction with or without fusion to albumin [81, 109, 264]. Furthermore, preclinical studies showed that EpCAMXCD3 and CD30XCD16 BsDbs completely inhibited outgrowth of xenografted tumor cells and induced a marked regression of established tumors in mouse models *via* recruitment and activation of CTLs [278] and human NK cells [272, 279], respectively. Moreover, CD19XCD16 and CD19XCD3 BsDbs were able to induce lysis of CD19-positive tumor cells in the presence of human Peripheral Blood Lymphocytes (PBLs) *in vitro*, and lead to partial tumor regression when applied alone and complete tumor eradication when combined, in 80% of SCID mice bearing an established human Burkitt's lymphoma. This was achieved by recruitment and activation of different populations of human effector cells to the target tumor site [272].

Currently, two BsAbs called BiTE (bispecific T-cell engager) antibodies, Blinatumomab (MT103) and MT110, are being tested in clinical trials. MT103, a CD19- and CD3-bispecific scDb, consistently caused lysis of human lymphoma cell lines *via* activation of granzyme-mediated apoptosis [267]. Blinatumomab is currently being tested in a phase I trial in patients with late stage, relapsed NHL [274] and in a phase II trial in patients with B-precursor acute lymphoblastic leukemia (B-ALL) [276]. Clinical studies showed that blinatumomab was able to engage all CTLs for lysis of cancer cells in NHL patients, leading to the elimination of tumor cells from blood, liver, and bone marrow, and resulted in partial and complete tumor regressions [274]. MT110, an EpCAM- and CD3-bispecific scDb, could eradicate established tumors in a NOD/SCID mouse model bearing human tumor xenografts and is currently being tested in a phase I trial in lung and gastrointestinal cancer patients [280, 281]. In some cases, scFv-based BsAbs have been shown to be more effective than the parent BsAbs at triggering T cell [267, 282] and NK cell [279] cytotoxicities of tumor cells *in vitro*. Recently, bispecific Fv tetramers (bis-tetrabodies) [283-285], $scFv_2$-Fv trimers [286], and a scFv triple body (sctb) [271] have also been generated. The trivalent bispecific $scFv_2$-Fv trimer and sctb were constructed by fusing a bivalent anti-HER2 $scFv_2$ or anti-CD19 $scFv_2$ to an anti-CD16 Fv, respectively, and were able to bind both target tumor cells and NK cells [271, 286] and further induced lysis of leukemic cell lines and primary cells from leukemia and lymphoma patients [271].

Fab-based BsAbs were also developed and performed well in preclinical studies. Divalent $F(ab')_2$ BsAbs have been generated by incorporating two different Fabs *via* either chemical coupling [287] or heterodimerization through fusion to adhesive heterodimeric domains, *i.e.*, leucine zippers [288] or C_H3 domains (Fig. **2D**) [286]. These divalent $F(ab')_2$ BsAbs, *i.e.*, anti-CD3XTac F(ab′-zipper)$_2$ and anti-p185HER2XCD3 $F(ab')_2$, showed significant enhancement in cytotoxic activities of T cells against specific tumor cells [286-288]. In addition, bispecific Fab-scFv (bibody) and trispecific Fab-$(scFv)_2$ heterodimers (triabody) have been constructed by fusion of two scFvs to Fd and L chains of a Fab (Fig. **2E**) [289, 290]. These molecules were able to bind both targets and recruit and activate T cells or NK cells at tumor sites, while the trispecific Fab-$(scFv)_2$ triabody exerted these activities on two different tumor cells.

BsAbs have also been developed to deliver chemo- or radio-therapeutic agents to tumor sites, with one arm being associated with the target cells and the other with a therapeutic agent (*e.g.* radioisotope or toxin) (Fig. **2C**) [217, 224, 226]. In this type of application, the BsAb is administered first, and then, after allowing sufficient time for it to bind tumor cells while unbound is cleared from circulation, the effector molecule is injected and rapidly accumulates in the target tissue through high affinity interaction with the tumor-bound BsAb [225]. Several such trivalent bispecific Fab-based fusion proteins, each consisting of two identical Fabs fused to a different Fab, have been constructed as targeting molecules for improved tumor imaging and therapy [228]. For example, a bispecific tri-Fab, generated by linking two anti-CEA Fabs to a Fab specific for a hapten peptide and coupled to either a diagnostic or therapeutic radionuclide, was very effective at targeting CEA-expressing tumors for diagnostic imaging [228] and radioimmunotherapy [224], respectively. In the latter case, *i.e.*, in radioimmunotherapy, this bispecific tri-Fab displayed improved therapeutic efficacy in a pancreatic cancer xenograft mouse model [224]. In another case, cross-linking of a divalent hapten histamine-succinyl-glycine (HSG)-peptide with one of BsAbs, including IgGXFab′, $F(ab')_2$XFab′, and Fab′XFab′ BsAbs, which were prepared by coupling the IgG, $F(ab')_2$, or Fab′ of a humanized anti-CD20 antibody to a Fab′ of a murine antibody directed against HSG, induced significantly enhanced apoptosis in several lymphoma cells as compared with antibody alone [291]. Moreover, pretargeting with a tri-Fab BsAb (TF4), which contains two Fabs that bind CD20 and another Fab that bind HSG and bears radionuclides, improved tumor uptake of ^{111}In-HSG-peptide by 1.6-fold and enhanced tumor-to-blood ratios by 1600-fold, when compared with radiolabeled anti-CD20 IgG [217]. TF4 pretargeting resulted in significant improvement in survival, curing 33% to 90% of the animals even at relatively low doses, whereas most tumors progressed quickly without cures with ^{90}Y-anti-CD20 IgG.

The significant successes in experimental and preclinical studies indicate the great potential of BsAbs as therapeutics in tumor therapy because of their ability to recruit a variety of effector functions, *i.e.*, effector cells, radionuclides, drugs, and toxins, to the target sites. As therapeutic agents, the development of BsAbs mainly relies on the advances in the design of recombinant BsAb constructs and production efficiency. Despite the difficulty in production of sufficient quantities of BsAbs of high quality, they may provide an innovative therapeutic alternative for cancer therapy in the future.

5.3. IgG-Like Molecules

In some applications, antibody-based therapeutic efficacy relies on the recruitment of an array of antibody-dependent immune effector functions. In this respect, intact mAbs with appropriate constant region isotypes, mainly human IgG_1 and IgG_3, are favored because of their ability to trigger multiple immune activities, including stimulation of phagocytosis and induction of cell- and complement-dependent cytotoxicities. By contrast, rAbFs lack the functional Fc region and thus are unable to mediate natural effector functions. To circumvent such therapeutic limitations, rAbFs have been rebuilt into IgG-like molecules by fusing them to the Fc fragment or C_H3 domain of an IgG, with an isotype capable of mediating all the effector functions (Fig. **2F**; Table **1D**) [292, 293]. These IgG-like molecules restored the properties of an intact IgG, such as a prolonged serum half-life, high binding avidity, and the ability to mediate ADCC against target tumor cells. For instance, a human anti-ErbB2 scFv fused to the Fc region of a human IgG_1 was selectively cytotoxic to ErbB2-positive cancer cells both *in vitro* and *in vivo*. It was also toxic to trastuzumab-resistant tumor cells and able to inhibit the signaling pathway downstream of ErbB2 [293].

scFv-based IgG-like bispecific molecules are the most studied format in which two scFvs with different specificities are genetically fused to the C_H3 domain or Fc fragment of an IgG to create an IgG-like bispecific $(scFv)_2$-C_H3 or $(scFv)_2$-Fc fusion protein [113, 292, 294-296]. In general, these proteins have binding affinities identical to that of their corresponding parent IgGs and retain Fc-associated effector functions. For example, $(scFv)_2$-Fc bispecific fusion proteins, constructed by fusing the human IgG_1 Fc fragment to an anti-CEA or anti-HER2 scFv and also to the H60 murine ligand of NKG2D, promoted an NKG2D-dependent and antibody-specific tumor cell lysis by murine NK cells [294]. Similar results were obtained with an anti-EGFRXCD3 $(scDb)_2$-Fc fusion protein, which had a binding affinity greater than that of the parent scDbs and comparable to that of the corresponding IgG; it also induced a high level of cytotoxicity in peripheral blood mononuclear cells [296]. scFv-based IgG-like proteins are also developed by fusing scFvs to the entire constant regions of an IgG (Fig. **2D** and **2F**). For example, two scFvs with different specificities were separately fused to the constant region (C_H1-C_H2-C_H3) of human heavy gamma chain and to the constant region (C_L) of human kappa light chain, resulting in the formation of two polypeptides, $(scFv)_A$-C_H1-C_H2-C_H3 and $(scFv)_B$-C_L, respectively [297]. Coexpression of these two polypeptides in mammalian cells produced a tetravalent bispecific $(scFv)_4$-IgG heterotetramer (Fig. **2F**). This $(scFv)_4$-IgG has the potential to be engineered against two different epitopes on a single antigen [297] or different molecules on a single cell [298]. By using these techniques, two bispecfic $(scFv)_4$-IgG molecules, $scFv_{anti\text{-}EGFR}$-C_LX$scFv_{anti\text{-}IGFR}$-C_H1-C_H2-C_H3 and $scFv_{anti\text{-}IGFR}$-C_LX$scFv_{anti\text{-}EGFR}$-C_H1-C_H2-C_H3, which are directed against both EGFR (epithelial growth factor receptor) and IGFR (insulin-like growth factor receptor), were able to inhibit signal transduction mediated by both EGF and IGF by preventing their interactions with the corresponding receptors [298]. Furthermore, these molecules also inhibited proliferation of tumor cells *in vitro* at a degree similar to that of the combined parental IgGs from which the V_L and V_H were derived.

Tetravalent bispecific IgG-like molecules can also be generated by fusion of bispecific scDb either to the Fc fragment or to the C_H3 domain of human IgG, forming IgG-like $(scDb)_2$-Fc or $(scDb)_2$-C_H3 fusion proteins, respectively [296, 299]. In this format, two scDbs with defined specificities were genetically fused to the constant region (C_H1-C_H2-C_H3) of human heavy chain, resulting in the formation of a V_HA-V_LB-V_HB-V_LA-C_H1-C_H2-C_H3 polypeptide, which then assembles into IgG-like $(scDb)_2$-Fc dimers through the Fc domains [299]. An alternative Db-Fc fusion format, called "di-diabody", was also created. In this setting, one "cross-over" scFv is fused to the C_H2-C_H3 domain of a human heavy chain, producing a heavier chain V_LA-V_HB-C_H2-C_H3, which assembles with the other "cross-over" scFv, *i.e.* the lighter chain V_LA-V_HB, through the V_H/V_L interfaces, and then two heavier chains homodimerize through the C_H2-C_H3 regions to form an IgG-like tetravalent bispecific $(scFv)_4$-Fc molecules [300]. For example, a $(scFv)_4$-Fc di-diabody, engineered to target EGFR and IGFR and constructed using this method, showed high affinity to both target antigens [300]. This di-diabody also induced IGFR internalization and degradation, effectively mediated ADCC towards different tumor cells, and inhibited the outgrowth of two different human tumor xenografts in mice. A similar di-diabody, namely V_LB-V_HAXV_LA-V_HB-C_H3, was generated by fusing a divalent bispecific diabody to the C_H3 domain of an IgG *via* the hinge region [301].

Other rAbF-based multivalent IgG-like molecules were also designed and constructed in a similar manner. A hexavalent anti-CD20 Fab-Fc fusion protein, called Hex-hA20, constructed by fusing six Fabs to one Fc region, retained the binding activities of all six Fabs, was able to mediate ADCC but not CDC, and showed inhibitory effects on tumor cell proliferation *in vitro* and antitumor efficacy in tumor-bearing mice [302]. In addition, tetravalent bispecific sVD-IgG fusion proteins were developed by genetically fusing a sVD with a defined specificity to either the N-terminus of the light chain or the C-terminus of the heavy chain of an IgG with a different specificity [303, 304]. These bispecific sVD-IgG fusion proteins, including anti-PDGFRαXEGFR2 and anti-PDGFRαXPDGFRβ, retained their antigen binding specificities and the receptor neutralizing activities of both of parent antibodies [303, 304]. More importantly, the anti-PGFRαXPGFRβ sVD-IgG fusion protein inhibited the activation of both its target receptors in tumor cells stimulated by both platelet-derived growth factor (PDGF) AA and BB [304].

Compared to monomeric rAbFs, multivalent IgG-like fusion proteins are very stable, have an *in vivo* half-life equivalent to that of an intact human IgG, and more importantly are capable of triggering Fc-dependent effector functions. However, the use of multiple non-human polypeptide linkers within these molecules may potentially induce an immune response, thus possibly reducing their therapeutic efficiency. The other drawbacks are the multiple cloning steps involved and the requirement of mammalian cells for their production. In addition, expression level of IgG-like molecules is usually low, which may also affect their practical application as therapeutic agents. Despite these challenges, IgG-like multivalent proteins have become a promising alternative to mAbs.

5.4. Intrabody

The targeted expression of intracellular antibodies (intrabodies) using a well characterized signal peptide is another advance in antibody engineering. Intrabodies have been used as a biotechnological tool to define, modulate, or interrupt the functions of a wide range of targeted molecules in a specific cellular compartment, *e.g.* in the nucleus by a SV40 T antigen-derived nuclear localization signal, in the ER by a SEKDEL retention signal, or in cytosol by deletion of the signal peptide, as well as in mitochondria, peroxisomes, plasma membrane and trans-Golgi network *via* fusion with intracellular localization peptide sequences (Table **1E**) [305-308]. In theory, upon interaction with its target, an intrabody is expected to modulate the function of a targeted molecule by one of the following mechanisms: 1) down-regulating the expression of the targeted protein by interfering with its transcription or translation; 2) blocking the subcellular translocation of the target protein from its normal site of action; 3) modulating the enzymatic activity of the target protein by either inhibiting its activity or maintaining its catalytic site in an active conformation; 4) disrupting the signaling transduction mediated by the target protein through interference with its interaction with other molecules [305-308].

The therapeutic efficacy of intrabodies is highly dependent on their intracellular stability, especially when they are directed to the cytosol, which is a reducing environment and thereby, does not support the formation of intrachain disulfide bonds and often leads to protein aggregation. Therefore, among rAbFs, V_Hs and scFvs are the most commonly used intrabody formats because their assembly does not require disulfide bond formation unlike Fabs [307, 309, 310]. When compared to intrabodies, the limitations associated with extracellular antibodies, such as immunogenicity, short serum persistence, poor tissue penetration, low tumor-to-normal tissue ratios, and poor specificity are reduced or eliminated [121]. In comparison with other approaches used intracellularly, such as antisense RNA-based therapies, intrabodies are more versatile because antisense RNA can only be used to target mRNA, whereas intrabodies can be directed to modulate the functions of a variety of molecules, including nucleic acids, proteins, carbohydrates, and lipids [311].

Intrabodies have been intensively investigated in preclinical studies for preventing viral infections and the treatment of cancer. Several intrabodies directed against viral proteins have been demonstrated to have potent antiviral activities, *e.g.* sVD intrabodies against HIV by reducing late reverse transcripts and proviral integration [312], scFvs against Kaposi Sarcoma-Associated Herpes Virus (KSHV) by inhibiting its maintanence in host cells [313], and scFvs against Human Papilloma Virus (HPV) by blocking its interactions with host cellular proteins in host cells [310, 314]. The antiviral activities can be achieved by directing intrabodies to inhibit the functions of mandatory viral proteins (*i.e.*, Vif, LANA1, Tat, Rev, and E6), viral envelop proteins (*i.e.*, gp41 and gp160) [315, 316], or receptors on the surface of host cells (*i.e.*, CCR5) [310, 313, 317, 318]. For example, the expression of scFv intrabodies, specific for KSHV-associated nuclear antigen-1 (LANA 1) that is critical for the maintenance and segregation of viral episomes in infected host cells, caused a reduction or loss of the typical LANA1 punctate and KSHV episome in infected lymphoma cells [313]. The loss of KSHV episome in these cells resulted in cell death without inducing viral lytic reactivation. These results suggest that intrabodies can be useful candidates for preventing viral infections.

Intrabodies are also targeted to inhibit tumor growth or induce tumor cell death by down-regulating protein expression, blocking protein subcellular translocation, inhibiting angiogenesis, inducing apoptosis, or recruiting cytotoxic cells. For example, the targeted intracellular expression of rAbFs significantly down-regulated the expression of VEGFR-2/KDR [319], erbB2 [320], Tie-2 [321], MHC [322], p65 [323] and hTERT (human telomerase reverse transcriptase) [324] in cancer cells. The expression of a scFv intrabody directed against hTERT specifically neutralized over 70% of telomere synthesis activity, thereby inhibiting the viability and proliferation of target cancer cells [324]. Intrabodies are also designed to block the translocation of secreted or membrane proteins to their function sites, thereby inhibiting tumor growth through interfering with signal transduction and angiogenesis [321, 325]. The expression of an ER-directed intradiabody led to a 92.2% and 74.4% inhibition of tumor growth and angiogenesis in mice, respectively, by simultaneously blocking both VEGFR-2 and Tie-2 pathways [325]. Moreover, the nuclear expression of anti-p65 scFv suppressed tumor invasion and angiogenesis in glioma cells and resulted in complete regression of established tumors in nude mice as a result of inhibition of p65 expression and blockage of NF-kB nuclear translocation and its transcriptional activity [323]. Intrabodies are also directed to target apoptosis-associated proteins, and thus induce cell death *via* activation of the apoptosis pathway. The ER-targeted expression of an anti-ErbB2 scFv caused cell death of different cancer cell lines *in vitro* and suppressed tumor growth in mice inoculated with cancer cells expressing the intrabody [320]. This intrabody is currently being tested in a phase I trial for recurrent ovarian cancer gene therapy [326]. The cytosolic expression of an anti-Ras scFv specifically induced apoptosis in targeted cancer cells *in vitro* and elicited sustained tumor regression in nude mice [327, 328], while expression of a secreted anti-CEAXCD3 bispecific diabody inhibited the tumor growth *in vivo via* the recruitment and activation of CTLs to the target site [329]. Intrabodies have also been designed to express in the nucleus and act against cell-cycle proteins whose functions are dysregulated in tumor cells. The nuclear expression of an anti-c-Myc scFv inhibited transactivating activity of c-Myc and proliferation of human leukemia cell lines [330] and an anti-cyclin E scFv-Fc intrabody suppressed the growth of breast cancer cell lines [331]. In addition, intrabodies are also used for the inactivation of specific cytotoxic drugs in normal cells, thereby increasing the therapeutic efficacy against tumor cells and preventing the possibility of induction of multidrug resistant tumor cells in chemotherapy [332]. The intracellular expression of a scFv, specific for the intracellular domain of the multidrug resistance (MDR) protein, enhanced uptake and retention of different drugs in target human cancer cell lines.

Table 1: Examples of Important rAbFs and rAbF-Based Fusion Proteins.

A. Multimeric rAbFs

Generic Name	Antibody Format	Molecular Target	Cellular Target	Potential Application	Production Systems	Clinical Phase	Ref.
C6.5 scFv	$scFv_2$	HER2/neu	Ovarian cancer cells	Tumor diagnosis and imaging	*E. coli*	NA	[71]
4D5-p53 miniantibody	$scFv_4$-p53	p185HER-2	Ovarian cancer cells	Delivery of effector molecules for tumor imaging and therapy	*E. coli*	Preclinical	[69]
scFv-10 diabody scFv-1 tetrabody scFv-0 triabody	$scFv_2$ $scFv_4$ $scFv_3$	CD19	Malignant B cells	Tumor imaging and immunotherapy	*E. coli*	NA	[72]
741F8 $(sFv')_2$	$dsFv'_2$	HER2/neu	Ovarian cancer cells	Tumor diagnosis and therapy	*E. coli*	NA	[73]
A5B7 humanised divalent-Fab' maleimide	Fab'_2	CEA	Colorectal cancer cells	Tumor imaging and radioimmunotherapy	*E. coli*	I, II	[67]
$[sc(Fv)_2]_2$	$[sc(Fv)_2]_2$	TAG-72	Colorectal tumor cells	Tumor imaging	*P. pastoris*	Preclinical	[38]
T84.66 diabody T84.66 minibody	$scFv_2$ $(scFv-C_H3)_2$	CEA	Colorectal tumor cells	Tumor targeting	NS0 cells	Preclinical	[51]

B. rAbF-based fusion proteins

Generic Name	Antibody Format	Molecular Target	Cellular Target	Potential Application	Production Systems	Clinical Phase	Ref.
Certolizumab pegol (CDP-870)	Fab′-PEG	TNF-α	NA	Treatment for rheumatoid arthritis and Crohn's disease	*E. coli*	II, III	[85][91]
CDP791	Fab'_2-PEG	VEGFR-2/KDR	Non-small cell lung cancer	Tumor therapy *via* blocking VEGFR-2 signaling pathway	*E. coli*	II	[86]
M18	scFv-PEG	*Bacillus anthracis* exotoxin	*B. anthracis*	Treatment for prophylactic anthrax	*E. coli*	Preclinical	[88]
Abciximab* (c7E3Fab′)	Fab′-PEG	gpIIb/IIIa	Platelets	Inhibition of platelet aggregation	*E. coli*	Clinical	[89]

AlbudAb/IL-1ra	dAb	SA	NA	Treatment of rheumatoid arthritis	*E. coli*	Preclinic al	[110]
Cys-diabody	$scFv_2$	CEA	Colon carcinoma cells	Tumor imaging	NS0 cells	Preclinic al	[115]
T84.66/212 LD minibody T84.66/212Flex minibody	$(scFv\text{-}C_H3)_2$ $(scFv\text{-}C_H3)_2$	CEA	Colon carcinoma cells	Tumor imaging	Sp2/0 cells	Preclinic al	[77]
A-dmDT(390)-bisFv(UCHT1)	scFv-DT	CD3	Malignant T cells	Treatment for cutaneous T cell lymphoma		I	[122]
LMB-2	scFv-PE38	CD25	T-regulatory cells	Cancer vaccine, cell transfer immunotherapy	*E. coli*	II	[129][133]
scFv(MUC1)-ETA	scFv-ETA	MUC1	Primary breast cancer cells, Breast carcinoma cells	Therapy of primary breast tumor	*E. coli*	NA	[130]
SGN-10 (BR96sFv-PE40)	scFv-PE40	$Lewis^Y$	Multiple carcinoma cells	Tumor therapy	*E. coli*	I	[131]
BL22 RFB4(dsFv)-PE38	dsFv-PE38	CD22	B acute lymphoblastic leukemia cells, B Non–Hodgkin lymphoma cells	Treatment of B cell malignancies	*E. coli*	I	[135]
B1(Fv)PE38 B1(dsFv)PE38	Fv-PE38 dsFv-PE38	$Lewis^Y$	Adenocarcino ma cells	Tumor therapy	*E. coli*	Preclinic al	[150]
B3(Fv)-PE38	Fv-PE38	B3	Epidermoid carcinoma cells	Epidermoid carcinoma therapy	*E. coli*	Preclinic al	[144]
$(Fab\text{-}PE38)_2$	$(Fab\text{-}PE38)_2$	$Lewis^Y$	Breast cancer cells	Tumor therapy	*E. coli*	NA	[147]
F16IL2	scFv-IL-2	Tenascin-C	Breast cancer cells	Tumor therapy	CHO cells	I, II	[179]
C215Fab-IL-2	Fab-IL-2	C215	B16 melanoma cells	Tumor therapy *via* recruitment of CTLs	*E. coli*	Preclinic al	[180]
L19-IL12 L19-IFN-γ L19-IL-15	scFv-p40, scFv-p35 scFv-IFN-γ scFv-IL-15	Fibronect in	F9 teratocarcino ma cells	Tumor therapy	HEK 293 cells	Preclinic al	[184] [188] [189]
scFvMEL/TNF	scFv-TNF	gp240	Melanoma cells	Tumor therapy	*E. coli*	Preclinic al	[190]
scHLA-A2/aTac(scFv) scHLA-A2/SS1(scFv)	scFv-MHC-peptide	α-subunit of p55 mesothelin	Epidermoid cancer cells	Tumor therapy *via* activation of CTLs	*E. coli*	Preclinic al	[194]
$F(ab')_2$ x H-$2D^b$/GP33	$F(ab')_2$-H-2D/GP33	CEA	Carcinoma cells	Tumor therapy	Pepsin digestio n	Preclinic al	[198]
CD1d-scFv	scFv-CD1d	HER2/ne u	Melanoma cells	Inhibition of lung metastasis *via* recruitment of iNKT, NK, and T cells	HEK 293 cells	Preclinic al	[199]

PE-HER-liposomes	Fab′-PE38-liposomes	HER2/neu	Breast cancer cells	Targeted delivery of anticancer drugs	Pepsin digestion	NA	[212]
SIL-Dox	scFv-doxorubicin-liposomes	Ep-CAM	Breast and lung cancer cells	Targeted delivery of anticancer drugs	*E. coli*	Preclinical	[214]
H310A, H435Q	$scFv_2$-Fc	CEA	Colon carcinoma cells	Tumor targeting	NS0 cells	Preclinical	[218]
C6.5diabody	$scFv_2$	HER2/*neu*	Ovarian carcinoma cells, Breast cancer cells	Tumor targeting	*E. coli*	Preclinical	[220]
^{90}Y-CHX-A"-C6.5K-A diabody	$scFv_2$	HER2/*neu*	Breast cancer cells	Targeted radioimmunotherapy	*E. coli*	Preclinical	[223]
AP39 x m679	scFv-Fab′	Fibronectin X HSG	Glioblastoma cancer cells	Targeted radioimmunotherapy	Cross-linking	Preclinical	[227]
B9E9FP	$(scFv)_4$-streptavidin	Cd20	B non-Hodgkin's lymphoma cells	Pretargeted radioimmunotherapy	*E. coli*	I	[230]
Db-RLuc (T84.66anti-CEA diabody)	$(scFv)_2$-RLuc8	CEA	Colon carcinoma cells	Tumor imaging (ADEPT)	*E. coli*	Preclinical	[236]
GrB-5 GrB-scFv(FRP5)	GrB-scFv	ErbB2	Breast carcinoma cells	Tumor therapy (ADEPT)	*P. pastoris*	NA	[237]
A33scFv::CDy	scFv-CDy	gpA33	Colon carcinoma cells	Tumor therapy (ADEPT)	*P. pastoris*	Preclinical	[238] [240]
MFECP1	scFv-carboxypeptidase G2	CEA	Metastatic cancer cells	Tumor therapy (ADEPT)	P. pastoris	I	[241]
EDIAs (anti-ErbB2immunoagents)	scFv-RNase, scFv-Fc	ErbB2	Breast carcinoma cells	Tumor therapy	CHO cells	Preclinical	[293]
s-tP	scFv-protamine	HBsAg	Hepatoma cells	Targeted delivery of siRNA against HBV	*E. coli*	Preclinical	[252]
F105-P	Fab-protamine	gp160	HIV-infected primary T cells	Targeted delivery of siRNA against HIV	COS cells	Preclinical	[253]
Fab immunoporter	Fab-polylysine	EGFR	Squamous carcinoma tumor cells	Targeted delivery of siRNA to tumor cells	Pepsin digestion	NA	[257]

C. Bispecific rAbFs

Generic Name	**Antibody Format**	**Molecular Target**	**Cellular Target**	**Potential Application**	**Production Systems**	**Clinical Phase**	**Ref.**
$scFv_2$-HAS scDb-HAS taFv-HAS	$scFv_2$-HAS scDb-HAS taFv-HAS	CEA X CD3	CEA^+ Tumor cells X CTLs	Tumor therapy *via* engagement of CTLs	HEK 293 cells	NA	[104]

αHEL-αLAM	$scFv_2$	Ig X HEL	Colon carcinoma cells	Serotherapy *via* CDC and ADCC	*E. coli*	NA	[105]
scDb-ABD	scDb-ABD	CEA X CD3	CEA^+ tumor cells X CTLs	Tumor-specific retargeting of T cells	HEK 293 cells	Preclinical	[109]
bsscFv ds[CD19 X CD16]	$scFv_2$	CD19 X CD16	Malignant B lymphoid cells	Tumor therapy *via* engagement of effector cells	293T cells	NA	[269]
CD19 X CD16 BsDb	$scFv_2$	CD19 X CD16	Burkitt's lymphoma cells	Tumor therapy *via* engagement of NK cells	*E. coli*	Preclinical	[272]
CD19 X CD3 BsDb	$scFv_2$	CD19 X CD3	Burkitt's lymphoma cells	Tumor therapy *via* engagement of CTLs	*E. coli*	Preclinical	[272]
BS1.5H	$F(ab')_2$	CEA X HSG	Colon tumor cells	Pretargeted radioimmunotherapy	*E. coli*	Preclinical	[79]
TF4	Fab_3	CD20 X HSG	B lymphoma cells	Pretargeted radioimmunotherapy	Mammalian	Preclinical	[217]
Blinatumomab (MT103/MEDI-538)	$scFv_2$	CD19 X CD3	B acute lymphoblastic leukemia cells, Non-Hodgkin lymphoma cells	Tumor therapy *via* engagement of CTLs	*P. pastoris*	I, II	[274][276]
MT110	$scFv_2$	Ep-CAM X CD3	Colon carcinoma cells	Tumor therapy *via* engagement of CTLs	CHO cells	Preclinical	[278][280]
anti-ErbB2/anti-CD16 BsAb	$scFv_2$-Fab	ErbB2 X CD16	Breast cancer cells	Tumor therapy *via* engagement of effector cells	*E. coli*	Preclinical	[290]

D. IgG-like molecules

Generic Name	Antibody Format	Molecular Target	Cellular Target	Potential Application	Production Systems	Clinical Phase	Ref.
C6.5-Fc	$scFv_2$-Fc	HER2/*neu*	Breast cancer cells	Tumor therapy *via* ADCC	*P. pastoris*	Preclinical	[113]
(scFv4D5/rH60)-Fc	scFv-rH60-Fc	HER2 X NKG2D	Breast cancer cells	Tumor therapy *via* engagement of NK cells	HEK 293 cells	NA	[294]
hEx3-scFv-Fc	$scFv_4$-Fc	EGFR X CD3	Extrahepatic bile duct carcinoma cells	Tumor therapy *via* ADCC	CHO cells	NA	[296]
Anti-EGFR x Anti-IGFR BsAb	scFv-C_H1-Fc	EGFR X IGFR	Colorectal adenocarcinoma cancer, Pancreatic carcinoma cells	Tumor therapy *via* blocking GFR signaling pathways	NS0 cells	NA	[298]
Di-diabody	$scFv_4$-Fc	EGFR X IGFR	Breast cancer cells, Pancreatic carcinoma cells. Epidermoid	Tumor therapy *via* blocking GFR signaling pathways and mediating	NS0 cells	Preclinical	[300]

			carcinoma cells	ADCC			
Hex-hA20	Fab_6-Fc	CD20	B lymphoblast T cells, Burkitt's lymphoma cells	Tumor therapy *via* ADCC	Sp/ESF cells	Preclinical	[302]
1F2-1B3IgG 1B3IgG-1F2	sVD_2-IgG IgG-sVD_2	PDGFRα X PDGFRβ	Lewis lung cancer cells	Tumor therapy *via* blocking GFR signaling pathways	COS-7cells	NA	[304]

E. Intrabody

Generic Name	Antibody Format	Molecular Target	Subcelluar Location	Cellular Target	Potential Application	Clinical Phase	Ref.
GTE6-scFv GTE6-diabody GTE6-diabody	scFv $scFv_2$ $scFv_2$	E6	Cytoplasm/ nucleus	Cervical cancer cells	Therapy against HPV *via* with protein-protein interactions	NA	[310]
Anti-Vif V_H	V_H	Vif	Cytoplasm	Non-permissive cells	Therapy against HIV *via* neutralizing infectivity enhancing function of Vif	NA	[312]
BM9, BM10 (anti-LANA1scFvs)	scFv	LANA1	Cytoplasm	Primary effusion lymphoma cells	Therapy against KSHV *via* neutralizing episome maintenance function of LANA 1	NA	[313]
1F4, 1F4-P41L	scFv	16E6	Cytoplasm	Cervical cancer cell	Therapy against HPV *via* inducing apoptosis of host cells	NA	[314]
F240 scFv	scFv	gp41	Cytoplasm	HIV-infected $CD4^+$ T cells	Therapy against HIV *via* inhibiting viral assembly and transport	NA	[316]
Anti-Vif scFv	scFv	Vif	Cytoplasm	Non-permissive cells, Peripheral blood mononuclear cells	Therapy against HIV *via* neutralizing infectivity-enhancing function of Vif	NA	[317]
CCR5-intrabody	scFv	CCR5	ER	Primary $CD4^+$ T cells	Therapy against HIV *via* disrupting CCR5 cell surface expression	NA	[318]
scFv A7	scFv	VEGFR-	ER	Aorticendothelial	Tumor therapy	NA	[31

		2/KDR		cells	*via* inhibiting KDR surface expression and angiogenesis		9]
pAd-2S03	scFv	Tie-2	ER	Human umbilical vein endothelial cells, Kaposi's sarcoma cells Colon carcinoma cells	Tumor therapy *via* inhibiting Tie-2 surface expression and angiogenesis	Preclinical	[321]
pFv/nu	scFv	p65	Nucleus	Glioma cells	Tumor therapy *via* inhibiting transcriptional activity of NF-κB	Preclinical	[323]
Anti-hTERT scFv	scFv	hTERT	Nucleus	Uterine cervix and hepatoma cells	Tumor therapy *via* neutralizing telomere synthesis activity of hTERT	NA	[324]
VEGF-R2/Tie-2 BsAb	$scFv_2$	VEGF-R2 X Tie-2	ER	Endothelial cells and melanoma cells	Tumor therapy *via* blockade of both VEGF-R2 and Tie-2 pathways	Preclinical	[325]
Anti-erbB-2 scFv	scFv	erbB-2	ER	Ovarian cancer	Tumor therapy *via* down regulation of erB2 expression and induction of apoptosis	I	[326]
Anti-Ras scFv	scFv	Ras	Cytoplasm	Fibroblasts	Tumor therapy *via* sequestering Ras and impairing proteasome activity	NA	[327]
Y259-scFv	scFv	Ras	Cytoplasm	Fibroblasts and Colon carcinoma cells	Tumor therapy *via* inhibiting Ras signaling pathway and promoting apoptosis	Preclinical	[328]
Anti-c-Myb scFv	scFv	c-Myb	Nucleus	Chronic myelogenous leukemia cells	Tumor therapy *via* inhibition of transactivating	NA	[330]

Legend: *, approved by FDA; ABD= albumin-binding domain, ADCC= antibody-dependent cellular cytotoxicity, ADEPT= antibody-directed enzyme-prodrug therapy, CEA= carcinoembryonic antigen, CDC= complement-dependent cytotoxicity, CDy= cytosine deaminase from yeast, CTL= cytolytic T lymphocyte, DT= Diphtheria toxin, EGFR= epidermal growth factor receptor, Ep-CAM= epithelial cell adhesion molecule, ER= endoplasmic reticulum, GrB2= growth factor receptor bound protein 2, HAS= human serum albumin, HBsAg= hepatitis B surface antigen, HBV= hepatitis B virus, HEL= hen egg lysozyme, HER2= human epidermal growth factor receptor 2, HIV= Human immunodeficiency virus, HPV= genital human papillomavirus, HSG= histamine-succinyl-glycine, hTERT= human telomerase reverse transcriptase, IFN-γ= interferon-gamma, IGFR= insulin-like growth factor receptor, LANA1= latency-associated nuclear antigen 1, MHC= major histocompatibility complex, MUC1= mucin 1, cell surface associated, NA= not applicable, NKG2D= natural-killer group 2 member D, PDGFR= platelet-derived growth factor receptor, PEG= polyethylene glycol, RLuc8= *Renilla* luciferase 8, SA= serum albumin, TAG-72= tumor-associated glycoprotein 72, TNF-α= tumour necrosis factor α, VEGFR-2= vascular endothelial growth factor receptor-2, Vif= viral infectivity factor.

Fundamentally, intrabody-based therapy is a gene-based approach with antibodies being expressed inside of target cells and functioning in specific cellular compartments. In comparison with antisence RNA approach, the generation of intrabodies is more technically challenging, time consuming, and labor intensive, but the intrabody-mediated knockdown of protein function is more target-specific. At present, the major obstacle for the clinical application of intrabodies is the delivery of the intrabody-coding gene into target cells. To date, the most commonly used delivery strategies for gene transfer include viral (*e.g.* retroviruses, adenoviruses, and adeno-associated viruses) or non-viral (*e.g.* liposomes, molecular conjugates) transduction systems [333]. Although progress is being made in the development of delivery approaches, there are still concerns about the delivery efficiency, target specificity, immunogenicity, toxicity, and safety. In spite of these challenges, intrabodies are emerging as a promising agent for the generation of phenotypic knockouts, manipulation of biological processes, and a more thorough understanding of functional genomics. Moreover, they have great potential to be used as therapeutics in a large array of applications.

6. ANTIBODY LIBRARIES

6.1. Immune Libraries

More than 20 years have passed since the first immune library was constructed by Huse *et al.* [334]. Immune libraries are constructed using IgG mRNA isolated from B cells of animals (*e.g.* mice, rabbit, sheep, llama) hyper-immunized with an Antigen (Ag), or cocktail of Ags, of interest [335]. Alternatively, B cells from naturally infected, vaccinated or diseased humans have been used to create valuable human antibody libraries [336-338]. Furthermore, transgenic mice carrying human Ig genes (Xenomice^{TM}) can be immunized to generate a 'human' immune library [339].

Several tissues can be used as a source of B cells and include peripheral blood lymphocytes (PBL), bone marrow, tonsils and spleen. Total RNA or mRNA is harvested from these cells (ca. 10^7 cells) and reverse transcribed into the first strand of cDNA using oligo (dT), random hexamers and/or constant/framweork region primers. Depending on the type of rAb being engineered, the appropriate coding sequences are PCR amplified from the cDNA using family-based primer sets that anneal to the framework or constant regions. Since Ig genes have been sequenced and are available through databases [*e.g.*, V BASE Database (http://vbase.mrc-cpe.cam.ac.uk); Kabat Database (http:// http://www.kabatdatabase.com)], it is straightforward to design sets of primers that amplify all human [336, 340, 341] V genes.

For the construction of Fab libraries, the V_H-C_H1 and light chain (V_L-C_L) are amplified; while only the V_H and V_L chain are amplified to create Fv and scFv libraries. To create a scFv library, the rearranged V_H and V_L gene repertoires are covalently linked with a short flexible polypeptide linker such as $(Gly_4Ser)_3$ using splicing by overlap extension (PCR assembly) or by sequential cloning [342]. The cloning strategy to create a scFv library has been discussed extensively in the literature, and hence, is not discussed in details here. Since camelid V_HHs are becoming increasingly popular as therapeutic reagents, a detailed description of V_HH library construction is given under subheading 5.1.1.

After amplification and assembly into the desired rAbF format, the rAbF gene repertoire is batch-cloned into a suitable display vector (*e.g.* pHEN phagemid vector) and transformed into highly competent bacterial cells (*e.g. E. coli* TG1) to create a diverse library with $\sim10^{7\text{-}10}$ individual clones. Antigen-specific rAbFs are subsequently selected from the library using any of the available display technologies (*e.g.* phage-, cell-, ribosomal-displays) discussed under subheading 0.

The main advantage of immune libraries over non-immune libraries is that antigen-specific antibodies have undergone natural affinity maturation *via* the immune system of the host, thereby allowing the isolation of rAbFs with high affinity and specificity to the target antigen. rAbFs to a wide variety of antigens, including protein toxins *e.g.* scFv: [343]; diabody: [344]; V_HH, bivalent-V_HH: [345], glycoproteins [V_HH: 346], haptens (*e.g.*, scFv: [347], VHH [348]), and carbohydrates (*e.g.*, scFv: [349, 350]) have been isolated from immune libraries.

There are several disadvantages to using immune libraries. First, antibodies to self-antigens cannot be generated using immune libraries. This severely limits the use of immune libraries for therapeutic application since most of the mAbs in the clinic are antibodies against self-antigens [351]. Other shortcomings of creating immune libraries include the long time required for animal immunization and the unpredictability of immune response to the antigen of interest [352]. Finally, creating immune libraries can be a costly and laborious process since a new library must be generated for each antigen.

6.1.1. V_HH Library Construction

In addition to conventional IgGs, species of *Camelidae* (camels, llamas, alpacas) produce functional heavy-chain antibodies (HCAbs) that are naturally devoid of light chains and the C_H1 domains [353]. Thus, in contrast to conventional IgGs, the antigen-binding site of these HCAbs are reduced to a single variable domain, also known as a V_HH, and are the smallest natural antigen binding domain (~15 kDa). Camelid V_HHs have been attracting attention as therapeutic reagents since they are relatively non-immunogenic, are highly soluble and stable (to heat and pH), and because of their small size are highly tissue penetrable [242, 354-356].

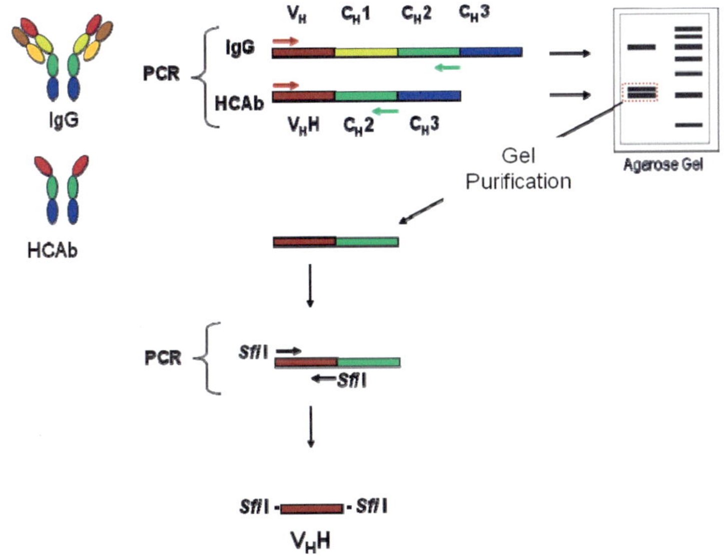

Figure 5: Summary of the camelid V_HH cloning strategy. See text for details.

Since *Camelidae* possess both HCAbs and convention IgG, and the V_H share high sequence identity with V_HHs, one must take care to prepare a V_HH library free of conventional V_H contaminants. To eliminate this contamination, two sequential PCR amplifications are required as outlined in (Fig. **5**). In the first set of PCR reactions, framework-1 specific sense primers and C_H2-specific anti-sense primers are used to amplify the V_HH-C_H2 and V_H-C_H1-C_H2 regions of HCAb and convIgG genes, respectively. Since HCAbs lack the C_H1 domain, the amplicon product of V_HH-C_H2 (~600 bp) can be separated and purified from conventional V_H-C_H1-C_H2 product (~900 bp) by gel electrophoresis. Subsequently, the V_HH-C_H2 product from the first PCR is used as template DNA for nested PCR using primers specific for the extremities of framework-1 (sense) and framework-4 (anti-sense), resulting in an amplified V_HH fragment without the C_H2 gene segment. Restriction sites (*e.g. Sfi* I) are also introduced at the 5' and 3' end of the V_HH sequence for cloning purposes. Subsequently, the V_HH gene repertoire is cloned into a phagemid vector (*e.g.*, pMED1, [357]) and transformed into highly, efficient bacterial host (*e.g. E. coli*) to create a diverse library containing billions of clones.

6.2. Naïve Libraries

Naïve libraries are derived from the natural primary (unselected) antibody repertoire of unimmunized animals or humans. For the construction of naïve libraries, naïve B cells are used as they have not yet encountered a specific antigen. These B cells are predominantly found in PBLs and bone marrow, but can also be found in spleen and tonsils [358-360]. IgMs are the preferred source of V genes as they are highly diverse, are produced by B cells that have not previously encountered a specific antigen, and are unscreened for tolerance by the immune system [361]. The rearranged V genes are amplified from IgM cDNA using IgM-derived oligonucleotide primers.

Since non-immune (*i.e.* naïve, synthetic and semi-synthetic) libraries are antigen-unbiased and are not restricted to immunological tolerance, rAbFs to a wide variety of antigens, including non-immunogenic, self, cell surface, toxic and chemically unstable antigens, can be generated [362-364]. In fact, non-immune libraries represent an important source of therapeutic antibodies in the clinic since most are against self antigens [351]. Furthermore, using these libraries can save time and money since they avoid animal immunization, and a single library can be used to select antibodies against a variety of antigens [352].

The major disadvantage of naïve libraries is that, compared to an immune library of the same size ($\sim 10^7$-10^8 individual clones), which can generate rAbFs with affinities in the nanomolar range and even lower, the antibodies isolated from a naïve library usually have much lower affinities [10^{-6} to 10^{-7} M^{-1}] [340, 365, 366]. Such low affinity antibodies are impractical for most applications including therapeutic use and *in vitro* affinity maturation is often required to improve their antigen binding affinity. However, there are specific cases where antibodies with low nanomolar to even sub-nanomolar [10^{-8} to 10^{-10} M^{-1}] affinities against a wide variety of antigens have been recovered from large naïve libraries ($>10^{10}$ individual clones) [359]; these affinities are similar as those created by a secondary immune response [366]. Thus, creating very large non-immune libraries may reduce the need for laborious *in vitro* affinity maturation [352].

Large naïve libraries can be constructed by improving bacterial transformation efficiencies and increasing the number of transformations [359], by optimizing the cloning efficiencies [358], or by taking advantage of bacteria for *in vivo* recombination of the V genes [363, 367]. In addition, the size and diversity of the library can be improved by using naïve B cells from multiple tissues (*e.g.* PBLs, bone marrow, *etc.*), by collecting B cells from multiple donors (*e.g.* >100 donors), and/or by using multiple Ig classes (IgG, IgM, IgA, and IgD) as sources of V genes [367].

6.3. Synthetic and Semi Synthetic Libraries

The availability of detailed structural and functional knowledge of the antibody molecule has fuelled the rational design of synthetic and semi-synthetic antibody libraries with tailored characteristics [368]. Synthetic antibody libraries are artificially built by incorporating diversity using degenerate synthetic oligonucleotides on selected template scaffold(s) [369]. By using this method, the position and degree of randomization can be precisely controlled [369]. Numerous synthetic libraries have been generated and reviewed [368-370].

Semi-synthetic libraries are constructed by assembling natural and synthetic antibody variable gene segments. The first semi-synthetic scFv library was created by using 49 natural human V_H germline gene segments which contained fully randomized synthetic heavy-chain CDR3 regions (designed to contain 5 or 8 residues), and combined with a single natural V_L chain [371]. This library was rather small, *i.e.*, $\sim 10^7$ clones, and generated scFvs with moderate affinities (μM range) to haptens but performed poorly against protein antigens [369, 371]. Over the years, different design strategies were explored to create larger (up to 10^{11} clones) and more diverse semi-synthetic and synthetic libraries by varying the length and composition of the heavy-chain CDR3 region, *e.g.* 4-12 residues [372] or 6-15 residues [373], by targeting multiple CDR regions [374-376], and/or by using a set of V_L genes [363, 373, 377].

Synthetic and semi-synthetic libraries share many of the same advantages discussed for naïve libraries. Since these libraries are not biased to a particular antigen, antibodies with high affinity (low to sub nM) and specificity to a variety of antigens have been generated from these libraries [363, 372, 378-380].

7. MOLECULAR DISPLAY TECHNOLOGIES

Over the past two decades, a number of display platforms have been developed for the selection of antigen-specific rAbFs from large rAbFs repertoires. These technologies include phage display, cell surface displays (*e.g.* yeast, *E. coli*, mammalian), and cell-free displays (*e.g.* ribosomal, mRNA). The principle underlying all these display technologies is the direct physical link between the phenotype (displayed rAbF) and the genotype (DNA or RNA encoding the rAbF) of each clone. Coupling the phenotype and genotype of individual rAbFs enables the identification, isolation and amplification of rAbFs with the desired properties from libraries with large repertoires. Here, we discuss the most popular display formats which include phage, ribosomal, *E. coli*, and yeast displays (Fig. **6**).

7.1. Phage-Display

Phage-display technology has been by far the most widely used display platform for antibody discovery. The concept of displaying functional foreign peptides on the surface of filamentous bacteriophage was first demonstrated by George Smith in 1985 [381]. Shortly afterwards, McCafferty *et al.* [382] showed that a scFv fused to the phage coat minor protein pIII retained its antigen binding ability and specificity. Since the time of these groundbreaking reports, phage-display of antibody fragments has proven to be a powerful tool for the isolation of antigen-specific clones from libraries with large antibody repertoires.

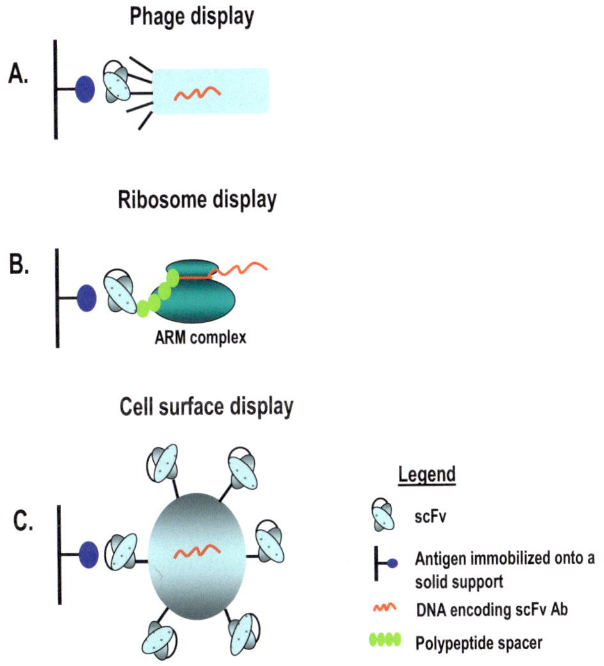

Figure 6: Molecular display technologies for rAbF selecktion; **(A)** phage display, **(B)** ribosome display, **(C)** cell surface display [394].

Phage-displayed Ab libraries are created by cloning the assembled rAbF gene repertoire into either a phage [363, 382] or phagemid vector [383, 384]; these libraries have extensively been reviewed elsewhere [385-387]. The distinct difference between these two systems is that with phage vectors there is multivalent display of the rAbF, which is fused to all available pIII minor coat proteins (usually 3-5 copies) on the phage, whereas with phagemid vectors there is only monovalent display of the rAbF. Due to the absence of avidity effects, higher affinity rAbFs are usually generated from phagemid libraries [385]. Furthermore, using phagemid vectors creates larger libraries since they have higher bacterial transformation efficiencies compared to phage vectors.

To display rAbFs on the surface of phage, the rAbF gene is fused to the N-terminal coding sequence of the gene encoding a minor phage coat protein (*e.g.* pIII) or, in some cases, to a major coat protein (*e.g.* pVIII). An amber stop codon (TAG) is generally engineered between the coding sequences of the antibody and the phage coat protein. Upon phage infection of an *E. coli* non-suppressor strain (*e.g.* TG1), this amber stop codon is read as a glutamine. As a result, the phage displays a unique rAbF protein (phenotype) on its surface, while its respective gene is encapsulated in the phage particle (Fig. **6A**). This direct link between phenotype and genotype enables the enrichment of each Ag-specific phage clone from large phage-rAbF libraries (~10^{10} members) by selection using an immobilized Ag target.

The selection of antigen-specific rAbFs from large phage display libraries occurs through a relatively standard procedure called 'panning'. The target antigen is first immobilized on a solid support, such as wells of a microtitre plate [340], immunotubes [388], nitrocellulose [389], or magnetic beads [390]. The phage-rAbF library is incubated with the immobilized antigen and unspecific phage-rAbF are removed by thorough washing. Bound phage-Ab are eluted by changing the binding conditions, *e.g.*, with low [391] or high pH buffers [392], proteolytic cleavage [384], or by competition with free Ag [393]. The recovered phage are amplified by infection of a suppressor strain of *E. coli* (*e.g.* TG1) prior to a subsequent round of selection. In general, 2-4 rounds of selection with increased stringency are necessary to enrich antigen-specific clones. Stringency can be increased by, for example, decreasing the concentration of immobilized Ag and/or by increasing the number of washes per round of panning [394].

Phage-display technology has enabled the generation of rAbFs with both high affinity and specificity against virtually any type of antigen [362, 363, 395]. Despite the development of alternative display formats (*e.g.*, ribosome and cell surface displays), phage-display remains the most popular display system as it is a robust, simple to use, and highly versatile technique [396].

7.2. Ribosome Display

Ribosome display is a completely cell-free system for the *in vitro* selection of antibodies, or other polypeptides, from large libraries. The key feature of ribosome display is the formation of a stable complex between the mRNA encoding the rAbF, the ribosome, and the newly translated rAbF (Fig. **6B**) [397]. The stable complex, also known as an ARM (Antibody-Ribosome-mRNA) complex, is formed by removing the stop codon at the 3′ end of the mRNA which consequently prevents the release of the nascent polypeptide and the mRNA from the ribosome. The rAbFs displayed on the complexes can be subjected to functional screening against an immobilized antigen or against biotinylated antigen in solution. After selection, the recovered mRNA is amplified by Reverse-Transcriptase-Polymerase Chain Reaction (RT-PCR) and either used for subsequent rounds of selection, for cloning purposes or mutated for affinity maturation [398].

Ribosome display has a number of advantages over phage and cell-base display technologies. Since this methodology is not limited by cloning and bacterial transformation efficiencies, very large libraries with up to 10^{14} members can be created and screened [397, 399]. Screening such large libraries increases the probability of selecting rare sequences of high-affinity antibodies [400]. Furthermore, since ribosome display is PCR-based, affinity maturation using, *e.g.* error-prone PCR [401] or DNA shuffling [402], can be performed between rounds of selection. Antibodies with nanomolar to even picomolar affinities have been generated using ribosome display technology [380, 403].

Despite these advantages, ribosome display has mostly been used for the *in vitro* affinity maturation of rAbFs [380, 398, 404]. The use of ribosome display for screening large rAbF libraries has been limited by the perceived technical challenges and by the unavailability of tailored commercial reagents [399]. More recently, Thom [399] has provided technical updates, including an improved method for the preparation of S-30 extracts, which make this technology more easily accessible. As many of the limitations of ribosome display are overcome, this technology may become one of the simplest and most robust of the display technologies [394].

7.2.1. E. coli Display

Since the early 1990s, several approaches to display antibodies on bacterial cells (Gram-positive and Gram-negative) have been described and a detailed review can be found elsewhere [405] (Fig. **6C**). Of particular interest is the work done by Mazor *et al.* [406] who devised the first system to display full-length IgG, whereas previous systems have been restricted to smaller antibody fragments (*e.g.* scFv, Fab) [396, 406]. In their methodology, IgG heavy and light chains are expressed and secreted into the periplasmic space of *E.*

coli. The assembled IgG were then bound, non-covalently, by an engineered Fc-binding protein that anchors the IgG to the inner membrane facing the periplasmic space to prevent diffusion of the Ab out of the cell. Following outer membrane permeabilization, the cell-bound IgGs are available to bind fluorescently-labeled Ag, and fluorescent cells are sorted by FACS. Several clones with low nM affinities have been isolated using this technology (Mazor *et al.*, 2007). In addition, this system is unique as it avoids the physical attachment of antibodies to fusion partners which could impair their stabilities and/or activities (Harvey *et al.*, 2004; Van Blarcom and Harvey, 2009). While phage and ribosome display technologies are restricted to display rAbFs composed of a single polypeptide chain (*e.g.* scFv, Fab), this system could provide a unique means to display engineered IgG-like Abs, *e.g.* scFv-Fc fusion protein and $scDb_2$-IgG, which are composed of two polypeptide chains.

One of the main advantage of utilizing cell-based display technologies, including bacterial, yeast and mammalian cell displays over phage display, is that they can be screened using Fluorescence Activated Cell Sorting (FACS) [405, 407]. FACS is a powerful, high-throughput tool suitable for quantitative screening of large libraries [407].

Although the proof-of-concept of this bacterial display technology and other similar technologies have been described, further evidence is needed to validate their utility as antibody engineering platforms [405].

7.3. Yeast Display

Yeast-surface display shares many of the same advantages as bacterial display; however, it has the added advantage of providing eukaryotic post-translational processing and modification of mammalian proteins [408]. In comparison with phage display, yeast display has been shown to generate twice as many novel antibodies when the same immune scFv library was screened using these two methods [409]. In yeast display, rAbFs are displayed on the cell surface of yeast (*e.g. Saccharomyces cerevisiae*) *via* fusion to α-agglutinin (Aga), a yeast mating adhesion receptor which is anchored to the cell wall of yeast [408]. As in *E. coli* display, yeast cells displaying rAbFs are incubated with fluorescently-labeled Ag and sorted by Fluorescence-Activated Cell Sorting (FACS).

In addition to antibody discovery, yeast-surface display has proven to be a very powerful method for engineering antibodies with improved affinity and specificity [410-412]. By coupling yeast display with directed evolution, Boder *et al.* (2000) produced a scFv with the highest affinity (48 fM) recorded to date. Another notable report effectively evolved an scFv with a dissociation half-time >4 days at 37 °C using yeast display [412]. Moreover, yeast display has also been used to enhance the stability and soluble expression of antibodies [413], as well as for antibody epitope mapping and characterization [414]. Owing to its noteworthy success, yeast display has been gaining popularity in recent years.

8. EXPRESSION SYSTEMS

Several expression systems have been developed for the production of rAbFs and their derivatives. These include bacteria, yeast, plants, and mammalian cells. Each has advantages, potential applications, and limitations.

8.1. Bacteria

Bacteria are a prokaryotic expression system favored for the production of small non-glycosylated rAbFs, mostly scFv, dsFv, Fab, and sVD fragments as well as some of their multimer and fusion products [283, 415-418]. Among bacteria, *E. coli* is the most widely used host for the production of heterologous proteins. In addition to rapid and economic production of heterogeneous proteins, bacteria have advantages of ease of culture, genetic manipulation, and high yields [419]. However, they cannot assemble functional Fc-fusion proteins and full-length antibodies because they lack the cellular machinery required for sophisticated post-translation modifications, *i.e.*, protein glycosylation and multiple disulfide bond formation [415].

In general, rAbFs expressed in bacteria are targeted for secretion into the media or periplasm, or expressed and retained in the cytoplasm, which is a reducing environment that prevents proper formation of disulfide bonds essential for antibody stability In most cases, antibodies are produced in bacteria as cytoplasmic inclusion bodies without a signal sequence at a high expression level (*i.e.*, 40 mg/L for a scFv-IP10 fusion protein), which requires additional solubilization and subsequent refolding process to obtain soluble and functional proteins [420-422]. By using this expression pathway, functional multivalent fusion proteins, *i.e.*, divalent $(Fab\text{-}SWn\text{-}PE38)_2$ and $(Fab\text{-}PE38fl)_2$ fusion proteins [147, 148], tetravalent TNF-TeAb mini-antibodies [423], and dimeric and trimeric 4D5 scFv-barnase-His_5 or 4D5 scFv-dibarnase-His_5 complexes [424], have been produced. Alternatively, by using *E. coli* strains capable of processing proper folding and oxidation *in vivo*, soluble rAbFs, including bivalent formats, can be produced in the cytoplasm at a level similar to or greater than that achieved with periplasmic expression [425-428]. Cytoplasmic expression is particularly recommended for the production of immunotoxins that may be toxic for bacteria or sensitive to intracellular degradation when expressed in a soluble form in the periplasmic space.

In addition, bacteria can also produce and secret soluble rAbFs into the media or to the periplasm when a specific signal sequence is used. For example, functional V_HH, scFv and Fab can be correctly processed and secreted into the periplasm of *E. coli* [23, 415, 416, 421]. Furthermore, more complicated antibody fragments, including fusion proteins (*i.e.*, a single-domain antibody (sdAb)-intein fusion protein [418] and scFv-toxin immunoconjugates [130]] and multivalent complexes [*i.e.*, bivalent $(scFv')_2$ [283, 429], bispecific Fab-scFv [430], and multivalent Fab fusion proteins [431]), have been produced in the periplasm and proven to be functional. However, in some cases, high-level expression of rAbFs can result in the accumulation of insoluble antibody fragments in the periplasm [74]; thus, extra steps are needed to recover the antigen binding activity by solubilization and refolding of the aggregated proteins [429]. In addition to the simple, rapid and low-cost production of antibody fragments in *E. coli*, our thorough understanding of *E. coli* transcription, translation, and protein processing together with the advances in DNA recombination technology makes this expression system valuable for the production of non-glycosylated antibody fragments.

8.2. Yeasts

Yeasts are a common expression system for the large-scale production ofproteins for industrial and biopharmaceutical use. Among yeasts, *Candida boidinii*, *Hansenula polymorpha*, *Pichia methanolica*, *Pichia pastoris* and *Saccharomyces cerevisiae* are well known hosts for the production of heterologous proteins, with *S. cerevisiae* and *P. pastoris* being the most used [24, 432, 433]. These yeast strains are genetically well characterized and able to perform many post-translational modifications. The main advantages of yeasts over other expression systems are that they are both a microorganism and a eukaryote. Unlike mammalian expression systems, yeast can rapidly grow in simple defined media, require short processing time, and are as easy to genetically manipulate as *E. coli*. In comparison to *E. coli*, yeasts produce proteins using a eukaryotic protein-synthesis machinery, and thereby, have the ability to produce large correctly folded and processed eukaryotic proteins and further to secret them into culture media when a proper signal sequence is used; therfore, yeasts are useful in producing properly folded active and soluble multisubunit proteins [24, 432, 434]. Proteins that are insoluble in *E. coli* are often soluble when expressed in yeast [435]. Due to these advantages, yeasts have been widely used as an expression system for the cost-effective and large-scale production of rAbFs, particularly multivalent and multispecific antibody molecules and Fc fusion proteins.

There are three types of vectors that have been used for the expression of recombinant proteins in yeasts: integration vectors (YIp), episomal plasmids (YEp), and centromeric plasmids (YCp) [433]. The YIp integrative vectors do not replicate autonomously, but integrate into the genome of hosts by homologous recombination and thus are used for high-level expression. By contrast, the YEp and YCp plasmid vectors propagate extrachromosomally, but are relatively unstable. Therefore, the YEp vector is more often used for small scale expression due to the high copy number ranging from 10 to 40 copies per cell, whereas the YCp plasmid is used as a regular cloning vector because it is typically present at very low copy numbers from 1 to 3 per cell [433, 436].

The post-translational modification machinery of yeast is eukaryotic and thus, it is able to glycosylate proteins at Asn-X-Ser/Thr motifs and to produce full-length antibodies and Fc fusion proteins [437]. However, these molecules contain high-mannose and multiple-branched oligosaccharides and in some cases are defective in effector functions, *i.e.*, complement-mediated lysis [438]. Despite the significant differences in the composition and structures of carbohydrates, the binding activity of whole antibodies produced in yeasts are similar to [439] or even better [437] than that of their counterparts derived from mammalian cells. A number of full-length antibodies [437] and monomeric rAbFs [440] as well as their fusion proteins (*i.e.*, toxin and enzyme immunoconjugates) [7, 238, 239], scFv-Fc fusion proteins [441], bispecific Fab-scFv and Fab-$(scFv)_2$ multimers [434]), have been successfully produced in yeasts at high yields (*i.e.*, 36.8 mg pure bibody and 12 mg pure tribody per liter supernatant) and function well both *in vitro* and *in vivo*. The eukaryotic protein-synthesis machinery and high yields of heterologous protein production make yeasts an attractive option for the expression of antibody molecules for clinical use.

8.3. Plants

Plants have been explored over the past two decades for the production of therapeutic drugs because they can be grown easily and inexpensively in large quantities and harvested, stored and processed using existing agricultural infrastructure, and are safe and free of human pathogens [442]. Plants have been considered to be a potential alternative bioreactor for the cost-effective, highly scalable, and safe production of therapeutic antibodies. This system offers several advantages over other currently used expression systems, which include the lack of animal pathogenic contaminants, low cost of production, and ease of agricultural scale-up. Moreover, plants as an eukaryotic organism have the ability to execute normal post-translational modifications, such as signal peptide cleavage, disulfide bond formation, and addition of O- and N-linked carbohydrates, thereby being able to produce correctly folded, processed, and glycosylated full-length antibodies [22, 443, 444] as well as multivalent Fc fusion proteins [445].

Recombinant antibodies can be produced in plants using stable expression systems by integrating their coding genes into the plant genome using the Ti plasmid of *Agrobacterium tumefaciens* as a vector for introducing recombinant DNA into the plant cell nucleus [22, 446]. Alternatively, they can also be produced using a transient expression system *via* vacuum infiltration of plant leaves with a recombinant *Agrobacterium* strain transformed with a vector carrying the gene of interest [447, 448], or *via* infection of plants with RNA transcribed *in vitro* from an potato virus X-based episomal vector [446, 449] or a bean yellow dwarf virus (BeYDV)-derived multi-replicon system [444]. Several transgenic plants, including tobacco, maize, soybean, and alfalfa, have been successfully used for the expression of full-length antibodies [22, 444, 450] and monomeric and multimeric rAbFs (*i.e.*, scFv, diabody, and scFv-Fc fusion protein) [442, 445, 451, 452]. IgGs have been produced at a level of 0.35-1.3% of the total soluble protein and scFvs at 0.01-6.8% in tobacco [451]. To obtain high levels of expression, antibodies are targeted for expression in the Endoplasmic Reticulum (ER) [453], apoplast [454], or seeds [445, 455] by using a appropriate signal sequence, with ER most favored, or using a multi-replicon vector [444].

The long time required to build a new expression system, the difficulty associated with plant protein purification, and the concerns on the suitability of plant-derived antibodies for therapeutic use have limited the broad application of plants as a bioreactor for the production of therapeutic proteins. One of the major concerns is the significant difference in glycan structures generated in plants, which lack the essential sugars galactose and sialic acid, and contain the potentially immunogenic sugars xylose and α1,3-fucose [456, 457]. The differences in glycosylation may influence *in vivo* biologic properties of plant-derived antibodies, such as immunogenicity, biodistribution, half-life, and effector functions [457-459]. To date, efforts have been made to humanize the glycosylation patterns of plant-derived antibodies by coexpressing the specific human glycosyltransferases [460, 461], by using specific knockout transgenic lines that lack xylosyltransferase and α1,3-fucosyltransferase [462], or by modulating plant glycosylation with RNA interference [463, 464]. Despite the difference in glycosylation pattern, plant-derived antibodies have been demonstrated to have a high binding affinity [446, 453, 465]; Fc-associated functions *in vitro* [22, 466] and retain their activity *in vivo* [466, 467]. The ability of plants to produce large amounts of rAbFs and Fc fusion proteins offers an economical alternative for the production of therapeutic and diagnostic agents.

However, the major drawbacks to plant-based systems are low expression and difficulty in offering inexpensive separation of antibodies from the large biomass (*i.e.* purification).

8.4. Mammalian Cells

Mammalian cells including mouse myeloma (NS0, SP2/0), Chinese Hamster Ovary (CHO), and human embryonic kidney cells (HEK-293) are the dominant cell types used in production systems for the generation of therapeutic antibodies, especially mAbs and Fc fusion proteins. These systems possess the mechanisms required for correct protein assembly, proper folding, and post-translational modification, which are equivalent to those of humans [465, 468]. The post-translational modifications include folding, aggregation, proteolysis, oxidation of methionine, deamidation of asparagine and glutamine, and glycosylation; these modifications are essential for efficient secretion, stability, and therapeutic efficacy of antibody molecules [469]. Mammalian cells are more likely to produce N-glycans similar to those found on human antibodies, and thus are the appropriate expression system for the production of antibodies capable of mediating all Fc-associated effector functions. However, they also have several limitations, including high cost of production, probability of contamination with infectious agents (*i.e.*, viruses and prions), time required to develop a desired cell line, and differences in N-glycan pattern. For example, CHO cell-derived mAbs contain fucosylated glycans [470, 471]. Therefore, to improve antibody-mediated effector functions, several approaches have been utilized to modify the glycans, including addition of bisecting GlcNAc that is absent in antibodies generated in CHO cells [472], reduction of fucose content [473, 474], or use of fucose-deficient strains [475].

Mammalian cell-derived mAbs have serum half-lives and effector functions comparable to those of naturally occurring antibodies [465, 468]. Numerous multivalent, bispecific antibodies (*i.e.*, Fab-scFv, and Fab-$(scFv)_2$) [289] and Fc fusion proteins (*i.e.*, IgG-like molecules) with capacity to mediate all Fc-dependent effector functions [296-298, 300, 303, 304] have also been produced using mammalian cells. Despite the high cost associated with the manufacturing process [476], this system is easily transfected andgrows naturally *in vitro*, which allows large-scale production of desired antibody molecules [468].

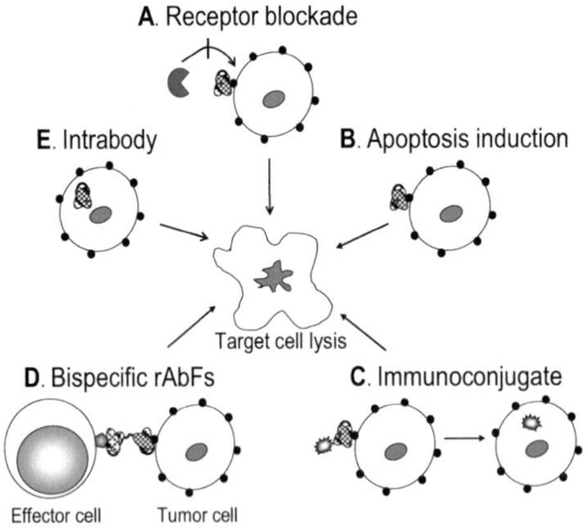

Figure 7: Therapeutic applications of rAbFs in cancer therapy. In cancer immunotherapy, rAbFs can be utilized to block the binding of ligands (*i.e.*, growth factors) to their receptors on tumor cells (A), induce apoptosis *via* interaction with specific receptors associated with apoptotic pathway activation (B), deliver an effective moiety (*i.e.*, radionucleotide, cytotoxic drug, toxin, cytokine, enzyme, or siRNA) that performs a specific function, resulting in tumor cell death, in the form of immunoconjugates (C), recruit and activate effector cells (*i.e.*, NK cells or CTLs) that kill the tumor cells *via* antibody-dependent cell-mediated cytotoxicity (ADCC), in the form of bispecific rAbFs with one side binding to a tumor cell and another side binding to an effector cell (D), or target intracellular molecules in a specific cellular compartment (*i.e.*, ER, nucleus, or cytosol mitochondria, peroxisomes, plasma membrane and trans-Golgi network) through intracellular expression *via* a specific signal peptide (E).

In summary, bacteria and yeasts are generally the most useful systems for the expression of non-glycosylated (*E. coli* only) antibody fragments and immunoconjugates (*i.e.*, immunotoxins and rAbF-enzyme conjugates), whereas mammalian cells and transgenic plants are favored for high-yield expression of intact antibodies and monomeric rAbFs as well as their derivatives (*i.e.*, diabodies, minibodies, and multivalent IgG-like molecules).

9. CONCLUSIONS

To date, antibodies and their related molecules are being increasingly explored as biotherapeutics, especially in cancer therapy (Fig. 7). The advances in recombinant DNA technology and protein engineering have made rAbFs a powerful alternative to intact mAbs in many applications, especially in the treatment of cancers and viral infections, because of their high specificity for target antigens, improved tissue penetration, cost-effective scale-up production, and easy manipulation to create the desired properties for clinical applications. Furthermore, the progress in designing and constructing different formats of rAbFs with unique properties (*e.g.* diabodies, minibodies, fusion proteins, facilitate the development of rAbFs for different applications. Many of the engineered rAbFs and related molecules discussed in this chapter are currently undergoing clinic trials. However, immunogenicity and safety are the major concerns associated with antibody applications in the medical field. New technologies are still urged to allow the rapid development of rAbFs with desired bispecific antibodies, and intrabodies), the advances of displaying and screening technologies (*e.g.* phage-, ribosome-, and microbial surface-display), and the emergence of various production systems (*e.g.* bacteria, yeast, plants, and mammalian cells) also significantly properties for efficient applications. In spite of these challenges, recombinant antibodies and antibody fragments will continue to play an increasingly important role in disease management in the near future.

REFERENCES

[1] Kohler G, Milstein C. Continuous cultures of fused cells secreting antibody of redefined specificity. Nature 1975; 256: 495-97.

[2] Jain RK, Baxter LT. Mechanisms of heterogeneous distribution of monoclonal antibodies and other macromolecules in tumors: significance of elevated interstitial pressure. Cancer Res 1988; 48: 7022-32.

[3] Carter P. Bispecific human IgG by design. J Immunol Methods 2001; 248: 7-15.

[4] Maynard JA, Maassen CB, Leppla SH, *et al.* Protection against anthrax toxin by recombinant antibody fragments correlates with antigen affinity. Nat Biotechnol 2002; 20: 597-601.

[5] Mozdzanowska K, Feng J, W. WG. Virus-neutralizing activity mediated by the Fab fragment of a hemagglutinin-specific antibody is sufficient for the resolution of influenza virus infection in SCID mice. J Virol 2003; 77: 8322-28.

[6] Song E, Zhu P, Lee SK, *et al.* Antibody mediated *in vivo* delivery of small interfering RNAs *via* cell-surface receptors. Nat Biotechnol 2005; 23: 709-17.

[7] Sharma SK, Pedley RB, Bhatia J, *et al.* Sustained tumor regression of human colorectal cancer xenografts using a multifunctional mannosylated fusion protein in antibody-directed enzyme prodrug therapy. Clin Cancer Res 2005; 11: 814-25.

[8] Owens RJ, Young RJ. The genetic engineering of monoclonal antibodies. J Immunol Methods 1994; 168: 149-65.

[9] Chowdhury PS, Wu H. Tailor-made antibody therapeutics. Methods 2005; 36: 11-24.

[10] van Dijk MA, van de Winkel JGJ. Human antibodies as next generation therapeutics. Curr Opin Chem Biol 2001; 5: 368-74.

[11] Janeway CA, Travers P, Walport M, Shlomachik MJ, Eds. Innate immunity. Immunobiology, 2001: 35-91.

[12] Presta LG. Molecular engineering and design of therapeutic antibodies. Curr Opin Immunol 2008; 20: 460-70.

[13] Roopenian DC, Akilesh S. FcRn: the neonatal Fc receptor comes of age. Nat Rev Immunol 2007; 7: 715-25.

[14] Abès R, Teillaud JL. Impact of glycosylation on effector functions of therapeutic IgG. Pharmaceuticals 2010; 3: 146-57.

[15] Mueller BM, Reisfeld RA, Gillies SD. Serum half-life and tumor localization of a chimeric antibody deleted of the CH2 domain and directed against the disialoganglioside GD2. Proc Natl Acad Sci USA 1990; 87: 5702-05.

[16] Ralph P, Nakoinz I, Diamond B, Yelton D. All classes of murine IgG antibody mediate macrophage phagocytosis and lysis of erythrocytes. J Immunol 1980; 125: 1885-88.

[17] Michaelsen TE, Kolberg J, Aase A, Herstad TK, Hoiby EA. The four mouse IgG isotypes differ extensively in bactericidal and opsonophagocytic activity when reacting with the P1.16 epitope on the outer membrane PorA protein of Neisseria meningitidis. Scand J Immunol 2004; 59: 34-9.

[18] Preston JM, Gerceker AA, Reff ME, Pier GB. Production and characterization of a set of mouse-human chimeric immunoglobulin G (IgG) subclass and IgA monoclonal antibodies with identical variable regions specific for Pseudomonas aeruginosa serogroup O6 lipopolysaccharide. Infect Immun 1998; 66: 4137-42.

[19] Bruggemann M, Williams GT, Bindon CI, *et al.* Comparison of the effector functions of human immunoglobulins using a matched set of chimeric antibodies. J Exp Med 1987; 166: 1351-61.

[20] Green LL. Antibody engineering *via* genetic engineering of the mouse: XenoMouse strains are a vehicle for the facile generation of therapeutic human monoclonal antibodies. J Immunol Methods 1999; 231: 11-23.

[21] Takauchi A, Kobayashi T, Tahara T, *et al.* The trans-chromosomic mouse-derived human monoclonal antibody promotes phagocytosis of Porphyromonas gingivalis by neutrophils. J Periodontol 2005; 76: 680-5.

[22] McLean MD, Almquist KC, Niu Y, *et al.* A human anti-Pseudomonas aeruginosa serotype O6ad immunoglobulin G1 expressed in transgenic tobacco is capable of recruiting immune system effector function *in vitro*. Antimicrob Agents Chemother 2007; 51: 3322-8.

[23] Humphreys DP. Production of antibodies and antibody fragments in Escherichia coli and a comparison of their functions, uses and modification. Curr Opin Drug Discov Devel 2003; 6: 188-96.

[24] Joosten V, Lokman C, Van Den Hondel CA, Punt PJ. The production of antibody fragments and antibody fusion proteins by yeasts and filamentous fungi. Microb Cell Fact 2003; 2: 1-15.

[25] Colcher D, Pavlinkova G, Beresford G, *et al.* Pharmacokinetics and biodistribution of genetically-engineered antibodies. Q J Nucl Med 1998; 42: 225-41.

[26] Batra SK, Jain M, Wittel UA, Chauhan SC, Colcher D. Pharmacokinetics and biodistribution of genetically engineered antibodies. Curr Opin Biotechnol 2002; 13: 603-8.

[27] Mariani G, and Strober, W. Fc receptors and the action of antibodies. Washington DC: American Society of Microbiology 1990.

[28] King DJ, Turmer A, Farnsworthe APH, *et al.* Improved tumor targeting with chemically cross-linked recombinant antibody fragments. Cancer Res 1994; 54: 6176-85.

[29] Kim J, Bronson CL, Wani MA, *et al.* Beta 2-microglobulin deficient mice catabolize IgG more rapidly than FcRn- alpha-chain deficient mice. Exp Biol Med (Maywood) 2008; 233: 603-9.

[30] Krinner EM, Hepp J, Hoffmann P, *et al.* A highly stable polyethylene glycol-conjugated human single-chain antibody neutralizing granulocyte-macrophage colony stimulating factor at low nanomolar concentration. Protein Eng Des Sel 2006; 19: 461-70.

[31] Weir ANC, Nesbitt A, Chapman AP, *et al.* Formatting antibody fragments to mediate specific therapeutic functions Biochem Soc Trans 2002; 30: 512-6.

[32] Ghetie V, Hubbard JG, Kim JK, *et al.* Abnormally short serum half-lives of IgG in beta 2-microglobulin-deficient mice. Eur J Immunol 1996; 26: 690-6.

[33] Shawler DL, Bartholomew RM, Smith LM, Dillman RO. Human immune response to multiple injections of murine monoclonal IgG. J Immunol 1985; 135: 1530-5.

[34] Jain RK, Baxter LT. Mechanisms of heterogeneous distribution of monoclonal antibodies and other macromolecules in tumors: significance of elevated interstitial pressure. Cancer Res 1988; 48: 7022-32.

[35] Pavlinkova G, Beresford GW, Booth BJM, Batra SK, Colcher D. Pharmacokinetics and biodistribution of engineered single-chain antibody constructs of MAb CC49 in colon carcinoma xenografts. J Nucl Med 1999; 40: 1536-46.

[36] Hudson PJ, Souriau C. Engineered antibodies. Nat Med 2003; 9: 129-34.

[37] Adams GP, Schier R, McCall AM, *et al.* High affinity restricts the localization and tumor penetration of single-chain fv antibody molecules. Cancer Res 2001; 61: 4750-5.

[38] Goel A, Baranowska-Kortylewicz J, Hinrichs SH, *et al.* 99mTc-labeled divalent and tetravalent CC49 single-chain Fvs: novel imaging agents for rapid *in vivo* localization of human colon carcinoma. J Nucl Med 2001; 42: 1519-27.

[39] Endo K, Kamma H, Ogata T. Radiolabeled monoclonal antibody 15 and its fragments for localization and imaging of xenografts of human lung cancer. J Natl Cancer Inst 1988; 80: 835-42.

[40] Kortt AA, Dolezal O, Power BE, Hudson PJ. Dimeric and trimeric antibodies: high avidity scFvs for cancer targeting. Biomol Eng 2001; 18: 95-108.

[41] Booy EP, Johar D, Maddika S, *et al.* Monoclonal and bispecific antibodies as novel therapeutics. Arch Immunol Ther Exp (Warsz) 2006; 54: 85-101.

[42] Kuss-Reichel K, Grauer L, Karavodin LM, *et al.* Will immunogenicity limit the use, efficacy, and future development of therapeutic monoclonal antibodies. Clin Diagn Lab Immunol 1994; 1: 365-72.

[43] Chatenoud L, Baudrihaye MF, Chkoff N, *et al.* Restriction of the human *in vivo* immune response against the mouse monoclonal antibody OKT3. J Immunol 1986; 137: 830-8.

[44] Stockwin LH, Holmes S. Antibodies as therapeutic agents: vive la renaissance. Expert Opin Biol Ther 2003; 3: 1133-52.

[45] Alegre ML, Gastaldello K, Abramowicz D, *et al.* Evidence that pentoxifylline reduces anti-CD3 monoclonal antibody-induced cytokine release syndrome. Transplantation 1991; 52: 674-9.

[46] Bugelski PJ, Achuthanandam R, Capocasale RJ, Treacy G, Bouman-Thio E. Monoclonal antibody-induced cytokine-release syndrome. Expert Rev Clin Immunol 2009; 5: 499-521.

[47] Hudson PJ, Souriau C. Engineered antibodies. Nat Med, 2003; 9: 129-34.

[48] Behr TM, Goldenbery DM, Becker W. Reducing the renal uptake of radiolabeled antibody fragments and peptides for diagnosis and therapy: present status, future prospects and limitations. Eur J Nucl Med 1998; 25: 201-12.

[49] Wu AM, Wiliams LE, Zieran L, *et al.* Anti-carcirnoembryonic antigen (CEA) diabody for rapid tumor imaging. Tumor Target 1999; 4: 47-54.

[50] Tahtis K, Lee F-T, Smyth FE, *et al.* Biodistribution properties of indium-111-labeled C-functionalized trans-cyclohexyl diethylenetriaminepentaacetic acid humanized 3S193 diabody and F(ab')2 constructs in a breast carcinoma xenograft model. Clin Cancer Res 2001; 7: 1061-72.

[51] Yazaki PJ, Wu AM, Tsai SW, *et al.* Tumor targeting of radiometal-labeled anti-CEA recombinant T84.66 diabody and t84.66 minibody: comparison to radioiodinated fragments. Bioconjug Chem 2001; 12: 220-8.

[52] Lamminmaki U, Pauperio S, Westerlund-Karlsson A, Karvinen J, Virtanen PL. Expanding the conformational diversity by random insertions into CDRH2 results in improved anti-estradiol antibodies. J Mol Biol 1999; 291: 589-602.

[53] Sheedy C, MacKenzie CR, Hall JC. Isolation and affinity maturation of hapten-specific antibodies. Biotechnol Adv 2007; 25: 333-52.

[54] Tachibana H, Matsumoto N, Cheng XJ, Tsukamoto H, Yoshihara E. Improved affinity of a human anti-Entamoeba histolytica Gal/GalNAc lectin Fab fragment by a single amino acid modification of the light chain. Clin Diagn Lab Immunol 2004; 11: 1085-8.

[55] Short MK, Krykbaev RA, Jeffrey PD, Margolies MN. Complementary combining site contact residue mutations of the anti-digoxin Fab 26-10 permit high affinity wild-type binding. J Biol Chem 2002; 277: 16365-70.

[56] Hawkins RE, Russell SJ, Winter G. Selection of phage antibodies by binding affinity. Mimicking affinity maturation. J Mol Biol 1992; 226: 889-96.

[57] Schlapschy M, Gruber H, Gresch O, *et al.* Functional humanization of an anti-CD30 Fab fragment for the immunotherapy of Hodgkin's lymphoma using an *in vitro* evolution approach. Protein Eng Des Sel 2004; 17: 847-60.

[58] Irving RA, Kortt AA, Hudson PJ. Affinity maturation of recombinant antibodies using E. coli mutator cells. Immunotechnology 1996; 2: 127-43.

[59] Kobayashi N, Oyama H, Kato Y, *et al.* Two-step *in vitro* antibody affinity maturation enables estradiol-17beta assays with more than 10-fold higher sensitivity. Anal Chem 2010; 82: 1027-38.

[60] Gram H, Marconi LA, Barbas CF, 3rd, *et al. In vitro* selection and affinity maturation of antibodies from a naive combinatorial immunoglobulin library. Proc Natl Acad Sci USA 1992; 89: 3576-80.

[61] Irving RA, Coia G, Raicevic A, Hudson PJ. Use of Escherichia coli mutator cells to mature antibodies. Methods Mol Biol 2002; 178: 295-302.

[62] Boder ET, Wittrup KD. Yeast surface display for directed evolution of protein expression, affinity, and stability. Methods Enzymol 2000; 328: 430-44.

[63] Jia L, Yu J, Song H, *et al.* Screening of human antibody Fab fragment against HBsAg and the construction of its dsFv form. Int J Biol Sci 2008; 4: 103-10.

[64] Fukuda I, Kojoh K, Tabata N, *et al. In vitro* evolution of single-chain antibodies using mRNA display. Nucleic Acids Res 2006; 34: 1-8.

[65] Finlay WJ, Cunningham O, Lambert MA, *et al.* Affinity maturation of a humanized rat antibody for anti-RAGE therapy: Comprehensive mutagenesis reveals a high level of mutational plasticity both inside and outside the CDRs. J Mol Biol 2009; 388: 541-58.

[66] Ness JE, Kim S, Gottman A, *et al.* Synthetic shuffling expands functional protein diversity by allowing amino acids to recombine independently. Nat Biotechnol 2002; 20: 1251-5.

[67] Casey JL, Napier MP, King DJ, *et al.* Tumour targeting of humanised cross-linked divalent-Fab' antibody fragments: a clinical phase I/II study. Br J Cancer 2002; 86: 1401-10.

[68] Hust M, Jostock T, Menzel C, *et al.* Single chain Fab (scFab) fragment. BMC Biotechnol 2007; 8: 1-15.

[69] Kubetzko S, Balic E, Waibel R, Zangemeister-Wittke U, Plückthun A. PEGylation and Multimerization of the Anti-p185-HER-2 Single Chain Fv Fragment 4D5. J Biol Chem 2006; 281: 35186-201.

[70] Todorovska A, Roovers RC, Dolezal O, *et al.* Design and application of diabodies, triabodies and tetrabodies for cancer targeting. J Immunol Methods 2001; 248: 47-66.

[71] Adams GP, Schier R, McCall AM, *et al.* Prolonged *in vivo* tumour retention of a human diabody targeting the extracellular domain of human HER2/neu. Br J Cancer 1998; 77: 1405-12.

[72] Le Gall F, Kipriyanov SM, Moldenhauer G, Little M. Di-, tri- and tetrameric single chain Fv antibody fragments against human CD19: Effect of valency on cell binding. FEBS Lett 1999; 453: 164-68.

[73] Adams GP, McCartney JE, Tai MS, *et al.* Highly specific *in vivo* tumor targeting by monovalent and divalent forms of 741F8 anti-c-erbB-2 single-chain Fv. Cancer Res 1993; 53: 4026-34.

[74] Kipriyanov SM, Dubel S, Breitling F, Kontermann RE, Little M. Recombinant single-chain Fv fragments carrying C-terminal cysteine residues: production of bivalent and biotinylated miniantibodies. Mol Immunol 1994; 31: 1047-58.

[75] Adams GP, Tai M-S, McCartney JE, *et al.* Avidity-mediated enhancement of *in vivo* tumor targeting by single-chain Fv dimers. Clin Cancer Res 2006; 12: 1599-605

[76] Liu B. Exploring cell type-specific internalizing antibodies for targeted delivery of siRNA. Brief Funct Genomic Proteomic 2007; 6: 112-9.

[77] Hu S, Shively L, Raubitschek A, *et al.* Minibody: A novel engineered anti-carcinoembryonic antigen antibody fragment (single-chain Fv-CH3) which exhibits rapid, high-level targeting of xenografts. Cancer Res 1996; 56: 3055-61.

[78] Müller D, Trunk G, Sichelstiel A, *et al.* Murine endoglin-specific single-chain Fv fragments for the analysis of vascular targeting strategies in mice. J Immunol Methods 2008; 339: 90-8.

[79] Griffiths GL, Chang CH, McBride WJ, *et al.* Reagents and methods for PET using bispecific antibody pretargeting and 68Ga-radiolabeled bivalent hapten-peptide-chelate conjugates. J Nucl Med 2004; 45: 30-9.

[80] Arndt MA, Krauss J, Rybak SM. Antigen binding and stability properties of non-covalently linked anti-CD22 single-chain Fv dimers. FEBS Lett 2004; 578: 257-61.

[81] Le Gall F, Reusch U, Little M. Kipriyanov SM. Effect of linker sequences between the antibody variable domains on the formation, stability and biological activity of a bispecific tandem diabody. Protein Eng Des Sel 2004; 17: 357-66.

[82] Gregoriadis G, Jain S, Papaioannou I, Laing P. Improving the therapeutic efficacy of peptides and proteins: A role for polysialic acids. Int J Pharm 2005; 300: 125-30.

[83] Fishburn CS. The pharmacology of pegylation: balancing pd with pk to generate novel therapeutics. J Pharm Sci 2007: 1-17.

[84] Chapman AP. PEGylated antibodies and antibody fragments for improved therapy: a review. Adv Drug Deliv Rev 2002; 54: 531-45.

[85] Kaushik V, Moots RJ. CDP-870 (certolizumab) in rheumatoid arthritis. Expert Opin Biol Ther 2005; 5: 601-6.

[86] Ton NC, Parker GJ, Jackson A, *et al.* Phase I evaluation of CDP791, a PEGylated di-Fab' conjugate that binds vascular endothelial growth factor receptor 2. Clin Cancer Res 2007; 13: 7113-8.

[87] Yang K, Basu A, Wang M, *et al.* Tailoring structure-function and pharmacokinetic properties of single-chain Fv proteins by site-specfic PEGylation. Protein Eng 2003; 16: 761-70.

[88] Mabry R, Rani M, Geiger R, *et al.* Passive protection against anthrax by using a high-affinity antitoxin antibody fragment lacking an Fc region. Infect Immun 2005; 73: 8362-68.

[89] Knight DMea. Pharmacodynamic enhancement of the anti-platelet antibody fab abciximab by site-specific pegylation. Platelets 2004; 15: 409-18.

[90] Choy EH, Hazleman B, Smith M, *et al.* Efficacy of a novel PEGylated humanized anti-TNF fragment (CDP870) in patients with rheumatoid arthritis: a phase II double-blinded, randomized, dose-escalating trial. Rheumatology (Oxford) 2002; 41: 1133-7.

[91] Schreiber S, Rutgeerts P, Fedorak RN, *et al.* A randomized, placebo-controlled trial of certolizumab pegol (CDP870) for treatment of Crohn's disease. Gastroenterology 2005; 129: 807-18.

[92] Baum P, Müller, D., Rüger, R., and Kontermann, R.E. Single-chain Fv immunoliposomes for the targeting of fibroblast activation protein-expressing tumor stromal cells. J Drug Target 2007; 15: 399-406.

[93] Messerschmidt SK, Kolbe A, Müller D, *et al.* Novel single-chain Fv' formats for the generation of immunoliposomes by site-directed coupling. Bioconjug Chem 2008; 19: 362-69.

[94] Hayes ME, Drummond DC, Hong K, *et al.* Increased target specificity of anti-HER2 genospheres by modification of surface charge and degree of PEGylation Mol Pharm 2006; 3: 726-36.

[95] Kirpotin DB, Drummond DC, Shao Y, *et al.* Antibody targeting of long circulating lipidic nanoparticles does not increase tumor localization but does increase internalization in animal models. Cancer Res 2006; 66: 6732-40.

[96] Caliceti P, Veronese FM. Pharmacokinetic and biodistribution properties of poly(ethylene glycol)-protein conjugates. Adv Drug Deliv Rev 2003; 55: 1261-77.

[97] Wunderlich DA, Macdougall M, Mierz DV, *et al.* Generation and characterization of a monoclonal IgG antibody to polyethylene glycol. Hybridoma (Larchmt) 2007; 26: 168-72.

[98] Gregoriadis G, McCormack B, Wang Z, Lifely R. Polysialic acids: potential in drug delivery. FEBS Lett 1993; 315: 271-6.

[99] Gregoriadis G, Fernandes A, Mital M, McCormack B. Polysialic acids: potential in improving the stability and pharmacokinetics of proteins and other therapeutics. Cell Mol Life Sci 2000; 57: 1964-9.

[100] Epenetos AA, Hreczuk-Hirst DH, McCormack B, Gregoriadis G. Polysialylated proteins: a potential role in cancer therapy. Clin Pharm 2002; 21: 2186.

[101] Constantinou A, Epenetos AA, Hreczuk-Hirst D, Jain S, Deonarain MP. Modulation of antibody pharmacokinetics by chemical polysialylation. Bioconjug Chem 2008; 19: 643-50.

[102] Rehlaender BN, Cho MJ. Antibodies as drug carriers. II. For proteins. Pharm Res 2001; 18: 753-60.

[103] Chaudhury C, Brooks CL, Carter DC, *et al.* Albumin Binding to FcRn: Distinct from the FcRn-IgG Interaction. Biochem 2006; 45: 4983-90.

[104] Müller D, Karle A, Meissburger B, *et al.* Improved pharmacokinetics of recombinant bispecific antibody molecules by fusion to human serum albumin. J Biol Chem 2007; 282: 12650-60.

[105] Holliger P, Wing M, Pound JD, Bohlen H, Winter G. Retargeting serum immunoglobulin with bispecific diabodies. Nat Biotechnol 1997; 15: 632 - 6.

[106] Yazaki PJ, Kassa T, Cheung CW, *et al.* Biodistribution and tumor imaging of an anti-CEA single-chain antibody-albumin fusion protein. Nucl Med Biol 2008; 35: 151-8.

[107] Dennis MS, Zhang M, Meng YG, *et al.* Albumin binding as a general strategy for improving the pharmacokinetics of proteins. J Biol Chem 2002: 35035-43.

[108] Nguyen A, Reyes AE, 2nd, Zhang M, *et al.* The pharmacokinetics of an albumin-binding Fab (AB.Fab) can be modulated as a function of affinity for albumin. Protein Eng Des Sel 2006; 19: 291-7.

[109] Stork R, Müller D, Kontermann RE. A novel tri-functional antibody fusion protein with improved pharmacokinetic properties generated by fusing a bispecific single-chain diabody with an albumin-binding domain from streptococcal protein G. Protein Eng Des Sel 2007; 20: 569-76.

[110] Holt LJ, Basran A, Jones K, *et al.* Anti-serum albumin domain antibodies for extending the half-lives of short lived drugs. Protein Eng Des Sel 2008; 21: 283-8.

[111] Smith BJ, Popplewell A, Athwal D, *et al.* Prolonged *in vivo* residence times of antibody fragments associated with albumin. Bioconjug Chem 2001; 12: 750-6.

[112] Palma E, Cho MJ. Improved systemic pharmacokinetics, biodistribution, and antitumor activity of CpG oligodeoxynucleotides complexed to endogenous antibodies *in vivo*. J Control Release 2007; 120: 95-103.

[113] Powers DB, Amersdorfer P, Poul M, *et al.* Expression of single-chain Fv-Fc fusions in Pichia pastoris. J Immunol Methods 2001; 251: 123-35.

[114] Kenanova V, Olafsen T, Crow DM, *et al.* Tailoring the pharmacokinetics and positron emission tomography imaging properties of anti-carcinoembryonic antigen single-chain fv-fc antibody fragments. Cancer Res 2005; 65: 622-31.

[115] Olafsen T, Cheung CW, Yazaki PJ, *et al.* Covalent disulfide-linked anti-CEA diabody allows site-specific conjugation and radiolabeling for tumor targeting applications. Protein Eng Des Sel 2004; 17: 21-7.

[116] Stork R, Zettlitz KA, Müller D, *et al.* N-glycosylation as novel strategy to improve pharmacokinetic properties of bispecific single-chain diabodies. J Biol Chem 2008; 283: 7804-12.

[117] Kim MK, Jeong HJ, CH K, *et al.* Improved renal clearance and tumor targeting of 99mTc-labeled anti-Tac monoclonal antibody Fab by chemical modifications. Nucl Med Biol 2002; 29: 139-46.

[118] Kim IS, Yoo TM, Kobayashi H, *et al.* Chemical modification to reduce renal uptake of disulfide-bonded variable region fragment of anti-Tac monoclonal antibody labeled with 99mTc. Bioconjug Chem 1999; 10: 447-53.

[119] Pavlinkova G, Beresford G, Booth BJ, Batra SK, Colcher D. Charge-modified single chain antibody constructs of monoclonal antibody CC49: generation, characterization, pharmacokinetics, and biodistribution analysis. Nucl Med Biol 1999; 26: 27-34.

[120] Onda M, Nagata S, Tsutsumi Y, *et al.* Lowering the isoelectric point of the Fv portion of recombinant immunotoxins leads to decreased nonspecific animal toxicity without affecting antitumor activity. Cancer Res 2001; 61: 5070-7.

[121] Holliger P, Hudson PJ. Engineered antibody fragments and the rise of single domains. Nat Biotechnol 2005; 23: 1126 -36.

[122] Frankel AE, Zuckero SL, Mankin AA, *et al.* Anti-CD3 recombinant diphtheria immunotoxin therapy of cutaneous T cell lymphoma. Curr Drug Targets 2009; 10: 104-9.

[123] Kreitman RJ. Immunotoxins for targeted cancer therapy. Aaps J 2006; 8:E532-51.

[124] Olsnes S, van Deurs B, Sandvig K. Protein toxins acting on intracellular targets: cellular uptake and translocation to the cytosol. Med Microbiol Immunol 1993; 182: 51-61.

[125] Frankel AE, McCubrey JA, Miller MS, *et al.* Diphtheria toxin fused to human interleukin-3 is toxic to blasts from patients with myeloid leukemias. Leukemia 2000; 14: 576-85.

[126] Thorpe PE, Wallace PM, Knowles PP, *et al.* Improved antitumor effects of immunotoxins prepared with deglycosylated ricin A-chain and hindered disulfide linkages. Cancer Res 1988; 48: 6396-403.

[127] Schrama D, Reisfeld RA, Becker JC. Antibody targeted drugs as cancer therapeutics. Nat Rev Drug Discov 2006; 5: 147-59.

[128] Pastan I, Hassan R, FitzGerald DJ, Kreitman RJ. Immunotoxin treatment of cancer. Annu Rev Med 2007; 58: 221-37.

[129] Attia P, Powell DJ, Jr., Maker AV, *et al.* Selective elimination of human regulatory T lymphocytes *in vitro* with the recombinant immunotoxin LMB-2. J Immunother 2006; 29: 208-14.

[130] Singh R, Samant U, Hyland S, *et al.* Target-specific cytotoxic activity of recombinant immunotoxin scFv(MUC1)-ETA on breast carcinoma cells and primary breast tumors. Mol Cancer Ther 2007; 6: 562-9.

[131] Posey JA, Khazaeli MB, Bookman MA, *et al.* A phase I trial of the single-chain immunotoxin SGN-10 (BR96 sFv-PE40) in patients with advanced solid tumors. Clin Cancer Res 2002; 8: 3092-9.

[132] Kim GB, Wang Z, Liu YY, *et al.* A fold-back single-chain diabody format enhances the bioactivity of an anti-monkey CD3 recombinant diphtheria toxin-based immunotoxin. Protein Eng Des Sel 2007; 20: 425-32.

[133] Kreitman RJ, Wilson WH, White JD, *et al.* Phase I trial of recombinant immunotoxin anti-tac(Fv)-PE38 (LMB-2) in patients with hematologic malignancies. J Clin Oncol 2000b; 18.

[134] Kreitman RJ, Squires DR, Stetler-Stevenson M, *et al.* Phase I trial of recombinant immunotoxin RFB4(dsFv)-PE38 (BL22) in patients with B-cell malignancies. J Clin Oncol 2005; 23: 6719-29.

[135] Kreitman RJ, Margulies I, Stetler-Stevenson M, *et al.* Cytotoxic Activity of Disulfide-stabilized Recombinant Immunotoxin RFB4(dsFv)-PE38 (BL22) toward Fresh Malignant Cells from Patients with B-Cell Leukemias. Clin Cancer Res 2000; 6: 1476-87.

[136] Ohno N, Kreitman RJ, Saito T. Augmentation of the activity of an immunotoxin, anti-Tac(Fv)-PE40KDEL, in T cell lines infected with human T cell leukemia virus type-I. Leuk Lymphoma 2002; 43: 885-88.

[137] Kreitman RJ, Pastan I. Accumulation of a recombinant immunotoxin in a tumor *in vivo*: fewer than 1000 molecules per cell are sufficient for complete responses. Cancer Res 1998; 58: 968-75.

[138] Kreitman RJ, Bailon P, Chaudhary VK, FitzGerald DJ, Pastan I. Recombinant immunotoxins containing anti-Tac(Fv) and derivatives of Pseudomonas exotoxin produce complete regression in mice of an interleukin-2 receptor-expressing human carcinoma. Blood 1994; 83: 426-34.

[139] Kreitman RJ. Immunotoxins in cancer therapy. Curr Opin Immunol 1999; 11: 570-78.

[140] Mansfield E, Amlot P, Pastan I, FitzGerald DJ. Recombinant RFB4 immunotoxins exhibit potent cytotoxic activity for CD22-bearing cells and tumors. Blood 1997; 90: 2020-26.

[141] Kreitman RJ, Wang QC, FitzGerald DJ, Pastan I. Complete regression of human B-cell lymphoma xenografts in mice treated with recombinant anti-CD22 immunotoxin RFB4(dsFv)-PE38 at doses tolerated by cynomolgus monkeys. Int J Cancer 1999; 81: 148-55.

[142] Kreitman RJ. Quantification of immunotoxin number for complete therapeutic response. Methods Mol Biol 2001; 166: 111-23.

[143] Brinkmann U, Buchner J, Pastan I. Independent domain folding of Pseudomonas exotoxin and single-chain immunotoxins: influence of interdomain connections. Proc Natl Acad Sci USA 1992; 89: 3075-9.

[144] Brinkmann U, Pai LH, FitzGerald DJ, Willingham M, Pastan I. B3(Fv)-PE38KDEL, a single-chain immunotoxin that causes complete regression of a human carcinoma in mice. Proc Natl Acad Sci USA 1991; 88: 8616-20.

[145] Reiter Y, Brinkmann U, Jung SH, *et al.* Improved binding and antitumor activity of a recombinant anti-erbB2 immunotoxin by disulfide stabilization of the Fv fragment. J Biol Chem 1994; 269: 18327-31.

[146] Reiter Y, Brinkmann U, Webber KO, *et al.* Engineering interchain disulfide bonds into conserved framework regions of Fv fragments: improved biochemical characteristics of recombinant immunotoxins containing disulfide-stabilized Fv. Protein Eng 1994; 7: 697-704.

[147] Won J, Choe M. Disulfide bond bridged divalent antibody-toxin, (Fab-PE38fl)2, with the toxin PE38 fused to the light chain. J Microbiol Biotechnol 2008; 18: 1475-81.

[148] Won J, Nam P, Lee Y, Choe M. Higher cytotoxicity of divalent antibody-toxins than monovalent antibody-toxins. Biochem Biophys Res Commun 2009; 382: 15-20.

[149] Buchner J, Rudolph R. Renaturation, purification and characterization of recombinant Fab-fragments produced in Escherichia coli. Biotechnology (N Y) 1991; 9: 157-62.

[150] Benhar I, Pastan I. Characterization of B1(Fv)PE38 and B1(dsFv)PE38: single-chain and disulfide-stabilized Fv immunotoxins with increased activity that cause complete remissions of established human carcinoma xenografts in nude mice. Clin Cancer Res 1995; 1: 1023-9.

[151] Choe M, Webber KO, Pastan I. B3(Fab)-PE38M: a recombinant immunotoxin in which a mutant form of Pseudomonas exotoxin is fused to the Fab fragment of monoclonal antibody B3. Cancer Res 1994; 54: 3460-7.

[152] Derocq JM, Casellas P, Laurent G, *et al.* Comparison of the cytotoxic potency of T101 Fab, F(ab')2 and whole IgG immunotoxins. J Immunol 1988; 141: 2837-43.

[153] Saito T, Kreitman RJ, Hanada S, *et al.* Cytotoxicity of recombinant Fab and Fv immunotoxins on adult T-cell leukemia lymph node and blood cells in the presence of soluble interleukin-2 receptor. Cancer Res 1994; 54: 1059-64.

[154] Kreitman RJ, Chang CN, Hudson DV, *et al.* Anti-Tac(Fab)-PE40, a recombinant double-chain immunotoxin which kills interleukin-2-receptor-bearing cells and induces complete remission in an *in vivo* tumor model. Int J Cancer 1994; 57: 856-64.

[155] Hexham JM, Dudas D, Hugo R, *et al.* Influence of relative binding affinity on efficacy in a panel of anti-CD3 scFv immunotoxins. Mol Immunol 2001; 38: 397-408.

[156] Wargalla UC, Reisfeld RA. Rate of internalization of an immunotoxin correlates with cytotoxic activity against human tumor cells. Proc Natl Acad Sci USA 1989; 86: 5146-50.

[157] Frankel AE. Reducing the immune response to immunotoxin. Clin Cancer Res 2004; 10: 13-5.

[158] Hetzel C, Bachran C, Fischer R, *et al.* Small cleavable adapters enhance the specific cytotoxicity of a humanized immunotoxin directed against CD64-positive cells. J Immunother 2008; 31: 370-6.

[159] Xiang J. Targeting cytokines to tumors to induce active antitumor immune responses by recombinant fusion proteins. Hum Antibodies 1999; 9: 23-36.

[160] Khawli LA, Hu P, Epstein AL. Cytokine, chemokine, and co-stimulatory fusion proteins for the immunotherapy of solid tumors. Handb Exp Pharmacol 2008; 181: 291-328.

[161] Kirkwood JM, Tarhini AA, Panelli MC, *et al.* Next generation of immunotherapy for melanoma. J Clin Oncol 2008; 26: 3445-55.

[162] Rossi EA, Goldenberg DM, Cardillo TM, Stein R, Chang CH. CD20-targeted tetrameric interferon-alpha, a novel and potent immunocytokine for the therapy of B-cell lymphomas. Blood 2009; 114: 3864-71.

[163] Lode HN, Xiang R, Becker JC, Gillies SD, Reisfeld RA. Immunocytokines: a promising approach to cancer immunotherapy. Pharmacol Ther 1998; 80: 277-92.

[164] Ortiz-Sanchez E, Helguera G, Daniels TR, Penichet ML. Antibody-cytokine fusion proteins: applications in cancer therapy. Expert Opin Biol Ther 2008; 8: 609-32.

[165] Davis CB, Gillies SD. Immunocytokines: amplification of anti-cancer immunity. Cancer Immunol Immunother 2003; 52: 297-308.

[166] Seruga B, Zhang H, Bernstein LJ, Tannock IF. Cytokines and their relationship to the symptoms and outcome of cancer. Nat Rev Cancer 2008; 8: 887-99.

[167] Borish LC, Steinke JW. 2. Cytokines and chemokines. J Allergy Clin Immunol 2003; 111:S460-75.

[168] Steinke JW, Borish L. 3. Cytokines and chemokines. J Allergy Clin Immunol 2006; 117:S441-5.

[169] Mattijssen V, Balemans LT, Steerenberg PA, De Mulder PH. Polyethylene-glycol-modified interleukin-2 is superior to interleukin-2 in locoregional immunotherapy of established guinea-pig tumors. Int J Cancer 1992; 51: 812-7.

[170] Grunhagen DJ, de Wilt JH, van Geel AN, Eggermont AM. Isolated limb perfusion for melanoma patients--a review of its indications and the role of tumour necrosis factor-alpha. Eur J Surg Oncol 2006; 32: 371-80.

[171] Grunhagen DJ, de Wilt JH, Graveland WJ, *et al.* Outcome and prognostic factor analysis of 217 consecutive isolated limb perfusions with tumor necrosis factor-alpha and melphalan for limb-threatening soft tissue sarcoma. Cancer 2006; 106: 1776-84.

[172] Schliemann C, Neri D. Antibody-based targeting of the tumor vasculature. Biochim Biophys Acta 2007; 1776: 175-92.

[173] Den Otter W, Jacobs JJ, Battermann JJ, *et al.* Local therapy of cancer with free IL-2. Cancer Immunol Immunother 2008; 57: 931-50.

[174] Heuser C, Guhlke S, Matthies A, *et al.* Anti-CD30-scFv-Fc-IL-2 antibody-cytokine fusion protein that induces resting NK cells to highly efficient cytolysis of Hodgkin's lymphoma derived tumour cells. Int J Cancer 2004; 110: 386-94.

[175] Hombach A, Heuser C, Abken H. Simultaneous targeting of IL2 and IL12 to Hodgkin's lymphoma cells enhances activation of resting NK cells and tumor cell lysis. Int J Cancer 2005; 115: 241-7.

[176] Helguera G, Penichet ML. Antibody-cytokine fusion proteins for the therapy of cancer. Methods Mol Med 2005; 109: 347-74.

[177] Schanzer JM, Baeuerle PA, Dreier T, Kufer P. A human cytokine/single-chain antibody fusion protein for simultaneous delivery of GM-CSF and IL-2 to Ep-CAM overexpressing tumor cells. Cancer Immun 2006; 6: 4.

[178] Halin C, Rondini S, Nilsson F, *et al.* Enhancement of the antitumor activity of interleukin-12 by targeted delivery to neovasculature. Nat Biotechnol 2002; 20: 264-9.

[179] Marlind J, Kaspar M, Trachsel E, *et al.* Antibody-mediated delivery of interleukin-2 to the stroma of breast cancer strongly enhances the potency of chemotherapy. Clin Cancer Res 2008; 14: 6515-24.

[180] Sogaard M, Ohlsson L, Kristensson K, *et al.* Treatment with tumor-reactive Fab-IL-2 and Fab-staphylococcal enterotoxin A fusion proteins leads to sustained T cell activation, and long-term survival of mice with established tumors. Int J Oncol 1999; 15: 873-82.

[181] Yamane BH, Hank JA, Albertini MR, Sondel PM. The development of antibody-IL-2 based immunotherapy with hu14.18-IL2 (EMD-273063) in melanoma and neuroblastoma. Expert Opin Investig Drugs 2009; 18: 991-1000.

[182] Osenga KL, Hank JA, Albertini MR, *et al.* A phase I clinical trial of the hu14.18-IL2 (EMD 273063) as a treatment for children with refractory or recurrent neuroblastoma and melanoma: a study of the Children's Oncology Group. Clin Cancer Res 2006; 12: 1750-9.

[183] King DM, Albertini MR, Schalch H, *et al.* Phase I clinical trial of the immunocytokine EMD 273063 in melanoma patients. J Clin Oncol 2004; 22: 4463-73.

[184] Gafner V, Trachsel E, Neri D. An engineered antibody-interleukin-12 fusion protein with enhanced tumor vascular targeting properties. Int J Cancer 2006; 119: 2205-12.

[185] Borsi L, Balza E, Carnemolla B, *et al.* Selective targeted delivery of TNFalpha to tumor blood vessels. Blood 2003; 102: 4384-92.

[186] Castellani P, Borsi L, Carnemolla B, *et al.* Differentiation between high- and low-grade astrocytoma using a human recombinant antibody to the extra domain-B of fibronectin. Am J Pathol 2002; 161: 1695-700.

[187] Carnemolla B, Borsi L, Balza E, *et al.* Enhancement of the antitumor properties of interleukin-2 by its targeted delivery to the tumor blood vessel extracellular matrix. Blood 2002; 99: 1659-65.

[188] Ebbinghaus C, Ronca R, Kaspar M, *et al.* Engineered vascular-targeting antibody-interferon-gamma fusion protein for cancer therapy. Int J Cancer 2005; 116: 304-13.

[189] Kaspar M, Trachsel E, Neri D. The antibody-mediated targeted delivery of interleukin-15 and GM-CSF to the tumor neovasculature inhibits tumor growth and metastasis. Cancer Res 2007; 67: 4940-8.

[190] Liu Y, Zhang W, Cheung LH, *et al.* The antimelanoma immunocytokine scFvMEL/TNF shows reduced toxicity and potent antitumor activity against human tumor xenografts. Neoplasia 2006; 8: 384-93.

[191] Huang TH, Morrison SL. A trimeric anti-HER2/neu ScFv and tumor necrosis factor-alpha fusion protein induces HER2/neu signaling and facilitates repair of injured epithelia. J Pharmacol Exp Ther 2006; 316: 983-91.

[192] Halin C, Gafner V, Villani ME, *et al.* Synergistic therapeutic effects of a tumor targeting antibody fragment, fused to interleukin 12 and to tumor necrosis factor alpha. Cancer Res 2003; 63: 3202-10.

[193] Robert B, Guillaume P, Luescher I, *et al.* Redirecting anti-viral CTL against cancer cells by surface targeting of monomeric MHC class I-viral peptide conjugated to antibody fragments. Cancer Immun 2001; 1: 2.

[194] Lev A, Noy R, Oved K, *et al.* Tumor-specific Ab-mediated targeting of MHC-peptide complexes induces regression of human tumor xenografts *in vivo*. Proc Natl Acad Sci USA 2004; 101: 9051-6.

[195] Gallimore A, Glithero A, Godkin A, *et al.* Induction and exhaustion of lymphocytic choriomeningitis virus-specific cytotoxic T lymphocytes visualized using soluble tetrameric major histocompatibility complex class I-peptide complexes. J Exp Med 1998; 187: 1383-93.

[196] Murali-Krishna K, Altman JD, Suresh M, *et al.* Counting antigen-specific CD8 T cells: a reevaluation of bystander activation during viral infection. Immunity 1998; 8: 177-87.

[197] Flynn KJ, Belz GT, Altman JD, *et al.* Virus-specific CD8+ T cells in primary and secondary influenza pneumonia. Immunity 1998; 8: 683-91.
[198] Cesson V, Stirnemann K, Robert B, *et al.* Active antiviral T-lymphocyte response can be redirected against tumor cells by antitumor antibody x MHC/viral peptide conjugates. Clin Cancer Res 2006; 12: 7422-30.
[199] Stirnemann K, Romero JF, Baldi L, *et al.* Sustained activation and tumor targeting of NKT cells using a CD1d-anti-HER2-scFv fusion protein induce antitumor effects in mice. J Clin Invest 2008; 118: 994-1005.
[200] Schnyder A, Huwyler J. Drug transport to brain with targeted liposomes. NeuroRx 2005; 2: 99-107.
[201] Park JW, Benz CC, Martin FJ. Future directions of liposome- and immunoliposome-based cancer therapeutics. Semin Oncol 2004; 31: 196-205.
[202] Gabizon A. Emerging role of liposomal drug carrier systems in cancer chemotherapy. J Liposome Res 2003; 13: 17-20.
[203] Moghimi SM, Patel HM. Opsonophagocytosis of liposomes by peritoneal macrophages and bone marrow reticuloendothelial cells. Biochim Biophys Acta 1992; 1135: 269-74.
[204] Frank MM. The reticuloendothelial system and bloodstream clearance. J Lab Clin Med 1993; 122: 487-8.
[205] Maruyama K. PEG-immunoliposome. Biosci Rep 2002; 22: 251-66.
[206] Messerschmidt SK, Musyanovych A, Altvater M, *et al.* Targeted lipid-coated nanoparticles: delivery of tumor necrosis factor-functionalized particles to tumor cells. J Control Release 2009; 137: 69-77.
[207] Gabizon A, Horowitz AT, Goren D, *et al.* *In vivo* fate of folate-targeted polyethylene-glycol liposomes in tumor-bearing mice. Clin Cancer Res 2003; 9: 6551-9.
[208] Allen TM. Long-circulating (sterically stabilized) liposomes for targeted drug delivery. Trends Pharmacol Sci 1994; 15: 215-20.
[209] Gabizon A, Shmeeda H, Barenholz Y. Pharmacokinetics of pegylated liposomal Doxorubicin: review of animal and human studies. Clin Pharmacokinet 2003; 42: 419-36.
[210] Hermanson GT. Bioconjugate techniques: San Diego: Academic Press, 1996.
[211] Mamot C, Drummond DC, Greiser U, *et al.* Epidermal growth factor receptor (EGFR)-targeted immunoliposomes mediate specific and efficient drug delivery to EGFR- and EGFRvIII-overexpressing tumor cells. Cancer Res 2003; 63: 3154-61.
[212] Gao J, Zhong W, He J, *et al.* Tumor-targeted PE38KDEL delivery *via* PEGylated anti-HER2 immunoliposomes. Int J Pharm 2009; 374: 145-52.
[213] Kitamura N, Shigematsu N, Nakahara T, *et al.* Biodistribution of immunoliposome labeled with Tc-99m in tumor xenografted mice. Ann Nucl Med 2009; 23: 149-53.
[214] Hussain S, Pluckthun A, Allen TM, Zangemeister-Wittke U. Antitumor activity of an epithelial cell adhesion molecule targeted nanovesicular drug delivery system. Mol Cancer Ther 2007; 6: 3019-27.
[215] Volkel T, Holig P, Merdan T, Muller R, Kontermann RE. Targeting of immunoliposomes to endothelial cells using a single-chain Fv fragment directed against human endoglin (CD105). Biochim Biophys Acta 2004; 1663: 158-66.
[216] Holliger P, Hudson PJ. Engineered antibody fragments and the rise of single domains. Nat Biotechnol 2005; 23: 1126-36.
[217] Sharkey RM, Karacay H, Litwin S, *et al.* Improved therapeutic results by pretargeted radioimmunotherapy of non-Hodgkin's lymphoma with a new recombinant, trivalent, anti-CD20, bispecific antibody. Cancer Res 2008; 68: 5282-90.
[218] Kenanova V, Olafsen T, Crow DM, *et al.* Tailoring the pharmacokinetics and positron emission tomography imaging properties of anti-carcinoembryonic antigen single-chain Fv-Fc antibody fragments. Cancer Res 2005; 65: 622-31.
[219] Olafsen T, Tan GJ, Cheung CW, *et al.* Characterization of engineered anti-p185HER-2 (scFv-CH3)2 antibody fragments (minibodies) for tumor targeting. Protein Eng Des Sel 2004; 17: 315-23.
[220] Robinson MK, Doss M, Shaller C, *et al.* Quantitative immuno-positron emission tomography imaging of HER2-positive tumor xenografts with an iodine-124 labeled anti-HER2 diabody. Cancer Res 2005; 65: 1471-8.
[221] Brack SS, Dinkelborg LM, Neri D. Molecular targeting of angiogenesis for imaging and therapy. Eur J Nucl Med Mol Imaging 2004; 31: 1327-41.
[222] Matter CM, Schuler PK, Alessi P, *et al.* Molecular imaging of atherosclerotic plaques using a human antibody against the extra-domain B of fibronectin. . Circ Res 2004; 95: 1225-33.
[223] Adams GP, Shaller CC, Dadachova E, *et al.* A single treatment of yttrium-90-labeled CHX-A"-C6.5 diabody inhibits the growth of established human tumor xenografts in immunodeficient mice. Cancer Res 2004; 64: 6200-6.

[224] Karacay H, Brard PY, Sharkey RM, *et al.* Therapeutic advantage of pretargeted radioimmunotherapy using a recombinant bispecific antibody in a human colon cancer xenograft. Clin Cancer Res 2005; 11: 7879-85.
[225] Meredith RF, Buchsbaum DJ. Pretargeted radioimmunotherapy. Int J Radiat Oncol Biol Phys 2006; 66:S57-9.
[226] McBride WJ, Zanzonico P, Sharkey RM, *et al.* Bispecific antibody pretargeting PET (immunoPET) with an 124I-labeled hapten-peptide. J Nucl Med 2006; 47: 1678-88.
[227] Moosmayer D, Berndorff D, Chang CH, *et al.* Bispecific antibody pretargeting of tumor neovasculature for improved systemic radiotherapy of solid tumors. Clin Cancer Res 2006; 12: 5587-95.
[228] Goldenberg DM, Rossi EA, Sharkey RM, McBride WJ, Chang CH. Multifunctional antibodies by the Dock-and-Lock method for improved cancer imaging and therapy by pretargeting. J Nucl Med 2008; 49: 158-63.
[229] Pagel JM, Lin Y, Hedin N, *et al.* Comparison of a tetravalent single-chain antibody-streptavidin fusion protein and an antibody-streptavidin chemical conjugate for pretargeted anti-CD20 radioimmunotherapy of B-cell lymphomas. Blood 2006; 108: 328-36.
[230] Forero A, Weiden PL, Vose JM, *et al.* Phase 1 trial of a novel anti-CD20 fusion protein in pretargeted radioimmunotherapy for B-cell non-Hodgkin lymphoma. Blood 2004; 104: 227-36.
[231] Hong H, Sun J, Cai W. Radionuclide-based cancer imaging targeting the carcinoembryonic antigen. Biomark Insights 2008; 3: 435-51.
[232] Bagshawe KD. Targeting: the ADEPT story so far. Curr Drug Targets 2009; 10: 152-7.
[233] Bagshawe KD. Antibody-directed enzyme prodrug therapy (ADEPT) for cancer. Expert Rev Anticancer Ther 2006; 6: 1421-31.
[234] Denny WA. Tumor-activated prodrugs--a new approach to cancer therapy. Cancer Invest 2004; 22: 604-19.
[235] Senter PD, Springer CJ. Selective activation of anticancer prodrugs by monoclonal antibody-enzyme conjugates. Adv Drug Deliv Rev 2001; 53: 247-64.
[236] Venisnik KM, Olafsen T, Loening AM, *et al.* Bifunctional antibody-Renilla luciferase fusion protein for *in vivo* optical detection of tumors. Protein Eng Des Sel 2006; 19: 453-60.
[237] Dalken B, Giesubel U, Knauer SK, Wels WS. Targeted induction of apoptosis by chimeric granzyme B fusion proteins carrying antibody and growth factor domains for cell recognition. Cell Death Differ 2006; 13: 576-85.
[238] Coelho V, Dernedde J, Petrausch U, *et al.* Design, construction, and *in vitro* analysis of A33scFv::CDy, a recombinant fusion protein for antibody-directed enzyme prodrug therapy in colon cancer. Int J Oncol 2007; 31: 951-7.
[239] Panjideh H, Coelho V, Dernedde J, *et al.* Production of bifunctional single-chain antibody-based fusion proteins in Pichia pastoris supernatants. Bioprocess Biosyst Eng 2008; 31: 559-68.
[240] Panjideh H, Da Silva Coelho VC, Dernedde J, *et al.* Biodistribution and efficacy of [131I]A33scFv::CDy, a recombinant antibody-enzyme protein for colon cancer. Int J Oncol 2008; 32: 925-30.
[241] Mayer A, Francis RJ, Sharma SK, *et al.* A phase I study of single administration of antibody-directed enzyme prodrug therapy with the recombinant anti-carcinoembryonic antigen antibody-enzyme fusion protein MFECP1 and a bis-iodo phenol mustard prodrug. Clin Cancer Res 2006; 12: 6509-16.
[242] Cortez-Retamozo V, Backmann N, Senter PD, *et al.* Efficient cancer therapy with a nanobody-based conjugate. Cancer Res 2004; 64: 2853-7.
[243] Rothbauer U, Zolghadr K, Tillib S, *et al.* Targeting and tracing antigens in live cells with fluorescent nanobodies. Nat Methods 2006; 3: 887-9.
[244] Mayer A, Sharma SK, Tolner B, *et al.* Modifying an immunogenic epitope on a therapeutic protein: a step towards an improved system for antibody-directed enzyme prodrug therapy (ADEPT). Br J Cancer 2004; 90: 2402-10.
[245] Afshar S, Olafsen T, Wu AM, Morrison SL. Characterization of an engineered human purine nucleoside phosphorylase fused to an anti-her2/neu single chain Fv for use in ADEPT. J Exp Clin Cancer Res 2009; 28: 147.
[246] Pirollo KF, Chang EH. Targeted delivery of small interfering RNA: approaching effective cancer therapies. Cancer Res 2008; 68: 1247-50.
[247] Kumar A. RNA interference: a multifaceted innate antiviral defense. Retrovirology 2008; 5: 17.
[248] Schiffelers RM, Woodle MC, Scaria P. Pharmaceutical prospects for RNA interference. Pharm Res 2004; 21: 1-7.
[249] Schiffelers RM, Ansari A, Xu J, *et al.* Cancer siRNA therapy by tumor selective delivery with ligand-targeted sterically stabilized nanoparticle. Nucleic Acids Res 2004; 32:e149.
[250] Morrissey DV, Blanchard K, Shaw L, *et al.* Activity of stabilized short interfering RNA in a mouse model of hepatitis B virus replication. Hepatology 2005; 41: 1349-56.

[251] Andreakos E, Rauchhaus U, Stavropoulos A, *et al.* Amphoteric liposomes enable systemic antigen-presenting cell-directed delivery of CD40 antisense and are therapeutically effective in experimental arthritis. Arthritis Rheum 2009; 60: 994-1005.

[252] Wen WH, Liu JY, Qin WJ, *et al.* Targeted inhibition of HBV gene expression by single-chain antibody mediated small interfering RNA delivery. Hepatology 2007; 46: 84-94.

[253] Song E, Zhu P, Lee SK, *et al.* Antibody mediated *in vivo* delivery of small interfering RNAs *via* cell-surface receptors. Nat Biotechnol 2005; 23: 709-17.

[254] Nakayama K, Pergolizzi RG, Crystal RG. 670. Intracellular shigatoxin 1A1 delivered by adenovirus-mediated segmental trans-splicing causes apototic cell death *in vitro* and *in vivo*. 2004; 9:S253.

[255] Vallera DA, Jin N, Baldrica JM, *et al.* Retroviral immunotoxin gene therapy of acute myelogenous leukemia in mice using cytotoxic T cells transduced with an interleukin 4/diphtheria toxin gene. Cancer Res 2000; 60: 976-84.

[256] Kouraklis G. Gene therapy for cancer: from the laboratory to the patient. Dig Dis Sci 2000; 45: 1045-52.

[257] Chen J, Gamou S, Takayanagi A, *et al.* Receptor-mediated gene delivery using the Fab fragments of anti-epidermal growth factor receptor antibodies: improved immunogene approach. Cancer Gene Ther 1998; 5: 357-64.

[258] Zhong XG, Yin W, Huang SR, *et al.* Construction and expression of recombinant adenovirus containing secreted endostatin in liver stem cell as a vector for gene therapy. Zhonghua Gan Zang Bing Za Zhi 2009; 17: 628-9.

[259] Fumoto S. [Organ-, region- and cell-selective gene transfer using non-viral vectors]. Yakugaku Zasshi 2009; 129: 1055-61.

[260] Somia NV, Zoppe M, Verma IM. Generation of targeted retroviral vectors by using single-chain variable fragment: an approach to *in vivo* gene delivery. Proc Natl Acad Sci USA 1995; 92: 7570-4.

[261] Fominaya J, Wels W. Target cell-specific DNA transfer mediated by a chimeric multidomain protein. Novel non-viral gene delivery system. J Biol Chem 1996; 271: 10560-8.

[262] Song SU, Marasco WA. Rapid establishment of myeloma cell lines expressing Fab(Tac)-Protamine, a targetable protein vector, directed against high-affinity α-chain of human interleukin-2 receptor. Gene Targeting Protocols, Vol. 133:Humana Press, 2000: 157-66.

[263] Stankovics J, Crane AM, Andrews E, *et al.* Overexpression of human methylmalonyl CoA mutase in mice after *in vivo* gene transfer with asialoglycoprotein/polylysine/DNA complexes. Hum Gene Ther 1994; 5: 1095-104.

[264] Müller D, and Kontermann, R.E. Recombinant bispecific antibodies for cellular cancer immunotherapy. Curr Opin Mol Ther 2007; 9: 319-26.

[265] Marvin JS, Zhu Z. Bispecific antibodies for dual-modality cancer therapy: killing two signaling cascades with one stone. Curr Opin Drug Discov Devel 2006; 9: 184-93.

[266] Nieri P, Donadio E, Rossi S, Adinolfi B, Podestà A. Antibodies for therapeutic uses and the evolution of biotechniques. Curr Med Chem 2009; 16: 753-79.

[267] d'Argouges S, Wissing S, Brandl C, *et al.* Combination of rituximab with blinatumomab (MT103/MEDI-538), a T cell-engaging CD19-/CD3-bispecific antibody, for highly efficient lysis of human B lymphoma cells. Leuk Res 2009; 33: 465-73.

[268] Milstein C, Cuello AC. Hybrid hybridomas and their use in immunohistochemistry. Nature 1983; 305: 537-40.

[269] Bruenke J, Barbin K, Kunert S, *et al.* Effective lysis of lymphoma cells with a stabilised bispecific single-chain Fv antibody against CD19 and FcgammaRIII (CD16). Br J Haematol 2005; 130: 218-28.

[270] Cao Y, Suresh MR. Bispecific Antibodies as Novel Bioconjugates. Bioconjug Chem 1998; 9: 635-44.

[271] Kellner C, Bruenke J, Stieglmaier J, *et al.* A novel CD19-directed recombinant bispecific antibody derivative with enhanced immune effector functions for human leukemic cells. J Immunother 2008; 31: 871-84.

[272] Kipriyanov SM, Cochlovius B, Schafer HJ, *et al.* Synergistic antitumor effect of bispecific CD19 x CD3 and CD19 x CD16 diabodies in a preclinical model of non-Hodgkin's lymphoma. J Immunol 2002; 169: 137-44.

[273] Schlenzka J, Moehler TM, Kipriyanov SM, *et al.* Combined effect of recombinant CD19 CD16 diabody and thalidomide in a preclinical model of human B cell lymphoma. Anticancer Drugs 2004; 15: 915-9.

[274] Bargou R, Leo E, Zugmaier G, *et al.* Tumor regression in cancer patients by very low doses of a T cell-engaging antibody. Science 2008; 321: 974-7.

[275] Haas C, Lulei M, Fournier P, Arnold A, Schirrmacher V. T-cell triggering by CD3- and CD28-binding molecules linked to a human virus-modified tumor cell vaccine. Vaccine 2005; 23: 2439-53.

[276] Topp M, Goekbuget N, Kufer P, *et al.* Treatment with anti-CD19 BiTE antibody blinatumomab (MT103/MEDI-538) is able to eliminate minimal residual disease (MRD) in patients with B-precursor acute lmphoblastic

leukemia (ALL): First results of ongoing phase 2 study [ASH Annual Meeting Abstract]. Blood 2008; 112: 1926.

[277] Hoffmann P, Hofmeister R, Brischwein K, *et al.* Serial killing of tumor cells by cytotoxic T cells redirected with a CD19-/CD3-bispecific single-chain antibody construct. Int J Cancer 2005; 115: 98-104.

[278] Schlereth B, Fichtner I, Lorenczewski G, *et al.* Eradication of tumors from a human colon cancer cell line and from ovarian cancer metastases in immunodeficient mice by a single-chain Ep-CAM-/CD3-bispecific antibody construct. Cancer Res 2005; 65: 2882-9.

[279] Arndt MA, Krauss J, Kipriyanov SM, al. e. A bispecific diabody that mediates natural killer cell cytotoxicity against xenotransplanted human Hodgkin's tumors. Blood 1999; 94: 2562-8.

[280] Brischwein K, Schlereth B, Guller B, *et al.* MT110: a novel bispecific single-chain antibody construct with high efficacy in eradicating established tumors. Mol Immunol 2006; 43: 1129-43.

[281] Maetzel D, Denzel S, Mack B, *et al.* Nuclear signalling by tumour-associated antigen EpCAM. Nat Cell Biol 2009; 11: 162-71.

[282] Cochlovius B, Kipriyanov SM, Stassar MJ, *et al.* Treatment of human B cell lymphoma xenografts with a CD3 × CD19 diabody and T cells. J Immunol 2000; 165: 888-95.

[283] Schmiedl A, Breitling F, Dübel S. Expression of a bispecific dsFv-dsFv' antibody fragment in Escherichia coli. Protein Eng 2000; 13: 725-34.

[284] Wolf E, Hofmeister R, Kufer P, Schlereth B, Baeuerle PA. BiTEs: bispecific antibody constructs with unique anti-tumor activity. Drug Discov Today 2005; 10: 1237-44.

[285] Offner S, Hofmeister R, Romaniuk A, Kufer P, Baeuerle PA. Induction of regular cytolytic T cell synapses by bispecific single-chain antibody constructs on MHC class I-negative tumor cells. Mol Immunol 2006; 43: 763-71.

[286] Shalaby MR, Shepard HM, Presta L, *et al.* Development of humanized bispecific antibodies reactive with cytotoxic lymphocytes and tumor cells overexpressing the HER2 protooncogene. J Exp Med 1992; 175: 217-25.

[287] Kornacker M, Verneris M, Kornacker B, *et al.* The apoptotic and proliferative fate of cytokine-induced killer cells after redirection to tumor cells with bispecific Ab. Cytotherapy 2006; 8: 13-23.

[288] Kostelny SA, Cole MS, Tso JY. Formation of a bispecific antibody by the use of leucine zippers. J Immunol 1992; 148: 1547-53.

[289] Schoonjans R, Willems A, Grooten J, Mertens N. Efficient heterodimerization of recombinant bi- and trispecific antibodies. Bioseparation 2000; 9: 179-83.

[290] Lu H, Shi M, Wang M, *et al. In vitro* and *in vivo* antitumor effect of a trivalent bispecific antibody targeting ErbB2 and CD16. Cancer Biol Ther 2008; 7.

[291] Brard PY, Karacay H, Stein R, *et al.* A divalent hapten-peptide induces apoptosis in human non hodgkin lymphoma cell lines targeted by anti-CD20xanti-hapten bispecific antibodies. Clin Cancer Res 2007; 13: 5564s-71s.

[292] Lu D, Zhu Z. Construction and production of an IgG-like tetravalent bispecific antibody for enhanced therapeutic efficacy. Methods Mol Biol 2009; 525: 377-404, xiv.

[293] Gelardi T, Damiano V, Rosa R, *et al.* Two novel human anti-ErbB2 immunoagents are active on trastuzumab-resistant tumours. Br J Cancer 2010; 102: 513-9.

[294] Germain C, Campigna E, Salhi I, *et al.* Redirecting NK cells mediated tumor cell lysis by a new recombinant bifunctional protein. Protein Eng Des Sel 2008; 21: 665-72.

[295] Coloma MJ, Morrison SL. Design and production of novel tetravalent bispecific antibodies. Nat Biotechnol 1997; 15: 159-63.

[296] Asano R, Watanabe Y, Kawaguchi H, *et al.* Highly effective recombinant format of a humanized IgG-like bispecific antibody for cancer immunotherapy with retargeting of lymphocytes to tumor cells. J Biol Chem 2007; 282: 27659-65.

[297] Zuo Z, Jimenez X, Witte L, Zhu Z. An efficient route to the production of an IgG-like bispecific antibody. Protein Eng 2000; 13: 361-7.

[298] Lu D, Zhang H, Ludwig D, *et al.* Simultaneous blockade of both the epidermal growth factor receptor and the insulin-like growth factor receptor signaling pathways in cancer cells with a fully human recombinant bispecific antibody. J Biol Chem 2004; 279: 2856-65.

[299] Alt M, Müller R, Kontermann RE. Novel tetravalent and bispecific IgG-like antibody molecules combining single-chain diabodies with the immunoglobulin gamma1 Fc or CH3 region. FEBS Lett 1999; 454: 90-4.

[300] Lu D, Zhang H, Koo H, *et al.* A fully human recombinant IgG-like bispecific antibody to both the epidermal growth factor receptor and the insulin-like growth factor receptor for enhanced antitumor activity J Biol Chem 2005; 280: 19665-72.

[301] Lu D, X. J, H. Z, *et al.* Di-diabody: a novel tetravalent bispecific antibody molecule by design. J Immunol Methods 2003; 279: 219-32.

[302] Rossi EA, Goldenberg DM, Cardillo TM, *et al.* Novel designs of multivalent anti-CD20 humanized antibodies as improved lymphoma therapeutics.Cancer Res 2008; 68: 8384-92.

[303] Shen J, Vil MD, Jimenez X, *et al.* Single variable domain-IgG fusion. A novel recombinant approach to Fc domain-containing bispecific antibodies. J Biol Chem 2006; 281: 10706-14.

[304] Shen J, Vil MD, Jimenez X, *et al.* Single variable domain antibody as a versatile building block for the construction of IgG-like bispecific antibodies. J Immunol Methods 2007; 318: 65-74.

[305] Boldicke T. Blocking translocation of cell surface molecules from the ER to the cell surface by intracellular antibodies targeted to the ER. J Cell Mol Med 2007; 11: 54-70.

[306] Sanz L, Blanco B, Álvarez-Vallina L. Antibodies and gene therapy: teaching old `magic bullets´ new tricks. Trends Immunol 2004; 25: 85-91.

[307] Lo AS, Zhu Q, Marasco WA. Intracellular antibodies (intrabodies) and their therapeutic potential. Handb Exp Pharmacol 2008; 181: 343-73.

[308] Tragoolpua K, Intasai N, Kasinrerk W, *et al.* Generation of functional scFv intrabody to abate the expression of CD147 surface molecule of 293A cells. BMC Biotechnol 2008; 8: 5.

[309] Lynch SM, Zhou C, Messer A. An scFv intrabody against the nonamyloid component of alpha-synuclein reduces intracellular aggregation and toxicity. J Mol Biol 2008; 377: 136-47.

[310] Griffin H, Elston R, Jackson D, *et al.* Inhibition of papillomavirus protein function in cervical cancer cells by intrabody targeting. J Mol Biol 2006; 355: 360-78.

[311] Marasco WA, Dana Jones S. Antibodies for targeted gene therapy: extracellular gene targeting and intracellular expression. Adv Drug Deliv Rev 1998; 31: 153-70.

[312] Aires da Silva F, Santa-Marta M, Freitas-Vieira A, *et al.* Camelized rabbit-derived VH single-domain intrabodies against Vif strongly neutralize HIV-1 infectivity. J Mol Biol 2004; 340: 525-42.

[313] Corte-Real S, Collins C, Aires da Silva F, *et al.* Intrabodies targeting the Kaposi sarcoma-associated herpesvirus latency antigen inhibit viral persistence in lymphoma cells. Blood 2005; 106: 3797-802.

[314] Lagrange M, Boulade-Ladame C, Mailly L, *et al.* Intracellular scFvs against the viral E6 oncoprotein provoke apoptosis in human papillomavirus-positive cancer cells. Biochem Biophys Res Commun 2007; 361: 487-92.

[315] Zhou P, Goldstein S, Devadas K, Tewari D, Notkins AL. Cells transfected with a non-neutralizing antibody gene are resistant to HIV infection: targeting the endoplasmic reticulum and trans-Golgi network. J Immunol 1998; 160: 1489-96.

[316] Liu F, Kumar M, Ma Q, *et al.* Human single-chain antibodies inhibit replication of human immunodeficiency virus type 1 (HIV-1). AIDS Res Hum Retroviruses 2005; 21: 876-81.

[317] Goncalves J, Silva F, Freitas-Vieira A, *et al.* Functional neutralization of HIV-1 Vif protein by intracellular immunization inhibits reverse transcription and viral replication. J Biol Chem 2002; 277: 32036-45.

[318] Swan CH, Fischer KM, Bühler B, *et al.* 973. Targeting of CCR5 through intrabody mediated HIV-1 vector gene delivery is sufficient for blocking HIV-1-infection and confers a T-Cell survival and growth advantage. Mol Ther 2005; 11:S376-S.

[319] Boldicke T, Weber H, Mueller PP, Barleon B, Bernal M. Novel highly efficient intrabody mediates complete inhibition of cell surface expression of the human vascular endothelial growth factor receptor-2 (VEGFR-2/KDR). J Immunol Methods 2005; 300: 146-59.

[320] Arafat W, Gomez-Navarro J, Xiang J, *et al.* Antineoplastic effect of anti-erbB-2 intrabody is not correlated with scFv affinity for its target. Cancer Gene Ther 2000; 7: 1250-6.

[321] Popkov M, Jendreyko N, McGavern DB, Rader C, Barbas CF, 3rd. Targeting tumor angiogenesis with adenovirus-delivered anti-Tie-2 intrabody. Cancer Res 2005; 65: 972-81.

[322] Mhashilkar AM, Doebis C, Seifert M, *et al.* Intrabody-mediated phenotypic knockout of major histocompatibility complex class I expression in human and monkey cell lines and in primary human keratinocytes. Gene Ther 2002; 9: 307-19.

[323] Li L, Gondi CS, Dinh DH, *et al.* Transfection with anti-p65 intrabody suppresses invasion and angiogenesis in glioma cells by blocking nuclear factor-kappaB transcriptional activity. Clin Cancer Res 2007; 13: 2178-90.

[324] Zhu X, Yang N, Cai J, *et al.* The intrabody targeting of hTERT attenuates the immortality of cancer cells. Cell Mol Biol Lett; 15: 32-45.

[325] Jendreyko N, Popkov M, Rader C, Barbas CF, 3rd. Phenotypic knockout of VEGF-R2 and Tie-2 with an intradiabody reduces tumor growth and angiogenesis *in vivo*. Proc Natl Acad Sci USA 2005; 102: 8293-8.

[326] Alvarez RD, Barnes MN, Gomez-Navarro J, *et al.* A cancer gene therapy approach utilizing an anti-erbB-2 single-chain antibody-encoding adenovirus (AD21): a phase I trial. Clin Cancer Res 2000; 6: 3081-7.

[327] Cardinale A, Filesi I, Mattei S, Biocca S. Evidence for proteasome dysfunction in cytotoxicity mediated by anti-Ras intracellular antibodies. Eur J Biochem 2003; 270: 3389-97.

[328] Cochet O, Kenigsberg M, Delumeau I, *et al.* Intracellular expression of an antibody fragment-neutralizing p21 ras promotes tumor regression. Cancer Res 1998; 58: 1170-6.

[329] Blanco B, Holliger P, Vile RG, Alvarez-Vallina L. Induction of human T lymphocyte cytotoxicity and inhibition of tumor growth by tumor-specific diabody-based molecules secreted from gene-modified bystander cells. J Immunol 2003; 171: 1070-7.

[330] Kasono K, Heike Y, Xiang J, *et al.* Tetracycline-induced expression of an anti-c-Myb single-chain antibody and its inhibitory effect on proliferation of the human leukemia cell line K562. Cancer Gene Ther 2000; 7: 151-9.

[331] Strube RW, Chen SY. Characterization of anti-cyclin E single-chain Fv antibodies and intrabodies in breast cancer cells: enhanced intracellular stability of novel sFv-F(c) intrabodies. J Immunol Methods 2002; 263: 149-67.

[332] Heike Y, Kasono K, Kunisaki C, *et al.* Overcoming multi-drug resistance using an intracellular anti-MDR1 sFv. Int J Cancer 2001; 92: 115-22.

[333] Stocks M. Intrabodies as drug discovery tools and therapeutics. Curr Opin Chem Biol 2005; 9: 359-65.

[334] Huse WD, Sastry L, Iverson SA, *et al.* Generation of a large combinatorial library of the immunoglobulin repertoire in phage lambda. Science 1989; 246: 1275-81.

[335] Clackson T, Hoogenboom HR, Griffiths AD, Winter G. Making antibody fragments using phage display libraries. Nature 1991; 352: 624-8.

[336] Burton DR, Barbas CF, 3rd, Persson MA, *et al.* A large array of human monoclonal antibodies to type 1 human immunodeficiency virus from combinatorial libraries of asymptomatic seropositive individuals. Proc Natl Acad Sci USA 1991; 88: 10134-7.

[337] Kramer RA, Marissen WE, Goudsmit J, *et al.* The human antibody repertoire specific for rabies virus glycoprotein as selected from immune libraries. Eur J Immunol 2005; 35: 2131-45.

[338] Wrammert J, Smith K, Miller J, *et al.* Rapid cloning of high-affinity human monoclonal antibodies against influenza virus. Nature 2008; 453: 667-71.

[339] Green LL, Hardy MC, Maynard-Currie CE, *et al.* Antigen-specific human monoclonal antibodies from mice engineered with human Ig heavy and light chain YACs. Nat Genet 1994; 7: 13-21.

[340] Marks JD, Hoogenboom HR, Bonnert TP, *et al.* By-passing immunization : Human antibodies from V-gene libraries displayed on phage. J Mol Biol 1991; 222: 581-97.

[341] Marks JD, Tristem M, Karpas A, Winter G. Oligonucleotide primers for polymerase chain reaction amplification of human immunoglobulin variable genes and design of family-specific oligonucleotide probes. Eur J Immunol 1991; 21: 985-91.

[342] Marks JD, Bradbury A. PCR cloning of human immunoglobulin genes. In: Lo BKC, ed. Methods in molecular biology, Vol. 248. Totowa, NJ:Humana Press Inc., 2004: 117-34.

[343] Razai A, Garcia-Rodriguez C, Lou J, *et al.* Molecular evolution of antibody affinity for sensitive detection of botulinum neurotoxin type A. J Mol Biol 2005; 351: 158-69.

[344] Aubrey N, Devaux C, Sizaret PY, *et al.* Design and evaluation of a diabody to improve protection against a potent scorpion neurotoxin. Cell Mol Life Sci 2003; 60: 617-28.

[345] Hmila I, Abdallah RB, Saerens D, *et al.* VHH, bivalent domains and chimeric Heavy chain-only antibodies with high neutralizing efficacy for scorpion toxin AahI'. Mol Immunol 2008; 45: 3847-56.

[346] Forsman A, Beirnaert E, Aasa-Chapman MM, *et al.* Llama antibody fragments with cross-subtype human immunodeficiency virus type 1 (HIV-1)-neutralizing properties and high affinity for HIV-1 gp120. J Virol 2008; 82: 12069-81.

[347] Tout NL, Yau KY, Trevors JT, Lee H, Hall JC. Synthesis of ligand-specific phage-display ScFv against the herbicide picloram by direct cloning from hyperimmunized mouse. J Agric Food Chem 2001; 49: 3628-37.

[348] Doyle PJ, Arbabi-Ghahroudi M, Gaudette N, *et al.* Cloning, expression, and characterization of a single-domain antibody fragment with affinity for 15-acetyl-deoxynivalenol. Mol Immunol 2008; 45: 3703-13.

[349] Mao S, Gao C, Lo CH, *et al.* Phage-display library selection of high-affinity human single-chain antibodies to tumor-associated carbohydrate antigens sialyl Lewisx and Lewisx. Proc Natl Acad Sci USA 1999; 96: 6953-8.

[350] Gerstenbruch S, Brooks CL, Kosma P, *et al.* Analysis of cross-reactive and specific anti-carbohydrate antibodies against lipopolysaccharide from Chlamydophila psittaci. Glycobiology 2010; 20: 461-72.

[351] Dwek R. Antibodies and antigens: it's all about the numbers game. Proc Natl Acad Sci USA 2009; 106: 2087-8.
[352] Azzazy HME, Highsmith WE. Phage display technology: clinical applications and recent innovations. Clin Biochem 2002; 35: 425-45.
[353] Hamers-Casterman C, Atarhouch T, Muyldermans S, *et al.* Naturally occurring antibodies devoid of light chains. Nature 1993; 363: 446-8.
[354] Vu KB, Ghahroudi MA, Wyns L, Muyldermans S. Comparison of llama VH sequences from conventional and heavy chain antibodies. Mol Immunol 1997; 34: 1121-31.
[355] Conrath K, Vincke C, Stijlemans B, *et al.* Antigen binding and solubility effects upon the veneering of a camel VHH in framework-2 to mimic a VH. J Mol Biol 2005; 350: 112-25.
[356] Arbabi Ghahroudi M, Desmyter A, Wyns L, Hamers R, Muyldermans S. Selection and identification of single domain antibody fragments from camel heavy-chain antibodies. FEBS Letters 1997; 414: 521-6.
[357] Arbabi-Ghahroudi M, MacKenzie R, Tanha J. Selection of non-aggregating VH binders from synthetic VH phage-display libraries. Methods Mol Biol 2009; 525: 187-216, xiii.
[358] de Haard HJ, van Neer N, Reurs A, *et al.* A large non-immunized human Fab fragment phage library that permits rapid isolation and kinetic analysis of high affinity antibodies. J Biol Chem 1999; 274: 18218-30.
[359] Vaughan TJ, Williams AJ, Pritchard K, *et al.* Human antibodies with sub-nanomolar affinities isolated from a large non-immunized phage display library. Nat Biotech 1996; 14: 309-14.
[360] Klein U, Rajewsky K, Kuppers R. Human immunoglobulin (Ig)M+IgD+ peripheral blood B cells expressing the CD27 cell surface antigen carry somatically mutated variable region genes: CD27 as a general marker for somatically mutated (memory) B cells. J Exp Med 1998; 188: 1679-89.
[361] de Haard HJ. Construction of large naive Fab libraries. Methods Mol Biol 2002; 178: 87-100.
[362] Winter G, Griffiths AD, Hawkins RE, Hoogenboom HR. Making antibodies by phage display technology. Annu Rev Immunol 1994; 12: 433-55.
[363] Griffiths AD, Williams SC, Hartley O, *et al.* Isolation of high affinity human antibodies directly from large synthetic repertoires. EMBO J 1994; 13: 3245-60.
[364] Stewart CS, MacKenzie CR, Hall CJ. Isolation, characterization and pentamerization of [alpha]-cobrotoxin specific single-domain antibodies from a naïve phage display library: Preliminary findings for antivenom development. Toxicon 2007; 49: 699-709.
[365] Griffiths AD, Malmqvist M, Marks JD, *et al.* Human anti-self antibodies with high specificity from phage display libraries. EMBO J 1993; 12: 725-34.
[366] Hoogenboom HR. Designing and optimizing library selection strategies for generating high-affinity antibodies. Trends Biotechnol 1997; 15: 62-70.
[367] Lowe D, Vaughan TJ. Human antibody repertoire libraries. In: An Z, ed. Therapeutic monocloal antibodies: from bench to clinic. Hoboken, N.J.:John Wiley & Sons 2009: 169-88.
[368] Sidhu SS, Fellouse FA. Synthetic therapeutic antibodies. Nat Chem Biol 2006; 2: 682-8.
[369] Fuh G. Synthetic antibodies as therapeutics. Expert Opin Biol Ther 2007; 7: 73-87.
[370] Holt LJ, Enever C, de Wildt RMT, Tomlinson IM. The use of recombinant antibodies in proteomics. Curr Opin Biotech 2000; 11: 445-9.
[371] Hoogenboom HR, Winter G. By-passing immunisation : Human antibodies from synthetic repertoires of germline VH gene segments rearranged *in vitro*. J Mol Biol 1992; 227: 381-8.
[372] Nissim A, Hoogenboom HR, Tomlinson IM, *et al.* Antibody fragments from a 'single pot' phage display library as immunochemical reagents. Embo J 1994; 13: 692-8.
[373] de Kruif J, Boel E, Logtenberg T. Selection and application of human single chain fv antibody fragments from a semi-synthetic phage antibody display library with designed cdr3 regions. J Mol Biol 1995; 248: 97-105.
[374] Knappik A, Ge L, Honegger A, *et al.* Fully synthetic human combinatorial antibody libraries (HuCAL) based on modular consensus frameworks and CDRs randomized with trinucleotides. J Mol Biol 2000; 296: 57-86.
[375] Persson H, Lantto J, Ohlin M. A focused antibody library for improved hapten recognition. J Mol Biol 2006; 357: 607-20.
[376] Rothe C, Urlinger S, Löhning C, *et al.* The human combinatorial antibody library HuCAL GOLD combines diversification of all six CDRs according to the natural immune system with a novel display method for efficient selection of high-affinity antibodies. J Mol Biol 2008; 376: 1182-200.
[377] Hoet RM, Cohen EH, Kent RB, *et al.* Generation of high-affinity human antibodies by combining donor-derived and synthetic complementarity-determining-region diversity. Nat Biotech 2005; 23: 344-8.

[378] Lee CV, Liang W-C, Dennis MS, *et al.* High-affinity human antibodies from phage-displayed synthetic Fab libraries with a single framework scaffold. J Mol Biol 2004; 340: 1073-93.
[379] Fellouse FA, Wiesmann C, Sidhu SS. Synthetic antibodies from a four-amino-acid code: a dominant role for tyrosine in antigen recognition. Proc Natl Acad Sci USA 2004; 101: 12467-72.
[380] Hanes J, Schaffitzel C, Knappik A, Pluckthun A. Picomolar affinity antibodies from a fully synthetic naive library selected and evolved by ribosome display. Nat Biotech 2000; 18: 1287-92.
[381] Smith GP. Filamentous fusion phage: novel expression vectors that display cloned antigens on the virion surface. Science 1985; 228: 1315-7.
[382] McCafferty J, Griffiths AD, Winter G, Chiswell DJ. Phage antibodies: filamentous phage displaying antibody variable domains. Nature 1990; 348: 552-4.
[383] Hoogenboom HR, Griffiths AD, Johnson KS, *et al.* Multi-subunit proteins on the surface of filamentous phage: methodologies for displaying antibody (Fab) heavy and light chains. Nucleic Acids Res 1991; 19: 4133-7.
[384] Goletz S, Christensen PA, Kristensen P, *et al.* Selection of large diversities of antiidiotypic antibody fragments by phage display. J Mol Biol 2002; 315: 1087-97.
[385] O'Connell D, Becerril B, Roy-Burman A, Daws M, Marks JD. Phage versus phagemid libraries for generation of human monoclonal antibodies. J Mol Biol 2002; 321: 49-56.
[386] Hust M, Thie H, Schirrmann T, Dübel S. Antibody phage display. In: An Z, ed. Therapeutic monocloal antibodies: from bench to clinic. Hoboken, N.J.:John Wiley & Sons, 2009: 191-211.
[387] Arbabi-Ghahroudi M, Tanha J, MacKenzie R. Isolation of monoclonal antibody fragments from phage display libraries. Methods Mol Biol 2009; 502: 341-64.
[388] Weisser NE, Almquist KC, Hall JC. A rAb screening method for improving the probability of identifying peptide mimotopes of carbohydrate antigens. Vaccine 2007; 25: 4611-22.
[389] Hawlisch H, Müller M, Frank R, *et al.* Site-specific anti-c3a receptor single-chain antibodies selected by differential panning on cellulose sheets. Anal Biochem 2001; 293: 142-5.
[390] Matsumoto S, Yamashita M, Katakura Y, *et al.* A rapid and efficient strategy to generate antigen-specific human monoclonal antibody by *in vitro* immunization and the phage display method. J Immunol Methods 2008; 332: 2-9.
[391] MacKenzie R, To R. The role of valency in the selection of anti-carbohydrate single-chain Fvs from phage display libraries. J Immunol Methods 1998; 220: 39-49.
[392] Davies EL, Smith JS, Birkett CR, *et al.* Selection of specific phage-display antibodies using libraries derived from chicken immunoglobulin genes. J Immunol Methods 1995; 186: 125-35.
[393] Meulemans EV, Slobbe R, Wasterval P, Ramaekers FCS, van Eys GJJM. Selection of phage-displayed antibodies specific for a cytoskeletal antigen by competitive elution with a monoclonal antibody. J Mol Biol 1994; 244: 353-60.
[394] Weisser NE, Hall JC. Applications of single-chain variable fragment antibodies in therapeutics and diagnostics. Biotechnol Adv 2009; 27: 502-20.
[395] Hoogenboom HR, Chames P. Natural and designer binding sites made by phage display technology. Immunol Today 2000; 21: 371-8.
[396] Hoogenboom HR. Selecting and screening recombinant antibody libraries. Nat Biotech 2005; 23: 1105-16.
[397] He M, Taussig MJ. Antibody-ribosome-mRNA (ARM) complexes as efficient selection particles for *in vitro* display and evolution of antibody combining sites. Nucleic Acids Res 1997; 25: 5132-4.
[398] Jermutus L, Honegger A, Schwesinger F, Hanes J, Pluckthun A. Tailoring *in vitro* evolution for protein affinity or stability. Proc Natl Acad Sci USA 2001; 98: 75-80.
[399] Thom G. Ribosomal display. In: An Z, ed. Therapeutic monocloal antibodies: from bench to clinic. Hoboken, N.J. John Wiley & Sons 2009: 239-53.
[400] He M, Taussig MJ. Ribosome display: Cell-free protein display technology. Brief Funct Genomics 2002; 1: 204-12.
[401] Cadwell RC, Joyce GF. Mutagenic PCR. PCR Methods Appl 1994; 3:S136-40.
[402] Stemmer WP. Rapid evolution of a protein *in vitro* by DNA shuffling. Nature 1994; 370: 389-91.
[403] Hanes J, Jermutus L, Weber-Bornhauser S, Bosshard HR, Pluckthun A. Ribosome display efficiently selects and evolves high-affinity antibodies *in vitro* from immune libraries. Proc Natl Acad Sci USA 1998; 95: 14130-5.
[404] Schaffitzel C, Berger I, Postberg J, *et al. In vitro* generated antibodies specific for telomeric guanine-quadruplex DNA react with Stylonychia lemnae macronuclei. Proc Natl Acad Sci USA 2001; 98: 8572-77.
[405] Van Blarcom TJ, Harvey BR. Bacterial display of antibodies. In: An Z, ed. Therapeutic monocloal antibodies: from bench to clinic Hoboken, N.J.:John Wiley & Sons 2009: 255-81.

[406] Mazor Y, Blarcom T, Mabry R, Iverson BL, Georgiou G. Isolation of engineered, full-length antibodies from libraries expressed in *Escherichia coli*. Nat Biotech 2007; 25: 563-65.

[407] Daugherty PS, Iverson BL, Georgiou G. Flow cytometric screening of cell-based libraries. J Immunol Methods 2000; 243: 211-27.

[408] Boder ET, Wittrup KD. Yeast surface display for screening combinatorial polypeptide libraries. Nat Biotech 1997; 15: 553-7.

[409] Bowley DR, Labrijn AF, Zwick MB, Burton DR. Antigen selection from an HIV-1 immune antibody library displayed on yeast yields many novel antibodies compared to selection from the same library displayed on phage. Protein Eng Des Sel 2007; 20: 81-90.

[410] Boder ET, Midelfort KS, Wittrup KD. Directed evolution of antibody fragments with monovalent femtomolar antigen-binding affinity. Proc Natl Acad Sci USA 2000; 97: 10701-5.

[411] Colby DW, Kellogg BA, Graff CP, *et al.* Engineering antibody affinity by yeast surface display. Methods in enzymology, Vol. Volume 388: Academic Press, 2004: 348-58.

[412] Graff CP, Chester K, Begent R, Wittrup KD. Directed evolution of an anti-carcinoembryonic antigen scFv with a 4-day monovalent dissociation half-time at 37 degrees C. Protein Eng Des Sel 2004; 17: 293-304.

[413] Shusta EV, Kieke MC, Parke E, Kranz DM, Wittrup DK. Yeast polypeptide fusion surface display levels predict thermal stability and soluble secretion efficiency. J Mol Biol 1999; 292: 949-56.

[414] Chao G, Cochran JR, Dane Wittrup K. Fine epitope mapping of anti-epidermal growth factor receptor antibodies through random mutagenesis and yeast surface display. J Mol Biol 2004; 342: 539-50.

[415] Laden JC, Philibert P, Torreilles F, Pugnière M, Martineau P. Expression and folding of an antibody fragment selected *in vivo* for high expression levels in Escherichia coli cytoplasm. Res Microbiol 2002; 153: 469-74.

[416] Zhao Q, Chan YW, Lee SS, Cheung WT. One-step expression and purification of single-chain variable antibody fragment using an improved hexahistidine tag phagemid vector. Protein Expr Purif 2009; 68: 190-5.

[417] Graumann K, Premstaller A. Manufacturing of recombinant therapeutic proteins in microbial systems. Biotechnol J 2006; 1: 164-86.

[418] Reulen SW, van Baal I, Raats JM, Merkx M. Efficient, chemoselective synthesis of immunomicelles using single-domain antibodies with a C-terminal thioester. BMC Biotechnol 2009; 9: 66.

[419] Jana S, Deb JK. Strategies for efficient production of heterologous proteins in Escherichia coli. Appl Microbiol Biotechnol 2005; 67: 289-98.

[420] Kipriyanov SM, Little M. Generation of recombinant antibodies. Mol Biotechnol 1999; 12: 173-201.

[421] Kwong KY, Rader C. E. coli expression and purification of Fab antibody fragments. Curr Protoc Protein Sci 2009;Chapter 6:Unit 6 10.

[422] Min WK, Cho YJ, Park JB, *et al.* Production and characterization of monoclonal antibody and its recombinant single chain variable fragment specific for a food-born mycotoxin, fumonisin B1. Bioprocess Biosyst Eng 2009; 33: 109-15.

[423] Liu M, Wang X, Yin C, *et al.* Targeting TNF-alpha with a tetravalent mini-antibody TNF-TeAb. Biochem J 2007; 406: 237-46.

[424] Deyev SM, Waibel R, Lebedenko EN, Schubiger AP, Pluckthun A. Design of multivalent complexes using the barnase*barstar module. Nat Biotechnol 2003; 21: 1486-92.

[425] Levy R, Weiss R, Chen G, Iverson BL, Georgiou G. Production of correctly folded Fab antibody fragment in the cytoplasm of Escherichia coli trxB gor mutants *via* the coexpression of molecular chaperones. Protein Expr Purif 2001; 23: 338-47.

[426] Philibert P, Martineau P. Directed evolution of single-chain Fv for cytoplasmic expression using the beta-galactosidase complementation assay results in proteins highly susceptible to protease degradation and aggregation. Microb Cell Fact 2004; 3: 16.

[427] Philibert P, Stoessel A, Wang W, *et al.* A focused antibody library for selecting scFvs expressed at high levels in the cytoplasm. BMC Biotechnol 2007; 7: 81.

[428] Ni M, Yu B, Huang Y, *et al.* Homology modelling and bivalent single-chain Fv construction of anti-HepG2 single-chain immunoglobulin Fv fragments from a phage display library. J Biosci 2008; 33: 691-7.

[429] Kurucz I, Titus JA, Jost CR, Jacobus CM, Segal DM. Retargeting of CTL by an efficiently refolded bispecific single-chain Fv dimer produced in bacteria. J Immunol 1995; 154: 4576-82.

[430] Lu D, Jimenez X, Zhang H, *et al.* Fab-scFv fusion protein: an efficient approach to production of bispecific antibody fragments. J Immunol Methods 2002; 267: 213-26.

[431] Charles CH, Luo GX, Kohlstaedt LA, *et al.* Prevention of human rhinovirus infection by multivalent fab molecules directed against ICAM-1. Antimicrob Agents Chemother 2003; 47: 1503-8.

[432] Gerngross TU. Advances in the production of human therapeutic proteins in yeasts and filamentous fungi. Nat Biotechnol 2004; 22: 1409-14.

[433] Boer E, Steinborn G, Kunze G, Gellissen G. Yeast expression platforms. Appl Microbiol Biotechnol 2007; 77: 513-23.

[434] Schoonooghe S, Kaigorodov V, Zawisza M, *et al.* Efficient production of human bivalent and trivalent anti-MUC1 Fab-scFv antibodies in Pichia pastoris. BMC Biotechnol 2009; 9: 70.

[435] Ridder R, Schmitz R, Legay F, Gram H. Generation of rabbit monoclonal antibody fragments from a combinatorial phage display library and their production in the yeast Pichia pastoris. Biotechnol 1995; 13: 255-60.

[436] Gasser B, Mattanovich D. Antibody production with yeasts and filamentous fungi: on the road to large scale? Biotechnol Lett 2007; 29: 201-12.

[437] Kuroda K, Kobayashi K, Kitagawa Y, *et al.* Efficient antibody production upon suppression of O mannosylation in the yeast Ogataea minuta. Appl Environ Microbiol 2008; 74: 446-53.

[438] Kukuruzinska MA, Bergh ML, Jackson BJ. Protein glycosylation in yeast. Annu Rev Biochem 1987; 56: 915-44.

[439] Horwitz AH, Chang CP, Better M, Hellstrom KE, Robinson RR. Secretion of functional antibody and Fab fragment from yeast cells. Proc Natl Acad Sci USA 1988; 85: 8678-82.

[440] Burtet RT, Santos-Silva MA, Buss GA, *et al.* Production of a recombinant Fab in Pichia pastoris from a Monocistronic expression vector. J Biochem 2007; 142: 665-9.

[441] Ren F, Li BC, Zhang NN, *et al.* Expression, purification and characterization of anti-BAFF antibody secreted from the yeast Pichia pastoris. Biotechnol Lett 2008; 30: 1075-80.

[442] Floss DM, Falkenburg D, Conrad U. Production of vaccines and therapeutic antibodies for veterinary applications in transgenic plants: an overview. Transgenic Res 2007; 16: 315-32.

[443] Schirrmann T, Al-Halabi L, Dubel S, Hust M. Production systems for recombinant antibodies. Front Biosci 2008; 13: 4576-94.

[444] Huang Z, Phoolcharoen W, Lai H, *et al.* High-level rapid production of full-size monoclonal antibodies in plants by a single-vector DNA replicon system. Biotechnol Bioeng 2009.

[445] Van Droogenbroeck B, Cao J, Stadlmann J, *et al.* Aberrant localization and underglycosylation of highly accumulating single-chain Fv-Fc antibodies in transgenic Arabidopsis seeds. Proc Natl Acad Sci USA 2007; 104: 1430-5.

[446] Villani ME, Morgun B, Brunetti P, *et al.* Plant pharming of a full-sized, tumour-targeting antibody using different expression strategies. Plant Biotechnol J 2009; 7: 59-72.

[447] Vaquero C, Sack M, Schuster F, *et al.* A carcinoembryonic antigen-specific diabody produced in tobacco. FASEB J 2002; 16: 408-10.

[448] Vezina LP, Faye L, Lerouge P, *et al.* Transient co-expression for fast and high-yield production of antibodies with human-like N-glycans in plants. Plant Biotechnol J 2009; 7: 442-55.

[449] Wagner B, Fuchs H, Adhami F, *et al.* Plant virus expression systems for transient production of recombinant allergens in Nicotiana benthamiana. Methods 2004; 32: 227-34.

[450] Ko K, Brodzik R, Steplewski Z. Production of antibodies in plants: approaches and perspectives. Curr Top Microbiol Immunol 2009; 332: 55-78.

[451] Peeters K, De Wilde C, De Jaeger G, Angenon G, Depicker A. Production of antibodies and antibody fragments in plants. Vaccine 2001; 19: 2756-61.

[452] Semenyuk EG, Stremovskiy OA, Edelweiss EF, *et al.* Expression of single-chain antibody-barstar fusion in plants. Biochimie 2007; 89: 31-8.

[453] Makvandi-Nejad S, McLean MD, Hirama T, *et al.* Transgenic tobacco plants expressing a dimeric single-chain variable fragment (scfv) antibody against Salmonella enterica serotype Paratyphi B. Transgenic Res 2005; 14: 785-92.

[454] Schillberg S, Zimmermann S, Voss A, Fischer R. Apoplastic and cytosolic expression of full-size antibodies and antibody fragments in Nicotiana tabacum. Transgenic Res 1999; 8: 255-63.

[455] Brereton HM, Chamberlain D, Yang R, *et al.* Single chain antibody fragments for ocular use produced at high levels in a commercial wheat variety. J Biotechnol 2007; 129: 539-46.

[456] Gomord V, Faye L. Posttranslational modification of therapeutic proteins in plants. Curr Opin Plant Biol 2004; 7: 171-81.

[457] Jin C, Altmann F, Strasser R, *et al.* A plant-derived human monoclonal antibody induces an anti-carbohydrate immune response in rabbits. Glycobiology 2008; 18: 235-41.
[458] Wright A, Morrison SL. Effect of glycosylation on antibody function: implications for genetic engineering. Trends Biotechnol 1997; 15: 26-32.
[459] Sethuraman N, Stadheim TA. Challenges in therapeutic glycoprotein production. Curr Opin Biotechnol 2006; 17: 341-6.
[460] Bakker H, Rouwendal GJ, Karnoup AS, *et al.* An antibody produced in tobacco expressing a hybrid beta-1,4-galactosyltransferase is essentially devoid of plant carbohydrate epitopes. Proc Natl Acad Sci USA 2006; 103: 7577-82.
[461] Fujiyama K, Furukawa A, Katsura A, *et al.* Production of mouse monoclonal antibody with galactose-extended sugar chain by suspension cultured tobacco BY2 cells expressing human beta(1,4)-galactosyltransferase. Biochem Biophys Res Commun 2007; 358: 85-91.
[462] Schahs M, Strasser R, Stadlmann J, *et al.* Production of a monoclonal antibody in plants with a humanized N-glycosylation pattern. Plant Biotechnol J 2007; 5: 657-63.
[463] Cox KM, Sterling JD, Regan JT, *et al.* Glycan optimization of a human monoclonal antibody in the aquatic plant Lemna minor. Nat Biotechnol 2006; 24: 1591-7.
[464] Strasser R, Stadlmann J, Schahs M, *et al.* Generation of glyco-engineered Nicotiana benthamiana for the production of monoclonal antibodies with a homogeneous human-like N-glycan structure. Plant Biotechnol J 2008; 6: 392-402.
[465] Birch JR, Racher AJ. Antibody production. Adv Drug Deliv Rev 2006; 58: 671-85.
[466] Brodzik R, Glogowska M, Bandurska K, *et al.* Plant-derived anti-Lewis Y mAb exhibits biological activities for efficient immunotherapy against human cancer cells. Proc Natl Acad Sci USA 2006; 103: 8804-9.
[467] Hong SY, Lee TS, Kim J, *et al.* Tumor targeting of humanized fragment antibody secreted from transgenic rice cell suspension culture. Plant Mol Biol 2008; 68: 413-22.
[468] Yoo EM, Chintalacharuvu KR, Penichet ML, Morrison SL. Myeloma expression systems. J Immunol Methods 2002; 261: 1-20.
[469] Jenkins N, Murphy L, Tyther R. Post-translational modifications of recombinant proteins: significance for biopharmaceuticals. Mol Biotechnol 2008; 39: 113-8.
[470] Kumpel BM, Rademacher TW, Rook GA, Williams PJ, Wilson IB. Galactosylation of human IgG monoclonal anti-D produced by EBV-transformed B-lymphoblastoid cell lines is dependent on culture method and affects Fc receptor-mediated functional activity. Hum Antibodies Hybridomas 1994; 5: 143-51.
[471] Shields RL, Lai J, Keck R, *et al.* Lack of fucose on human IgG1 N-linked oligosaccharide improves binding to human Fcgamma RIII and antibody-dependent cellular toxicity. J Biol Chem 2002; 277: 26733-40.
[472] Umana P, Jean-Mairet J, Moudry R, Amstutz H, Bailey JE. Engineered glycoforms of an antineuroblastoma IgG1 with optimized antibody-dependent cellular cytotoxic activity. Nat Biotechnol 1999; 17: 176-80.
[473] Rothman RJ, Perussia B, Herlyn D, Warren L. Antibody-dependent cytotoxicity mediated by natural killer cells is enhanced by castanospermine-induced alterations of IgG glycosylation. Mol Immunol 1989; 26: 1113-23.
[474] Jefferis R, Lund J, Mizutani H, *et al.* A comparative study of the N-linked oligosaccharide structures of human IgG subclass proteins. Biochem J 1990; 268: 529-37.
[475] Shinkawa T, Nakamura K, Yamane N, *et al.* The absence of fucose but not the presence of galactose or bisecting N-acetylglucosamine of human IgG1 complex-type oligosaccharides shows the critical role of enhancing antibody-dependent cellular cytotoxicity. J Biol Chem 2003; 278: 3466-73.
[476] Farid SS. Process economics of industrial monoclonal antibody manufacture. J Chromatogr B Analyt Technol Biomed Life Sci 2007; 848: 8-18.

CHAPTER 15

Therapeutic Antibodies: State of the Art and Promises

Patrick Chames* and Daniel Baty

INSERM U624, GDR2352, 163 avenue de Luminy - case 915, 13288 Marseille Cedex 09, France

Abstract: With more than 25 molecules in clinical use, monoclonal antibodies have finally come of age as therapeutics, generating a market value of $11 billion in 2004, expected to reach $26 billion by 2010. While delivering interesting results in the treatment of several major diseases including autoimmune, cardiovascular and infectious diseases, cancer and inflammation, clinical trials and research are generating a wealth of useful information, for instance about associations of clinical responses with Fc receptor polymorphisms and the infiltration and recruitment of effector cells into targeted tissues. Some functional limitations of therapeutic antibodies have come to light such as inadequate pharmacokinetics and tissue accessibility as well as impaired interactions with the immune system. This review aims at giving an overview of the current state of the art and describes the most promising avenues that are followed for generating the next generation of antibody-based cancer therapeutics, with a special emphasis on bispecific antibodies.

Keywords: Immunotherapy, Monoclonal antibodies, Pharmacokinetics, Cancer, Antibody engineering, glycosylation, Fc receptors, Therapeutic antibodies, Intrabodies.

1. THERAPEUTIC ANTIBODIES: COMING OF AGE

1.1. First Hopes and Disappointments

Since 1975, when Kohler and Milstein developed a procedure to efficiently produce monoclonal antibodies [1], it has been widely believed that these molecules would be ideal reagents for imaging and therapy, similar to the magic bullets imagined by Paul Ehrlich at the beginning of the 20th century. Antibodies have been selected during evolution for their ability to bind with high specificity and affinity to a wide variety of molecules, and since they are stable molecules, they seemed to be ideal molecules to be used as targeting reagents. However, the early excitement was rapidly replaced by disappointment when it became clear that these molecules were facing serious problems when used as therapeutics. The first monoclonal antibodies (mAbs) were murine molecules and were recognized as foreign when injected into patients, leading to their elimination by the patient's immune system. Moreover, in order to be effective, antibodies often need to interact with certain elements of the immune system such as receptors displayed on effector cells or the complement cascade. Because of their murine nature, these early antibodies did not interact properly with components of the human immune system and their biological efficacy was severely restricted.

1.2. Antibody Engineering

Developments in molecular biology made it possible in the early 90's to clone the genes of IgG variable domains [2] and, as a result, the genes of mAbs of interest could be cloned in eukaryotic expression vectors. In this way, recombinant versions of any mAb could be obtained from diverse cell lines in a reproducible fashion, and this solved production issues caused by the instability of many hybridoma lines [3]. Cloning antibody genes was the first step toward the modification of antibodies by subcloning, random or directed mutagenesis and molecular evolution procedures, which made it possible to optimise recombinant antibodies at will and ushered the age of antibody engineering [4].

1.3. Chimeric, Humanized and Human Antibodies

A major application of antibody engineering was the possibility to create chimeric antibodies (Fig. **1**). The

***Address correspondence to Patrick Chames:** INSERM U624, GDR2352, 163 avenue de Luminy - case 915, 13288 Marseille Cedex 09; France: Tel: +33491828833; Fax +33491826083; E-mail: patrick.chames@inserm.fr binding activity of IgG molecules is generated by the variable domains of the heavy and light chains. Since antibodies are well conserved through evolution, it was possible to create chimeras by fusing murine variable domains, responsible for the binding activity, with human constant domains [5] leading to the development of a new generation of therapeutic candidates [6] (Fig. **1**). These chimeric antibodies are 70% human and possess a fully human Fc portion, which makes them considerably less immunogenic in humans and allows them to interact with human effector cells and the complement cascade. With the development of antibody engineering techniques, it became possible to decrease even further the murine part of monoclonal antibodies by replacing the hypervariable loops of a fully human antibody with the hypervariable loops of the murine antibody of interest, using an approach called Complementarity Determining Region (CDR) grafting [7]. These antibodies, called "humanized", are 85 to 90% human and are even less immunogenic than chimeric antibodies (Fig. **1**). However, CDR grafting is more technically demanding than a mere fusion and directed mutagenesis approaches are often needed to restore the affinity present in the murine parental antibody. Most of the approved monoclonal antibodies in current use are either chimeric or humanized (Table **1**).

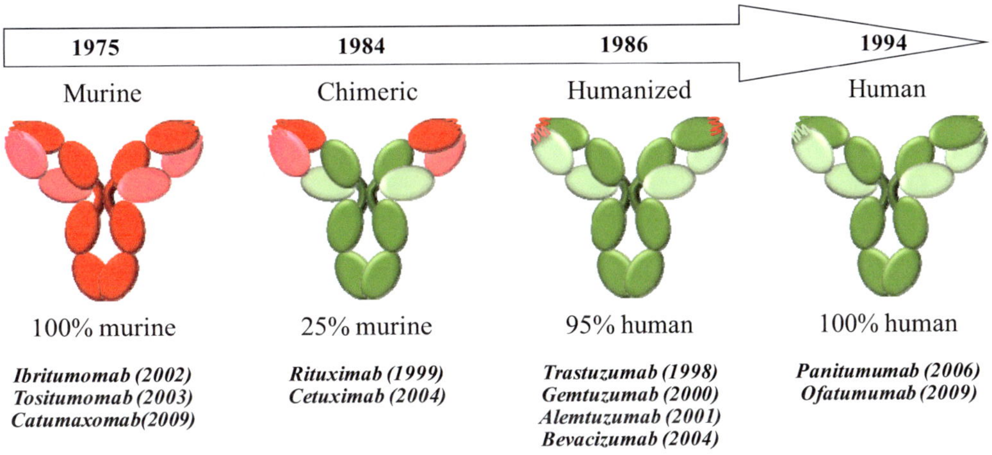

Figure 1: Chimeric and humanized antibodies. Murine sequences are depicted in red, and human sequences in green, using light colors for light chain and dark colors for heavy chains.

Table 1: Monoclonal antibodies approved for therapeutic use.

Generic Name	Trade Name	Antibody Format	Antigen	Approved Indication	FDA Approval	EMEA Approval
Muromomab	Orthoclone	murine, IgG2a	CD3	Allograft rejection in allogeneic renal transplantation	86/06/19	NA
Abciximab[1]	ReoPro	chimeric, IgG1	GPIIb/IIIa r	Maintenance of coronary patency	94/12/22	NA
Rituximab[2]	Mabthera	chimeric, IgG1	CD20	CD20-positive B-cell non-Hodgkin's lymphoma	97/11/26	98/06/02
Daclizumab	Zenapax	humanized, IgG1	CD25 (Il2r)	Allograft rejection	97/12/10	99/02/26
Basiliximab	Simulect	chimeric, IgG1	CD25 (Il2r)	Allograft rejection	98/05/12	98/10/09
Palivizumab	Synagis	humanized, IgG1	protéine F	Respiratory syncytial virus (RSV inhibitor) in children	98/06/19	99/08/13
Infliximab	Remicade	chimeric, IgG1	TNF□	Crohn's Disease and rheumatoid arthritis	98/08/24	99/08/13
Trastuzumab	Herceptin	humanized, IgG1	HER-2/Neu	Metastatic breast cancer	98/09/25	00/08/28
Etanercept[3]	Enbrel	huFcγ1/TNFr	TNFα and β	Autoimmune diseases such as ankylosing	98/11/02	00/02/03

				spondylitis		
Gemtuzumab[4]	Mylotarg	humanized, IgG4	CD33	CD33 positive acute myeloid leukemia	00/05/17	NA
Alemtuzumab[5]	Mabcampath	humanized, IgG1	CD52	B-cell chronic lymphocytic leukemia	01/05/07	01/07/06
Ibritomomab[6]	Zevalin ^{90}Y	mouse, IgG1	CD20	B-cell non-Hodgkin's lymphoma	02/02/19	04/01/16
Adalimumab[7]	Trudexa	human, IgG1 (PD)	TNFα	Crohn's Disease and rheumatoid arthritis	02/12/31	03/09/01
Alefacept[3]	Amevive	huFcγ1/LFA-3	CD2	Chronic plaque psoriasis	03/01/30	NA
Omalizumab	Xolair	humanized, IgG1	IgE	Treatment of asthma	03/06/20	05/10/25
Tositumomab[6,8]	Bexxar ^{131}I	murine, IgG2a	CD20	CD20-positive B-cell non-Hodgkin's lymphoma	03/06/27	NA
Efalizumab[13]	Raptiva	humanized, IgG1	CD11a	Moderate to severe plaque psoriasis	03/10/27	04/09/20
Cetuximab	Erbitux	chimeric, IgG1	EGFr	metastatic colorectal and head and neck carcinoma	04/02/12	04/06/29
Bevacizumab	Avastin	humanized, IgG1	VEGF-A	Metastatic colon and rectum and non-small cell lung cancer	04/02/26	05/01/12
Natalizumab[9]	Tysabri	humanized, IgG4	integrin α4	Multiple sclerosis	04/11/23	06/06/27
Ranibizumab	Lucentis	humanized, IgG1	VEGF-A	Wet-type age-related macular degeneration	06/06/30	07/01/22
Panitumumab[10]	Vectibis	human, IgG2	EGFr	Metastatic colorectal carcinoma	06/09/27	07/12/19
Eculizumab[11]	Soliris	humanized,IgG2/4	C5	Paroxysmal nocturnal hemoglobinuria	07/03/16	07/06/20
Certolizumab[12]	Cimzia	humanized, IgG1	TNFα	Crohn's disease and rheumatoid arthritis	08/04/22	09/10/01
Golimumab	Simponi	Human, IgG1	TNF□	Rheumatoid arthritis	09/04/24	09/10/01
Catumaxomab	Removа	mouse IgG2a/rat IgG2b	EpCam/CD3	Malignant ascites	NA	09/04/20
Canakinumab	Ilaris	Human, IgG1	IL-1□	Cryopyrin-associated periodic syndrome	09/06/17	09/10/23
Ustekinumab	Stelara	Human, IgG1	IL-12/IL-23	Plaque psoriasis	09/09/25	09/02/09
Ofatumumab	Arzerra	Human, IgG1	CD20	B-cell chronic lymphocytic leukemia	09/10/26	NA
Tocilizumab	Actemra	Humanized, IgG1	IL-6R	Rheumatoid arthritis	10/01/08	09/01/16

1 Abciximab is a Fab fragment.

2 Rituximab is commercialized under the trade name Rituxan in USA.

3 These molecules are fusions between the IgG1 Fc portion and a receptor. On May 2nd, 2008, the FDA placed a black box warning on Etanercept due to a number of serious infections associated with the drug.

4 Gemtuzumab "ozogamicine" is coupled to calicheamicin, an antitumoral antibiotic.

5 Alemtuzumab is commercialized under the trade name Campath in USA.

6 Ibritomomab "tiuxetan" and Tositumomab are coupled to radioisotopes.

7 Adalimumab is commercialized under the trade name Humira in USA.

8 All approved antibodies have a kappa light chain kappa except Tositumomab which has a lambda light chain.

9 Natalizumab was voluntary withdrawn from the market in February 2005. The 5th June 2006, FDA approved a special restricted distribution program.

10 Panitumumab is the first human antibody obtained from humanized mice.

11 Eculizumab contains a CH1 domain and hinge from IgG2, and CH2-CH3 domains from IgG4.

12 Certolizumab pegol is a PEGylated humanized Fab' fragment.

13 In April, 2009, Genentech Inc. announced a phased voluntary withdrawal of Raptiva from the U.S.and E.U. market.

Another major improvement came with the development of *in vitro* selection methods, the most successful one being phage display. With the ever increasing power of antibody engineering, it became possible to clone entire repertoires of antibody fragment genes, from immunized or non-immunized animals, including humans. A powerful selection method was therefore needed to select from this large number of potential binders the ones able to bind the antigen of choice. The first technique, and still by far the most common one was mainly developed in the laboratory of Greg Winter [8], and was inspired by earlier work by George Smith [9]. Like all *in vitro* selection methods, this technique relies on the ability to establish a physical link between a protein and the gene encoding this protein, in this case between a protein fused to a filamentous phage capsid protein (p3 or p8) displayed at the surface of phage M13 and its corresponding gene contained in the encapsidated DNA. If the molecule is immunopurified by binding to the antigen of interest, its gene is immediately available, allowing sequencing and further multiplication of the specific clone. Thanks to these *in vitro* selection methods, it is now possible to rapidly and efficiently select fully human antibody fragments against virtually any antigen using "universal" large non-immunized libraries [4]. Moreover, the same approach can be used to mature the affinity of a valuable antibody by creating a secondary library consisting of mutants of the first candidate, and performing stringent *in vitro* selection against the antigen of choice. Phage display and more recently ribosome display have been used to obtain binders with sub-picomolar affinities for the relevant antigen, outperforming the affinities of most conventional monoclonal antibodies [10].

During the same decade, a complementary approach was developed to create fully human antibodies. Transgenic "humanized" mice were created by replacing the entire mouse IgG repertoire with a human repertoire [11]. Upon immunization, these humanized mice produce human IgGs and conventional hybridoma techniques can be used to clone human antibodies with the required properties. This approach has the advantage to give *in vivo* matured antibodies, circumventing the need for additional affinity maturation. Moreover, they directly lead to full length IgG, which is often the preferred format for therapy. However, humanized mice cannot be used effectively when the immunogen is toxic or when the targeted antigen shares a high degree of homology with its murine ortholog. This latter problem represents a real limitation since it could sometimes be highly convenient to use a murine model for preclinical characterization and the murine ortholog of a therapeutic target.

2. CURRENT LIMITATIONS

The creation of chimeric, humanized or fully human antibodies was a major breakthrough and led to a wave of FDA-approved antibodies. Currently, more than 25 antibodies are approved in the US and other countries as therapeutics, mainly for cancer and immune disorders (Table **1**) (see [12] for review). Impressive results have been achieved in cancer therapy, as exemplified by the success met by Rituximab in the treatment of several cancer types. However, mAb-based treatments are nevertheless facing several limitations which limit their widespread use as therapeutics.

2.1. Production Costs

Monoclonal antibodies are large (150 kDa) multimeric proteins containing numerous disulfide bonds and post-translational modifications such as glycosylation. They need a sophisticated eukaryotic machinery to be produced in active form. Moreover, most studies have shown that these molecules have to be injected in large amounts to achieve clinical efficacy (*e.g.* 8 to 16 doses of 375 mg/m^2 *i.e.* a total amount of 6 to 12 g per patient for Rituximab; see http://www.rituxan.com). Consequently, the production of therapeutic antibodies necessitates the use of very large cultures of mammalian cells followed by extensive purification steps under Good Manufacturing Practice, leading to extremely high production costs and limiting the wide use of these drugs. Several alternative production systems in microorganisms and plants are being evaluated at the moment, which might lead to significant progress in the near future [13, 14].

2.2. Pharmacokinetics *vs.* Tissue Penetration

In murine xenograft models, mAbs directed against tumor-specific antigens largely remain in the blood and no more than 20% of the administered dose typically interacts with the tumor [15]. This represents probably one of the major limitations faced by mAbs. Antibody uptake by the tumor depends on a subtle balance between favorable pharmacokinetics and efficient penetration and retention in the targeted tissue and various characteristics of mAbs, such as molecular size, shape, affinity and valency control these properties. Monoclonal antibodies are large molecules that are characterized by very long serum half lives (Table **2**). They far exceed the renal clearance threshold (~ 70 kDa), preventing them from being eliminated through the kidney glomeruli. Moreover, the Fc portion of IgG molecules can interact with various receptors expressed at the surface of several cell types, which increase their retention in the circulation. Most importantly, the Fc portion can interact with the neonatal Fc receptor (FcRn) expressed at the surface of several cell types, including vascular endothelium cells, monocytes and macrophages as well as with barrier sites such as the blood–brain interface, the glomerular filter in the kidneys and the intestinal epithelium [16]. Beside its role in the transport of antinatal maternal antibody to the fetus, across the placenta, FcRn plays an important role in IgG homeostasis. Indeed it has been shown that FcRn extends the serum half life of IgG and albumin (*i.e.* ~ 90 % of serum protein content) from one day (the typical half life of serum protein not freely filtered by the kidneys) to up to several weeks. Most serum proteins are pinocytosed and undergo gradual acidification in endosomes, followed by fusion with lysosomes and hydrolysis. However, IgGs bind to FcRn at low pH and the complex is carried back to the cell surface, whereupon it dissociates at neutral pH. FcRn therefore serves as a protective carrier that shuttles IgG molecules away from the lysosome and back into the serum, conferring to them an even longer serum half-life.

Table 2: Properties of antibody isotypes and antibody fragments[1].

Isotype	Serum Level (mean adult mg/ml)	Biological half-life (days)	Biological Functions	MW (kDa)
IgA1	6	6	Pathogen neutralization in mucosal secretions	160
IgA2	6	6	Pathogen neutralization in mucosal secretions	160
IgD	3	3	Membrane B cell receptor	184
IgE	2	2	Mast cell histamine release	188
IgG1	21	21	Pathogen neutralization in tissues Classical complement activation Opsonization NK cell ADCC Transplacental transfer	146
IgG2	20	20	Pathogen neutralization in tissues	146
IgG3	7	7	Pathogen neutralization in tissues Classical complement activation Opsonization NK cell ADCC Transplacental transfer	165
IgG4	21	21	Pathogen neutralization in tissues Transplacental transfer	146
IgM	10	10	Classical complement activation Membrane B cell receptor (monomer)	970
Fab		0.3-0.8		50
scFv		0.1		27
sdAb		< 0.05		13

[1]Adapted from Janeway CA, Travers P, Walport M and Shlomchick. Immunobiology. Garland publishing, NY, 2001.

While the large size of mAbs and the presence of the Fc region can be advantageous in terms of pharmacokinetics, they can also be a serious handicap. Except in the case of hematologic malignancies and diseases, therapeutic antibodies have to penetrate tissues and the extracellular matrix to reach their target cells. Tissue penetration, especially in the case of solid tumors, is a crucial parameter, most of the time severely limiting the overall efficiency of the treatment. Tumors are characterized by heterogeneous and tortuous vasculature, high interstitial fluid pressure, and high viscosity of the tumor blood supply. Consequently, mAbs must diffuse against this pressure gradient to penetrate tumors [15]. A major determinant of speed of diffusion through tumors is molecular size. The rate of diffusion is approximately inversely proportional to the cube root of molecular weight. Consequently, large macromolecules such as mAbs diffuse poorly explaining why larger tumor masses may be more difficult to treat by monoclonal antibody therapy. Strikingly, among the ten mAbs approved for cancer therapy in the US, only three (Trastuzumab, Cetuximab, Panitumumab) are targeting membrane antigens expressed on solid tumors, whereas over 85% of human cancers are solid tumors, clearly reflecting the current limitation of mAb treatment.

Moreover, another issue called the "binding site barrier effect" can further decrease the penetration of tumors by mAbs [17]. Whereas one might presume that tighter binding is always better, several studies have shown that very high affinities can be suboptimal for therapeutic antibodies that target solid tumors [18]. Since high affinity antibodies tightly bind their antigen upon the first encounter, *i.e.* at the periphery of the tumor, they do not penetrate deeper inside the tumor until all antigen molecules are saturated in the periphery. By contrast, moderate binders are released from these first encountered antigens and penetrate deeper into the tumor, ultimately leading to uniform intratumoral distribution, and higher tumor uptake. The right balance in terms of affinity will lead to an efficient tumor targeting and tumor retention, and will also allow some diffusion inside the tumor. Because these properties depend on several factors, including antigen density, internalization, association and dissociation rates, the optimal affinity is not always easy to engineer.

2.3. Mode of Action and Associated Limitations

Monoclonal antibodies can have various modes of actions *in vitro*, and the actual mode of action once injected in patients is not always clear [19]. The simplest mode of action is mere binding of the antibody to its antigen, thereby interfering with its activity and interaction with binding partners. The antigen can be a soluble ligand, and examples of such antibodies include Infliximab, Adalimumab and Certolizumab (anti-TNFα) or Bevacizumab (anti-VEGF). On the other hand, the antibody may target a receptor displayed at the cell surface, block its interaction with a ligand, interfere with a multimerisation process or trigger internalization of receptors or apoptosis of targeted cells. Examples of such antibodies include cetuximab and panitumumab (anti-EGFR or HER1) and trastuzumab (anti-HER2) (Table **1**).

In addition, once bound to their antigen, antibodies can also interact in several ways with the immune system of the recipient through their Fc portion. They can recruit the complement cascade through interaction with C1q, ultimately leading to the formation of pores in the targeted cell membrane, or they can recruit effector cells through interaction with the C4b/C2b/C3b complex bound to the target cell surface and the receptor CR1. However, although most therapeutic antibodies can trigger complement dependent cytotoxicity *in vitro*, this has not been demonstrated *in vivo* so far.

One of the most important mechanisms by which IgG antibodies engage the cellular immune system is *via* interaction of the Fc domain with Fc gamma receptors (FcγRs) [20]. The human FcγR family contains six known members in three subgroups, including FcγRI (CD64), FcγRIIa,b,c (CD32a,b,c), and FcγRIIIa,b (CD16a,b), expressed by various effector cells of the immune system, including macrophages, neutrophils, dendritic cells and natural killer (NK) cells. The latter cell type is the main actor of the antibody dependent cell-mediated cytotoxicity (ADCC). These cells can be recruited and activated through the interaction between FcγRIIIa and the Fc region, leading to the formation of an immunological synapse, the release of perforin/granzyme, and the establishment of the Fas/FasL interaction, both leading to apoptosis of the target cells. The other cell types mainly lead to the phagocytosis of target cells.

Several pieces of evidence demonstrate that ADCC plays a major role in the *in vivo* efficacy of mAbs. Several investigators have examined the relationship between FcγR polymorphisms and clinical responses to antibody therapy [21, 22]. Around 20% of the Caucasian population possess a valine in position 158 of FcγRIIIa, while the rest of the population has a phenylalanine. *In vitro*, a fivefold higher affinity between FcγRIIIa-V158 and IgG1 Fc compared to FcγRIII-F158 has been reported, leading to a more efficient *in vivo* ADCC using PBMCs or purified NKs. Interestingly, several studies demonstrated that Rituximab-treated follicular lymphoma patients who were homozygous for the higher affinity form of FcγRIIIa (V/V158) had significantly prolonged periods of progression-free survival relative to patients heterozygous or homozygous for the lower affinity F158 form. This finding is probably the strongest available demonstration of a major role of ADCC in patients.

Unfortunately the triggering of ADCC by therapeutic antibodies faces several limitations. First of all, as described above, the affinity between the Fc and its receptors plays a crucial role, and the fact that 80% of the population expresses a low affinity variant of the receptor is a major issue. Secondly, IgG1 molecules are glycosylated in the CH2 domain (Asn 297) of the Fc region. This modification is extremely important since it modulates the affinity of the Fc for FcγRIIIa, thereby modifying the *in vivo* efficacy of antibodies. More specifically, the presence of fucose residues in the carbohydrate has been shown to decrease ADCC efficiency [23]. The nature of the carbohydrate moiety is dependent on which enzymes are expressed by the cell line used for antibody production [24]. For example, an anti-CD20 chimeric IgG1 produced by the rat hybridoma YB2/0 cell line showed more than 50-fold higher ADCC using purified human peripheral blood mononuclear cells as effector than the same antibody produced by the Chinese Hamster Ovary (CHO) cell line, the cell line traditionally used for the production of therapeutic proteins. This difference was attributed to the elevated expression of *FUT8*, the gene coding for α1,6-fucosyltransferase, in the CHO line [23].

The affinity between the antibody and its antigen is not the only issue. A third limitation lies in the fact that therapeutic antibodies have to compete with a high concentration of patient's IgGs for binding to FcγRIIIa. Indeed, the serum concentration of IgG is 8-17 mg/ml, and around 66% of those molecules are IgG1 capable of interacting with FcγRIIIa. Strikingly, most antibodies, in order to show a therapeutic effect, have to be injected at high doses to reach a serum concentration between 10 to 100 µg/ml, whereas these antibodies lead to a saturating ADCC at 10 ng/ml *in vitro*, *i.e.* in the absence of competing IgGs. Competition with patients' IgGs has been proposed to account for this huge concentration difference [25].

Finally, a fourth limitation of the use of therapeutic antibodies may be their affinity for inhibitory Fc receptors such as FcγRIIb, expressed by B cells, macrophages, dendritic cells and neutrophils [20]. Unlike activating receptors possessing a cytoplasmic Immuno-Receptor Tyrosine Based Activation Motif (ITAM), which is either encoded directly (FcγRIIa,c) or gained by association with a common ITAM γ-chain (FcγRI and FcγRIIIa), FcγRIIb possesses an inhibitory motif (ITIM) in its cytoplasmic domain, and signaling through this receptor negatively regulates effector functions. This signaling leads to a balance between activating and inhibitory signals which is used by the immune system to control the immune reaction. Like other IgG1, therapeutic antibodies do interact with this receptor, which decreases their overall efficiency.

So far, all approved therapeutic antibodies are IgG, capable of interacting with effector cells through FcγRs. However, FcαRI, also called CD89, and capable of binding to IgA, should deserve more attention. Indeed, FcαRI is constitutively expressed on myeloid effector cells, including neutrophils, monocytes, macrophages, eosinophils, and dendritic cells, but not on non-cytolytic cell populations [26]. Neutrophils are of special interest since several studies support their *in vitro* and *in vivo* role in tumor cell lysis and tumor rejection [27-30]. Moreover, they represent the most abundant FcR-expressing leukocyte subset in blood, and their numbers can be increased by treatment with G-CSF. Since FcαRI is capable of efficiently activating immature neutrophils, its targeting by the use of IgA therapeutic antibodies [31, 32] or bispecific antibodies [33] has considerable potential and that will certainly be explored in depth in the near future.

3. NEW AVENUES

Antibody engineering has played a major role in the development of the first generation of therapeutic antibodies. It is now being used in several ways to obtain a new generation of optimized antibodies with a modified Fc region capable of circumventing some of the limitations described above. However, the potential offered by antibody engineering can go further than optimization, and is a way to create entirely new Ig domain-based molecules, not found in nature, that can be tailored to match desired characteristics.

3.1. Fc Engineering and Glycoengineering of Therapeutic mAbs

Because mAbs depend on their Fc region for eliciting certain immune reactions, a way to improve their action is to engineer this portion of the antibody. For instance, for most therapeutic applications, a long serum half life is desirable since it would decrease the need for repetitive injections of the molecule to achieve a therapeutically relevant serum concentration. Accordingly, several groups are attempting to use mutagenesis to increase the affinity of the IgG Fc portion for FcRn at acidic pH (in the endosome) without raising the affinity of the interaction at physiological pH (to allow an efficient release of the antibody in the circulation). On the other hand, some applications such as imaging necessitate very high contrasts which depend on rapid clearance of the excess of unbound molecules. Some studies have demonstrated the possibility to engineer the Fc portion in order to decrease its affinity for FcRn, leading to shorter serum half-lives and thus better contrast [34]. Worthy of note, the IgG3 isotype is not efficiently bound by FcRn and consequently, its serum half-life is naturally short (1 week instead of 3 for IgG1) (Table **2**).

More importantly, the affinity of the Fc region for various Fc receptors also plays a major role in the effectiveness of therapies. A way to increase the efficiency of therapeutic antibodies would be to increase their binding to activating receptors, namely FcγRI, FcγRIIa and more importantly FcγRIIIa, and decrease their interaction with inhibitory FcγRIIb receptors [35-37].

Since NK cells are known to be responsible for most if not all tumor cell lysis observed when PBMCs are used as effector cells and as this cell type typically expresses a unique activating receptor, FcγRIIIa, most mutagenesis studies have tried to increase the affinity of the Fc region for this receptor. Several approaches have been used to reach this goal, including alanine scanning, site-directed mutagenesis, computational structure-based design, and selection-based methods. Impressive results have been achieved, with variants possessing up to 100-fold greater affinity for FcγRIIIa, resulting in 100-fold enhanced *in vitro* ADCC [24, 37].

The second receptor of importance for therapy is FcγRIIa. This receptor is important for the function of neutrophils, monocytes, macrophages, and dendritic cells, although macrophages and dendritic cells also express FcγRIIIa. Macrophages and monocytes can phagocytose opsonized target cells through engagement of FcγRs. They can also induce apoptosis of target cells through the release of reactive nitrogen and oxygen intermediates, or lyse them through the release of cytolytic granules. Perhaps more importantly, macrophages and dendritic cells, being professional antigen presenting cells, facilitate a potentially more robust anti-tumor effect known as cross-priming, by which these cells process and present tumor-derived antigens on their surface class I MHC molecules, thus acquiring the ability to activate T cells. Cross-priming can activate cytotoxic T lymphocytes that recognize MHC/tumor antigen complexes, ultimately leading to T cell attack on the tumor cells [38]. Remarkably, this process has the potential to lead to a long lasting adaptive immune response that could protect patients from relapses. Increasing the affinity of human Fc for FcγRIIa is therefore of considerable interest. Unfortunately, the same cells also express the inhibitory FcγRIIb receptor, whose extracellular domain shares 93% of homology with that of FcγRIIa, and the task of selectively increasing the Fc affinity for the activating receptor remains a challenge that has not yet been solved [39].

It must be stressed that the clinical relevance of FcγRIIa activation is still not clear, the most compelling piece of evidence being the correlation between the FcγRIIa (R/R131) genotype and progression-free survival in an anti-GD2 antibody and GM-CSF cotherapy of neuroblastoma using a murine IgG3 [40]. Most clinical trials use human IgG1 molecules which bind the two alleles (H131 and R131) with a similar affinity and thus cannot shed any light on the clinical relevance of FcγRIIa polymorphism. By contrast human IgG2 binds with a tenfold higher affinity to the H131 allele. Polymorphism studies with Panitumumab, an IgG2 anti-EGFR antibody for treatment of cancer of the colon, would therefore be of considerable interest.

The high affinity of the third main receptor, FcγRI, for monomeric IgG ($K_D = 10^{-9}$ M) probably precludes the capacity to distinguish between unbound antibody and immune complexes, suggesting that this receptor is not a key player in anti-tumor antibody activity; no engineering studies have been done on this receptor.

Mutagenesis of the Fc region is not the only way to improve its affinity for Fc receptors. As mentioned earlier, the nature of carbohydrates linked to Asn297 of the CH2 domain has a major influence on the affinity of the Fc for FcγRs. Several studies demonstrated that the presence of fucose residues can lead to severely reduced ADCC efficiency. Several academic groups and pharmaceutical companies are presently focusing on the development of new cell lines capable of producing defucosylated mAbs, such as CHO cell lines deleted of the *FUT8* gene coding for the enzyme α-1,6-fucosyltransferase, or overexpressing a recombinant β-1,4-N-acetylglucosaminyltransferase III leading to antibodies enriched in bisected and non-fucosylated oligosaccharides [41]. The same kind of studies have also been conducted on non-mammalian expression systems such as yeast, plant and moss [42-44]. Although the effects of such modifications on FcγR interaction need further characterization, it is assumed that defucosylated antibodies have increased affinity for FcγRIIIa/b, and the same affinity for other receptors, including FcγRIIb.

Many of these optimized antibodies have entered clinical trials [12]. The near future will tell us what will be the impact of these modifications.

3.2. Antibody Fragments

Antibody engineering has been used to chimerize or humanize mAbs, and more recently to optimize the Fc portion of mAbs. However, many studies have demonstrated that it is possible to produce various antibody fragments that retain the binding activity of the full length molecule (Fig. **2**), and to use these new formats in certain specific applications [45]. As mentioned earlier, the large size of antibodies limits tumor penetration, and their long serum half life is not suitable for applications such as radioimmunotherapy or imaging since it would lead to irradiation of healthy tissues and high background, respectively. Antibody fragments such as Fab fragments, although they lack an effector function, can be an attractive alternative since they are monovalent, and are rapidly eliminated by renal clearance. To compensate for these shortcomings, several groups have proposed new engineered antibody formats (Fig. **2**).

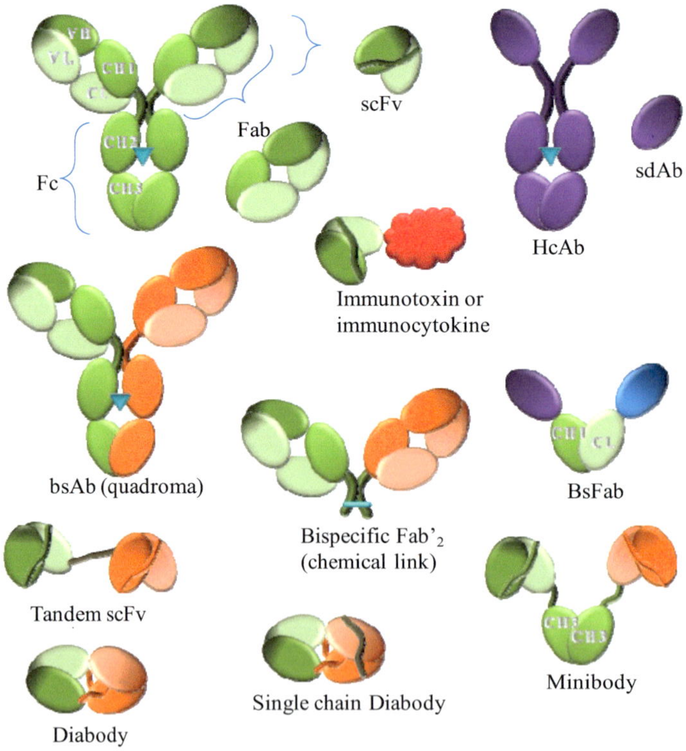

Figure 2: Antibody formats. Depicting a conventional antibody in green (light for light chain, dark for heavy chain, blue triangle indicate the glycosylation site) and the derived fragments (shaded areas represent the binding sites). The orange color symbolizes a different specificity. Heavy chain only antibodies (HcAb) from camelids and their fragments (sdAb for single domain antibodies) are depicted in mauve or blue. The red molecule is depicting a cytokine or a toxin. bsFab: bispecific Fab fragment.

ScFv fragments (variable domains of the heavy and light chains linked by a flexible linker) were described very early as small fragments capable of retaining the binding activity of the full IgG molecule, albeit in a monovalent fashion [46]. Because of its very short half life in serum (~ 2 hr) this fragment cannot be used as such, although it has been extensively used as a binding moiety when incorporated in more complex molecules (see next section). However, the team of Greg Winter discovered that decreasing the length of the linker between the two domains induced the formation of a dimer, named diabody [47] (Fig. **2**). Diabodies are compact, medium-size (60 kDa) molecules and can be an interesting choice for imaging purposes or radioimmunotherapy. Besides increasing the molecular weigth, the dimerization provides bivalency, which leads to a higher avidity and higher tumor retention. Thus, diabodies provide rapid tissue penetration, high target retention and rapid blood clearance. Because they are rapidly eliminated through the kidneys, they limit the exposure to the bone marrow, which is most often the dose-limiting organ with intact radiolabeled mAbs. Diabodies possess an excellent combination of rapid tumor uptake and clearance for *in vivo* imaging when labeled with ^{123}I or ^{111}In, or for rapid xenograft visualization by PET when labeled with positron emitters such as ^{64}Cu or ^{124}I [48]. Diabodies therefore have a high potential for radiotherapy. Indeed, a single intravenous dose of 90Y-labeled diabody inhibited growth rates of established HER-2 tumor xenografts in athymic nude mice (Adams, G.P 2004), and even more promising results have been reported with an anti HER2 diabody coupled to α-emitting radioisotope 211At, with 60% tumor-free animals one year after a single injection of the conjugate in immunodeficient nude mice bearing established HER2/neu-positive tumors [48].

More recently, several teams have shown that it is possible to obtain high affinities using a single variable domain. In 1989, the group of Greg Winter demonstrated that mouse variable domains could be used as binding units [49], but this was not further developed because the vast majority of these domains aggregate spontaneously. However, it was later found that camelids and sharks express a type of antibodies devoid of light chains (Fig. **2**), called Heavy chain Antibodies (HcAbs) [50] and new antigen receptor antibodies (IgNAR) [51], respectively. These antibodies have a single variable domain (called VHH for camelids and V-NAR for sharks) which generates high affinities toward a large spectrum of antigens. These small domains (13 kDa) can be easily produced in bacteria or yeast and are then called domain antibodies (dAbs), single domain antibodies (sdAbs) or nanobodies. Interestingly, these sdAbs are naturally endowed with very useful characteristics [45], for instance a very high stability, even when the intradomain disulfide bond characteristic of Ig domains is not present, the possibility to strongly bind to epitopes not accessible to conventional antibodies such as enzyme active sites, and a high homology of sequence with the human VHIII gene family in the case of VHH. Since then, several studies have demonstrated the possibility to develop human variable domains into stable dAbs [45]. These fragments combine the high affinity and specificity of antibodies with the stability and ease of production of small molecules, and have the potential to be administered by means other than injection. Several dAbs are being tested in Phase I and Phase II clinical trials at the moment, including two anti-TNFα against rheumatoid arthritis and Crohn disease, and an anti-Von Willebrand factor used as an anti-thrombotic. Furthermore, dAbs can be very efficiently engineered as targeting moiety of more complex molecular constructions (see next section).

Because of their reduced size, antibody fragments usually penetrate tumors much more rapidly and efficiently than full IgG, but this benefit is counterbalanced by a very short serum half life which decreases the overall tumor uptake of these small molecules (Table **2**). Several academic groups and companies are investigating alternative approaches to increase the serum half life of antibody fragments, the most promising one being the chemical addition of PEG residues which considerably increase the size of the fragments. An example is the Certolizumab pegol [52], a recently approved anti-TNFα pegylated Fab' fragment which has a 14 days serum half-life. PEG linkage (PEGylation) is very efficient for increasing the half-life and scFv stability, conferring improved anti-tumor activity and apparently also reducing immunogenicity [45]. Improved circulation time and accumulation in tumors has been demonstrated with PEGylated scFv fragments, tandem scFv (two scFvs linked with a flexible linker) and diabodies. However, these chemical modifications sometimes lead to partial inactivation or decreased affinity of the fragment and several alternatives are currently being explored. For example, fusion of recombinant antibody fragments to Human Serum Albumin (HSA) can be used to increase the serum half life without affecting the binding and activity of the fragments, unlike PEGylation. HSA is not eliminated by the kidneys and is actively recycled by its interaction with neonatal receptor FcRn. Fusion proteins containing HSA have been obtained with scFv, tandem scFv and diabodies and showed a large increase in circulation time [53].

Interestingly, similar results were obtained by fusing antibody fragments to HSA-binding peptides or proteins. The half life of an anti-HER2 Fab fragment (derived from Trastuzumab) could be increased 10 to 15 folds by fusing it to short HSA binding peptides selected by phage display. The resulting Fab fragments outperformed the parental IgG *in vivo*, in terms of efficacy, targeting, tumor accumulation and retention, and tumor to blood ratio [54]. Similarly, the group of Ian Tomlinson isolated human domain antibodies of 12 kDa directed against albumin (albudAbs) [55]. The serum half life of these fragments was extended from 45 min to the half-life of their targets (53h for rats, 35 h in mice) and this extended half-life was conferred to a fused partner such as IL-1. The group of Roland Kontermann improved the circulation time of a single-chain diabody by a factor of 6 by fusing it to an albumin-binding domain from streptococcal protein G [56]. The same laboratory also fused a tag displaying several N-glycosylation motifs to a single chain diabody and produced glycosylated diabodies after expression in transfected HEK293 cells [57]. The half life of these molecules was increased by a factor 2-3, albeit at the cost of reduced activity of the fragment in a target cell-dependent IL-2 release assay.

More generally, multimerisation has been proposed in order to obtain a good compromise between serum half life, tumor penetration and multivalency. In addition to diabodies, triabodies or tetrabodies have also been produced by multimerisation of scFvs harboring a short or no linker, leading to high molecular weight and multivalent fragments with increased serum half lifes [45].

3.3. Fusions with Effector Proteins

Since they are small and easy to produce in *E. coli* or in yeast, antibody fragments have also been used as the binding moiety in newly created molecules endowed with new functions. Various proteins have been fused to antibody fragments (Fig. **2**). For instance, interesting results have been obtained with immunotoxins, consisting of a toxin, such as a fragment of *Pseudomonas* exotoxin (PE38) without its cell-binding domain, diphtheria toxin or the A chain of ricin, fused to a scFv [58]. However, such molecules are immunogenic and are rapidly neutralized by the immune system of recipients. More potent immunotoxins have been created by fusing a human RNase to a human scFv targeting a tumor antigen such as HER2 receptor, leading to a dramatic reduction in tumor volume in animal models [59]. Several immunotoxins are being tested in clinical trials at the moment [58].

Antibody-Directed Enzyme Prodrug Therapy (ADEPT) uses a fusion between a scFv and an enzyme to convert a relatively non-toxic prodrug into a potent cytotoxic drug in the vicinity of the targeted cells, thereby avoiding the effects of the drug on healthy cells. Examples of such molecules include a fusion between a scFv with specificity for TAG-72, a carbohydrate epitope that is overexpressed and exposed on the cell surface in a large fraction of solid malignancies, and β-lactamase. This fusion can convert C-Mel, a nitrogen mustard prodrug, into melphalan, a very potent drug [60].

Antibody fragments were also fused to cytokines (immunocytokines). These molecules have the potential to activate the immune system of patients in the vicinity of the tumor, thereby avoiding important side effects traditionally associated with systemic administration of activating cytokines. Tumor specific scFvs have been fused to various cytokines, including IL2, IL15, GM-CSF, IFN γ, leading to impressive results [61-63] and several of these constructs are now tested in the clinic.

Finally, scFv can also be fused to membrane proteins, to create chimeric receptors. "T-bodies" are genetically retargeted T cells armed with chimeric receptors whose extracellular recognition unit is an antibody fragment such as a scFv and whose intracellular region is derived from lymphocyte stimulating moieties, including CD3ζ and FcεRI-gamma [64]. These chimeric receptor constructs are introduced *ex vivo* into T cells from peripheral lymphocytes of a given patient using retroviral vectors. The retargeted T-cells are then infused back into the patient. This approach has been used with success against several targets, including tumors, HIV-infected cells and autoimmune effector cells [65]. Interestingly, this approach is not HLA-restricted and can thus be used for a wide spectrum of patients and tumors, and thus holds promise for future immunotherapies.

3.4. Bispecific Antibodies (bsAb)

As hypothesized very early [66], many mAb shortcomings could be overcome by creating bispecific antibodies (bsAbs) capable of simultaneous binding to two different targets. Such molecules would be capable of retargeting a large variety of payloads to cancer cells. The potential of this approach has been demonstrated by several studies over the years, but the difficulty of producing large amounts of homogenous bsAbs using the available techniques (*e.g.*, hybrid hybridomas, chemical cross-linking) hindered wider adoption and development of this approach. However, using advanced antibody engineering, new recombinant formats have been designed and validated to a certain extent. These formats include tandem scFv, diabodies, tandem diabodies, dual variable domain antibodies, and heterodimerization using a motif such as CH1/Ck domain or the Dock and Lock motif (reviewed in Ref. [67]). The development of single domain antibodies from Camelid antibodies or engineered VH domain should also facilitate design of improved antibody therapeutics. [68] However, few candidates based on these formats have reached the clinic.

The most studied recombinant formats include tandem scFv, minibodies (using "knob into hole" CH3 domains engineered to decrease homodimerization), or bispecific diabodies (Fig. **2**). The very compact structure of diabodies gives them attractive properties such as good tumor penetration, expression and solubility as well as enhanced stability. Although several preclinical studies have shown the efficiency of these molecules, no clinical trials have yet been reported [69]. Another format is the single chain diabody where the two chains of the fragment are linked *via* an additional linker, thereby combining all domains in a single polypeptide (Fig. **2**). Several preclinical studies have demonstrated the potency of this format [70]. All described recombinant bispecific antibodies rely on the use of flexible peptide linkers and although these linkers have obvious advantages in terms of antibody engineering, they also have some disadvantages due to their foreign nature, which leads to an unwanted immune response. Furthermore, their flexible nature makes linkers prone to proteolytic cleavage in serum, potentially leading to production issues, poor antibody stability, aggregation and increased immunogenicity [69]. Domain antibodies can overcome these limitations since they do not require the use of two separate variable domains. Our laboratory has recently developed a format obtained by the direct fusion of two different llama domain antibodies to human CH1 and Cκ constant domains (Fig. **2**). The resulting linker-free molecule closely resembles a human Fab fragment but is capable of simultaneously binding to two different antigens, such as a tumor marker (*e.g.* CEA, [71]) and an activating receptor (*e.g.* CD16a [72]). This new format and a bivalent bispecific derivative are currently being evaluated as a NK cell retargeting agent (see below).

Very recently, Wozniak-Knopp abnd colleagues have demonstrated the possibility to introduce antigen-binding sites in structural loops of CH3 domains of human Fc fragments leading to 50 kDa antigen binding fragments called Fcab [73]. Interestingly, these fragments kept their ability to elicit ADCC and to bind to FcRn. Obviously, these fragments can be fused to regular Fab fragments of a different specificity, thereby yielding a bivalent and bispecific full length IgG. This promising technology should be rapidly applied to the generation of new therapeutic antibodies.

3.4.1. Mode of Action of Bispecific Antibodies

3.4.1.1. Dual Targeting

Inhibition of signaling pathways is one of the main modes of action of therapeutic antibodies. Combinations of small molecule-based treatments were shown to lead to additive or even synergetic effect [74], can block redundant signaling pathways and minimize the possibility of escape from therapy, but are often excluded due to high toxicity. Human or humanized mAb are often very well tolerated and are thus very good candidates for combined therapies. Consequently, several companies are actively testing these combinations, including Genentech with Trastuzumab (anti-Her2) plus Bevacizumab (anti-VEGF) or Immunomedics with Epratuzumab (anti-CD22) plus Rituximab (anti-CD20) [75]. However, combining therapeutic antibodies faces several limitations, including intellectual property issues and high costs involved in research, manufacturing and regulatory affairs. An elegant answer to these hurdles might be the simultaneous inactivation of two targets by a single (bispecific) antibody, as exemplified by two studies

[76, 77] targeting simultaneously EGF and IGF receptors showing that simultaneous targeting is more efficient than monotherapies against the same targets.

3.4.1.2. T Cell Retargeting

Perhaps the most obvious applications of bsAb is T cell retargeting. Indeed, cytotoxic T cells are considered the most potent killer cells of the immune system. They are abundant; they can efficiently proliferate upon activation, they can kill multiple times [78], and efficiently infiltrate tumors but do not express Fcγ receptors. Very early, the idea to make T cells kill tumor cells more potently using bsAb emerged [66]. Bispecific antibodies directed against a tumor marker and CD3 have the potential to redirect and activate any circulating T cells against tumors. However, T cells have a major drawback. Without secondary signal given by the interaction between CD28 and one of its ligand such as B7, T cells are not fully activated and might even become anergic [79]. The first anti-CD3 bsAbs were thus applied in combination with anti CD28 antibodies, with mixed results [80]. Other alternatives are being explored, such as the massive *ex vivo* expansion (>300x109) and activation of patient's T cells using low concentration of anti CD3 and IL-2, and reinjection of these polyclonally activated T cells decorated with an anti CD3 bsAb [81]. Interestingly, armed activated T cells have been shown to be resistant to activation induced cell death and are able to proliferate and kill tumor cells repeatedly [82]. Surprisingly, a small recombinant bsAb format appears to bypass the need for costimulation. Baeuerle and collaborators are developing murine TaFv called BiTE [83]. An anti CD19 x CD3 BiTE was used to obtain a very efficient inhibition of tumor growth in a subcutaneous or leukemic human B cell lymphoma xenograft models, at low concentrations and low effector-to-target ratios [84]. Similar impressive results including eradication of tumors from a human colon cancer cell line and ovarian cancer metastasis in immunodeficient mice were obtained with an anti EpCAM x CD3 BiTE [85]. Interestingly, another BiTE directed this time against the murine CD3 could be used in immunocompetent mice and led to a strong anti tumor effect in the absence of costimulation [86]. The proposed explanation for this outstanding efficacy without costimulation includes a very efficient formation of immunologic synapses [87] due to the very short linker (5 residues) linking the two scFv fragments. Recently, the high potential of these molecules has been cleary demonstrated in clinical trials [88]. Blinatumomab, an anti CD3 x CD19 BiTE (MT103) was shown to induce partial and complete regression in non–Hodgkin's lymphoma patients at extremely low doses (15 $\mu g/m^2$/day), about 5 orders of magnitude below serum levels reported for Rituximab (375 mg/m^2/week). All seven patients treated with 60 $\mu g/m^2$/day experienced a tumor regression. Another clinical trial (NCT00635596), targeting this time solid tumors, has recently been initiated MT110 (anti EpCAM x CD3) [89, 90].

On the other hand, T cell stimulation *via* CD28 has been shown to be very efficient and self sufficient. rM28, a TaFv dimer directed to a melanoma-associated proteoglycan (NG2) and to the costimulatory CD28 molecule on human T cells was indeed shown to induce pronounced T cell activation in PBMC preparations without additional TCR/CD3 stimulation being required *via* supraagonistic T-cell activation. Interestingly it was demonstrated that cytokines produced by CD28-stimulated T cells activate NK cells, which then significantly contribute to tumor-cell lysis [91, 92]. The molecule safety and efficiency of intralesional application of this murine bispecific TaFv rM28 and autologous PBMCs in patients with metastatic melanoma stage III/IV and unresectable metastasis is currently being studied in a phase I/II trial.

Perhaps the most unexpected successes come from rat/mouse chimeric full IgG anti CD3 bsAbs named triomabs, designed by Lindhofer and collaborators. This resulting chimeric Fc was shown to efficiently interact with activating human Fc receptors (FcγRI and FcγRIII) but not inhibitory ones (FcγRIIB), thereby achieving the goal of several academic and industrial laboratories using human Fc engineering. Furthermore, triomabs were shown capable of activating DCs, inducing NK-dependent ADCC and stimulating tumor cell phagocytosis by macrophages [93, 94]. Consequently, this Fc adds two crucial functions to this anti CD3 x target bsAb: additive tumor killing capabilities through the recruitment of macrophages and NK cells, but most importantly, efficient co stimulation of T cells through direct contact with accessory cells such as macrophages and DC (B7/CD28, CD40/CD40L, LFA3/CD2) or cytokine secretion (IL-2 IL-6 IL-12). In fact, the only limitation of these exciting molecules resides in their immunogenicity, precluding repetitive injections of large quantities of bsAb. Nevertheless triomabs have led to impressive preclinical results and clinical results with reduction of up to 5 logs in number of tumor cells in ovarian carcinoma patients, despite the use of low doses of bsAb due to reversible adverse effects [95] for catumaxomab, an EpCAM x CD3 bispecific antibody. By early 2009, the results of a large international Phase 2/3 pivotal study involving 258 patients demonstrated a statistically significant improvement of the primary endpoint, puncture-free survival. Consequently, the European commission approved catumaxomab in April 2009 for the treatment of malignant ascites in patients with EpCAM positive carcinomas in cases where standard therapy is not available or no longer feasible. This first marketing approval clearly represents an important milestone in the field of bispecific antibodies. Two other molecules, ertumaxomab (anti Her2 x CD3) and Lymphomun™ (anti CD20 x CD3) are currently in clinical trials (II and I, respectively).

3.4.1.3. FcγR Bearing Cell Retargeting

Whereas T cells are very attractive effector cells, NK cells have also been shown to be very efficient at destroying tumor cells. ADCC is thought to be one of the main modes of action of therapeutic antibodies, as demonstrated by associations of functionally relevant FcγRIIIA polymorphisms with clinical responses observed with Rituximab [21]. It is known that NK cells mediate essentially all of the ADCC measured *in vitro* using PBMCs as effector cells. Worth of note, neutrophils, the most numerous leukocyte type, do express FcγRIIIB (extremely homologous to FcγRIIIA) but cannot be activated to induce ADCC through this receptor. *In vitro*, neutrophils were shown not to interfere with ADCC efficiency [96]. Compared with T cells, NK cells have the advantage that pre-activation is not required since they constitutively exhibit cytolytic functions [97]. On the other hand, these cells represent less than 10% of lymphocytes and very small numbers of NK cells are found in direct contact with tumor cells, suggesting that NK cells poorly infiltrate tumors [70]. Therefore, many ongoing studies aim at optimizing NK cell killing through engineering of the Fc/FcγRIIIA interaction [37]. Indeed, therapeutic antibodies suffers from several limitations including the influence of FcγR polymorphisms as described earlier but also the influence of the glycans post-translationally added to the IgG CH2 domain, competition with high concentration of circulating IgG for binding to FcγRIIIA, and co-activation of inhibitory receptors such as FcγRIIB decreasing the overall immune response [98]. As postulated very early, a way to overcome all of these limitations would be to redirect and activate NK cells using anti target x FcγRIIIA bispecific antibodies targeting an epitope not involved in IgG binding [99, 100]. The potential of this approach was validated in clinical trials [101, 102]. However, high human anti mouse responses prevented further evaluation of these quadromas. One of these promising bsAb (HRS-3/A9) was converted to a bispecific diabody format and the resulting molecule was shown to induce tumor lysis by NK cells more efficiently than the parental molecules [97] and should be less immunogenic due to the absence of Fc portion. Yet, this antibody fragment still carries the framework sequences of murine origin. The clinical potential of bsAb-based NK cell retargeting still has to be demonstrated. For this goal, we have isolated activating anti FcγRIIIA domain antibodies [72] and anti CEA dAbs [103] that were used to produce anti CEA x FcγRIIIA bsFab molecules. These stable and efficiently produced bsAbs, capable of inducing very potent ADCC at subpicomolar concentrations (Cornillon *et al.*, unpublished), currently undergo preclinical studies.

A third class of interesting effector cells is represented by neutrophils. These cells are of special interest since several studies support their *in vitro* and *in vivo* role in tumor cell lysis and tumor rejection [27-30]. Moreover, they represent by far the most abundant FcR-expressing leukocyte subset in blood, and their numbers can be increased by treatment with G-CSF. FcαRI is constitutively expressed on myeloid effector cells, including neutrophils, monocytes, macrophages, eosinophils, and dendritic cells, but not on non-cytolytic cell populations [26]. Since this receptor is capable of efficiently activating immature neutrophils, its targeting by the use of bsAbs has considerable potential [33], that should be explored more extensively in the future.

Finally receptor FcγRI (CD64) has also been targeted by bsAbs. This receptor is constitutively expressed by monocytes and macrophages. Moreover, its expression can by induced at the surface of neutrophils upon stimulation with interferon-γ or G-CSF. Most notably two bsAbs, an anti Her2 x CD64 and an anti EGFR x CD64, built by chemical conjugation of Fab' fragments, were extensively studied for the treatment of advanced breast cancer and head and neck cancer, respectively. These bsAbs were even used in phase I clinical trials [104]. These molecules were well tolerated but unfortunately did not lead to consistent anti tumor activity. This lack of efficacy was suggested to be due to too low effector to target ratio and bsAb concentration. An anti EpCAM x CD64 bsAb also demonstrated efficient carcinoma cell killing using G-CSF and interferon-gamma stimulated neutrophils [105], supporting the idea that activated neutrophils might represent efficient tumor killing cells.

3.4.1.4. Pretargeting

Radioimmunotherapy approaches have several advantages. One of the most attractive one is the bystander effect. Indeed, in a given tumor, cells often tend to lose antigen expression to escape therapy. However, radiolabeled antibodies can bind to antigen-positive tumor cells and irradiate cells in its close proximity, including antigen negative tumor cells, tumor stromal fibroblasts and tumor vasculature. Unfortunately, despite promising results obtained during the last 25 years with directly labeled antibodies, few convincing clinical results have been achieved, mainly due to the fact that IgG remains in the circulation for days, thereby causing unacceptable toxicities to normal tissues [106]. On the other hand, antibody fragments rapidly clear from the circulation and often show better tumor penetration and faster maximum tumor uptake but overall lead to very poor tumor uptake leading to insufficient radiation doses delivered. As proposed nearly 20 years ago, one way to resolve this dilemma would be to separate the antibody targeting moiety from the radiolabeled effector [107]. A bsAb could be injected in a first step, leading to an optimal tumor uptake and wait for the clearance of the bsAb before injecting in a second step the small radiolabeled effector that is then captured at the tumor site and rapidly cleared, thereby sparing the rest of the organism. Although the potential of the bsAb pretargeting technology was shown to be successful in both preclinical and clinical experiments [108], the use of chemical constructs leading to poor production yield has so far limited its expansion. However, by using the dock-and-lock approach, Goldenberg and collaborators have produced trivalent bsAbs, composed of two anti MUC1 Fabs linked to Fab TF2 binding to the hapten HSG. This molecules used in pretargeting of 90Y-labeled hapten led to more than 100:1 tumor-to-non-tumor ratios for normal tissues and tumor-to-blood ratios averages of 1000:1 in animal model studies. A single injection could lead to complete regression of 8 of 10 tumors, demonstrating the high clinical potential of this efficiently produced bsAb [109].

4. CONCLUSION

The second generation of recombinant antibodies has already led to the approval of more than 20 monoclonal antibodies used for therapy (Table **1**), leading to valuable clinical data. Clinical results are now being used to guide antibody engineers to new approaches for making these antibodies even more efficient. At present, a third generation of antibody-derived molecules, potentially much more efficient than conventional monoclonal antibodies, are being evaluated in early clinical trials. This is an exciting time which should see the emergence of ever more efficient immunotherapeutic molecules, vindicating earlier expectations that antibody engineering will deliver considerable medical benefits.

DISCLOSURE

Part of this chapter corresponds to an update of a previously published review (see ref. 98).

Abbreviations: mAb: monoclonal antibody; CEA: carcinoembryonic antigen; CR: complement receptor; GM-CSF: Granulocyte-macrophage colony-stimulating factor; IFN: interferon; FDA: U.S. Food and Drug Administration; EMEA: European Medicines Agency; TNF: Tumor necrosis factor; VEGF: Vascular endothelial growth factor; EGFR: Epidermal growth factor receptor; HER: human epidermal growth factor receptor; PBMC: Peripheral Blood Mononuclear Cell; ITIM: Immunoreceptor tyrosine-based inhibitory motif; ITAM: immunoreceptor tyrosine-based activation motif

REFERENCES

[1] Kohler G, Milstein C. Continuous cultures of fused cells secreting antibody of predefined specificity. Nature 1975; 256(5517): 495-7.

[2] Winter G, Milstein C. Man-made antibodies. Nature 1991; 349(6307): 293-9.
[3] Chames P, Baty D. Antibody engineering and its applications in tumor targeting and intracellular immunization. FEMS Microbiol Lett 2000; 189(1): 1-8.
[4] Hoogenboom H R, Chames P. Natural and designer binding sites made by phage display technology. Immunol Today 2000; 21(8): 371-8.
[5] Neuberger MS, Williams GT, Mitchell EB, *et al.* A hapten-specific chimaeric IgE antibody with human physiological effector function. Nature 1985; 314(6008): 268-70.
[6] Reichert JM, Rosensweig CJ, Faden LB, Dewitz M C. Monoclonal antibody successes in the clinic. Nat Biotechnol 2005; 23(9): 1073-8.
[7] Jones PT, Dear PH, Foote J, Neuberger, MS, Winter G. Replacing the complementarity-determining regions in a human antibody with those from a mouse. Nature 1986; 321(6069): 522-5.
[8] McCafferty J, Griffiths AD, Winter G, Chiswell DJ. Phage antibodies: filamentous phage displaying antibody variable domains. Nature 1990; 348(6301): 552-4.
[9] Smith GP. Filamentous fusion phage: novel expression vectors that display cloned antigens on the virion surface. Science 1985; 228: 1315-7.
[10] Luginbuhl B, Kanyo Z, Jones RM, *et al.* Directed evolution of an anti-prion protein scFv fragment to an affinity of 1 pM and its structural interpretation. J Mol Biol 2006 Oct 13; 363(1): 75-97.
[11] Lonberg N. Human monoclonal antibodies from transgenic mice. Handb Exp Pharmacol 2008(181): 69-97.
[12] Dübel S. Handbook of Therapeutic Antibodies. first ed.; Wiley-VCH: Weinheim, 2007; Vol. 1,2&3, p 1190.
[13] Graumann K, Premstaller A. Manufacturing of recombinant therapeutic proteins in microbial systems. Biotechnol J 2006; 1(2): 164-86.
[14] Giritch A, Marillonnet S, Engler C, van Eldik G, Botterman J, Klimyuk V, Gleba Y. Rapid high-yield expression of full-size IgG antibodies in plants coinfected with noncompeting viral vectors. Proc Natl Acad Sci USA 2006; 103(40): 14701-6.
[15] Beckman RA, Weiner LM, Davis HM. Antibody constructs in cancer therapy: protein engineering strategies to improve exposure in solid tumors. Cancer 2007; 109(2): 170-9.
[16] Roopenian, DC, Akilesh S. FcRn: the neonatal Fc receptor comes of age. Nat Rev Immunol 2007; 7(9): 715-25.
[17] Fujimori K, Covell DG, Fletcher JE, Weinstein JN. A modeling analysis of monoclonal antibody percolation through tumors: a binding-site barrier. J Nucl Med 1990; 31(7): 1191-8.
[18] Adams GP, Schier R, McCall AM, Simmons HH, Horak EM, Alpaugh RK, Marks JD, Weiner LM. High affinity restricts the localization and tumor penetration of single-chain fv antibody molecules. Cancer Res 2001; 61(12): 4750-5.
[19] Borrebaeck CA, Carlsson R. Human therapeutic antibodies. Curr Opin Pharmacol 2001; 1(4): 404- 8.
[20] Nimmerjahn F, Ravetch JV. Antibodies, Fc receptors and cancer. Curr Opin Immunol 2007; 19(2): 239-45.
[21] Cartron G, Dacheux L, Salles G, *et al.* Therapeutic activity of humanized anti-CD20 monoclonal antibody and polymorphism in IgG Fc receptor FcgammaRIIIa gene. Blood 2002; 99(3): 754-8.
[22] Weng WK, Levy R. Two immunoglobulin G fragment C receptor polymorphisms independently predict response to rituximab in patients with follicular lymphoma. J Clin Oncol 2003; 21(21):3940-7.
[23] Shinkawa T, Nakamura K, Yamane N, *et al.* The absence of fucose but not the presence of galactose or bisecting N-acetylglucosamine of human IgG1 complex-type oligosaccharides shows the critical role of enhancing antibody-dependent cellular cytotoxicity. J Biol Chem 2003; 278(5): 3466-73.
[24] Siberil S, Dutertre CA, Boix C, *et al.* Molecular aspects of human FcgammaR interactions with IgG: functional and therapeutic consequences. Immunol Lett 2006; 106(2): 111-8.
[25] Preithner S, Elm S, Lippold S, *et al.* High concentrations of therapeutic IgG1 antibodies are needed to compensate for inhibition of antibody-dependent cellular cytotoxicity by excess endogenous immunoglobulin G. Mol Immunol 2006; 43(8): 1183-93.
[26] Van Spriel AB, van de Winkel JG. CD89 (Fc alphaRI). J Biol Regul Homeost Agents 2001; 15(2): 179-81.
[27] Lichtenstein A, Kahle J. Anti-tumor effect of inflammatory neutrophils: characteristics of *in vivo* generation and *in vitro* tumor cell lysis. Int J Cancer 1985; 35(1): 121-7.
[28] Midorikawa Y, Yamashita T, Sendo F. Modulation of the immune response to transplanted tumors in rats by selective depletion of neutrophils *in vivo* using a monoclonal antibody: abrogation of specific transplantation resistance to chemical carcinogen-induced syngeneic tumors by selective depletion of neutrophils *in vivo*. Cancer Res 1990; 50(19): 6243-7.
[29] Seino K, Kayagaki N, Okumura K, Yagita H. Antitumor effect of locally produced CD95 ligand. Nat Med 1997; 3(2): 165-70.

[30] Di Carlo E, Forni G, Lollini P, *et al.* The intriguing role of polymorphonuclear neutrophils in antitumor reactions. Blood 2001; 97(2): 339-45.

[31] Huls G, Heijnen IA, Cuomo E, *et al.* Antitumor immune effector mechanisms recruited by phage display-derived fully human IgG1 and IgA1 monoclonal antibodies. Cancer Res 1999; 59(22):5778-84.

[32] Dechant M, Vidarsson G, Stockmeyer B, *et al.* Chimeric IgA antibodies against HLA class II effectively trigger lymphoma cell killing. Blood 2002; 100(13): 4574- 80.

[33] Stockmeyer B, Dechant M, van Egmond M, *et al.* Triggering Fc alpha-receptor I (CD89) recruits neutrophils as effector cells for CD20-directed antibody therapy. J Immunol 2000; 165(10): 5954-61.

[34] Vaccaro C, Zhou J, Ober RJ, Ward ES. Engineering the Fc region of immunoglobulin G to modulate *in vivo* antibody levels. Nat Biotechnol 2005; 23(10): 1283-8.

[35] Shields RL, Namenuk AK, Hong K, *et al.* High resolution mapping of the binding site on human IgG1 for Fc gamma RI, Fc gamma RII, Fc gamma RIII, and FcRn and design of IgG1 variants with improved binding to the Fc gamma R. J Biol Chem 2001; 276(9): 6591-604.

[36] Lazar GA, Dang W, Karki S, *et al.* Engineered antibody Fc variants with enhanced effector function. Proc Natl Acad Sci USA 2006; 103(11): 4005-10.

[37] Desjarlais JR, Lazar GA, Zhukovsky EA, Chu SY. Optimizing engagement of the immune system by anti-tumor antibodies: an engineer's perspective. Drug Discov Today 2007; 12(21-22): 898-910.

[38] Dhodapkar KM, Krasovsky J, Williamson B, Dhodapkar MV. Antitumor monoclonal antibodies enhance cross-presentation ofcCellular antigens and the generation of myeloma-specific killer T cells by dendritic cells. J Exp Med 2002; 195(1): 125-33.

[39] Armour KL, van de Winkel JG, Williamson LM, Clark MR. Differential binding to human FcgammaRIIa and FcgammaRIIb receptors by human IgG wildtype and mutant antibodies. Mol Immunol 2003; 40(9): 585-93.

[40] Cheung NK, Sowers R, Vickers AJ, *et al.* FCGR2A polymorphism is correlated with clinical outcome after immunotherapy of neuroblastoma with anti-GD2 antibody and granulocyte macrophage colony-stimulating factor. J Clin Oncol 2006; 24(18): 2885-90.

[41] Yamane-Ohnuki N, Kinoshita S, Inoue-Urakubo M, *et al.* Establishment of FUT8 knockout Chinese hamster ovary cells: an ideal host cell line for producing completely defucosylated antibodies with enhanced antibody-dependent cellular cytotoxicity. Biotechnol Bioeng 2004; 87(5): 614-22.

[42] Cox KM, Sterling JD, Regan JT, *et al.* Glycan optimization of a human monoclonal antibody in the aquatic plant Lemna minor. Nat Biotechnol 2006; 24(12): 1591-7.

[43] Li H, Sethuraman N, Stadheim TA, *et al.* Optimization of humanized IgGs in glycoengineered Pichia pastoris. Nat Biotechnol 2006; 24(2): 210-5.

[44] Nechansky A, Schuster M, Jost W, *et al.* Compensation of endogenous IgG mediated inhibition of antibody-dependent cellular cytotoxicity by glyco-engineering of therapeutic antibodies. Mol Immunol 2007; 44(7): 1815-7.

[45] Holliger P, Hudson PJ. Engineered antibody fragments and the rise of single domains. Nat Biotechnol 2005; 23(9): 1126-36.

[46] Bird RE, Hardman KD, Jacobson JW, *et al.* Single-chain antigen-binding proteins [published erratum appears in Science 1989 Apr 28;244(4903):409]. Science 1988; 242(4877): 423-6.

[47] Holliger P, Prospero T, Winter G."Diabodies": small bivalent and bispecific antibody fragments. Proc Natl Acad Sci USA 1993; 90(14): 6444-8.

[48] Robinson MK, Shaller C, Garmestani K, *et al.* Effective treatment of established human breast tumor xenografts in immunodeficient mice with a single dose of the alpha-emitting radioisotope astatine-211 conjugated to anti-HER2/neu diabodies. Clin Cancer Res 2008; 14(3): 875-82.

[49] Ward ES, Gussow D, Griffiths AD, Jones PT, Winter G. Binding activities of a repertoire of single immunoglobulin variable domains secreted from *Escherichia coli.* Nature 1989; 341(6242): 544-6.

[50] Hamers-Casterman C, Atarhouch T, Muyldermans S, *et al.* Naturally occurring antibodies devoid of light chains. Nature 1993; 363(6428): 446-8.

[51] Dooley H, Flajnik MF, Porter AJ. Selection and characterization of naturally occurring single-domain (IgNAR) antibody fragments from immunized sharks by phage display. Mol Immunol 2003; 40(1): 25-33.

[52] Blick SK, Curran MP. Certolizumab pegol: in Crohn's disease. BioDrugs 2007, 21(3): 195-201; discussion 2-3.

[53] Muller D, Karle A, Meissburger B, *et al.* Improved pharmacokinetics of recombinant bispecific antibody molecules by fusion to human serum albumin. J Biol Chem 2007; 282(17): 12650-60.

[54] Nguyen A, Reyes AE, 2nd, Zhang M, *et al.* The pharmacokinetics of an albumin-binding Fab (AB.Fab) can be modulated as a function of affinity for albumin. Protein Eng Des Sel 2006; 19(7): 291-7.

[55] Holt LJ, Basran A, Jones K, *et al.* Anti-serum albumin domain antibodies for extending the half-lives of short lived drugs. Protein Eng Des Sel 2008; 21(5): 283-8.
[56] Stork R, Muller D, Kontermann RE.A novel tri-functional antibody fusion protein with improved pharmacokinetic properties generated by fusing a bispecific single-chain diabody with an albumin-binding domain from streptococcal protein G. Protein Eng Des Sel 2007; 20(11): 569-76.
[57] Stork R, Zettlitz KA, Muller D, *et al.* N-glycosylation as novel strategy to improve pharmacokinetic properties of bispecific single-chain diabodies. J Biol Chem 2008; 283(12): 7804-12.
[58] Pastan I, Hassan R, FitzGerald DJ, Kreitman RJ. Immunotoxin treatment of cancer. Annu Rev Med 2007; 58: 221-37.
[59] De Lorenzo C, Arciello A, Cozzolino R, *et al.* A fully human antitumor immunoRNase selective for ErbB-2-positive carcinomas. Cancer Res 2004; 64(14): 4870-4.
[60] Alderson RF, Toki BE, Roberge M, *et al.* Characterization of a CC49-based single-chain fragment-beta-lactamase fusion protein for antibody-directed enzyme prodrug therapy (ADEPT). Bioconjug Chem 2006; 17(2): 410-8.
[61] Gillies SD, Lan Y, Williams S, *et al.* An anti-CD20-IL-2 immunocytokine is highly efficacious in a SCID mouse model of established human B lymphoma. Blood 2005; 105(10): 3972-8.
[62] Ebbinghaus C, Ronca R, Kaspar M, *et al.* Engineered vascular-targeting antibody-interferon-gamma fusion protein for cancer therapy. Int J Cancer 2005; 116(2): 304-13.
[63] Kaspar M, Trachsel E, Neri D. The antibody-mediated targeted delivery of interleukin-15 and GM-CSF to the tumor neovasculature inhibits tumor growth and metastasis. Cancer Res 2007; 67(10): 4940-8.
[64] Willemsen RA, Debets R, Chames P, Bolhuis RL. Genetic engineering of T cell specificity for immunotherapy of cancer. Hum Immunol 2003; 64(1): 56-68.
[65] Eshhar Z. The T-body approach: redirecting T cells with antibody specificity. Handb Exp Pharmacol 2008; (181): 329-42.
[66] Staerz UD, Kanagawa O, Bevan MJ. Hybrid antibodies can target sites for attack by T cells. Nature1985; 314: 628-31.
[67] Chames P, Baty D. Bispecific antibodies for cancer therapy: the light at the end of the tunnel? MAbs 2009; 1(6): 539-47.
[68] Saerens D, Ghassabeh GH, Muyldermans S. Single-domain antibodies as building blocks for novel therapeutics. Curr Opin Pharmacol 2008.
[69] Fischer N, Leger O. Bispecific antibodies: molecules that enable novel therapeutic strategies. Pathobiology 2007, 74(1):3-14.
[70] Muller D, Kontermann RE. Recombinant bispecific antibodies for cellular cancer immunotherapy. Curr Opin Mol Ther 2007; 9(4): 319-26.
[71] Baty D, BG, Chartier M, Pelegrin A, Teillaud JL, Teulon I. Production of antibody formats and immunological applications of said formats. 2006.
[72] Behar G, Siberil S, Groulet A, *et al.* Isolation and characterization of anti-Fc{gamma}RIII (CD16) llama single-domain antibodies that activate natural killer cells. Protein Eng Des Sel 2008; 21(1): 1-10.
[73] Wozniak-Knopp G, Bartl S, Bauer A, *et al.* Introducing antigen-binding sites in structural loops of immunoglobulin constant domains: Fc fragments with engineered HER2/neu-binding sites and antibody properties. Protein Eng Des Sel 2010.
[74] Takimoto CH, Awada A. Safety and anti-tumor activity of sorafenib (Nexavar) in combination with other anti-cancer agents: a review of clinical trials. Cancer Chemother Pharmacol 2008; 61(4): 535-48.
[75] Leonard JP, Coleman M, Ketas J, *et al.* Combination antibody therapy with epratuzumab and rituximab in relapsed or refractory non-Hodgkin's lymphoma. J Clin Oncol 2005; 23(22): 5044-51.
[76] Lu D, Zhang H, Ludwig D, *et al.* Simultaneous blockade of both the epidermal growth factor receptor and the insulin-like growth factor receptor signaling pathways in cancer cells with a fully human recombinant bispecific antibody. J Biol Chem 2004; 279(4): 2856-65.
[77] Lu D, Zhang H, Koo H, *et al.* A fully human recombinant IgG-like bispecific antibody to both the epidermal growth factor receptor and the insulin-like growth factor receptor for enhanced antitumor activity. J Biol Chem 2005; 280(20): 19665-72.
[78] Hoffmann P, Hofmeister R, Brischwein K, *et al.* Serial killing of tumor cells by cytotoxic T cells redirected with a CD19-/CD3-bispecific single-chain antibody construct. Int J Cancer 2005; 115(1): 98-104.
[79] Howland KC, Ausubel LJ, London CA, Abbas AK. The roles of CD28 and CD40 ligand in T cell activation and tolerance. *J* Immunol 2000; 164(9): 4465-70.

[80] Manzke O, Titzer S, Tesch H, Diehl V, Bohlen H. CD3 x CD19 bispecific antibodies and CD28 costimulation for locoregional treatment of low-malignancy non-Hodgkin's lymphoma. Cancer Immunol Immunother 1997; 45(3-4): 198-202.

[81] Lum LG, Davol PA, Lee RJ. The new face of bispecific antibodies: targeting cancer and much more. Exp Hematol 2006; 34(1): 1-6.

[82] Grabert RC, Cousens LP, Smith JA, *et al.* Human T cells armed with Her2/neu bispecific antibodies divide, are cytotoxic, and secrete cytokines with repeated stimulation. Clin Cancer Res 2006, 12(2):569-76.

[83] Baeuerle PA, Reinhardt C. Bispecific T-cell engaging antibodies for cancer therapy. Cancer Res 2009; 69(12): 4941-4.

[84] Dreier T, Baeuerle PA, Fichtner I, *et al.* T cell costimulus-independent and very efficacious inhibition of tumor growth in mice bearing subcutaneous or leukemic human B cell lymphoma xenografts by a CD19-/CD3-bispecific single-chain antibody construct. J Immunol 2003; 170(8): 4397-402.

[85] Schlereth B, Fichtner I, Lorenczewski G, *et al.* Eradication of tumors from a human colon cancer cell line and from ovarian cancer metastases in immunodeficient mice by a single-chain Ep-CAM-/CD3-bispecific antibody construct. Cancer Res 2005; 65(7): 2882-9.

[86] Schlereth B, Kleindienst P, Fichtner I, *et al.* Potent inhibition of local and disseminated tumor growth in immunocompetent mouse models by a bispecific antibody construct specific for Murine CD3. Cancer Immunol Immunother 2006; 55(7): 785-96.

[87] Offner S, Hofmeister R, Romaniuk A, Kufer P, Baeuerle PA. Induction of regular cytolytic T cell synapses by bispecific single-chain antibody constructs on MHC class I-negative tumor cells. Mol Immunol 2006; 43(6): 763-71.

[88] Bargou R, Leo E, Zugmaier G, *et al.* Tumor regression in cancer patients by very low doses of a T cell-engaging antibody. Science 2008; 321(5891): 974-7.

[89] Haas C, Krinner E, Brischwein K, *et al.* Mode of cytotoxic action of T cell-engaging BiTE antibody MT110. Immunobiology 2009; 214(6): 441-53.

[90] Brischwein K, Schlereth B, Guller B, *et al.* MT110: a novel bispecific single-chain antibody construct with high efficacy in eradicating established tumors. Mol Immunol 2006; 43(8): 1129-43.

[91] Grosse-Hovest L, Hartlapp I, Marwan W, *et al.* A recombinant bispecific single-chain antibody induces targeted, supra-agonistic CD28-stimulation and tumor cell killing. Eur J Immunol 2003; 33(5): 1334-40.

[92] Grosse-Hovest L, Wick W, Minoia R, *et al.* Supraagonistic, bispecific single-chain antibody purified from the serum of cloned, transgenic cows induces T-cell-mediated killing of glioblastoma cells *in vitro* and *in vivo*. Int J Cancer 2005; 117(6): 1060-4.

[93] Zeidler R, Mysliwietz J, Csanady M, *et al.* The Fc-region of a new class of intact bispecific antibody mediates activation of accessory cells and NK cells and induces direct phagocytosis of tumour cells. Br J Cancer 2000; 83(2): 261-6.

[94] Zeidler R, Reisbach G, Wollenberg B, *et al.* Simultaneous activation of T cells and accessory cells by a new class of intact bispecific antibody results in efficient tumor cell killing. J Immunol 1999; 163(3): 1246-52.

[95] Burges A, Wimberger P, Kumper C, *et al.* Effective relief of malignant ascites in patients with advanced ovarian cancer by a trifunctional anti-EpCAM x anti-CD3 antibody: a phase I/II study. Clin Cancer Res 2007; 13(13): 3899-905.

[96] Weiner LM, Alpaugh RK, Amoroso AR, *et al.* Human neutrophil interactions of a bispecific monoclonal antibody targeting tumor and human Fc gamma RIII. Cancer Immunol Immunother 1996; 42(3): 141-50.

[97] Arndt MA, Krauss J, Kipriyanov SM, Pfreundschuh M, Little M. A bispecific diabody that mediates natural killer cell cytotoxicity against xenotransplantated human Hodgkin's tumors. Blood 1999; 94(8): 2562-8.

[98] Chames P, Van Regenmortel M, Weiss E, Baty D. Therapeutic antibodies: successes, limitations and hopes for the future. Br J Pharmacol 2009; 157(2): 220-33.

[99] de Palazzo IG, Gercel-Taylor C, Kitson J, Weiner LM. Potentiation of tumor lysis by a bispecific antibody that binds to CA19-9 antigen and the Fc gamma receptor expressed by human large granular lymphocytes. Cancer Res 1990; 50(22): 7123-8.

[100] Hombach A, Jung W, Pohl C, *et al.* A CD16/CD30 bispecific monoclonal antibody induces lysis of Hodgkin's cells by unstimulated natural killer cells *in vitro* and *in vivo*. Int J Cancer 1993; 55(5): 830-6.

[101] Weiner LM, Clark JI, Davey M, Li WS, Garcia de Palazzo I, Ring DB, Alpaugh R K. Phase I trial of 2B1, a bispecific monoclonal antibody targeting c-erbB- 2 and Fc gamma RIII. Cancer Res 1995; 55(20): 4586-93.

[102] Hartmann F, Renner C, Jung W, *et al.* Anti-CD16/CD30 bispecific antibody treatment for Hodgkin's disease: role of infusion schedule and costimulation with cytokines. Clin Cancer Res 2001; 7(7): 1873-81.

[103] Behar G, Chames P, Teulon I, *et al.* Llama single-domain antibodies directed against nonconventional epitopes of tumor-associated carcinoembryonic antigen absent from nonspecific cross-reacting antigen. FEBS J 2009; 276(14): 3881-93.

[104] Repp R, van Ojik HH, Valerius T, *et al.* Phase I clinical trial of the bispecific antibody MDX-H210 (anti-FcgammaRI x anti-HER-2/neu) in combination with Filgrastim (G-CSF) for treatment of advanced breast cancer. Br J Cancer 2003; 89(12): 2234-43.

[105] Schweizer C, Strauss G, Lindner M, Marme A, Deo YM, Moldenhauer G.Efficient carcinoma cell killing by activated polymorphonuclear neutrophils targeted with an Ep-CAMxCD64 (HEA125x197) bispecific antibody. Cancer Immunol Immunother 2002, 51(11-12):621-9.

[106] Adams GP, Weiner LM. Radioimmunotherapy of solid tumors: from fairytale to reality. Cancer Biother Radiopharm 2001; 16(1): 9-11.

[107] Chang CH, Sharkey RM, Rossi EA, *et al.* Molecular advances in pretargeting radioimunotherapy with bispecific antibodies. Mol Cancer Ther 2002; 1(7): 553-63.

[108] Goldenberg DM, Chatal JF, Barbet J, Boerman O, Sharkey RM. Cancer Imaging and Therapy with Bispecific Antibody Pretargeting. Update Cancer Ther 2007; 2(1): 19-31.

[109] Goldenberg DM, Rossi EA, Sharkey RM, McBride WJ, Chang CH. Multifunctional antibodies by the Dock-and-Lock method for improved cancer imaging and therapy by pretargeting. J Nucl Med 2008; 49(1): 158-63.

CHAPTER 16

Aptamers the Chemical Antibodies

Frans P. Houwen[a*] and Andreas Kage[b]

[a]ScienceLynk B.V., Heuvelsestraat 5, 5976 NG Kronenberg, The Netherlands; [b]TU-Berlin, Institute of medical biotechnology, Berlin, Germany & Aptares AG, Am Scheunenviertel 1, 15749 Mittenwalde, Berlin, Germany

Abstract: Aptamers are small oligonucleotides (10 – 20 kD) that bind with high affinity and specificity to a large number of target molecules. K_d-values for the aptamer-target interactions vary from a few picomolar (pM) to a few nanomolar (nM), which is comparable to the binding of antibodies. They are selected from combinatorial libraries consisting of about 10^{15} different oligonucleotides in an entirely *in vitro* system. As no animal is used, the target molecule does not have to be immunogenic and is allowed to be (highly) toxic. After characterization, using standard molecular biological techniques, aptamers are chemically synthesized in small quantities or on large scale.

These "chemical antibodies" can easily be modified in a side directed way for different purposes, such as immobilization on a surface, addition of labels, or changing their pharmacodynamic and pharmacokinetic profiles. Over the last 20 years, aptamers have been widely used in diagnostic (sensors), biotechnology and therapeutic applications. To date, there is one marketed aptamer-based drug for the treatment of wet macula degeneration, and several aptamers are currently in the clinical pipeline.

Keywords: Chemical Antibodies, Aptamers, Development, Application.

1. INTRODUCTION

This chapter deals with the nucleic acid aptamers, including several comparisons with antibodies. No attempt was made to present an up-to-date review, but merely an introduction to the world of aptamers and their possible future role in medicine and science.

Aptare (Latin) could be translated by "to bind", or "to fit" and is the stem for the word "aptamer" [1]. Aptamers could therefore be translated as molecules that bind with high affinity and specificity to other structures, by which the adaptation occurs target-oriented.

Nucleic acids are molecules composed of linear sequences of nucleotides, each composed of a pentose sugar, a phosphate, and an organic base. The sugar in RNA is ribose, whereas in DNA this is deoxyribose. In RNA there are 4 nitrogenous bases: guanine, cytosine, adenine and uracil (in DNA uracil is replaced by thymine).

Aptamers are single stranded RNA or DNA oligonucleotides with a maximum length of about 120 nucleotides. In contrast to the common base-pair binding of other nucleic acid sequences, aptamers undergo conformational changes to form specific secondary and tertiairy structures that enable a non-base-pair or non-Watson-Crick type binding with high-affinity to a target. The structure interacts precisely and specifically with the target [2-3].

These interactions with the binding domain on the target molecule, the aptatope, are based on many contact points where not only the (polar) pentose-phosphate backbone is involved, but also van der Waals and hydrophilic interactions. In case of small target molecules a binding pocket is formed by the aptamers [2, 4].

These different types of interaction explain the fact that single stranded oligonucleotide sequences form a quite large number of thermodynamically stable structural binders. This is the basis for the remarkable

***Adress correspondence to Frans P. Houwen:** ScienceLynk B.V., Heuvelsestraat 5, 5976 NG Kronenberg, The Netherlands; Tel: +31-650234240; E-mail: info@sciencelynk.eu

Eline P. Meulenberg (Ed)

success of generating aptamers to a wide variety of target molecules [4].

To date, high affinity aptamers have widely been used for the recognition and detection of various targets including metal ions, organic dyes, drugs, cofactors, metabolites, aminoglycosides, antibiotics, nucleotides, nucleotide base analogues, amino acids, peptides (on cell surfaces), proteins or even whole cells, indicating their tremendous potential in biological applications [3-4]. Aptamers may distinguish between different conformational states of the same protein and chiral differences between molecules [3-6].

Although aptamers are not substitutes for antibodies in general, they can be used as their alternatives for many different applications. Thus, aptamers can be regarded as chemical antibodies.

A prerequisite for the biological production of monoclonal antibodies is the immunisation of an animal with the cognate antigen, followed by harvesting the antibodies that developed during the immune reaction. Consequently, isolation of antibodies in the traditional way is always problematic in case that the target molecule is tolerated by the animal, *i.e.* non-immunogenic or only slightly immunogenic, or not tolerated at all, *i.e.* too toxic.

Here lays one of the advantages of aptamer technology over antibody technology. The aptamer technology does not need a living system and is not depending on a binding reaction in a biological system. The method is an entirely *in vitro* selection system by which an oligonucleotide is selected with an affinity for a target molecule (aptatope). In the next section three methods for such selection, the SELEX method, the CE-SELEX method and the MonoLex method, are compared.

Aptamers are in the range of 10 to 20 kD. This is relatively small compared to antibodies (IgG 150 kD). Aptamers should, therefore, be better suited for effective therapy due to better penetration into target and extravascular tissue or the extracellular matrix. Introducing changes in their structure through defined chemical modifications will modify their pharmocokinetic properties [5].

In contrast to antibodies, there is no experimental evidence so far for aptamers being immunogenic, a very useful property for reagents that need to be administered repeatedly to the same individual for therapy or diagnostic when studying disease progression [7].

Because of their non-proteinaceous nature aptamers behave like robust chemicals rather than biologicals and are understood in pharmacy as large small molecules. They can be produced with constant quality and on a large scale in fully automated machines. Due to constantly higher demands the price for the nucleic acids are continuously dropping. After identification of the sequence, there is no further need for the antigen target. For instance, as soon as an aptamer has been selected with high affinity for the poison of a snake, the snake nor the poison are needed to produce the aptamer.

Further, modifications can be made at different places in the molecule for *e.g.* immobilization purposes, and (different) labels may be added efficiently and exactly for diagnostics [5].

Aptamers can be applied for many different purposes in biomedical and biotechnological fields. For the antibody industry aptamers are an interesting class of molecules, as they are alternatives for antibodies, based on their differences in structures but advantages compared to antibodies (section 3).

Aptamers are nowadays widely used in diagnostics (*e.g.* biosensors) and in therapeutics (section 4).

Table 1: Some terms related to aptamers.

Term	Explanation
Oligonucleotide	Linear sequence of of nucleotides, each composed of a pentose sugar, a phosphate and an organic base.

30-mer	Oligonucleotide or aptamer with a length of 30 nucleotides.
Aptatope	Binding domain on the target molecule with which the aptamer interacts (compare epitope).
Monoclonal aptamers	Oligonucleotides with the same sequence having the same property to bind to the aptatope (compare monoclonal antibodies).
Polyclonal aptamers	Mixture of oligonucleotides with different sequences having similar affinity for different aptatopes of a target (compare polyclonal antiserum).
K_d	Dissociation constant for the aptamer-target complex.
Combinatorial library	Mixture of oligonucleotides with the same length having different nucleic acid sequences in defined variable regions.
SELEX, CE-SELEX and MonoLex	Selection methods by which specific aptamers are obtained.
Aptasensor	Sensor where the recognition element is an aptamer.
Aptazyme	Ribozyme (RNA enzyme), which catalytic activity is regulated by binding of a small ligand (compare allosteric enzyme).
Eastern blotting	Detection of proteins immobilized on a membrane by an aptamer.

2. ACQUISITION OF APTAMERS

2.1. Background

The source of the selection of aptamers with specificities against a target is the combinatorial library, a mixture of oligonucleotides with the same length but different sequences. This combinatorial library is defined before the selection is started. By separation of oligonucleotides from the residual molecules which bind to the target, the high affinity oligonucleotide, *i.e.* the aptamer, can be identified. A main advantage of all aptamer isolation protocols is the fact that by using the Polymerase Chain Reaction (PCR) a very small number of specific binders can be amplified before the structural identification.

The first report on the potential of oligonucleotides as non-Watson-Crick-type binders was presented in 1988 by Joyce [8, 9] and Yarus [10, 11]. The latter imagined a new perspective having such aptamers binding to amino acids, peptides and proteins. It was shown for the first time that RNA can express a specific affinity for the free nucleotide guanidin [10, 11].

At the UCLA conference in 1988, a method was presented about selecting functional oligonucleotides from a pool of RNA oligonucleotides [8, 9]. Joyce distinguished three functional components of an RNA-based evolving system: mutation, selection and amplification (Fig. **1**). He reasoned that "the evolving system favors the emergence of individuals whose behavioral characteristics conform to the imposed selection constraints" [8]. He demonstrated separation of RNA molecules based on their reactivity (catabolic function).

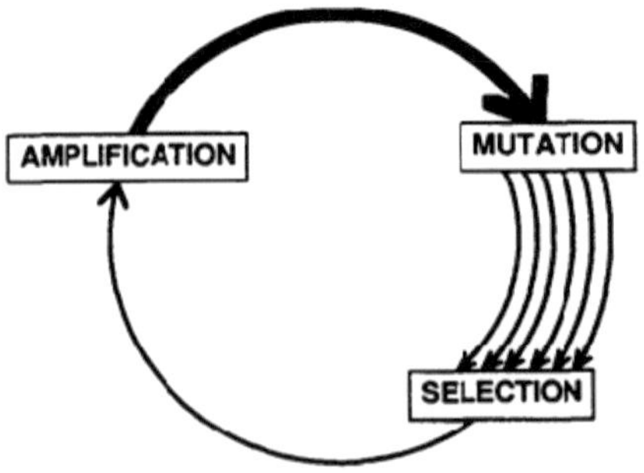

Figure 1: RNA-based evolving system made up of three components [8, 9].

Beyond these successes in scientific research, possible applications of aptamers were soon recognised.

The basic scheme (Fig. **1**) for the selection and isolation of RNA and DNA aptamers has been used for nearly 20 years now. The mutation step in the procedure has been added by the chemical synthesis of the aptamer library typically containing 10^{12} – 10^{15} or more nucleotide molecules of the same length with defined randomized positions [12].

Functional aptamers derived from a typical combinatorial library are about 100 nucleotides in length, consisting of 2 constant regions at both ends separated by a variable region of 25 – 60 nucleotides. The randomization of a sequence stretch of 25 – 60 nucleotides in length renders an enormous diversity of possible sequences and a vast number of different conformations with different binding properties.

Commonly, the target molecule is immobilized to a solid phase to isolate the specific binders from the combinatorial library. By choosing specific environmental conditions during the selection step, including temperature, pH, amount of cations, those aptamers with the desired properties will be selected and amplified [4, 5]. By including a selected small molecule or analyte in the reaction mixture offers the possibility to select for allosteric aptamers, which binding conformation is only stable or even possible in case a small molecule (or ion) adheres to the aptamer-target-complex. Furthermore, starting with a library of oligonucleotides with chemical modifications, might be useful in isolating aptamers that respond to different environmental stimuli. For example, inclusion of ionizable or metal chelating groups may render aptamers sensitive to pH or metal ions, respectively [4].

Selection and isolation has rendered many aptamers capable of binding different targets (aptatopes) with high affinity and specificity. K_d-values for the aptamer-target interactions vary from a few picomolar (pM) to a few nanomolar (nM). Therefore, the affinities and specificities of aptamers are comparable to, if not better than, those of antibodies that are used in diagnostic applications [4, 7, 13].

In the next section, the classical and improved methods for identification of aptamers are described.

2.2. Selection and Isolation

2.2.1. SELEX

Shortly after the first reports of identifying non-Watson-Crick-interacting oligonucleotides by Joyce and Yarus [8-11], a method for the selection of RNA and DNA aptamers by Systematic Evolution of Ligands by Exponential enrichment process (SELEX) was described by L. Gold [14] (Fig. **2**).

A random pool of RNA or DNA molecules (~ 10^{15} different sequences in a combinatorial library) is contacted to the target molecule, usually immobilized on a solid phase, and non-binding oligonucleotides are partitioned from binding oligonucleotides. By desorbing the binding oligonucleotides and amplification, a new oligonucleotide pool is formed which is used in the subsequent round. Here a different condition of the microenvironment can be applied. After five or more rounds of contacting, partitioning and amplification the high affinity binders to the target are enriched and can be identified [14].

The SELEX procedure is summarized in Fig. **2**. Starting from a combinatorial oligonucleotide library it comprises of several cycles of target binding, elution and amplification of putative aptamers. The presence of aptamers can be detected by the use of a quantitative PCR for the amplification or by oligonucleotide agarose electrophoresis.

The binding efficiency and selectivity of the aptamers improve with each round. The number of rounds of selection necessary is determined by both the type of library used as well as the specific enrichment achieved per selection cycle. However, small selection biases can have deleterious effects on the quality of the aptamers [16-18].

So, separation of the different aptamers is crucial regarding the efficiency of the selection procedure, which might be related to an impaired separation of target bound and unbound oligonucleotides. Aptamers with high affinity for their targets are also sometimes difficult to desorb from the column and the best binding aptamers are subsequently not always amplified [16]. Furthermore, as the target molecule has to be linked to the stationary support, a potential aptatope on the target molecule might be hidden or the aptamers can not fully interact with the target.

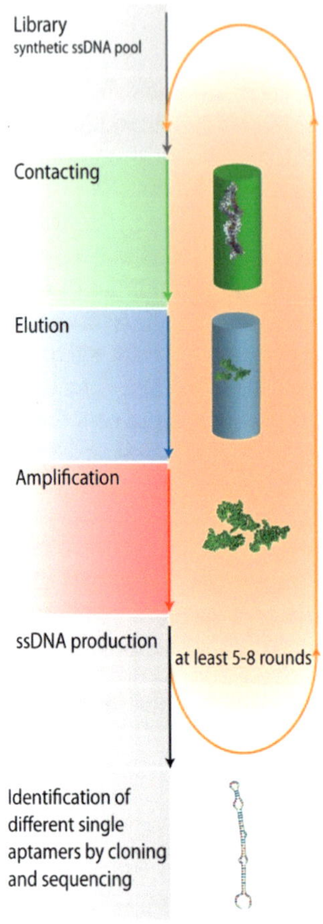

Figure 2: SELEX: Systematic Evolution of Ligands by Exponential Enrichment. Based on a combinatorial oligonucleotide library, SELEX comprises several cycles of target binding, elution and amplification of putative aptamers [15].

The selection/separation step in the SELEX approach can be compared to "inverse" Immuno-Affinity Chromatography (IAC). In SELEX the putative aptamers are (immuno) extracted by immobilized target moleucles.

To overcome some of the limitations above, selection strategies have been changed [19], and several separation methods were applied, adapted, and/or developed as part of the SELEX process to increase the efficiency and throughput of aptamer isolation, including filtration [20], micromagnetic separation [17, 18, 21], flow cytometry [22, 23], surface plasmon resonance [24], micro free flow electrophoresis [25], integration of microfluidic selection with high-throughput DNA sequencing technology [26], and capillary electrophoresis [6, 12, 13, 16, 27-30].

In particular, capillary electrophoresis based separation methods have shown remarkable selection efficiency (see next section).

In addition, the quality (affinity and specificity) of the aptamers can be improved by changing the experimental system. In counter selection (negative selection), aptamers are depleted from the pool by contacting the pool with specific target molecules (aptatopes) to which related but undesired aptamers bind. The classical example of counter selection is the elution of theophylline aptamers from a column using a solution of caffein. Both molecules differ from each other only by a methyl groupe at nitrogen atom N-7, and 99.7% of the "theophylline" aptamers were removed by caffein [31]. Another illustrative example is the isolation of a highly specific aptamer for ADP, during which ATP was used for counter selection [32]. Counter selection is also often applied during isolation of aptamers against cell surface proteins or whole cells [7, 19, 33-35], or for virus typing purposes [20]. Finally, in case the target molecule is bound on a solid surface, counter selection is often used to remove those aptamers that (a) specifically bind to the matrix [18, 36, 37].

2.2.2. CE-SELEX

The selection step in the aptamer selection procedure was highly improved by the introduction of capillary electrophoresis in the procedure. In CE-SELEX an aptamer library or pool of oligonucleotides is brought together in free solution with the target molecule (aptatope). After binding has taken place, selection of aptamers occurs during either Non-Equilibrium or Equilibrium Capillary Electrophoresis of the Equilibrium Mixtures (NECEEM or ECEEM). Binding and non-binding aptamers are collected separately in CE fractions [13, 16, 27]. The detection of the aptamer containing fraction can be identified by qPCR, analysis of the amplification product by oligonucleotide electrophoresis or by on-line photometry if *e.g.* a fluorescence labelled oligonucleotide library is used.

CE-SELEX-based selection has high efficiency, *i.e.* a much better separation occurs between binding and non-binding aptamers, which allows aptamer development with fewer rounds of selection [13, 16].

Furthermore, CE-SELEX eliminates the use of stationary support as selection occurs in free solution. This implies that putative aptatopes are not shielded but are free accessible.

Finally, as aptamers have uniform charge/mass ratios, and therefore have highly predictable behaviour in electrophoresis, CE-SELEX offers the possibility to accurately determine binding parameters of the aptamer-target interaction, and can potentially facilitate selection of aptamers with predefined kinetic characteristics (binding parameters) [13]. Since the introducttion of CE-SELEX in 2004, a number of aptamers has been selected by this method, specifically binding to *e.g.* human IgE, neuropeptide Y, farnesyltransferase and the *Escherichia coli* MutS protein [3].

The determination of kinetic parameters of aptamers during selection, has recently been greatly improved by the introduction of gradient micro free flow electrophoresis (μFFE) [25].

2.2.3. MonoLex

For a long time, the essential need of the multi-round SELEX protocol for the isolation of high affinity binders was expected. Recently, the so called MonoLex protocol was described and demonstrates a one-cycle approach for selection of aptamers [15]. The oligonucleotide ligands are isolated in one single cycle by exponential amplification after isolation of aptamers by affinity chromatography. The target-bound nucleotides are sorted along the affinity column with regard to their affinity.

Low affinity oligonucleotides are completely eluted from the column while the binding oligonucleotides are assorted along the column. To directly access the high affinity aptamers, the affinity column is physically segmented and the oligonucleotides are unspecifically desorbed from each individual column segment. Finally, the desorbed oligonucleotides are amplified by PCR for identification by cloning and sequencing.

Due to the affinity sorting, aptamers amplified from a single column segment show a similar affinity but the aptamers differ in binding to the domain of the target molecule (polyclonal aptamers). Such pools are comparable with a polyclonal antiserum.

Irrespective of the selection protocol, the sequence of the isolated aptamers can be obtained by the standard protocols of cloning and sequencing in order to have the complete master plan for production.

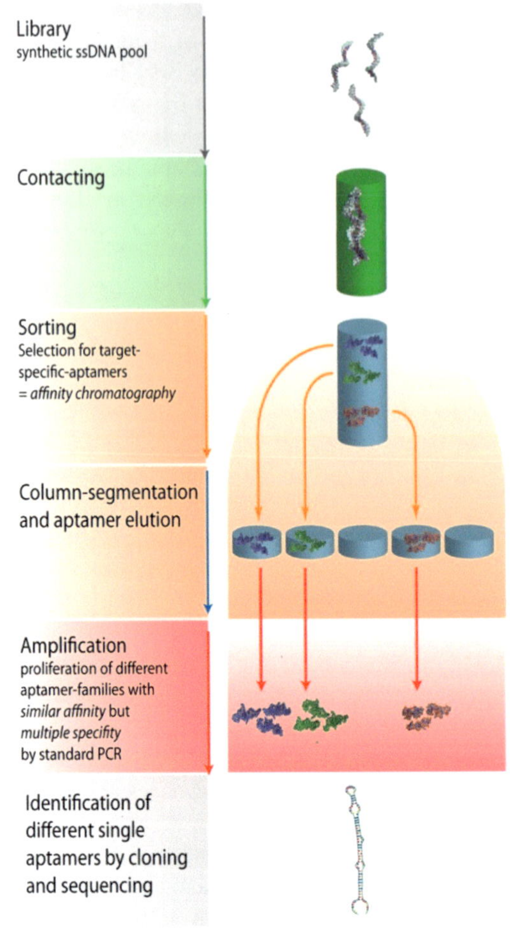

Figure 3: One cycle MonoLex approach. Based on a combinatorial oligonucleotide library, MonoLex starts with one affinity chromatography to sort non-binding oligonucleotides, low-affinity aptamers and high-affinity aptamers. Highly affine aptamers are amplified once and characterized [15].

2.3. Synthesis and modifications of aptamers

Based on the master plan of the aptamer, the aptamer can be chemically produced. Due to their principal behaviour as antibody equivalents and the possibility of chemical synthesis, aptamers are sometimes called chemical antibodies. The chemical synthesis enables a production in small quantities but also allows a quick scale up for large-scale production.

Before scale-up of the production, individual aptamers are synthetised and tested for specificity and selectivity. In order to improve their specific characteristics, aptamers are often engineered for several reasons [4, 38].

Being oligonucleotides, aptamers are potential substrates of nucleases in biological fluids, *e.g.* blood. Therefore, modification of the aptamers is required by medical chemistry especially for RNA. Nuclease activity is *e.g.* strongly inhibited if the 2'position in ribose, as part of the backbone in the RNA or DNA molecule is modified. Usually the –H (RNA) or the –OH (DNA) is replaced by a fluor atom (-F) or an amino group ($-NH_2$) [4]. However, non-modified DNA-aptamers were shown to be stable in biological fluids for extended periods of time [15] (section 4). Besides the post-selection modifications, also the riboses of the initial combinatorial aptamer library may be modified to reach a better stability. This strategy is also used to increase the molecular diversity within an aptamer library by adding different substituents to the nucleotide basis of the four monomers (guanine, cytosine, adenine and uracil (thymine in DNA)).

When aptamers derived from the combinatorial library bind to their aptatope, some nucleotides interact (directly) with the aptatope while other nucleotides are involved in the (thermodynamical) stabilization of the aptamer-target complex. However, some nucleotides or even stretches of nucleotides are not involved in the binding complex. These oligonucleotide can be trimmed from the original aptamer structure. The truncation and size reduction of the final aptamer saves production time and costs [4].

Optimization can be also obtained by *in silico*-strategies. Here, sequences corresponding to the initially variable region of the library are screened for conserved sequences and structural elements indicative for potential binding sites as the basis for consensus sequences. Such sequences can be subsequently tested for their ability to bind specifically to the target molecule or can be used as the basis for a new selection protocol [7].

In a variety of applications such as in diagnostics (section 4) aptamers need to be provided with reporter molecules or chemical active moieties. Such molecules can easily be chemically added in a site-directed way during the chemical synthesis procedure. The chemical modifications can be attached without a loss of binding properties. Still, it is necessary to check the desired characteristics of the aptamer after each (small) change in the molecule.

3. APTAMER CHARACTERISTICS (VERSUS ANTIBODIES)

Aptamers, the chemical antibodies, do not substitute for antibodies in general, but because of their different nature aptamers and antibodies show individual advantages and disadvantages, depending on the intended applications.

In this section several properties of both specific binding molecules and are summarized (Table **2**).

Table 2: Comparison of some properties of aptamers and antibodies.

Property	Aptamers	Antibodies
Acquisition	▪ selection ▪ *in vitro* process – no animals involved ▪ possible to obtain aptamers against targets that are non-immunogenic or toxic ▪ manipulate selection to obtain binding and kinetic properties desirable for specific assays ▪ non-physiological conditions acceptable ▪ expose different epitopes of the same target for selection ▪ identification easy – rapid process performed on automated platform ▪ the target used for selection can be a small portion in the target preparataion	▪ immunization ▪ *in vivo* proces -animals are involved ▪ difficult to obtain aptamers against targets that are non-immunogenic or toxic ▪ manipulation of selection hardly or not possible ▪ physiological conditions obligatory ▪ difficult to expose different epitopes of the same target for selection ▪ identification laborious ▪ the immunogen must be the major fraction in the immunization reagent
Stability	▪ susceptible to nucleases ▪ increased by modifications ▪ robust chemicals ▪ relatively stable over time (DNA aptamers) ▪ stability over a wide range of pH, ionic strength and temperature ▪ long room temperature shelf lives	▪ susceptible to proteinases ▪ biologicals ▪ narrow stability in terms of pH, ionic strength and temperature
Specificity and	▪ binding constants for target species	▪ binding constants for target species

selectivity	comparable with antibodies	comparable with aptamers
Production	▪ *in vitro* chemical synthesis ▪ highly reproducible without the use of living system ▪ master plan known (no batch-to-batch shift) ▪ automated synthesis in small production units	▪ *in vivo* synthesis ▪ living system (fermentation) needed ▪ tendency to vary from batch to batch (genetic shift) ▪ large production plants (more than 10.000 L) required (therapeutic monoclonals)
Modifications	▪ robust chemicals ▪ easy to engineer ▪ side specific attachment – efficient and exact - of reporter molecules - of spacers - of functional groups ▪ homogeneous product	▪ biologicals
Variability	▪ $> 10^{15}$ variants ▪ equal distribution ▪ design: chance and challenge	▪ $\sim 10^{7}$ variants per organism ▪ irregular distribution, modified by: - phylogenesis (evolutionary advantage) - embryogenesis (elimiantion of autoantibodies) - B-cell metamorphosis (selection of the most bioefffective)
Denaturation	▪ regeneration after denaturation possible ▪ easy to separate from aptamer-target-complex	▪ mild conditions needed to prevent irreversible denaturation ▪ sometimes difficult to separate from antibody-target-complex
Size	▪ 10 – 20 kD ▪ renal excretion possible ▪ able to penetrate well into target and extravascular tissue or the extracellular matrix	▪ ~ 150 kD
Characterization	▪ uniform charge/mass ratio's ▪ predictable behavior in electrophoresis	
Sensors	▪ immobilization at defined densities at precise locations on solid surfaces (microarrays) ▪ conformational changes on binding providing molecular-recognition functionalities ▪ irreversible cross-linking with target protein possible – second legand for detection not needed	▪ immobilization at defined densities and locations sometimes difficult ▪ molecular recognition functionalities hardly possible ▪ irreversible cross-linking usually not possible

Note: antibody fragments are not compared.

4. APTAMERS IN DIAGNOSTICS, THERAPY AND BIOTECHNOLOGY

Aptamers have been shown to discriminate between closely related molecules on the bases of subtle structural differences, such as the presence or absence of a methyl group at the example of theophylline and caffeine [31] or a hydroxyl group [39], and a urea versus a guanidino group [40]. They also exhibit a high degree of chiral discrimination of target molecules [41]. This level of specificity rivals that of monoclonal antibodies [4].

Since aptamers can be selected against most (protein) targets, the possible diagnostic and therapeutic applications range far and wide. Furthermore, aptamers are heat resistant, offering the possibility of sterilizing any device in which aptamers are applied.

4.1. Diagnostics

Using the above mentioned (and other) characteristics of aptamers, various analytical aptamer-based formats, assay types, have been developed (Table **3)** [4, 6].

Sensors are devices that respond to physical or chemical stimuli. A sensor contains at least two components, target recognition and signal transduction. The revolution of microtechnology and electronics led to a bunch of advanced biosensor technologies based on different transducing/reporter principles: fluorescence, colorimetry, electrochemistry, mass difference, liquid chromatography, capillary electrophoresis, mass spectroscopy, blotting, charge transfer, Fourier transform infrared attenuated total reflection, magnetic resonance imaging, or the allosteric properties of the aptamer [42].

The sensitivity of such sensors depends besides others on the density of specific binders at the sensor surface. The site-directed modification of aptamers enables a much higher density coverage than the coating with antibodies. This leads the building of aptasensors where the recognition element is an aptamer. These sensors can therefore be applied in detection of practically unlimited kind of compounds [43]. Extensive reviews on aptasensors were recently published [35, 42-47].

Sensors using either aptamers or antibodies as ligands for binding thrombin [48] and IgE [49] have been compared. However, an extensive comparison between both type of ligands in biosensors is beyond the scope of this paper. Instead, we refer to some recent reviews presenting information on detection limits and linearity ranges of aptasensors, for a large variety of targets [45, 50]. To date, no aptasensors have been tested (extensively) under field conditions.

Aptamers can be subjected to repeated cycles of denaturation and renaturation. For instance, an aptasensor for thrombin could be reused at least 25 times without loss of binding efficiency after regeneration with 1 M HCl or several other regenerating agents [51], or with 6 M guanidine HCl [52]. Another sensor was regenerated 8 times with 1 M NaOH at 50 °C without loss of sensitivity [53]. In contrast, mild and cheap conditions may be used to regenerate a sensor. A short wash with a physiological solution (without *e.g.* Mg^{2+}-ions) or with 10 % SDS at room temperature can be sufficient [45, 54]. Such regenerations of sensor surfaces is comparable to those used in the SPR technology. Herein the chip can be used many times under the right circumstances.

Capillary electrophoresis was used for isolating aptamers reacting to specific target molecules (see also section 2). The same technological platform is applied to specifically detect molecules in liquid samples. Affinity Probe Capillary Electrophoresis (APCE) refers to a collection of techniques in which affinity binding is used in conjunction with electrophoresis. Besides antibodies, aptamers are used as ligand in APCE [6, 28, 29].

Several platforms have been developed for diagnostic purposes in which aptamers are an important component (Table **3**).

Table 3: Some diagnostic formats in which aptamers (may) present a key role [4, 6].

Diagnostic Assay Format	Principle/Explanation
Sensors	Aptamer is recognition element.
Capillary electrophoresis	Affinity binding in conjugation with electrophoresis.
Two-site binding assay	Sandwich assay. Aptamers can act as capture or/and detector ligand.
Flow cytometry	Microsphere particles are coated with labelled aptamers.

Fluorescent polarization detection	Aptamers are small and fast tumbling. Labelled aptamers enable the performance of non-competitive assays.
Molecular beacons	A fluorophore and a quencher are attached to both termini of an aptamer. Binding of the aptamer to its cognate target results in fluorescence. Also other designs of aptamer beacons have been described.
Molecular switches	The folding of aptamers is susceptible to environmental factors. Binding of aptamers can therefore be manipulated and assays be influenced.
Eastern blotting	Detection of proteins immobilized on a membrane by an aptamer (molecular beacon).

4.1.1. Therapeutics

To date, there is one marketed aptamer-based product. Macugen™ is an inhibitory aptamer targeting Vascular Endothelial Growth Factor (VEGF). This aptamer was the first to be approved by the FDA (2004) for the treatment of age-related wet macula degeneration. Macugen™ is administered every 6 weeks, with a dose of 0.3 mg/eye [55]. A number of aptamers are currently in the clinical pipeline [38, 56].

The binding of an aptamer to a specific molecule is similar to that of monoclonal antibodies. The specific interaction with the target molecule can modulate its function in a competitive (and antagonistic) way if associated aptatopes are involved in the binding. Due to their properties, oligonucleotide-based drugs are normally free in circulation [7, 38].

Besides by binding to its target, aptamers can directly influence metabolic processes in a decoy-like way. They act by mimicking the target sequence of proteins (epitope) [38] and have been identified as powerful antagonists of protein interactions related to several diseases [7].

These properties of aptamers offer the possibility for pharmaceutical applications. A rapid blood clearance due to their small size (10 – 20 kD) in comparison to antibodies (150 kD) [5, 7] can be overcome *e.g.* by chemically complexing with polyethylene glycol (PEG). Other modification strategies to increase the molecular weight is the addition of a cholesterol moiety, embedding in liposomes and 3'-biotinylation, or 3' addition of a phosphopropyl amine group [5, 38, 57-61] (section 2). Further, half-lives ($t_{½}$) have been extended by using spiegelmer (mirror image) oligonucleotides [62] or circular aptamers [63]. Finally, the chemical substitutions may already be present in the oligonucleotide library used for the aptamer selection [64]. In contrast, there is experimental evidence that also unmodified aptamers may last serum incubation for up to 6 days, more than enough for *in vivo* and *ex vivo* applications [15].

RNA or DNA aptamers intended for clinical applications are usually modified in order to optimize their pharmacodynamic (PD) and pharmacokinetic (PK) profiles and to promote their safety. Beside the low side effects mentioned above, a specific advantage of aptamer as therapeutic agents is the high stability which simplifies the storage conditions.

Great efforts have been made to investigate possible toxic effects of aptamers in clinical applications. In studies performed according to the standard International Conference on Harmonization (ICH) genotoxicity and safety pharmacology studies, aptamers have turned out negative in all cases. This is in contrast with the (minor) toxic effects caused by non-aptamer oligonucleotides administered therapeutically. Overall, subchronic administration studies of therapeutic aptamers have demonstrated predictable toxicity profiles that are favourable. Further, based on No-Adverse-Effect Levels (NoAEL) it has been concluded that the expected pharmacologically applicable doses in animals and humans are safe [38]. There is no experimental evidence so far for aptamers being immunogenic, or activating complement or anticoagulation. These are very useful properties for reagents that need to be administered repeatedly to the same individual for therapy or diagnostic when studying disease progression [7, 38].

By addition of a second, complementary oligonucleotide, the function of the aptamer drug can be (almost) instantaneous deactivated, *i.e.* an individual antidote can be obtained. This aptamer-antidote principle was first demonstrated for the coagulation factor IX [65, 66] and is now under clinical investigation [38, 56]. Recently, universal (sequence-independent) antidotes were developed for extracellular (in blood and plasma) oligonucleotide-based drugs in animals and humans [67].

Another therapeutic function of aptamers is as targeted delivery tools. Aptamers have been developed to deliver siRNAs, toxins, radioisotopes, and chemotherapeutic agents encapsulated in nanoparticles [56]. Aptamers may be also linked together (multivalent aptamers) in order to increase the scope of their applications. This principle is comparable to that of oligomerization of antibodies [56].

In summary, as a new class of drugs, several therapeutic aptamers are tested now in clinical trials. They show excellent characteristics for local and acute systemic administration applications. Although, safety and efficacy under chronic systemic administration has yet to be demonstrated, strong preclinical profiles give good reason for optimism [38].

4.1.2. BioProcess Technology

The properties of aptamers enable their use in biotechnological applications and process technology. One recently presented example developed by AptaRes is their use in antibody affinity purification.

In the downstream process of monoclonal antibody production, Protein A is used in affinity chromatography, binding to the universal Fc-region of immunoglobulin G. For elution a highly acidic buffer is required, which might denature the immunoglobulins and therefore might limit the pharmaceutical application of the antibody. For more details, see the chapter in this book on therapeutic monoclonal antibodies.

To overcome the disadvantages of protein A an aptamer was selected against the Fc-fragment that can be used as an alternative to protein A. The aptamer binds the IgG with a molar ratio of 0.5 - 0.9 (IgG/aptamer) depending on the isotype, and allows an elution of the immunoglobulin under physiological conditions at pH 7.3.

There are different advantages of the aptamer usage compared to the protein A. These include: the absence of immnogenicity by the aptamer binder, which might leak from the affinity resin, the significantly lower stress of the immunoglobulin due to the acidic elution, which might also prodcure highly immunogenic immunoglobulin molecules, and the broader isotype specificity.

Exposing additionally intrinsic alkaline stability and high renaturation capability, DNA aptamers are expected to revolutionize biotechnology processes in the near future.

REFERENCES

[1] Ellington AD, Szostak JW. *In vitro* selection of RNA molecules that bind specific ligands. Nature 1990; 346: 818-22.

[2] Hermann T, Patel DJ. Adaptive recognition by nucleic acid aptamers. Science 2000; 287: 820-5.

[3] Li T, Li B, Dong S. Adaptive recognition of small molecules by nucleic acid aptamers through a label-free approach. Chem Eur J 2007; 13: 6718-23.

[4] Jayasena SD. Aptamers: an emerging class of molecules that rival antibodies in diagnostics. Clin Chem 1999; 45: 1628-50.

[5] Rimmele M. Nucleic acid aptamers as tools and drugs: recent developments. ChemBioChem 2003; 4: 963-71.

[6] Ruta J, Rabvelet C, Grosset C, *et al.* Enantiomeric separation using an L-RNA aptamer as chiral additive in partial-filling capillary electrophoresis. Anal Chem 2006; 78: 3032-39.

[7] Cercia L, Hamm J, Libri D, Tavitian B, de Franciscis, V. Nucleic acid aptamers in cancer medicine. FEBS Letters 2002; 528: 12-16.

[8] Joyce GF. Building the RNA world: evolution of catalytic RNA in the laboratory. In: Cech TR, Ed. Molecular biology of RNA, UCLA symposia on molecular and cellular biology, new series; 94 - proceedings of a director's

sponsors-UCLA symposium held at Keystone Colorado April 4 - 10 1988. New York, Alan R Liss Inc, 1989; pp. 361-71.
[9] Joyce GF. Amplification mutation and selection of catalytic RNA. Gene 1989; 82: 83-87.
[10] Yarus M. A specific amino acid binding site composed of RNA. Science 1988; 240: 1751-58.
[11] Yarus M. A stereoselective binding site for arginine on Tetrahymena self-splicing intron. In: Cech TR, Ed. Molecular biology of RNA, UCLA symposia on molecular and cellular biology, new series; 94 - proceedings of a director's sponsors-UCLA symposium held at Keystone Colorado April 4 - 10 1988. New York, Alan R Liss Inc, 1989; pp. 373-74.
[12] Mendonsa SD, Bowser MT. *In vitro* selection of aptamers with affinity for neuropeptide Y using capillary electrophoresis. J Am Chem Soc 2005; 127: 9382-83.
[13] Berezovski M, Drabovich A, Krylova SM, *et al.* Nonequilibrium capillary electrophoresis of equilibrium mixtures: a universal tool for development of aptamers. J Am Chem Soc 2005; 127: 3165-71.
[14] Tuerk C, Gold L. Systematic evolution of ligands by exponential enrichment: RNA ligands to bacteriophage T4 DNA polymerase. Science 1990; 249: 505-10.
[15] Nitsche A, Kurth A, Dunkhorst A, *et al.* One-step selection of Vaccinia virus-binding DNA aptamers by MonoLex. BMC Biotechnol 2007; 7: 48-59.
[16] Mendonsa SD, Bowser MT. *In vitro* evolution of functional DNA using capillary electrophoresis. J Am Chem Soc 2004; 126: 20-21.
[17] Qian J, Lou X, Zhang Y, Xiao Y, Soh HT. Generation of highly specific aptamers *via* micromagnetic selection. Anal Chem 2009; 81: 5490-95.
[18] Stoltenburg R, Reinemann C, Strehlitz B. FluMag-SELEX as an advantageous method for DNA aptamer selection. Anal Bioanal Chem 2005; 383: 83-91.
[19] Shamah SM, Healy JM, Cload ST. Complex target SELEX. Acc Chem Res 2008; 41:130-38.
[20] Gopinath SCB. Methods developed for SELEX. Anal Bioanal Chem 2007; 387: 171-82.
[21] Lou X, Qian J, XiaoY, *et al.* Micromagnetic selection of aptamers in microfluidic channels. Proc Natl Acad Sci USA 2009; 106: 2989-94.
[22] Blank M, Weinschenk T, Priemer M, Schluesener H. Systematic evolution of a DNA aptamer binding to rat brain tumor microvessels. J Biol Chem 2001; 276: 16464-68.
[23] Yang X, Li X, Prow T, *et al.* Immunofluorescence assay and flow-cytometry selection of bead-bound aptamers. Nucleic Acids Res 2003; 31: e54.
[24] Misono TS, Kumar PKR. Selection of RNA aptamers against human influenza virus hemagglutinin using surface plasmon resonance. Anal Biochem 2005; 342: 312-17.
[25] Turgeon RT, Fonslow BR, Jing M, Bowser MT. Measuring aptamer equilibria using gradient micro free flow electrophoresis. Anal Chem 2010; 82: 3636-41.
[26] Cho M, Xiao Y, Nie J, *et al.* Quantitative selection of DNA aptamers through microfluidic selection and high-throughput sequencing. Proc Nat Acad Sci USA 2010; 107: 15373-78.
[27] Drabovich A, Berezovski M, Krylov SN. Selection of smart aptamers by equilibrium capillary electrophoresis of equilibrium mixtures (ECEEM). J Am Chem Soc 2005; 127: 11224-25.
[28] German I, Buchanan DB, Kennedy RT. Aptamers as ligands in affinity probe capillary electrophoresis. Anal Chem 1998; 70: 4540-45.
[29] Haes AJ, Giordano BC, Collins GE. Aptamer-based detection and quantitative analysis of ricin using affinity probe capillary electrophoresis. Anal Chem 2006; 78: 3758-64.
[30] Mosing RK, Mendonsa SD, Bowser MT. Capillary electrophoresis-SELEX selection of aptamers with affinity for HIV-1 reverse transcriptase. Anal Chem 2005; 77: 6107-12.
[31] Jenison RD, Gill SC, Pardi A, Polisky B. High-resolution Molecular discrimination by RNA. Science 1994; 263: 1425-29.
[32] Srinivasan J, Cload ST, Hamaguchi N, *et al.* ADP-specific sensors enable universal assay of protein kinase activity. Chem Biol 2004; 11: 499-08.
[33] Shangguan D, Cao Z, Meng L, *et al.* Cell-specific aptamer probes for membrane protein elucidation in cancer cells. J Proteome Res 2008; 7: 2133-39.
[34] Ulrich H, Wrengler C. Disease-specific biomarker discovery by aptamers. Cytometry Part A 2009; 75A: 727-33.
[35] Torres-Chavolla E, Alocilja EC. Aptasensors for detection of microbial and viral pathogens. Biosens Bioelectron 2009; 24: 3175-82.

[36] Lau IPM, Ngan EKS, Loo JFC, Suen YK, Ho HP, Kong SK. Aptamer-based bio-barcode assay for the detection of cytochrome-c released from apoptotic cells. Biochem Biophys Res Com 2010: 395: 560-64.

[37] Morris KN, Jensen KB, Julin CM, Weil M, Gold L. High affinity ligands from *in vitro* selection: complex targets. Proc Nat Acad Sci USA 1998; 95: 2902-07.

[38] Bouchard PR, Hutabarat RM, Thompson KM. Discovery and development of therapeutic aptamers. Annu Rev Pharmacol Toxicol 2010; 50: 237-57.

[39] Sassanfar M, Szostak JW. An RNA motif that binds ATP. Nature 1993; 364: 550-53.

[40] Famulok M. Molecular recognition of amino acids by RNA-aptamers: an L-citrulline binding RNA motif and its evolution into an L-arginine binder. J Am Chem Soc 1994; 116: 1698-06.

[41] Geiger A, Burgstaller P, Eltz Hvd. RNA aptamers that bind L-arginine with sub-micromolar dissociation constants and high enantioselectivity. Nucleic Acids Res 1996; 24: 1029-36.

[42] Liu J, Cao Z, lu Y. Functional nucleic acid sensors. Chem Rev 2009; 109: 1948-98.

[43] Hianik T, Wang J. Electrochemical aptasensors - recent achievements and perspectives. Electroanalysis 2009; 11: 1223-35.

[44] Han K, Liang Z, Zhou N. Design strategies for aptamer-based bioensors. Sensors 2010; 10: 4541-57.

[45] Sassolas A, Blum LJ, Leca-Bouvier BD. Electrochemical aptasensors. Electroanalysis 2009; 21: 1237-50.

[46] Song S, Wang L, Li J, Zhao J, Fan CY. Aptamer-based biosensors. Trends Anal Chem 2008; 27: 108-17.

[47] Lee J-O, So H-M, Jeon E-K, Chang H, Won K, Kim YH. Aptamers as molecular recognition elements for electrical nanobiosensors. Anal Bioanal Chem 2008; 390: 1023-32.

[48] Schlecht U, Malavé A, Gronewold T, Tewes M, Löhndorf M. Comparison of antibody and aptamer receptors for the specific detection of thrombin with nanometer gap-sized impedance biosensors. Anal Chim Acta 2006; 573-574: 65-68.

[49] Yao C, Zhu T, Qi Y, Zhao Y, Xia H, Fu W. Development of a Quartz crystal microbalance biosensor with aptamers as bio-recognition element. Sensors 2010; 10: 5859-71.

[50] Strehlitz B, Nikolaus N, Stoltenburg R. Protein detection with aptamer biosensors. Sensors 2008; 8: 4296-07.

[51] Radi A-E, Sánchez JLA, Baldrich E, O'Sullivan CK. Reagentless reusable ultrasensitive electrochemical molecular beacon aptasensor. J Am Chem Soc 2006; 128: 117-24.

[52] So H-M, Won K, Kim YH, *et al.* Single-walled carbon nanotube biosensors using aptamers as molecular recognition elements. J Am Chem Soc 2005; 127: 11906-07.

[53] Zhang Y-L, Huang Y-F, Jiang J-H, Shen G.-L, Yu R-Q Electrochemical aptasensor based on proximity-dependent surface hybridization assay for single-step reusable, sensitive protein detection. J Am Chem Soc 2007; 129: 15448-49.

[54] Lai RY, Plaxco KW, Heeger AJ. Aptamer-based electrochemical detection of picomolar platelet-derived growth factor directly in blood serum. Anal Chem 2007; 79: 229-33.

[55] Ng EW, Shima DT, Calias P, Cunningham ET, Guyer DR, Adamis AP. Pegaptanib a targeted anti- VEGF aptamer for ocular vascular disease. Nature Rev Drug Discov 2006; 5: 123-32.

[56] Thiel KW, Giangrande PH. Therapeutic applications of DNA and RNA aptamers. Oligonucleotides 2009; 19: 209-22.

[57] Famulok M, Hartig JS, Mayer G. Functional aptamers and aptazymes in biotechnology diagnostics and therapy. Chem Rev 2007; 107: 3715-43.

[58] Healy JM, Lewis SD, Kurtz M, *et al.* Pharmacokinetics and biodistribution of novel aptamer compositions. Pharm Res 2004; 21: 2234-46.

[59] Hicke BJ, Watson SR, Koenig A, *et al.* DNA aptamers block L-selectin function *in vivo* Inhibition of human lymphocyte trafficking in SCID mice. J Clin Invest 1996; 98: 2688-92.

[60] Willis MC, Collins B, Zhang T, *et al.* Liposome-anchored vascular endothelial growth factors aptamers. Bioconjugate Chem 1998; 9: 573-82.

[61] Zendegui JG, Vasquez KM, Tinsley JH, Kessler DJ, Hogan ME. *In vivo* stability and kinetics of absorption and disposition of 3' phosphopropyl amine oligonucleotides. Nucleic Acids Res 1992; 20: 307-14.

[62] Eulberg D, Klussmann S. Spiegelmers: biostable aptamers. ChemBioChem 2003; 4: 979-83.

[63] Di Giusto DA, King GC. Construction stability and activity of multivalent circular anticoagulant aptamers. J Biol Chem 2004; 279: 46483-89.

[64] Keefe AD, Cload ST. SELEX with modified nucleotides. Curr Opin Chem Biol 2008; 12: 448-56.

[65] Rusconi CP, Scardino E, Layzer J, *et al.* RNA aptamers as reversible antagonists of coagulation factor IXa. Nature 2002; 419: 90-94.

[66] Rusconi CP, Roberts JD, Pitoc GA, *et al.* Antidote-mediated control of an anticoagulant aptamer *in vivo*. Nat Biotechnol 2004; 22: 1423-28.

[67] Oney S, Lam RTS, Bompiani KM, *et al.* Development of universal antidotes to control aptamer activity. Nat Med 2009; 15: 1224-28.h.

Index

Made in the USA
Las Vegas, NV
10 November 2026

57858719R00197